Reproduction and Social Organization in Sub-Saharan Africa

STUDIES IN DEMOGRAPHY
General Editors
Eugene A. Hammel
Ronald D. Lee
Kenneth W. Wachter

Reproduction and Social Organization in Sub-Saharan Africa

EDITED BY
RON J. LESTHAEGHE

UNIVERSITY OF CALIFORNIA PRESS
Berkeley   Los Angeles   London

University of California Press
Berkeley and Los Angeles, California

University of California Press, Ltd.
London, England

Copyright © 1989 by The Regents of the University of California

Library of Congress Cataloging-in-Publication Data

Reproduction and social organization in Sub-Saharan Africa/edited by
Ron J. Lesthaeghe.
   p. cm.—(Studies in demography; 4)
   Bibliography: p.
   Includes index.
   ISBN 0-520-06363-5 (alk. paper)
   1. Family—Africa, Sub-Saharan—Cross-cultural studies.
2. Marriage—Africa, Sub-Saharan—Cross-cultural studies.   3. Human
reproduction—Social aspects—Africa, Sub-Saharan—Cross-cultural
studies.   4. Fertility, Human—Social aspects—Africa, Sub-Saharan—
Cross-cultural studies.   I. Lesthaeghe, Ron J., 1945– .
II. Series: Studies in demography (Berkeley, Calif.); 4.
HQ691.R46   1989
306.8'0967—dc 19
                                  88-31501
                                  CIP

Printed in the United States of America

1   2   3   4   5   6   7   8   9

Contents

Contributors

Caroline Bledsoe is currently associate professor of anthropology at Northwestern University (Evanston, Illinois) and acting director of its program of African studies. At the time of writing she was a research associate at the Population Studies Center of the University of Pennsylvania (Philadelphia).

Ghislaine Delaine is at present resident advisor for the World Bank in Gambia. At the time of writing she was a demographer at the Direction de la Statistique in Abidjan, Ivory Coast, and *coopérant* of ORSTOM, Paris.

Frank Eelens is research associate at the Netherlands Interuniversity Demographic Institute in The Hague. At the time of writing he was a doctoral student in demography at the Vrije Universiteit in Brussels.

Samuel Gaisie is professor of demography at the University of Zambia (Lusaka) and formerly at the University of Ghana (Accra).

Noreen Goldman is research demographer at the Office of Population Research of Princeton University.

Wendy Graham (née Izzard) is research fellow at the Center for Population Studies of the London School of Hygiene and Tropical Medicine.

Uche Isiugo-Abanihe is currently professor of sociology at the University of Ibadan. At the time of writing he was affiliated with the Population Studies Center of the University of Pennsylvania in Philadelphia.

Georgia Kaufmann was research associate at the Interuniversity Programme in Demography of the Vrije Universiteit in Brussels. She is at present a doctoral student in anthropology at the University of Oxford.

Ulla Larsen is research associate in the department of statistics at the University of Lund, and at the time of writing she was a doctoral student in demography at Princeton University.

Ron Lesthaeghe is professor of sociology at the Vrije Universiteit of Brussels.

Wariara Mbugua is research staff member at the Population Studies and Research Institute of the University of Nairobi.

Dominique Meekers is at present a doctoral student in demography at the University of Pennsylvania. At the time of writing he was a research assistant at the Interuniversity Programme in Demography of the Vrije Universiteit of Brussels.

Hilary Page is professor in sociology at the Rijksuniversiteit of Ghent, and research associate at the Interuniversity Programme in Demography of the Vrije Universiteit in Brussels.

Anne Pebley is assistant director and research demographer at the Office of Population Research of Princeton University.

Ian Timaeus is lecturer at the London School of Tropical Medicine and Hygiene.

Camille Vanderhoeft is research associate at the Centrum voor Statistiek en Operationeel Onderzoek of the Vrije Universiteit in Brussels. At the time of writing he was affiliated with the Interuniversity Programme in Demography at the same university.

Acknowledgments

The production of this volume has been possible thanks to the support of several sponsors. The specific acknowledgments are found at the end of each chapter. But first and foremost, this project would have come to a quick halt if it were not for the kindness of the official offices of statistics in the various countries participating in the World Fertility Surveys (WFS) in Africa and the WFS staff itself in making the data available. Most of the financial resources were provided by USAID through the Population Council's International Awards Program. This support permitted several African colleagues to spend time overseas analyzing their own national WFS materials. Additional support was provided by the National Bank of Belgium, the Research Council of the Vrije Universiteit in Brussels, the National Institutes for Child Health and Development in Washington, the Andrew W. Mellon Foundation, the Rockefeller Foundation, and the Ford Foundation. Special thanks are also due to Etienne Vanden Balck in Brussels for typing much of the text and for preparing most of the tables and to Arille Tassin for computer file management.

R. Lesthaeghe
Brussels
June 1988

Introduction

Ron Lesthaeghe

There were several reasons for undertaking this project on reproduction and social organization in sub-Saharan Africa. Some were of a theoretical nature, whereas others stemmed from the need for a structuring of the recently increased flow of demographic information from the region. The book falls squarely in the tradition of cross-cultural comparative analysis. As such it addresses several limitations apparent in much of the existing comparative demographic literature.

A first issue concerns the inadequacies of worldwide comparisons based on a purely statistical analysis of the links between demographic variables and standard indicators of socioeconomic development. For instance, many Latin American and Asian populations have witnessed a substantial fall in fertility since the 1970s, whereas sub-Saharan populations have tended to have had constant or even rising fertility during the postcolonial period. It is tempting to compare the latter with the former in terms of a series of general development indicators, and to conclude from a set of regressions that sub-Saharan Africa has not produced a fertility transition simply because it has not yet reached adequate levels of income, schooling, urbanization, or family planning effort. This is essentially the conclusion of the World Bank report of 1986. Any worldwide comparison made today would indeed produce this statistical outcome. But, does this mean that Nigeria or Zaire will have a fertility decline as impressive as that of Thailand or Indonesia from the moment they reach the same income per capita, attain the same schooling level, or spend the same amount per capita on family planning? Such international statistical comparisons assume a socioeconomic threshold beyond which transitions in nuptiality and fertility take place. Unfortunately, such threshold hypotheses have failed to draw support from actual experience to date (see Knodel and van de Walle, 1979), and consequently, there must be

1

numerous other factors of social complexity mediating the process. In other words, the comparison of sub-Saharan Africa with other continents solely in terms of economic or programmatic indicators is a hazardous one today and will remain so in the future. The prime concern of this book is, therefore, to describe the link between the characteristics of reproduction in sub-Saharan Africa and the particular patterns of social organization in the region and to draw attention to the meaning of these context-specific links both for understanding the continent's recent demographic history and for speculating about the future of demographic change.

The next classic feature of many comparative analyses is the assumption that everything that is not "economic" must be "cultural." Economists and sociologists, who are about equally represented among the practitioners of demography, are often hopelessly divided on this issue. One commonly finds that measures of socioeconomic development operating at the macro level, or economic variables specifying the demand for children at the household level, account for only a small portion of the observed variance. The same also holds at the intermediate level, that is, for villages or communities, with respect to infrastructural variables, including medical and family planning facilities. John Casterline (1985, p. 73), for instance, concludes:

> Totalling up the statistically significant findings leaves one almost empty-handed. Measures of community development—agricultural modernization, non-agricultural economic activities, village modernization as measured by the presence of utilities and amenities—rarely show systematic relationships with fertility. . . . One cannot help but think that were community features—such as clinics, schools, availability of electricity and piped water, or paved roads—influencing reproductive behaviour through some means, this fact would be more apparent in the results.

By contrast, attention is often drawn by sociologists to the "explanatory power" of variables such as region, language, or ethnicity at the macro level, or to that of religion at the individual level. Such variables have indeed explained nonnegligible portions of the observed variance in fertility. This was essentially the outcome of the Princeton studies of the historical European fertility transitions. More recently, a host of similar findings have been commented upon by John Cleland and Christopher Wilson (1987) in their much broader survey of fertility transitions in both industrialized and developing nations. They too hold the view that ideational changes and the spread of new ideas are of major importance.

This "cultural" approach has major problems as well. First of all, economists quickly point out that these features do not constitute "policy variables." Cultural variables are at most interesting, but are irrelevant for planning and policy formulation. Second, "cultural" explanations are frequently residual explanations, or a messy bag into which everything is relegated that is not properly understood. It is very easy to introduce a nominal variable denoting ethnic group or language in any multivariate analysis and to assess its statistical significance and impact on the dependent variables. It is quite a different matter to explain on substantive grounds what such statistical results really mean. What is commonly lacking is a much more precise specification of these "cultural proxies."

The common explanation for linguistic effects, for example, is that language stands for communication density, which fosters the spread of new ideas: linguistic borders inhibit their diffusion. But language is invariably related to region and ethnicity, and therefore also to politics. In other words, used as an explanatory variable, language absorbs many other effects as well. Ethnicity is even more problematic, and specifications of its meaning (other than connecting it back to language and innovation or diffusion) are exceedingly rare in demographic analyses.

Even before starting this analysis of the existing and new demographic data for sub-Saharan Africa, we were sure that language, ethnicity, or region were going to play a major role, but that a mere statistical description of their effects would be devoid of any further meaning. This is the case, of course, unless, one can find a way of defining "cultural entities" in terms of other characteristics that need not be "cultural" in the narrow sense of the term (i.e., pertaining to normative systems). Our basic choice has, therefore, been to connect ethnicity to selected *characteristics of social organization*. Examples of such characteristics of variables are the productive value of women in the various types of traditional economies, the patterns of lineage organization and of exchange or rights in women between lineages, or the structural changes in social organization introduced by the penetration of non-African religions. In other words, ethnicity is translated into several features that pertain to the traditional modes of production and the structuring of gender relations. These are taken as the historical roots of sub-Saharan social organization, upon which later changes have been grafted. Such changes have stemmed from major alterations of the land tenure systems, the growth of wage sectors in the economy, rapid urbanization during the postcolonial period, or the general emergence of marked stratification by social class. All of these have been intricately interwoven during the course of history and the resulting picture is not only complex but also highly diversified.

As a result, we considered it necessary to offer a summary of the specific sub-Saharan features or social organization in chapter 1. Obviously, one cannot do justice to two centuries of economic and social change in all parts of this heterogeneous continent in just a single chapter. But we hope that this chapter gives the non-Africanist a feel for the basic organizational and socioeconomic differentiation and offers a justification for linking "reproduction" to "production."

This link owes tribute to the tradition of anthropological and ethnographic research and relies not only on their descriptions, but also on the interpretations that are given to all major features of ethnic-specific patterns of social organization. The best-known attempt at systematizing the massive amount of information is beyond doubt still G. P. Murdock's Ethnographic Atlas, also known as the Yale Human Relations Area files. Our "operationalization" of ethnicity is largely dependent on Murdock's classifications. These were supplemented by an independent scanning of ethnographic references, which resulted in alteration of a few codes and the construction of additional variables. Inasmuch as structural–functionalist anthropology drew elegant, holistic pictures of discrete societies, however, it tended not to engage in extensive comparative approaches. To compensate for that, we have drawn on the work of Ester Boserup (1970) and Jack Goody (1976) who offered precise and especially verifiable propositions with respect to the links between reproductive systems on the one hand, and modes of production, gender relations, and exchange of the productive and reproductive capacities of women on the other. Their propositions, along with those of several other authors, are also described in chapter 1. The empirical verification of these propositions on the basis of demographic and ethnographic information files is presented in chapter 2 (Lesthaeghe and Eelens), chapter 3 (Lesthaeghe, Vanderhoeft, Gaisie, and Delaine), and chapter 6 (Lesthaeghe, Kaufmann, and Meekers). As it will be seen, then, the anthropological tradition centering on modes of production and the economic value of women provides a starting point for this book.

Chapter 2 essentially links the components of the *spacing* pattern of reproduction (i.e., breastfeeding, lactational amenorrhea, postpartum abstinence, and contraception) to indicators of both traditional social organization and recent socioeconomic change. The demographic data base used here is derived from the World Fertility Surveys (WFS) that were held between 1976 and 1981 in ten sub-Saharan African countries: Mauritania, Senegal, the Ivory Coast, Ghana, Benin, Nigeria, Cameroon, Kenya, Sudan (northern part only), and Lesotho. These surveys had the advantage of using a common core-questionnaire facilitating standardized measurement. However, it should be borne in mind that the WFS was designed primarily as an instrument for demographic measurement and not as a tool for studying cultural variation or socioeconomic change. The WFS demographic data must therefore be linked to information from other sources, and both region and ethnicity as units are used for merging the demographic data with the cultural and socioeconomic data from other sources. Chapter 3 (Lesthaeghe, Vanderhoeft, Gaisie, and Delaine) also contains an elaboration of the WFS data files, but two additional features are introduced here. First, we were also interested in the combinatory effect of the so-called intermediate fertility variables upon overall fertility. This tradition in demography recognizes that economic, social, and cultural factors act upon the various components of fertility separately. In a subsequent phase these effects are aggregated in order to elucidate patterns of reinforcement or neutralization (e.g., shorter lactational amenorrhea compensated by more contraception). The first exhaustive layout of the "intermediate fertility variables"–scheme was given by Kingsley Davis and Judith Blake in 1956. Measurement of the various components remained fragmentary, however, until the 1970s. Subsequently, data gathering became more systematic as a result of renewed interest in both historical demography and Third World demography. John Bongaarts' statistical framework of 1978 in particular facilitated the integration of each of the components into overall fertility analysis. Since our own earlier work in African demography (Page and Lesthaeghe, 1981) falls in this tradition, we could not miss the opportunity to incorporate the new WFS information on the intermediate fertility variables in a broader African comparison. More specifically, we wanted to establish to what extent the initial fertility-increasing effect of female literacy and enhanced education, operating through reduced lactation and shortened postpartum abstinence, is currently being offset by increased contraceptive use. This involves a more technical "nuts and bolts" section in chapter 3 dealing with the measurement of what we have called "the postpartum abstinence bonus."

The assessment of the educational effect through the intermediate fertility variables leads us to the second part of chapter 3, which contains a multilevel analysis. Here the effect on the intermediate fertility variables of educational differences between individuals within each region is compared across regions. Contextual variables, that is, characteristics of the regions rather than of individuals, are used in this cross-regional analysis. The set of contextual variables employed contains features of traditional social organization (i.e., the economic value of women derived from their traditional involvement in trade), variables concerning the impact of historical Western and Islamic penetrations, and indicators of regional socioeconomic development.

The intellectual impact of Boserup and Goody is particularly obvious in chapter 6, which looks at the various patterns of nuptiality and their recent change. These authors originally formulated their propositions for the world as a whole, not just for sub-Saharan Africa. Their statistical tests were, therefore, performed on a global sample of ethnic groups. As a result, they essentially account for major differences in the nature of reproductive regimes between continents, especially those between Eurasia and sub-Saharan Africa. The question remains, however, whether their theses are equally capable of distinguishing between African societies, that is, in a setting characterized by much less heterogeneity than that found in a global sample.

Another intellectual tradition providing ample grist for our mill—and the basis of our next group of chapters—has been the sociological literature on social change and the family. Much of that literature centers on the concept of Westernization, that is, the penetration of Western ideals about the conjugal family which provide a direction for family change in the Third World. The shift towards nuclear residence patterns for households, and especially towards European-like conjugal marriage, is seen as taking place either because corporate kinship systems or extended families are too rigid and curtail individual freedom, or because their economic basis is gradually being withdrawn. In short, nonwestern family systems are presented as being sooner or later condemned, for both economic and ideological reasons. The literature of this nature is substantial and there exist many variations on the theme. But two authors have been particularly influential in family sociology and social demography, largely because of their erudition in studying worldwide patterns. We refer here to William Goode who published his *World Revolution and Family Patterns* in 1963 (second edition 1970) and John Caldwell who brought his most important articles together in his *Theory of Fertility Decline* of 1982. Goode's prediction of the direction of family change is very straightforward (1970, p. 368–369):

> We have stated as an initial point of view, validated throughout by data, that the direction of change for each characteristic of the family might be very different from one culture to another, even though the pattern of movement *for the system as a whole* is toward a *variant of the conjugal type* [our italics].

By separate characteristics of the family Goode refers to specific variables such as illegitimacy or divorce, which may be very different at the onset and which can therefore evolve in opposite directions in different cultural contexts as the general pattern evolves towards more conjugality. Goode attributes a major role to the ideological variables, that is, to the formation of a global community in the cultural sense (p. 369):

> We have asserted that we do not believe that the theoretical relations between a developing industrial system and the conjugal family system are entirely clear. On the empirical side we suggest that the changes that have taken place have been far more rapid than could be supposed or predicted from the degree of industrialization alone. We have insisted, instead, on the independent power of ideological variables. Everywhere the ideology of the conjugal family is spreading, even though a majority does not accept it. It appeals to the disadvantaged, to the young, to the women, and to the educated. It promises freedom and new alternatives as against the rigidities and controls of traditional systems. It is as effective as the appeal of freedom or land redistribution or an attack on the existing stratification system. It is radical, and it is arousing support in many areas where the rate of industrialization is very slight.

Goode is, however, equally convinced that the old systems will lose their functional rationale as peasant economies are replaced by industrial ones. The quotation cited above is immediately followed by (p. 369):

Yet, the ideology of the conjugal system would have only a minimal impact if each newly emerging system did not furnish some independent base for implementing the new choices implicit in the ideology.

For Africa, Goode's scenario is indeed revolutionary, especially as far as the proposed pace of the change is concerned (p. 201–202):

> If the new African nations follow the path of many other emerging nations, the *next decade* [our italics] will witness an accentuated move away from tribal family patterns, and toward a conjugal system. The resurgence of pride in the indigenous heritage will not buttress traditional family patterns, because the effort to be accepted by older nations as "modern" or "civilized" will create continuing social and legal forces in line with "progressive" family sentiments and behaviour.

Admittedly this quotation starts with a conditional "if," but in accordance with the optimism of the 1960s, Goode does not envisage the contrary, that is, that African nations would not follow the development path of newly industrializing Asian societies.

John Caldwell is considerably more cautious about the speed of the transformation, and this is undoubtedly due to his firsthand experience in tropical Africa. But he too stresses the role of Westernization, the formation of a global society (as distinct from a global economy) and the concomitant spread of the nuclear and conjugal family. The following quotation from his restatement of the theory of fertility transition speaks for itself (1982, p. 153):

> In the present situation, family nuclearization and the reversal of intergenerational wealth flow are likely to penetrate deeply into the Third World in the next half century, almost independently of the success of industrialization, and almost inevitably they will guarantee slower global population growth.

Also the source of this independent shift towards the conjugal and nuclear family is explicitly treated (1982, p. 153):

> An emphasis must be placed here on the export of the European social system as well as its economic system. It is absurd to deny that this is the central feature of our times as to deny the significance of the Hellinization of southwest Asia, the Romanization of the Mediterranean and western Europe, and the Sinoization of much of southeast and central Asia in other periods. . . . From the demographic viewpoint, the most important social exports have been the concept of the predominance of the nuclear family with its strong conjugal tie, and the concept of concentrating concern and expenditure on one's own children.

Caldwell's theory is remarkable in a number of ways. The main vehicle for Westernization is formal education. As such, education assumes a major cultural role along with the mere economic role assigned to it by the Chicago school of economists who define it in terms of greater direct and indirect costs of children. But even more important is that Caldwell views the emergence of the conjugal family as the *conditio sine qua non* for reversal of the traditional intergenerational "wealth flow" from young to old, and consequently as a *prerequisite* for a fertility transition.

To sum up, there is a remarkable congruence between Goode and Caldwell since both attribute a major role to the spread of a Western family model in triggering off changes in the social and economic relations in the family or between generations, and ultimately in producing a fertility transition.

The obvious questions now are whether such changes in the sub-Saharan family system have taken place and whether they will be necessary to produce a fertility decline. This issue is taken up in several chapters in this book, especially those that deal with nuptiality systems and child-fosterage. The Goode and Caldwell theories impinge directly upon demographic issues such as the survival of polygyny, the age gap between husbands and wives, the ages at first union formation, and the circulation of children. The issue of polygyny is taken up in chapter 5 (Goldman and Pebley), 6 (Lesthaeghe, Kaufmann, and Meekers), and 7 (Pebley and Mbugua), that of child circulation in chapters 9 (Page) and 10 (Bledsoe and Isiugo-Abanihe).

Chapter 5 treats the formal demographic aspects of polygyny. It is well known that widespread polygyny is possible only as a result of a large age gap between husbands and wives and hence as a consequence of early marriage for women, late marriage for men, and rapid remarriage of widows and divorcées. Polygyny and widow inheritance are features that are diametrical opposites of the Western conjugal family type, as Goode and numerous other authors have recognized. The importance of the chapter by Goldman and Pebley lies in the study of the demographic *potential* for polygyny rather than in its mere incidence. They show, for instance, how this potential is enhanced by a young age composition of the population resulting in relatively large generations of young women, and hence by fast population growth. As sub-Saharan demographic growth is currently breaking all records with rates of 2.5 to 4.0 percent in most areas, and since this is largely due to high fertility, additional support is being given to the maintenance of this potential for polygyny in the future. They show, furthermore, that feasible reductions in mortality and modest declines in fertility still leave sufficient potential for the institution to survive.

The same topic is also considered in the first part of chapter 6, showing the impact of different schedules of widowhood or divorce and remarriage and of different levels of fertility on a series of polygyny measures. The rest of chapter 6 is devoted largely to the measurement of regional and ethnic variations in the actual incidence of polygyny and to the analysis of the connections with the social organization features used in Boserup's and Goody's theories. Another section of chapter 6 tries to assess trends in ages at first marriage for both sexes and in polygyny levels. The outcome is that not only the formal demographic potential for polygyny, but also its actual incidence, show no major sign of decline despite the widespread trend toward later ages at first marriage for women. The reasons for the essentially horizontal trend in polygyny are the age structure effects resulting from accelerations of population growth and the increase in age at first marriage for men. In other words, the age gap between spouses has not undergone a fundamental change and polygyny is not being "squeezed out" by any significant convergence of the ages at first marriage for the two sexes. If we recall what Goode had to say in 1963 (p. 188),

> It seems unlikely that in the new nation-states emerging in Africa the generally favourable attitudes of African men toward polygyny will be changed quickly. Even so, it will, without question, eventually almost completely disappear as a pattern of behaviour. The new legal codes are gradually moving towards its abolition, women will avoid it where they can, and men will not generally be able to afford it.

then, the conclusion seems to be that men above ages 25 or 30 have been remarkably successful in maintaining their old prerogatives during the post-colonial period. In short, the evolution of the polygyny and age difference indicators provides no real support for the Westernization hypothesis to date.

The analysis of marriage and fertility in Lesotho and Botswana by Ian Timaeus and Wendy Graham (chapter 8) yields important insights on the evolution of these demographic factors in situations that are heavily conditioned by labor migration for both sexes. Marriages have become very late for men and women alike, large proportions of women never formally marry, widow remarriage is much less common than elsewhere in Africa, and households permanently headed by women have become a dominant trait. In these areas, Christian churches are strong and female literacy levels are among the highest on the continent. Despite the presence of such cultural props for the Westernization effect, domestic situations for women have become increasingly complex and varied, both in cross-sections and longitudinally. If the time a woman spends with a husband in a nuclear household is any indication of conjugality, then few person-years are spent in such conditions. The weakening of the traditional marriage pattern, which was not significantly different from that of other eastern and southern African patrilineal populations with a mixed agricultural and livestock economy, has led mainly to a longer reliance by women on their own kinship group, to greater self-reliance and subsequently to reliance on support from children, rather than to reliance on husbands. Labor migration is of major importance in many other African areas as well, and its association with marriage retardation implies that the changes in ages at first marriage should not be interpreted automatically as a sign of the coming of the conjugal family.

The last issue with direct connections to the Goode and Caldwell theses concerns child-fosterage. This topic is studied by Hilary Page at the macro level in chapter 9 and by Caroline Bledsoe and Uche Isiugo-Abanihe at the micro level in chapter 10. Page essentially measures the current incidence of child-fosterage with the WFS household data on the presence of own and other children. Her measurements thus pertain to "in-fostering" and not to "out-fostering." Bledsoe and Abanihe describe both ends of a particular form of child-fosterage, namely fosterage of young children by "grannies," together with its rationale and implications. As Caldwell remarked (see the preceding quotation), the conjugal family is characterized not only by close ties between husband and wife, but also by the concept of concentrating concern and expenditure on one's own children. African societies are, however, renowned for their stress of children as the human capital of lineages, and this has resulted in the socialization of new members by many agents other than the biological parents. Witness thereof is the distinction anthropologists had to make between pater and genitor, along with the role of East African age grades, the function of maternal uncles in matrilineal societies, circulation of children as domestic labor, or the "grannie" pattern. African child circulation is typical for a situation in which the wealth flow between generations has not been reversed since the present or anticipated economic benefits from children are at the core of child circulation. Child circulation creates a web of rights and obligations between the biological and foster parent(s), as is eloquently shown in chapter 10. Furthermore, fosterage is a means of spreading the costs and benefits of children much more widely than is possible in the nuclear family system. New patterns of fosterage centering on education involve exporting the costs of rural fertility to urban settings at certain ages, or the other way around at other stages of the child's life cycle. But the outcome is still that such cost devolution is to be matched by a transfer of rights to current or prospective child benefits. Finally, judging from Page's data, child circulation is not something restricted to a few areas or to the past; it is much more widespread than anticipated by Western social scientists. The picture emerging from these two chapters is that the current situation seems far removed from the close parent-child dyad fostered by Western ideals and from the "Eurasian model" involving two or three biologically related generations.

Last but not least, this book also contains chapters on two classic topics in African demography. Chapter 7, by Pebley and Mbugua, reassesses the impact of polygyny on fertility, and the second, by Larsen, considers trends and social differentials with respect to sterility. Both studies use the most recent information provided by the World Fertility Surveys for updating earlier insights gathered from more scattered information. Pebley and Mbugua show, for instance, that the polygyny-fertility link is a multistranded one involving compensating and reinforcing effects operating through the intermediate fertility variables. As such they leave little room for an overly simplified theory involving just one dominant mechanism. Chapter 4, by Larsen, on sterility also shows that easy extrapolations may be misleading. Until now, it was commonly believed that antibiotics have been able to reduce sterility levels, especially in the high sterility belt of Central Africa. Larsen finds, however, that sterility levels in Cameroon and Northern Sudan are surprisingly invariant across cohorts and over recent decades and that sterility even increased in Kenya during the 1960s and 1970s. This chapter calls attention to the problem of all sexually transmitted diseases in sub-Saharan Africa, and establishes, in view of the current and almost exclusive preoccupation with AIDS, that the older scourges of venereal disease still have not been brought under control, despite the existence of a cure. The persistence of sexually transmitted diseases in many areas of the continent shows that Western-style conjugal marriage and the concomitant limitation of extra-marital sexual behavior will take much longer to take root in Africa than was assumed by the sociological theories of the 1960s.

The concluding chapter goes beyond a critique of the Westernization hypothesis of family change and fertility transition. In its first part we explore Ester Boserup's proposition (1985) that a fertility transition could also be triggered off by the realization that expectations with respect to enhanced personal welfare and high returns to parents or community from greater investment in the education of children may not materialize. Two responses are possible: either investments in children drop and fertility remains unaltered, which is the continuation of or a return to an earlier situation, or investments are concentrated in a smaller number of children. Given the current heterogeneity of the continent with respect to economic trends and the recurrence of politically or ecologically induced disasters, both responses are likely to emerge depending on the region. But if fertility drops (and there is some evidence that a decline has started in the Kenyan Central Province, for instance) such a transition could conceivably level off at average parities that are still well above two or three children (see Cain, 1983; Bongaarts, 1986). As documented in this volume, many of the props for much higher than replacement fertility are likely to survive in sub-Saharan Africa. Moreover, we are not at all sure that family changes are occurring on the road traced by Goode or Caldwell. It seems rather that African populations are currently producing their own versions of new systems that are still far from being fully crystallized. But, as argued in the second half of the concluding chapter, this does not imply that there is at present no need for greater family planning effort. African leaders themselves have now realized, at least in political forums, that current population growth rates aggravate the economic and ecological crises, and that, in the face of reduced child-spacing through traditional means, contraception is required to restore the balance. Furthermore, African societies are not totally unarmed to meet this challenge. Many of them have a long tradition of communal solidarity which finds its expression in the existence of associations of various sorts. These associations, and particularly the women's groups, have on occasion been capable of addressing new problems and adopting their functions, most notably to include income-generating activities and initiatives concerning health care and social welfare in general. Although there are reasons for being cautious about the possibilities of such networks, we still feel that their potential in the fields of primary health care and family planning is undervalued. We therefore hope that the record for the 1980s and 1990s will show, as has happened in the past in other societies, that African communal solidarity too can be instrumental in solving the current demographic challenge.

BIBLIOGRAPHY

Bongaarts, J. 1978. A framework for analyzing the proximate determinants of fertility. *Population and Development Review* 4(1): 105–132.

———. 1986. The transition in reproductive behavior in the third world. *Working Papers of the Center for Policy Studies*, no. 125. New York: The Population Council.

Boserup, E. 1970. *Women's role in economic development*. London: Allen and Unwin, 283.

———. 1985. Economic and demographic interrelationships in sub-Saharan Africa. *Population and Development Review* 11(3): 383–398.

Cain, M. 1983. Fertility as an adjustment to risk. *Working Papers of the Center for Policy Studies*, no. 100. New York: The Population Council.

Casterline, J. 1985. Community effects on fertility. In: *The collection and analysis of community data*, ed. J. Casterline. Voorburg, Netherlands: International Statistical Institute.

Caldwell, J. C. 1982. *Theory of fertility decline*. New York: Academic Press.

Cleland, J., and C. Wilson. 1987. Demand theories of fertility transition: An iconoclastic view. *Population Studies* 41(1): 5–30.

Davis, K., and J. Blake. 1956. Social structure and fertility: An analytic framework. *Economic Development and Cultural Change* 4(4): 211–235.

Goode, W. 1963. *World revolution and family patterns*. New York: Free Press.

Goody, J. 1976. *Production and reproduction—A comparative study of the domestic domain*. Cambridge: Cambridge University Press.

Knodel, J., and E. van de Walle. 1979. Lessons from the past: policy implications of historical fertility studies. *Population and Development Review* 5: 217–245.

Murdock, G. P. 1967. Ethnographic atlas: A summary. *Ethnology* 6(2): 109–234.

Page, H. J., and R. Lesthaeghe, eds. 1981. *Child-spacing in tropical Africa—Traditions and change*. London: Academic Press.

World Bank. 1986. *Population policies and growth in sub-Saharan Africa: A World Bank policy study*. Washington, D.C.: World Bank.

CHAPTER ONE

Production and Reproduction in Sub-Saharan Africa: An Overview of Organizing Principles

Ron Lesthaeghe

INTRODUCTION

As the survival of any society hinges on (1) the technological adaptation to a given environment, (2) the demographic balance between births, deaths, and migration streams, and (3) the economic principles governing production and distribution, it is proper that this book on the various reproductive regimes of sub-Saharan Africa begins with the links between "production and reproduction." This is a classic starting point: Thomas Malthus integrated population dynamics into the context of the moral economies of peasant societies 200 years ago. His notions of preventive and positive checks still seem to have maintained their relevance, and although most of his applications dealt with the Western European system of the eighteenth century, it is by now evident that all populations, from the hunter-gatherer stage onwards, have generated arrangements through which the reproductive process is regulated. Moreover, these arrangements reflect the basic institutional setup that governs the functioning of the social system as a whole.

The links between the organizing principles of a society and the specific features of its reproductive regime, that is, the parameters of the starting, spacing, and stopping patterns of fertility, are not only of importance for gaining insights into demographic variations at a particular point in time, but they are of even greater value for the understanding of the various paths followed in the course of social change. More specifically, as changes in the spheres of political organization, division of labor, social stratification, economic exchange, cultural differentiation, and demographic regulation are not likely to proceed in a synchronized fashion, a clearer view of the relations between "production and reproduction" is essential to understand individual and group strategies, or, as McNicoll specified (1978, p. 89): "to locate emerging contradictions and to assess possibilities for their resolution."

This institutional approach to reproductive regimes calls for a comparative methodology. The classic multivariate statistical techniques will continue to occupy an important place, but in the institutional approach the accent shifts from the treatment of strictly individual-level data to a multilevel approach. For instance, it does not suffice to introduce the attribute "ethnic group" into a regression equation with individual-level characteristics such as schooling level or age at marriage. For one, ethnicity stands for organizational and cultural traits of a collectivity, and these traits require further specification. One way of clarifying the situation is to study the relationships between individual-level variables separately for each ethnic context, comparing the outcomes across such contexts. For instance, the impact of a rise in female education (a microvariable) on the length of postpartum abstinence may vary across ethnic groups or regions. This variation may then be explained in terms of characteristics measured for the group as a whole, such as religious composition (a macro- or contextual variable). This approach is not free from problems.

First, as just indicated, the meaning of any broad contextual variable such as ethnic group, region, language . . . , requires specification in terms of more precise and explicit cultural and organizational dimensions such as the type of religion, level of technology, pattern of division of labor, structure of the domestic group, form of wealth concentration or circulation, authority structure, and so forth. At this point choices with respect to the presumed importance of each of these underlying features cannot be avoided. Such choices are of necessity reductionist or subjective in nature, not only because of the merging of complex organizational forms into a few manageable dimensions, but also because of the subsumed causal ordering projected by any author onto the network of cultural and organizational features.

Second, the statistical tools and models used in measuring associations and effects require slight adaptations to fit multilevel theory, that is, theory operating on the levels of both individuals and aggregates. As a consequence, we shall adopt the basic design of "contextual analysis" by establishing the separate impact of individual-level variables (holding the context constant), of aggregate-level variables (fixing individual variable values), and, above all, of interactions between these two. These interaction terms most frequently address the question of *how* the relationships between individual-level variables vary in shape and strength across the various contexts. In the statistical parlance of multiple regression, for instance, the question is whether slopes and intercepts characterizing the relations between individual-level variables are themselves a function of characteristics of contexts (see Boyd and Iversen, 1979). This obviously leads into a question of comparative sociology: *why* are individual level elasticities differentiated with respect to contexts?

From this outline, it is clear that we cannot restrict ourselves to the variables measured in the recent round of African fertility surveys, but that additional source materials have to be integrated as well. In order not to lose the advantage of subsequent statistical testing, such qualitative materials have to be operationalized, but this involves approximation and some loss of validity. More specifically for this chapter, we shall attempt to re-express ethnicity as a few basic organizational dimensions on the basis of anthropological monographs and G. P. Murdock's (1967) classification of societies according to a set of organizational characteristics. Additional survey information on variables, such as female involvement in commerce, or on the shift from animism to Islam or Christianity, will also be of use. In short, in the next sections a choice of organizational dimensions believed to be both at the core of a society's functioning and relevant for its reproductive regime will be made. This leads into the construction of an operational typology useful for further work.

GENERAL CONNECTIONS BETWEEN SOCIAL ORGANIZATION AND REPRODUCTIVE REGIMES OF SUB-SAHARAN AFRICA

As the preventive checks of reproductive regimes are located at the level of "intermediate fertility variables," it is essential to understand why some societies rely predominantly on controls on the starting pattern of fertility (postponement of first sexual unions, celibacy), while others locate them within the spacing or stopping patterns (such as, through long postpartum nonsusceptible periods, reduced remarriage, or early "terminal" abstinence). An exploration of such differentiation leads us to a study of patterns of kinship organization and to an examination of systems of production and control over resources. At this point, various links can be made between aspects of "production" and features of "reproduction."

Several attempts have been made (1) to establish a list of variables through which the connections operate and (2) to measure the strength of the associations. In this respect, the Murdock Ethnographic Atlas (1967), which gives a relatively detailed coding of many organizational variables in over 800 societies, has often been used. The comparisons drawn from the Murdock atlas are highly illuminating for understanding the basics of African reproductive regimes, especially if contrasted to those of Eurasia. A brief account of the findings at a general level is offered here.

At the "production" end of the spectrum, all authors start from the means of subsistence and the degree of sophistication of agricultural technology in particular. The contrast is made between slash-and-burn forms of extensive agriculture, supportive only of low population densities, and intensive agriculture using the plough instead of the hoe as well as manuring and/or irrigation. Yet, already at this point, authors differ on whether to stress environmental factors such as nutrition and health or social organization factors such as landholding systems. Taken separately, these explanatory frameworks may give the impression of edging on monocausality, but their joint consideration provides the required set of core institutional and cultural variables.

The earliest explanations accounting for a crucial element of African reproductive regimes, namely the marked pattern of child-spacing, were essentially "environmentalist" in nature: child-spacing through prolonged lactation and postpartum abstinence was essentially seen as a cultural adaptation to environmental and technological constraints. As many African societies practice swidden agriculture, producing mainly tubers such as yams and cassava, and consume very limited amounts of dairy products, protein insufficiency is a major problem. Consequently, prolonged lactation is of paramount importance to curb infant and childhood mortality. In addition to the concern about child survival, the health of women, who constitute both the productive and reproductive capital of kinship groups, requires protection against exhaustion by rapid procreation. The implication of this environmental theory is then that the duration of the postpartum taboo on sexual intercourse during the lactation period is a function of the society's protein intake. At present, the duration of the taboo varies from 40 days to over 2 years. The theory furthermore expects a major split to emerge between societies with or without access to dairy products, between farmers and cattle raisers, or between the forest belt and the savannah.

The environmental theory was most popular in the period prior to World War II: when questioning Africans about the postpartum taboo, missionaries and medical personnel were obviously getting the classic answer that "semen poisons the mother's milk and causes illness to the suckling child." Virtually all African populations, including cattle keepers, explicitly recognize the health function of the taboo in these or similar terms.

The link between prolonged lactation or long postpartum abstinence and polygyny was also firmly recognized: polygyny facilitates abstinence for lactating women without causing sexual deprivation to polygynous men. It was therefore treated as a form of structural adaptation to an environmental constraint. Revealing in this context is the attitude of colonial authorities when faced with these practices. The example taken here is that of the Ryckmans Commission of 1930 which provided a blueprint for the Belgian colonial policy in the Congo. Constituted by lawyers, missionaries, agronomists, and medical doctors, the blueprint clearly intended to model the African family on the European one and based on Catholic principles. This meant in the first place that witchcraft and polygyny had to be eradicated. At this point, however, it was recognized that polygyny fulfilled a crucial function with respect to infant health via the postpartum taboo, and a more cautious plan was drafted: restrictions on polygyny needed to be accompanied by an improvement in infant diets, and plans were made for upgrading cattle farming in areas free of tse-tse flies with distribution of processed dairy produce over the entire territory (Ryckmans Commission, 1930, quoted by Schoenmaeckers et al., 1981, p. 37).

A worldwide test of the nutritional/environmental theory has been provided on the basis of the Murdock Ethnographic Atlas by G. P. Murdock himself (1967) and by J. W. M. Whiting (1964). The latter provides the following text (1964, p. 521):

> It seems then, that there is some evidence for a long causal chain leading from the rainy tropics to circumcision. Such a climate is conducive to the growing of low-protein roots and fruit crops. A diet based largely on such crops is assumed to lead to a high incidence of a protein deficiency called kwashiorkor. This in its turn, leads a mother to avoid getting pregnant while she is still lactating, since this might reduce the already low protein value of her milk below the danger point and might result in illness of the nursing child. The avoidance of pregnancy in these societies without an alternative means of contraception is generally accomplished by abstinence, which leads the husband to seek another wife, and hence to the acceptance of polygyny as a form of marriage. Finally, there is some indication that polygyny is more compatible with patrilocal than other forms of residence. Since both a long postpartum taboo and patrilocal residence have been shown to be associated with circumcision rites, a second reason for the tropical distribution of such rites is suggested.

Tables 1.1 and 1.2 provide the results of Murdock's test, involving 166 societies chosen in such a way as to cover a wide variety of societies evenly

TABLE 1.1   Type of Subsistence Economy and Length of the Postpartum Abstinence Period for 166 Societies as Chosen by G. P. Murdock

	Duration of Abstinence (in months)						
	less than 1	1–5	6–11	12–23	24+	Mean	N of Societies
Dairying Societies	13	14	3	5	5	7.5	40
Pastoralists	—	3	—	2	—	9.0	5
Agriculturists	11	10	3	3	5	7.6	32
Food collectors	2	1	—	—	—	1.3	3
Non Dairying Societies	27	40	12	28	19	10.0	126
Food Producers	9	14	6	15	10	11.7	54
Gatherers	4	5	2	3	3	10.0	17
Hunters	4	4	2	4	2	9.9	16
Incipient food producers	5	5	1	3	2	8.4	16
Fishers	5	12	1	3	2	6.6	23
All Societies in Sample	40	54	15	33	24	9.2	166

SOURCE: G. P. Mudock, 1967, p. 145.

TABLE 1.2   Form of Marriage and Length of the Postpartum Abstinence
Period for 166 Societies as Chosen by G. P. Murdock

	Duration of Abstinence (in months)						
	less than 1	1–5	6–11	12–23	24+	Mean	N of Societies
Monogamy or polyandry	10	12	1	6	1	6.2	20
Limited polygyny	12	27	7	11	8	8.7	65
General polygyny	18	15	7	16	15	11.4	71
All Societies in Sample	40	54	15	33	24	9.2	166

SOURCE: G. P. Murdock, 1967, p. 146.

distributed over the world. Although Murdock's coding of the length of the
postpartum taboo is subject to discussion itself (see for instance R. Schoenmaeckers et al., 1981, pp. 27–32 for sub-Saharan Africa), the tables clearly
provide support for the links between protein intake, length of postpartum
abstinence, and incidence of polygyny. Yet, aside from the general pattern,
the data in these two tables also describe a remarkable heterogeneity *within*
each type of subsistence economy or form of marriage. Among nondairying
food producers, which constitute the largest subgroup in Murdock's sample,
there are nearly as many societies with a postpartum abstinence duration of
less than 6 months as there are with a taboo of 2 years or more (twenty-three
versus twenty-five). Hence, factors other than protein intake must bear some
influence on the length of the taboo as well.

Very much the same holds with respect to Whiting's thesis that the long
taboo is essentially a feature encountered among forest dwellers. The test
performed by Schoenmaeckers et al. for 136 sub-Saharan societies showed
clearly that there is no major savannah-forest contrast, but rather a contrast
between West and Central versus East and Southern Africa (1981, pp. 32–
39). Moreover, early anthropological references to Eastern and Southern
populations or statements by older women in these societies often provide
durations that are not markedly different from those represented in Western
and Central Africa. This leads us to the alternative that the postpartum
taboo used to be least one year in almost every region of sub-Saharan Africa,
and that current variations are the result of some initial differences coupled
to major differences in the pace of erosion of the taboo (Lesthaeghe, 1984,
pp. 13–17). Although this proposition does not detract from the nutrition/
child health thesis—the statements of African women all over the continent
concur on this point and the presumed near universality of the taboo underscores the importance of lactation—one is nevertheless forced to look beyond
the strictly environmental explanation to account for the substantial variation in the practice as encountered in the period after World War II.

It is obviously not enough to detect a serious reason for the introduction of a particular practice or ingredient of the reproductive regime: there must also be a strong social support for its maintenance. Moreover, the concern over nutrition is by no means the sole reason for enhanced spacing and child-spacing is not the only distinctive feature of sub-Saharan reproductive regimes. Consequently, we shall explore the links between the organizing principles of sub-Saharan societies and a set of distinctive characteristics of the reproductive regime.

While on the topic of the postpartum taboo, some of the findings of J.-F. Saucier warrant reporting and discussion. Aside from the nutrition/wet tropics factor, the associations between the taboo and exclusive mother-child sleeping arrangements, initiation rites, kin avoidance, and sorcery had been discussed by authors such as Kluckhohn and Anthony (1958), Stephens (1962), and Young (1965) (quoted by Saucier), while Carr-Saunders had already pointed out the custom's demographic significance as early as 1922. Saucier, however, extended the hypotheses much further and proceeded with the statistical testing of twenty-three propositions using a worldwide sample of 172 societies from Murdock's files. The single best correlates of the taboo, as measured via the phi-coefficient, were the following:

1. Recruitment of women into marriage via bridewealth (or sister exchange): phi = 0.38.
2. Presence of extensive agriculture (slash-and-burn, hoe) rather than more sophisticated forms of intensive agriculture: phi = 0.36.
3. Customary polygyny: phi = 0.35.
4. A high degree of physical and psychological separation between the spouses: phi = 0.31.

The identification of the polygyny factor and of the predominance of swidden agriculture, often involving tuber cultivation, are perfectly in line with the nutrition theory. However, the two remaining factors in combination with those just mentioned point in the direction of a particular type of social organization. In Saucier's words (1972, p. 247):

> Briefly, the long postpartum taboo is found most frequently in small, compact communities which subsist mainly on extensive agriculture (with a low level of nutrition) and which are structured in terms of a localized unilineal kinship group. The adult women, obtained from outside via bridewealth, live in polygynous households, often in separate quarters, and perform extensive food-producing and food-processing work under the supervision of men. The inheritance of property is unequal. Daily life is controlled by rigid rules such as elaborate etiquette, kin-avoidance and joking relationships, segregation of boys at puberty, etc. The transition from adolescence to maturity is frequently marked by bodily mutilations. Although religion recognizes a high god, it describes him as unconcerned about human affairs. This description of the type of

society most likely to have a long taboo suggests some kind of *community gerontocracy* [Saucier's italics]. Through the command of land and cattle, the elders
control the acquisition of women, and through puberty rites they maintain
power over the young men.

Taking gerontocratic control of community and kinship group as a point of
departure rather than the nutrition/health factor reverses some of the earlier
causalities. In the Whiting framework, polygyny is an adaptation to the prerequisite of prolonged lactation and abstinence for women by giving the men
access to several partners, thereby solving at least the problem of male sexual
deprivation. In Saucier's framework the logic of the system works the other
way around: a gerontocracy implies appropriation and control over resources, that is, female labor and lineage land or cattle, to the detriment of
younger men. The political and economic aspects of polygyny (for example,
see Clignet's (1975) *Many Wives, Many Power*) are the core of the issue, whereas postpartum abstinence for women is a resulting characteristic, which,
from the demographic point of view, amounts to a major preventive check
operating through reduced fertility. Approached from this angle, the abstinence component of child-spacing constitutes not only a health- and
nutrition-related practice but it is also a direct consequence of a particular
type of appropriation of female labor, in much the same way as the Western
European late marriage pattern resulted from the concentration of wealth in
a system dominated by nuclear families with neolocal residence and requiring *independent* means of subsistence *prior* to marriage (Dupâquier, 1972; J.
Goody, 1976; Lesthaeghe, 1980).

The second factor encountered in Saucier's description is the relationship
between the long postpartum taboo and unilineal kinship organization.
Saucier provides no further specific explanation other than that bridewealth,
polygyny, unilineal kinship organization, and localized kin groups belong to
the same structural context (p. 243). Caldwell and Caldwell (1977) however
specify that the postpartum taboo can be seen as a device that prevents
"emotional nuclearization" between the spouses and therefore protects the
primacy of the individuals' kinship identification. In other words, the *allegiance* of adults to their respective lineages is protected by the maintenance of
a certain physical, social, and psychological distance between husband and
wife. This arrangement is the opposite of the one encountered in Western
Europe where husband and wife form a new economic entity on the basis of
conjugality. Consequently, Caldwell considers the decline of the long postpartum taboo as an indication of the success of the Western conjugal model
in sub-Saharan Africa.

Another factor revealed by Saucier's analysis of the Murdock files is the
relationship between a long postpartum taboo and the control of daily life by
rigid rules and rites. In this respect it is worth mentioning that the zone in

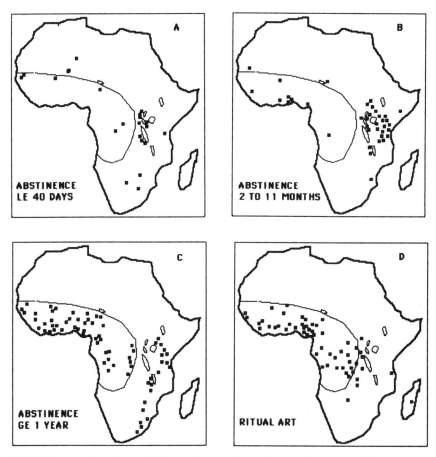

FIGURE 1.1. Location of Ethnic Groups According to Duration of Postpartum Abstinence as Stated in Ethnographic References; Comparison with Producion of Ritual Art (Source: R. Schoenmaeckers et al., 1980)

which the abstinence feature is most intact, that is, Western and Central Africa, is also the area inhabited by populations who have produced the vast majority of African ritual art (masks, fetishes, as opposed to jewelry or weaponry). This particular finding is illustrated by figure 1.1. Panels A, B, and C of this figure contain the plots of 136 societies according to the length of the postpartum taboo, ranging from 40 days to 1 year or more. The data are those used by Schoenmaeckers et al. (1981, pp. 59–65) and stem from a scanning of the anthropological literature not included by Murdock. As a result, most of the references pertain to the situation in the 1950s, 1960s, or early 1970s. If we accept the hypothesis that the postpartum taboo of at least one year is likely to have been typical for the whole of sub-Saharan Africa, then the maps must exhibit the progress of an erosion process. The greatest resistance to a reduction in abstinence durations is then found precisely in the zone that produced the ritual art (seen panel D). This underscores Saucier's finding that socialization and continued social control, both involving elaborate rituals (often based on fear), is essential in the maintenance of the moral code in general and of the postpartum taboo as a demographic preventive check in particular.

Gerontocratic control and its correlate, polygyny, not only lead to postpartum abstinence and child-spacing, but also account for specific characteristics of the use that is made of the overall reproductive age span. As already indicated, a gerontocracy restricts the rights of younger men who have to await their turn before being granted official access to the procreative and productive capacities of a women. Under conditions of balanced sex ratios, a high level of polygyny means that fewer (older) men exert a monopoly over nubile women. High polygyny ratios (number of married women per 100 married men) imply a large age difference between husbands and wives. The average age at first marriage is rasied for men and lowered for women. Hence, the mere mathematics of matching a small group of relatively old married men to a large group of married women of all ages contributes towards an early starting pattern of procreation in the sub-Saharan reproductive regime. This offsets, at least in part, the fertility-lowering effect of prolonged lactation and postpartum abstinence (Dorjahn, 1959).

The effects of polygyny do not end here. The large age gap between spouses has two further consequences. First, it reduces fecundity, or the monthly probability of conception, probably because of the joint effect of the following factors: the spread of sexual relations over several wives (sometimes regulated according to the periodicity of markets in West Africa), reduced male libido with age, and a similarly reduced semen count. Secondly, a portion of the overall exposure period for women is lost as large age differences between spouses lead to increased widowhood at any level of mortality. At low life expectancies widowhood can occur to women early in marriage and the amount of time lost for procreation could be substantial in the absence of remarriage. However, remarriage is common and the periods of widowhood are short. A marriage in the African context is not a contract between two individuals, but a *definitive* transfer of the rights *in uxorem* and *in genetricem* from one lineage or kinship group to another. There are substantial variations in the precise nature of rights that are transferred, but the deal between the two kinship groups often implies that a woman who is young enough to continue childbearing and/or to work in the fields will remain with the clan of the deceased husband. In this instance remarriage tends to take the form of widow-inheritance. Especially in East African patrilineal populations, the widow may even continue to bear children "for the deceased husband." Hence, remarriage for women in childbearing ages is generally very common and the period of widowhood short. Widow-inheritance in particular and fast remarriage in general therefore keep to a minimum the potential loss of exposure produced by a central characteristic of polygyny, namely, the large age gaps between spouses. In other words, the system provides its own corrections.

Prior to World War II, however, such an autocorrective feature almost led to demographic self-destruction. This happened when the bacilli of venereal disease (principally gonorrhea) were brought to many parts of Africa. Sterile women were being divorced, but as their labor was still valued, they usually became higher-order wives in polygynous unions. Monogamous men rejecting a childless woman married a younger one, and it is very likely that at one point the extent of polygyny rose while the age at first marriage for women fell. Consequently the infection spread rapidly and at its height, childlessness in parts of Central Africa rose to an extraordinary 40 to 50 percent of women still without offspring after 10 years of exposure. Clearly, polygyny is perfectly devised to cope with noninfectious causes of sterility and it reacted quite reasonably according to its own logic, thereby, unfortunately, setting into motion a positive feedback loop between polygyny and the spread of infection.

So far we have established two basic facts and their raison d'être: the reproductive regime of most of sub-Saharan Africa has a major preventive check operating through marked child-spacing, but this operates within a system that makes nearly complete use of the entire reproductive age span. In Western Europe, the regime of natural fertility operated the other way round: the starting of procreation was considerably delayed, but once married, birth intervals of women were generally much shorter. This led Caldwell and Caldwell (1977) to the metaphor that the African populations have taken the period of celibacy typical for Western Europe, cut it up in pieces, and inserted these in each successive birth interval. When they operationalized the implications of their metaphor by summing up the number of person-years of abstinence/celibacy in the two regimes, they came up with comparable amounts. Analyses using more sophisticated accounting schemes and parametrizations of the intermediate fertility variables (such as, using the Bongaarts decomposition of the birth interval) have also documented these findings (for example, Lesthaeghe et al., 1981, pp. 9–13; Gaisie, 1981, pp. 237–252; Lesthaeghe, Page, and Adegbola, 1981, pp. 172–174; Mosley, Werner, and Becker, 1982, pp. 19–22; Hill, 1985, pp. 59–63; Locoh, 1984, pp. 103–114).

Compared to Asian populations, however, there seems to be much less of a difference in reproductive pattern: Asian populations frequently exhibit early ages at marriage for girls and often have marked child-spacing accomplished through lactation and in several instances (for example, Hindus, Javanese) also through postpartum abstinence. The demographic survey of the Javanese village of Mojolama, for instance, produced a mean length of postpartum abstinence of 22 months (Singarimbun and Manning, 1976, pp. 175–176), which is definitely at the upper end of the distribution, even by African standards. Hence, the similarity of the Asian and African data on the starting and spacing patterns of reproduction clearly indicates how exceptional the Western European configuration was and implies that the exception was exported, together with Christianity, as if it were the global standard.

Yet, the Asian-African parallel does not go much beyond this point. This can probably be documented more fully by following the arguments of J. Goody (1976). The following list is at the core of Goody's theory of production and reproduction:

1. At the start, we find again the contrast between extensive agriculture based on the bush-fallow system, considerable land reserves, hoe cultivation, and a high input of female labor, versus more intensive forms of agriculture with more sophisticated technology and capital investment (plough, crop rotation, irrigation), fewer land reserves, and higher productivity. Up to this point, virtually all major theories still concur (such as Whiting, Murdock, Saucier, Boserup, Goody).

2. Grafted on this distinction is the contrast between a system where capital is *circulated* within a broader community or lineage on a relatively egalitarian basis and according to need, versus the system where relatively small factions or families have *concentrated* capital, and aim at consolidating their position, thereby institutionalizing class or caste inequality.

3. Directly related to this is the third distinction between systems with "diverging devolution" of property and systems without it. Goody's definition is as follows: "Under diverging devolution, the property which an individual disposes is not retained within the unilineal descent group of which he is a member, but is distributed to children of both sexes and hence diffused outside the clan or lineage" (1976, p. 7). Such diffusion or devolution of property can take the form of a dowry at marriage or it can occur through bilateral inheritance: in both instances capital is passed on to daughters and it leaves the family of origin. In a system of "homogeneous inheritance," by contrast, a man's property is transmitted solely to members of his own clan who belong to the same sex (a son, a brother's son in patrilineal societies, a sister's son, for instance, in matrilineal ones, or "male" property going to males and "female" property to females in African societies with duolateral descent). In societies where land is not inherited, since it was never appropriated by individuals but only temporarily granted to them by a corporate kinship group, there is obviously no diverging devolution.

4. In societies with appropriation and concentration of property com-

bined with bilateral inheritance systems or dowries, that is, *with* diverging devolution, there will be a marked tendency towards forms of "in-marriage," that is, endogamy (marriages among relatives), homogamy (marriages within the same social class or caste), and a preference for hypergamy (marriage to a partner of a higher social ranking). Such societies engage in marriage-politics along lines of class and caste and have a great preoccupation with locating suitable partners. As a result, prearranged child-marriages may occur. Even more important is the ban on premarital sex: uncontrolled alliances between the young could easily lead to a mismatch. In societies where there is no appropriation and concentration of property and/or no diverging devolution, there is much less preoccupation with partner selection along economic and social status lines, and hence much less fear of a *mésalliance*. Premarital sex is much more common and so are premarital births. In other words, marriage is not necessarily the point at which reproduction starts. Moreover, what counts for the child and for the lineage is the *pater*, and not so much the *genitor*, as long as the latter is not a lineage member (exogamy rule). With the exception of a tabooed (that is, incestuous) relationship, premarital and extramarital fertility may be encouraged in certain circumstances. If it is clear that a man cannot beget children, for instance, the rights *in uxorem*, which are not transferred solely to him, but also to his lineage upon the payment of bridewealth, can be taken up by a male relative of his or even an age mate in certain East African populations. The reason for this is that the payment of bridewealth also marks the transfer of rights *in genetricem*, and any offspring of a married woman, irrespective of who the genitor may be, is assumed to be her husband's and belongs therefore to his lineage in societies with unilineal descent. In West Africa the practice of "the sister's child" exists: here, a man without sons to continue the line and to perform the ancestral rites may choose an *unmarried* daughter to become pregnant and bear a son as a replacement of the male child he did not have. Such a "sister's child" may have an inferior social position, but the practice clearly shows that the continuation of the lineage may be of much greater importance than the picking of a socially or economically suitable partner.

In short, Goody's concentration on exogamy versus various forms of in-marriage, presence or lack of diverging devolution, and concentration of allodial property versus the circulation of land among lineage members according to need not only adds depth to some of Saucier's empirical findings (such as the strong relationship between the postpartum taboo and marriage via bridewealth rather than dowry), but explains why there is only a weak control on the starting pattern of reproduction and less preoccupation with children being born in or outside wedlock in sub-Saharan Africa. Asian populations may therefore also have an early starting pattern of fertility, but such a pattern stems from entirely different sources, namely the preoccupation with caste or class in-marriage, whereas in Africa it stems from the combination of polygyny, exogamy, and the lack of the strong need to control sex among the unmarried for purposes of wealth concentration. Note again that this should not be interpreted in an absolute sense: there *are* very strong taboos on sex between unmarried relatives or lineage members in sub-Saharan Africa, but the aim of such controls is to maintain *exogamy*, that is, the circulation of women across lineages, which is just the opposite of control aimed at implementing "in-marriage." As a result, Eurasian levels and patterns of premarital and extramarital fertility and the melting together of pater and genitor contrast strikingly with African levels of "illegitimate" fertility and the traditional lack of interest in biological fatherhood.

Goody tested his propositions in very much the same way as Saucier did: he too used the Murdock files but incorporated the full 863 entries rather than a sample. Furthermore, Goody's theoretical starting point was more clearly defined. The construction of dichotomies is therefore directly meaningful to his theory, whereas Saucier's dichotomies give at times the impression of being constructed for exploration only. On the other hand, Goody has little to say about the postpartum abstinence rule and child-spacing in general. His theory accounts far more satisfactorily for characteristics of the starting pattern of procreation and for rules governing marriage and partner selection in general.

This strongly abbreviated account of Goody's theoretical foundations requires at least a brief reporting of his major empirical findings as deduced from the Murdock Ethnographic Atlas. Goody presents linkage and path analyses results (1976, pp. 35–40), but the reporting of the simple phi-coefficients are enough. These coefficients have been reproduced in table 1.3, together with the operationalization of the dichotomies involved. We have, furthermore, added the phi-coefficients belonging to the dichotomy "male versus female dominance in agriculture" in accordance with Goody's incorporation of Ester Boserup's theoretical chain, which leads from swidden agriculture into heavy female labor input and other sex role differentiation characteristics (Boserup, 1970). These female roles will be taken up in later sections.

As table 1.3 shows, the two series of phi-coefficients are remarkably similar. Note, however, as indicated by the data of table 1.4, that sub-Saharan African societies are overwhelmingly concentrated in the categories *lacking* diverging devolution of property and *lacking* predominance of male farming. For them, the phi-coefficients have to be read as implying a tendancy towards a lack of premarital sex prohibitions, a lack of advanced agriculture, and so forth.

TABLE 1.3 Coefficients of Association (Phi) between Diverging Devolution or Division of Labor and Other Organizational Variables—Worldwide Sample of Societies

	Diverging Devolution[1]	Male Dominance in Farming[2]	Prohibited Premarital Sex[3]	Advanced Agriculture[4]	Complex Polity[5]	In-Marriage[6]	Monogamy[7]
Diverging Devolution	—	0.40	0.21	0.22	0.25	0.32	0.34
Male Dominance in Farming	0.40	—	0.19	0.42	0.26	0.33	0.26

SOURCE: J. Goody, 1976, pp. 34, 121–132.

1. *Diverging devolution*: all societies where daughters have a share in either land or movable property and all societies with dowry as main or alternative method of marriage transaction.

2. *Male farming*: dominance of male farming as coded by Murdock; equal participation is omitted from calculation of phi-coefficient; result based on 437 societies.

3. *Premarital sex*: prohibited and either weakly or strongly sanctioned, result for 321 societies.

4. *Advanced agriculture*: Intensive agriculture on permanent fields with fertilization, crop rotation, or dependent on irrigation; fallowing at most restricted to relatively short periods; animals used in cultivation, ploughing; results based on 592 societies.

5. *Complex polity*: presence of large states with multilevel jurisdictional hierarchy (excluding colonial courts) and/or complex stratification into social classes correlated with extensive differentiation of occupational statuses; 591 societies.

6. *In-marriage*: existence of demes, cross-cousin marriages, or caste stratification; results based on 590 societies.

7. *Monogamy*: Murdock's identification of monogamy, 590 societies.

So far, we have only dealt with starting and spacing characteristics. Several elements of sub-Saharan social organization also create the possibility for an additional fertility check located near the end of the reproductive age span. If procreation has an early start and if little time is lost in widowhood or divorce, a sizable proportion of women become grandmothers from their midthirties onward. For these women the birth of a grandchild signals that a new generation is assuming the task of procreation. Moreover, if polygyny is widespread, polygynous husbands can more easily forgo sexual relations with an older wife. This combination of early starting and polygyny therefore creates the possibility of permanent abstinence associated with grandmaternal status. In several African societies—the exact incidence of the practice is unknown—an explicit grandmaternal restriction on procreation has been defined: it is improper for an older woman to compete with a daughter or daughter-in-law with respect to childbirth; a grandmother who continues childbirth regardless is oversexed and confuses social roles.

Early stopping is not occasioned solely by grandmaternal status but may occur as a mere result of polygyny or even because a woman with several surviving children refuses sex. Such a blunt refusal, however, presupposes a relatively high degree of economic independence from the husband or a domestic organization involving bargaining between the spouses. A priori, one would expect earlier stopping to be more widespread in Western Africa than in the rest of the continent. An additional reason for such a distribution is the fact that abstinence is more readily accepted in West Africa, as indicated by the regional distribution of the long postpartum taboo.

On the whole, little research has been done on the subject of the incidence of voluntary stopping in high fertility populations. The work by Caldwell, Caldwell, and Ware in Ibadan (Southwest Nigeria) is one of the few exceptions, and they established that postpartum abstinence among Yoruba women aged 35 and older was frequently extended into definitive abstinence, especially in polygynous households. The lead provided by the Ibadan study was not sufficiently taken up by the fertility surveys of the WFS round, except in Benin where questions on grandmaternal status were explicitly asked. As a result, our knowledge of the stopping pattern and its social or cultural correlates falls considerably short of what is known for elements of starting and spacing.

The conclusion for this section is that the basic organizing principles of sub-Saharan reproductive regimes clearly reflect influences of the environment, technology, and pattern of social organization. Yet the associations discovered so far cannot be considered as "monolithic": on a worldwide scale, the highest phi-coefficient between any two variables of the ecological, production, organizational, or reproductive checklist used so far does not exceed 0.42, even after optimalization of the cutting points used in establishing the contrasting dichotomies. Also, the analysis of a matrix of bivariate associations may not be entirely adequate, since it leaves no room for *interaction* variables Z whose presence or absence strengthens or weakens the association between X and Y.

CAVEATS, VARIATIONS, AND ADDITIONAL DIMENSIONS

Contrasting traditional sub-Saharan reproductive regimes and their organizational bases with those found elsewhere yields some basic insights with respect to a general pattern, but the result is a skeletal picture that cannot account adequately for important variations within the region itself. Hence several caveats and additional dimensions need introducing.

First, there is a problem of discriminating power of the variables introduced so far. There is no continent where the prevalence of the organizational props of the fertility regime just outlined is as strong as in sub-Saharan Africa. For instance, Goody counts as many as 181 societies in the Murdock files out of 193 sub-Saharan entries, or 94 percent, where diverging devolution of property is lacking (see table 1.4). Very much the same holds for polygyny with 81 percent (this author's count for 299 entries in the Murdock sample of 1967) and for the lack of male dominance in farming with 80 percent (table 1.4). The latter percentage is furthermore the result of including nonagrarian populations such as hunter-gatherers and cattle-raising peoples. Hence, the key organizational characteristics used in the previous section are so widespread in sub-Saharan Africa that they lose their discriminating power when dealing with that part of the world only. Saucier came to an identical conclusion when trying to predict the presence of the long postpartum taboo on the basis of the twenty predictors identified from the world sample: the significant relationships disappeared entirely when the sample was restricted to sub-Saharan Africa only. Schoenmaeckers et al. tried an additional test: using eleven of the organizational props of the long taboo as identified by Saucier, they tried to construct a scale in the hope that either the number or the hierarchy of characteristics might be of additional relevance. They found, however, that the 131 sub-Saharan entries had mostly six to nine of these characteristics and that the particular combinations leading to such scores provided no prediction whatsoever. Furthermore, the few societies that fell short of a total of six items were about equally divided between societies with a long and with a short taboo. Admittedly, part of the problem is that the coding of the length of the taboo, both in Murdock's sample and in the one constructed by Schoenmaeckers et al., is sometimes debatable: the original references may contain conflicting evidence or only state broad durations. Moreover, figures are for different dates, which is a serious problem when a process of differential erosion of the postpartum taboo is involved. Yet despite these problems, the two experiments carried out so far with the abstinence custom as the dependent variable clearly show that crucial determi-

TABLE 1.4 Diverging Devolution and Dominance of Male Farming by Continent

	Africa	Eurasia Circum-Mediterranean	America	Pacific	Total
Presence of Diverging Devolution	12	84	32	32	160
Absence of Diverging Devolution or Lack of Individual Property Rights	181	77	128	46	422
Total	193	161	160	78	592
No information					271
Dominance of Male Farming	39	88	49	28	204
Dominance of Female Farming	125	11	61	36	233
Equal Participation	60	63	34	48	205
No Agriculture	8	16	155	9	188
Total	232	178	299	121	830
No information					33

SOURCE: J. Goody, 1976, pp. 12 and 131.

nants of pattern differentiation are still lacking. We shall take up this point in greater detail later on.

The second caveat pertains to the interpretation of the postpartum taboo as a preventive check in the strict Malthusian sense. As already indicated, a parallel can be drawn between the taboo and the Western European pattern of prolonged celibacy, basically because both subtract a substantial amount of person-years of exposure from the total biological reproductive age span. Yet, in the European system, later marriage not only resulted from constraints on the creation of new units of production, thereby limiting population growth, but it also provided a direct feedback mechanism of autoregulation. Subsequent to a mortality crisis, for instance, ages at marriage for women could decline as a result of vacancies in "ecological niches," and overall fertility could rapidly increase, thereby restoring earlier population densities. The African postpartum taboo does not have this property of allowing fast population recovery as its shortening is not clearly connected with an economic factor and as a reduction in abstinence could in fact be self-defeating. Such a shortening endangers lactation, which is so necessary for proper nourishment of infants. Furthermore, ages at marriage for women could be reduced only slightly given the existence of an early marriage pattern to start with. Moreover, there is again no clear link between the greater availability of land and earlier marriage, simply because there is no connection between the establishment of a new reproductive unit and the availability of independent means of subsistence. As a result, the effects of an exogenous shock that decimated population were presumably not that readily repaired in the sub-Saharan system. A much slower recovery of population may have led to more land remaining fallow for a longer period of time, thereby sustaining the pattern of production based on swidden agriculture with low population densities. Alternatively, other populations that had not experienced a mortality setback may have moved in to occupy the territory of their neighbors for a period of time, until they too suffered a population and territorial loss. Hence, in contrast with the European marriage valve, it seems to be the *lack* of a fast-acting reproductive reserve that prevented sub-Saharan societies from being pushed to the point where high population densities were pressing against constraints on resources and technology, which, according to E. Boserup's theory, would have been more conducive to technological innovation. Expressed succinctly, in Western Europe it is the fast recovery of population that leads to pattern maintenance, whereas in sub-Saharan Africa, it is rather slow recovery that fulfils this function.

The third caveat with respect to our earlier contrast of African with Eurasian systems is that it overlooked forms of cultural and economic exchange *between* African societies. These are of major importance since they produced variations with respect to patterns of social organization and therefore also with respect to the reproductive regimes.

The oldest form of cultural and economic exchange undoubtedly took place between African groups living in different ecosystems and using different technologies in producing complementary goods. Peaceful exchanges between hunter-gatherers and farmers, or even more, between farmers and herders probably stretch back very far into history. Moreover, moving frontiers, migrations, and the endemicity of tribal warfare also account for cultural and structural penetration, especially if an asymmetric relationship between the conquerors and the conquered is maintained in the form of a new stable political and economic conglomerate. As one could already judge from Saucier's cluster of structural correlates, polygyny and late marriage for men produce large numbers of young single men whose function in society is easily defined as that of hunters and warriors. Such a military reserve can be used in a variety of ways, ranging from the guarding of tribal frontiers and cattle or the organizing of raids against immediate neighbors, to the creation of a standing army involved in large-scale military conquests and the establishment of an empire. Such major military movements were not only associated with the relocation of populations in other ecological zones, for example, savannah populations into the forest belt or into mountainous regions, but they also decimated populations when they resulted in slave raids on behalf of European and Arab slave traders. Moreover, in the context of the formation of new patterns of social organization, military conquests have also carried major non-African influences, such as those associated with the Islamization of peoples living to the north of the forest or along the East African coast.

Since it is not our aim to produce a synopsis of African history, we shall discuss only those major dimensions whose inclusion is necessary for further studying of the reproductive regimes. They can be grouped under the following headings:

1. The impact of Islam and Christianity on cultural and organizational traits, which in their turn affect reproduction
2. The impact of variations in African kinship structures and more specifically of variations pertaining to the position of women, security, and the value of children
3. The effects of the growth of new economic sectors in both rural and urban areas, during and after the colonial era, and operating via factors such as individual property, labor migration, and education.

Islamic and Christian Penetration

The Judeo-Christian and Muslim traditions have their roots among Near Eastern and European populations whose forms of social organization were on several accounts diametrically opposed to those encountered in "primal" sub-Saharan situations. We shall deal with Islamization and Arabization first.

Goody (1976) has alreay pointed out three major factors that have been introduced with Islam and which are also typically Arab:

1. The presence of devolving devolution of property
2. The tendency toward endogamy with the presence of preferential cousin marriage of the "father's brother's daughter" (Fa Br Da) type (i.e., patrilateral parallel-cousin marriage)
3. The organization along the lines of caste stratification involving "holy men," warriors, artisans (i.e., the "free" groups) and conquered servants or farmers of different ethnic origin.

These three characteristics contrast with the sub-Saharan prototype with lineage ownership of land and strong exogamy rules. In fact, at a general level Islam has weakened lineage control. It has, for instance, redefined the lineage gerontocracy by providing the broader model of a theocratic gerontocracy which implies caste literacy and acceptance of a new universalistic and unifying religion. It has cut across ethnic division by introducing the notion of Umaa or the worldwide community of believers. Islam furthermore carried the trait of strong male dominance with models of the male-provider and the male-theologician, thereby running counter to female economic self-reliance and the roles of priestesses in certain animist traditions and female secret societies. Last but not least, Islam also weakened traits of matrilineal forms of kinship organization.

Yet, these contrasts between the Islamic and sub-Saharan principles of organization must not be carried too far. First, not all features of the two systems are in opposition, and second, symbiotic or syncretic forms of social organization are far more widespread in the region than cases of complete Arabization. Hence, there is a spectrum with respect to the depth of Islamization, often corresponding to the timing of Islamic penetration (that is, starting from the eighth century in the East and the eleventh century in the West) and to the contrast between conquering and conquered peoples.

The principle of appropriation of female labor by a gerontocracy and hence also the institution of polygyny probably constitutes the most important overlap between the two systems. Although polygyny is considerably less widespread in Muslim populations of Northern Africa and Asia than in sub-Saharan ones and limited to four wives by the Islamic definition, it seems that the combination of the Arab and sub-Saharan marriage patterns has produced a particularly forceful version of it. The Arab derivative of in-marriage, namely prearranged marriage involving very young women, and the sub-Saharan practice of widow-inheritance involving many older women, have been welded together and have jointly sustained a highly polygynous regime that brings women into almost continuous marriage from very early ages onward. Also the relative ease of divorcing women, a male prerogative in the Arab setup, and the possibilities for elopement, that is, a female initiative in the sub-Saharan one, seem to have found a common direction in the sense that they are both supportive of high frequencies of divorce. This in it turn enhances polygyny.

The duality between female seclusion typical of the Arab system and female economic independence of the sub-Saharan one is another domain of syncretic pattern formation, as illustrated by the following example. The Hausa of northern Nigeria are more Islamicized than most: Islamization started in the fourteenth century; they have Fa Br Da–preferential parallel-cousin marriage, occasionally diverging devolution of property, and wealthier men keep their wives in purdah. Yet, Enid Schildkrout (1983, pp. 106–126) found that Hausa women in Kano City, despite being secluded, continued to produce goods that were marketed by their children and managed to command *independent* economic means of major importance. In fact, Schildkrout argues that the custom of seclusion of women, being the expression of their husbands' economic success, has been on the increase in Kano as a result of increased prosperity in the region and as a consequence of the allowance made for continued participation of secluded women in the market economy (p. 107). Hence, purdah and control of independent resources can be fused together in a particular syncretic form and jointly specify a particular role for children. Note, however, that the case of the wealthier women in Kano is somewhat exceptional, not in the sense that Muslim women are permitted to maintain an independent source of revenue, but in that they succeed in accumulating capital (probably because of being married to more successful husbands). In many other circumstances capital accumulation is far less likely to occur given the great demands put on female incomes (see for instance Bisilliat, 1983, p. 105, for the Songhai).

Another duality exists between the dominance of husbands and patrikin versus the importance of matrikin. This duality is not particular to Islamized populations but is found in many regions of the world (for example, Southern India) where strong male-dominant and patrilineal forms of kinship organization have been superimposed on older matrilineal systems. But, Islamic organizing principles certainly are among those that have stressed the dominance of husband and patrikin to a considerable extent, so that the survival of important matrilineal allegiance is another salient element in the formation of new syntheses. Most frequently, matrikin remain important in fulfilling emotional needs. Patrikin see a child as a lineage member and interpret its socialization more in terms of producing a loyal and worthy addition to the group, whereas a freer and more affective bond is allowed to grow between a child and its matrikin. As said before, this form of "functional specialization" seems to be a frequently encountered *modus vivendi* wherever the two systems meet. The importance of matrikin can be much further reaching than that, even in societies that are by now thoroughly Islamized. Among the Wolof of Western Senegal, for instance, matrilateral ties may be used in soliciting support from powerful individuals, or conversely, in acquiring a political following. Matrilineal characteristics among the neighboring Serer are of even greater importance, still today. A Serer man inherits only personal belongings from his father, whereas rights to land and cattle stem from his maternal uncle. Serer girls also entrust their earnings to a maternal uncle or brother rather than to their father (H. Nelson et al., 1974, pp. 90–95). Not only traits of matrilineal but also of duolateral kinship organization have withstood the Islamic tendency toward more absolute supremacy of the paternal type of allegiance. Examples of this can be found among Islamized Guan of Central Ghana.

An example of a Muslim transformation of an older sub-Saharan institution is provided by the Muride *daara* in Senegal. A common practice in sub-Saharan populations is the socialization of children in groups, culminating in the institution of age grades. Both the Serer and Wolof of Senegal had such age grades, and those of the Serer have continued to function more or less in their original form. Among the Wolof, however, the Muridiya Islamic brotherhood has recruited young men into *daara* communities, which are at once farms and Koranic schools designed to form the character of boys and younger men (ages 9 to 25) by hard work and rather austere discipline. The first *daara* was founded in 1889 and Muridism played a vital role in the spread of groundnut cultivation. *Daaras* are led by marabouts (Sérigne) who are also managers of these "cooperatives" and who market the produce. One of the reasons why similar ventures did not succeed among the Serer is that they were farmers by tradition, whereas the Wolof were not. Poorer Wolof families needed apprenticeships in groundnut farming and these Muride communities provided just that. The net result was that the earlier age grades were transformed into an austere Islamic fraternity with a specific ethnic basis and fostering economic and political power. Later movements of reform, however, criticized this marabout-dominated system and urged believers to confront God directly, that is, without reliance on brotherhoods or marabouts. The other part of the criticism was that Muridism had cooperated with the colonial power and exploited religious naiveté (Nelson et al., 1974, pp. 132–136). Admittedly, the *daara* is a typical Muride and Wolof feature, and similar institutions are not commonly encountered elsewhere, but the example is rather illuminating in that it indicates how Islamization has developed historically through different syncretic forms of social organization adapted to the various ethnic settings.

The other major religious system that has reshaped sub-Saharan culture and social structure is obviously Christianity. For our purposes, the spread of Christianity is of particular importance because of its tendency to treat about any form of African family life as "sinful" and for its open combat against ritual expressions of authority, socialization, and exchange. Christianity—in contrast to Islam—had little or no tolerance of polygyny or divorce. Nor would it understand or endure marriages being contingent on payment of bridewealth, postpartum abstinence, or widow-inheritance. In contrast to a system that Christianity regarded as "promiscuous," it propagated the notions of premarital chastity, conjugality, and marital fidelity, thereby exporting a nineteenth-century version of a value system that stemmed directly from the late marriage pattern with neolocal residence, which was on all accounts highly idiosyncratic to Western Europe only.

The depth of Christian penetration is again quite varied and depends *inter alia* on the type of colonial rule and the type of church involved. In areas with indirect rule (but many were already Muslim) a head-on confrontation was often avoided by imposing restrictions on mission work. Here, Christianity relied less on mass conversion but rather on the subtle but powerful device of providing primary education for boys and girls. Generally speaking, Protestant churches were also more likely to take local customs and existing forms of social organization into account, but this expression of flexibility should be seen as a device for facilitating recruitment. In areas that had both direct colonial rule and a near monopoly by Catholic missions, Christianization was both more pervasive and uncompromising (for example, Zaire and especially Rwanda and Burundi).

The other contrast with Islam is the Christian reliance and stress on education and on the provision of medical services. Today, the boundary between regions with high versus medium or low illiteracy (especially for women) still corresponds largely to the historical demarcation zone between Islamic and Christian penetrations, despite schooling efforts in the least advantaged areas during the postcolonial period. As schooling for women is closely associated with changes in reproductive behavior all over Africa, one can expect a close relationship to emerge between the regional pattern of fertility transition and the geographic spread of Christianity, with education acting as a major intermediate variable.

The reactions against the colonial religion were manifold and frequently shared two important aspects: they were expressions of nascent nationalism and they restored African cultural and structural elements (such as the link between religion and health, tolerance of polygyny). To capture the present range, use can be made of several typologies. Here, we shall build on the one offered by H. W. Turner (1976, pp. 18–20):

1. *Neoprimal movements*, which are new forms of traditional African religions but are distinct from further developments within the old system. Despite the fact that neoprimal movements are often strongly opposed to older forms of animism, they are at the same time attempting to revitalize or remodel it by borrowing certain forms or ideas from Christianity in order to deal with inadequacies of the old system.
2. *Syncretic movements*, which have intentionally and consciously created a new system by borrowing from the African primal and the invasive traditions and intend to be neither traditional nor Christian.

3. *Independent churches*, which are already much closer to the Christian end of the spectrum. In fact, they consider themselves as Christian, mostly by retaining both New and Old Testament as the scriptures. A division can be made between "Ethiopian" and "Zionist" subtypes, with the former more closely resembling the parent orthodox churches and the latter being more Africanized, with faith healing and revelations through a prophet as their main emphasis. Polygyny is tolerated by both.

4. *African Protestant churches*, which have close ties to European and American Protestantism and are often formal members of the World Council of Churches in Geneva.

5. *Roman Catholicism.*

This spectrum, ranging from neoprimal to fully Christian faith corresponds largely with an educational continuum, both in terms of the educational attainments of their adherents as well as with respect to their organizing a network of schools. In the list given above, networks for primary education emerge from the independent churches onward, whereas secondary education is organized from African Protestant churches onward. This does not imply, however, that neoprimal and especially syncretic movements fail to recruit from the educated groups.

Finally, it should also be stressed that the impact of Christianity is often shallow: the conjugal family model is seldom realized, and faith-healing, divinations, presence of spirits, and, to some extent also, witchcraft are still very common expressions of an older tradition. Also polygyny has survived to a remarkable extent despite the Christian ban.

The Position of Women and Traditional Kinship Structures

In all societies women fulfill a plurality of functions and they consequently have a diversified role structure. If Oppong's classification (1981) is adopted, a distinction can be made between maternal, domestic, labor, conjugal, kin, community, and individual roles. Since all of these bear a direct relationship to processes of decision making at the individual and group levels, a more detailed discussion is warranted within the framework of this chapter.

In traditional sub-Saharan societies two of these functions can be singled out as most crucial: women are simultaneously major agricultural producers and procreators on behalf of corporate kinship groups. It is clear from the Murdock files that female labor inputs are frequently larger, and seldom lower, than those of men, and that rights *in genetricem* are usually conveyed to the husband's lineage through payments of bridewealth. This dual function is stressed by institutional arrangements and through normative prescriptions with respect to behavior. The reproductive function itself is so crucial to both the individual woman and to the two kinship groups concerned that the status of adulthood for women is almost completely contingent on motherhood and the last installments of bridewealth payments are often transferred upon the birth of the first child only.

The labor value of women, on the other hand, is not only underscored by high levels of polygyny and fast remarriage, even of childless women, but also by descriptions of the code of conduct for women. Irrespective of whether descriptions of expectations are formulated by men or women, two features are commonly stressed: apart from being a dedicated mother, a woman should neither be lazy nor quarrelsome (see A. Molnos, 1973, for a collection of such descriptions). It should be noted parenthetically that the aversion to "quarrelsome" women does not stem only from husbands who may like peace and quiet, but also from other women and especially from cowives. This hints, obviously, at the importance of domestic and community roles.

More important, however, is that a balance has to be found between the production and procreative functions of women, both in terms of time use and physical capacity. Several authors place the postpartum taboo in this context since too rapid childbearing endangers female labor productivity. This view draws support from popular sayings that "pregnant women become lazy," but even more from common notions that stress a proper balance between the two activities and stigmatize either too rapid or too slow a pace of childbearing. In other words, the traditional stress on the timing pattern of fertility in sub-Saharan Africa as a whole is in accordance with the duality between the productive and procreative functions of women.

The maternal and labor roles of women are intimately linked with those associated with the domestic group, kin, and community. It is predominantly with respect to these connections that a great deal of differentiation occurs. The first division that can be made pertains to groups that are organized along strictly patrilineal lines and those that have deviations from it in the direction of bilateral or matrilineal descent and organization. Most of the Eastern African populations are patrilineal (for example, Kikuyu, Kamba, Kisii, Luo, Chagga, Mijikenda, Embu-Meru, Kalenjin, Maasai), but this also holds for many West African ones (for example, Peul and Tukulor of Senegal; the Kru and southern and northern Mande groups of Ivory Coast and Mali; the Hausa and Kanuri of Northern Nigeria; the Yoruba, Ibo, and Ibibio-groups of Southern Nigeria; the Mandara, Chari-Logone, and Adamawa groups of Northern Cameroon). Deviations from the patrilineal pattern are most commonly found in West and Central Africa. Matrilateral descent can be of importance in the maintenance of exogamy and for minor functions, often falling within the emotional and sentimental domain but possibly extended toward the formation of political alliances as well. Usually different terms are used to distinguish between matrikin and patrikin, such as the Wolof *genyo* (= belt) versus *men* (= breast milk), and functional specifications are attached to each. Such "modest" deviations from strict patrilineal organization are, for instance, found among the Diola of Southern

Senegal, several Voltaic groups of Burkina Faso and Northern Ghana, the Songhai of Niger, the Adangbe and Anlo Ewe of Southern Ghana, and the Bamileke and Pangwe-groups of Western and Central Cameroon.

A major step away from the patrilineal pattern occurs when the matriliny assumes importance with respect to inheritance of movable goods or rights to land, and with respect to religious functions. This pattern is found *inter alia* among the Serer of Senegal, several Voltaic groups, the Lobi of Northern Ghana, the Senufo and Kulango of Mali and Northern Ivory Coast, and among the Bamileke nobility of Western Cameroon.

Fully corporate matrilineages are found along a Central African geographical band, that is, from Western Zaire and Northern Angola to Zambia, Malawi, and further to Northern Mozambique. A second cluster is located in Ghana and the western part of the Ivory Coast and includes the Akan group (including the Fante, Twi, Agni-Baoulé) and the neighboring Ga, Abron, and matrilineal Lagunaires groups. It should be stressed, however, that patrilineal descent still plays a significant role in these matrilineal societies and that many authors prefer to treat the Akan system, for instance, as being based on bilateral descent. The Akan make a clear distinction between the *Abusua* (that is, relationship through the mother's blood) and the *Ntoro* (that is, through the father's spirit) and again attach functional specifications to each (for a description, see for instance Manoukian, 1950). These specifications are such that the husband is not just a figurehead of the family, especially as far as his children are concerned. Furthermore, ascension to political office and land-use rights in cash crop areas are increasingly being passed on through the paternal line. The latter change occurred as a result of private appropriation of such land, and the former when several *Asantehene* of the nineteenth century created new offices or stools in an attempt to curtail the power of hereditary officials moving up through the matrilineal channel. The interplay between these two systems results in various forms of accomodation, but shifts are often in the direction of greater prominence for the patrilineal side, particularly with the advent of a more modern economy. Very much the same applies across the border in the Ivory Coast where Agni matrilineages are under severe strain in a typical plantation economy (Roberts et al., 1973, pp. 104–105).

Finally, the Guan groups of Central Ghana (Gonja) and along the Ghanaian coast (Efutu and Awutu) operate a system without corporate lineages. It is characterized by duolocal marriage, duolateral descent, and by the circulation of children through extensive child-fostering to either maternal or paternal kin.

The position of women is partially contingent upon these various patterns of kinship organization. In the strictly patrilineal societies of East Africa the rights *in genetricem* belong exclusively to the husband's clan, even in instances of adulterous offspring. Rights *in uxorem* can be extended to the husband's brothers or to his age mates, especially if it is clear that the husband himself cannot produce children for his lineage (for example, this occurs among the Maasai, Nandi, Kamba, Kikuyu, Kisii, Meru). Widow-inheritance in these societies used to be the rule and widows had only limited rights of appeal. In addition, any subsequent children born after the death of the husband and begotten by a new husband were counted for the deceased man. In several of these societies the husband's clan could claim a replacement wife from the kinship group of a deceased spouse. In other words, the full payment of bridewealth marked a definitive transfer of a rather impressive set of claims on a woman to the clan of the husband. The correlate of this strongly patrilineal and patrilocal form of kinship organization is a high degree of female encapsulation within the husband's domestic group. There is often a hierarchical ordering of females in the homestead starting from the husband's mother, senior cowives, the husband's sisters, and going down to younger wives of the husband's brothers. This hierarchy is not only of domestic importance but is also maintained in collective female work parties. A wife possesses, furthermore, only minor personal belongings and has no independent source of income. Female market activities are limited or nonexistent, and the husband provides for all the needs of his family. The "ideal woman" should not only be hardworking and a caring mother, she should also be obedient, pleasant, and hospitable to her husband's kin and friends. Childbearing occurs exclusively in the presence of affinal kin and the new mother does not return home during the postpartum period. A woman, however, retains visiting rights to her own kin; her father or brothers can complain if she is maltreated, but the initiation of divorce by the woman herself or by her kinsmen is difficult: the bridewealth—which is often used to finance the marriage of a younger brother—would then have to be returned to the husband's clan or another woman sent in replacement. Elopement is therefore the only alternative. Generally speaking, such kinship and domestic organization leaves all major decisions in the hands of a woman's affines and she can only increase her status and her security through her sons. This results in a preference for boys, which is, however, by no means comparable in strength to the sex preference found in many Asian societies. The principle of circulation of property—girls bring in bridewealth, boys spend it—acts as a major brake on son preference when considered from the point of view of the patriliny.

The social and economic position of women in West Africa revolves around three major dimensions:

1. Control over women is tightened with increased depth of Islamization, but even then there is no destruction of an essential and typically West African female prerogative, namely the participation in the market economy.

2. Female independence and reliance on own kin increase as one moves

away from stronger forms of patrilineal organization in the direction of corporate matrilineages or noncorporate kinship organization.

3. Female independence is positively correlated with increased economic complexity of traditional societies, or more specifically, with the growth of markets and trading.

The links between the position of women and forms of kinship organization can be described in greater detail for the ethnic groups that contribute demographic data in the subsequent chapters. Among groups with corporate matrilineages (such as the Akan) or without corporate kinship groups, rights *in genetricem* are evidently not directly transferred to the husband's lineage upon the payment of bridewealth. Among patrilineal and patrilocal societies that have such a transfer, deviations from the principle occur with respect to adulterous offspring and the custom of the "sister's child." An adulterous child can be rejected by the patriliny to whom the husband belongs and as a result, it can be reared by its matrikin (such as occurs among the Mole-Dagbani, Gonja, Anlo Ewe, Pangwe). In most West African societies a husband's sexual rights are never extended to his brothers, even if it is clear that he cannot beget children. He may accept an adulterous child or a foster child, or alternatively, the wife and her kin may initiate a divorce. Upon the death of a man, a widow often has the right of refusing the new partner, but even in instances of widow-inheritance, no further children are born "for the deceased husband." There is no replacement of the deceased wife by an unmarried sister or other female kin of hers, and several societies have no widow-inheritance (for example, the Gonja, Anlo Ewe).

The relationship between the women living in the same compound is also more egalitarian in West Africa than in East Africa. In the West, each woman has an individual plot for gardening or for more extensive cultivation and a good husband is defined as a man who avoids arousing jealousy among his cowives. His eating and sleeping arrangements may therefore rotate according to the market cycle. In West African patrilineal societies the link between a married woman and her own kin is often maintained: women can return home during the postpartum period and children (especially first ones) can be born away from her husband's compound. Child-fostering to matrikin is another possibility. In fact, child-fostering is *inter alia* a device for circumventing a husband's claim on the children in case of a divorce. Women can initiate divorce in a variety of circumstances and count on the support of their kin. Grounds for divorce are not only physical maltreatment but also a failure to support the wife economically or a failure to consult her when taking a junior wife. Also the notion of rape *within* marriage exists and is an additional ground for divorce (for example, among the Twi).

Even more important is the West African economic principle that any surplus goes to the producer in full ownership. As a result women participate intensively in the market economy and have their own revenue, even if the product is grown on the husband's land. In other societies the provision of starting capital is a relatively common ingredient of the bargaining associated with a marriage, which, in matrilineal societies, comes in addition to a wife retaining rights to her lineage land. In such situations, for example, many Akan women have become entrepreneurs in the sector of cocoa farming, and among the fishing populations of the Atlantic coast women own boats, paying their husbands for their labor with a part of the profit stemming from the sale of the catch. Moreover, female entrepreneurs control large segments of the market, including the black market, and wield political influence. In fact, throughout the colonial and postcolonial period, Akan, Yoruba, and Bamileke women have played very prominent political roles in Ghana, Nigeria, and Cameroon respectively. In this context, polygyny assumes a specific function, namely that of producing a joint commercial venture—the husband dealing with the fiducial aspects and the wives being responsible for production and marketing. Many small-scale industries in Lagos, for example, stem from such arrangements.

Another important feature of West African social organization is the presence of women's societies. The original function of these societies was to administer initiation rites, but in societies with a more complex economy and polity, both male and female associations grew in importance by assuming a plurality of administrative and commercial functions as well, such as tax collection, price control in markets, maintenance of public order, and organization of collective work. The *mandjon* societies of Bamileke men and women provide good examples of such traditional associations. The women's *mandjon* are presided over by the mother of the *fon* or chief—there are over a hundred of such chiefdoms in Bamileke territory—and its members help each other in agricultural work. The *mandjon* used to meet on a weekly basis to organize such work. In addition to associations that fit into the political structure of Bamileke society, there are also many autonomous associations based on neighborhood. Aside from ritual functions (such as divination and faith healing) they also act as saving groups and associations for mutual assistance. More recently, Bamileke associations (but for that matter also Pangwe age grades) have been adapted to the needs of urban living and have led to a proliferation of voluntary membership clubs that provide mutual aid, companionship for immigrants, and entertainment. The saving groups are maintained by members paying in fixed amounts at weekly meetings, taking turns in receiving the entire sum. Membership is not restricted to a single saving association and the Bamileke tend to join them as soon as they earn money (Nelson et al., 1973, pp. 86–87 and 94–95). Very similar evolutions have taken place in many other societies all along the Benin Gulf—for example, *esusu* in Lagos—and in Central Africa—for example, Kinshasa's *ikelemba* (saving societies) and *musiki* (mutual assistance associations). In Ghana and Nigeria men and women have turned to voluntary membership clubs and organizations composed of people with common interests. Mutual aid associations have an established tradition and the same holds for occupational societies (such as societies of market women which wield a considerable amount of influence in these countries). At least in Southern Ghana, men tend to dominate in the various ethnic clubs, but women by far outnumber men in mutual benefit and occupational associations (Kaplan et al., 1971, pp. 127–128).

The account given so far is highly condensed and fragmentary and may convey a general picture of the differences in institutional contexts within which the position of women is defined, but one should be wary of over-simplifications. Hence, a few caveats are in order.

First, the distinction between East and West Africa relative to the degree of economic independence of women should neither be exaggerated nor stereotyped. In a system with segregated budgets of husbands and wives, there are major demands on the women's incomes, and the possibilities for accumulation of savings are limited. Increasing costs of childrearing, for instance, have considerably increased the pressure on that income, while the revenue itself may not have grown in real terms. In fact, transformations of the traditional economy have frequently reduced female earning capacities for those who are not incorporated into the modern administrative or commercial sectors (Ware, 1981, pp. 19–22). Moreover, the corollary of a certain economic independence for women is that the husband's share in meeting daily expenditures of the household (food, clothing, shelter, education) is restricted and may not grow adequately in relation to the number of children or the rate of inflation. Younger children may therefore be a direct burden on their mother's income, but as they grow older and generate an income themselves, they will again be a major economic asset to women.

Second, the practice of child-fostering has to be taken into account, especially but not exclusively in West Africa. Child-fostering among kin spreads both costs of and benefits from children over a wider group of adults. A woman with young children may benefit from the services rendered by a teenage niece or nephew, while richer segments of a kinship group may help out with the education of a foster child. In societies with an expanding class structure following in the wake of differential economic development, the strength or weakness of such institutionalized forms of kinship solidarity is likely to be a major element in shaping any individual economic calculations of the costs and value of children (J. Sinclair, 1972; E. Goody, 1973; Isiugo-Abanihe, 1985).

Third, female economic independence in traditional societies is also a function of economic integration of large numbers of producers and consumers in a more complex economy and polity. As one moves away from the Benin Gulf in the direction of the Central African forest belt, population density decreases rapidly and so does economic complexity. In this environment economic exchange occurs less at large markets with a fixed periodicity and more in the form of occasional barter. In such situations with simpler

subsistence economies there is considerably less room for income generation and capital formation from trade. The corollary is that the position of
women in the domestic domain resembles the East African pattern more
closely and that the presence of women in the commercial sector has remained less marked in these areas, despite any recent development of a
market economy.

Fourth, several sub-Saharan societies contain a large number of female-
headed households. This is most clearly visible in Southern Africa where
relatively low levels of polygyny combined with very substantial labor
migration to the Republic of South Africa (RSA) have produced a high incidence of such households (for example, in Botswana, Lesotho, and African
populations within the RSA). Characteristically, female-headed households
are located at the disadvantaged end of the income distribution, which is
related to the fact that men and patrilineages control land and cattle even
if husbands are absent. A lack of capital assets in turn reduces the productive value of children (see for instance Mueller and Koussoudji, 1981, for
Botswana) and enhances the household's dependence on remittances from
a migrant worker. Female-headed households are not a feature typical of
Southern Africa alone. In addition, male labor outmigration is not the only
correlate: women in a polygynous union or urban "concubines" may have
charge of a separate household and the same often applies to older widows
as well (cf. Sala Diakanda, 1979, for Western Zaire).

The traditional position of women has undergone substantial changes
especially since World War II. We have already pointed out the impact of
male labor migration and the weakening of matrilineal kinship organization,
but these are both the result of major structural transformations with respect
to land tenure and the tendency toward private ownership, cash crop production, monetarization, modernization of technology, legal reforms, the
emergence of class stratification, and rapid urbanization (see Boserup, 1970,
and Ware, 1981, pp. 17–22). The position of women is further affected by
Islamization or Westernization of the value systems through religious institutions, schools, and media.

Several of these issues are taken up in the next section, but it is essential to
bear in mind that all these modern transformations have been grafted upon a
highly diversified set of older arrangements in the domains of kinship and economic
organization and on different cultural systems. As a result, the influence of
the heterogeneity of traditional organizing principles on *current* patterns of
reproduction is bound to be substantial, even in the wealthier countries of
sub-Saharan Africa.

Structural Changes: Land Tenure, Urban Growth, and Class Stratification

The general concept behind traditional sub-Saharan forms of " land
tenure" is that land constitutes an *inalienable ancestral trust* with rights of use

extended to members of a tribe, lineage, or localized kinship group. In other words, there is no "tenure" at all. This common inheritance is administered by a chief or by local headmen, and they hold it as representatives of both the living and the dead. Aside from its economic value, land is also the symbolic expression of group affiliation: it embodies a tribe's past, present, and future (Roberts et al., 1973, pp. 293–294; Kaplan et al., 1966, pp. 446–447). Many sub-Saharan societies link their social organization to the earth, not by fiefs, titles, or contracts, but by means of shrines (such as rain shrines among the Plateau Tonga), stools (such as among the Akan), or other ancestral marks (such as skulls among the Bamileke). If there were any mapping of land use, it would have been genealogical in nature (Bohannan, 1967, pp. 55–56) since the link is not between an individual and a particular plot, but between an individual and a social group that has traditionally farmed the area and protected it against encroachment by foreigners through uninterrupted crop-fallow rotation or migration within that area.

Land can be farmed (not owned) communally—hence the organization of working parties in some societies—but more often the head of each homestead or compound enjoys granted usufructuary rights to a specific area. The notion of a right has to be understood as legitimate use based on customary and factual occupancy and not in terms of a contractual right or alienable title. Such rights of usage can be inherited according to a variety of rules (such as a single chosen heir, primo- or ultimogeniture, sharing) depending on ethnic tradition. Usage rights can also be pledged to satisfy a lineage debt. Land, however, can never be sold or mortgaged by its occupant. Land "sales" by chiefs to other tribes or European settlers were hence not sales in the Western sense, but only long-term, and in principle revocable, permits of usage. If land is no longer used beyond the normal fallow period or if it is misused, it reverts to the community or to another segment of a kinship group. Furthermore, rights to cultivation do not exclude other community members from passage, gathering of wild products, or even from grazing cattle during the fallow period.

Farming methods range from shifting cultivation, involving a relocation of the entire settlement to a new farming zone, to sedentary cultivation based on rotating of plots around the settlement. Such a settlement may have an urban character (for example, the Yoruba towns) and farming plots can be located at quite a distance from it. In a few instances, farming without fallowing is practiced, but this tends to occur on narrow riverine flood strips (such as along the Senegal River) or on small manured plots only (such as among the Serer). In virtually all such instances of more intensive cultivation, farmers still practice fallowing on the rest of their land.

Substantial deviations from this traditional sub-Saharan system have come into existence in many areas. One of the earliest departures from it came into being as a result of military conquests of farmers by Islamized herders-warriors in the Sudanic region and by the expansion of the Shewan empire in Ethiopia. These conquests led to a reorganization of land tenure in accordance with the much more rigidly stratified political and social order prevailing among the conquerors.

The Fulani rule over Northern Nigeria during the early nineteenth century, for instance, was accompanied by the bestowal of fiefs to members of the higher caste and by the appointment of local overseers (the Fulani are not cultivators but pastoralists) who had the power to allocate unused and unoccupied land without regard for traditional community interests (Nelson et al., 1981, p. 148). The result was an influx of "foreigners" and the development of a dual system: the old customary rules applied to conquered populations accepting Islam, whereas the new system, based on occupancy permits granted by Muslim nobles against payment of tribute, applied to the new settlers. Such occupancy permits were formalized under British rule. *Kirdi* populations (that is, pagans) resisting Islamization were either enslaved and lost any claim to the usage of land, or were relocated in "farming colonies," owing tribute to the conquerors (such as was the fate of several Adamawa-speaking ethnic groups in Northern Cameroon).

The impact of caste stratification is also clearly visible in much of Senegal (except among the Diola of the Casamance region) and Northern Sudan. Among the Wolof and Serer every freeman not belonging to the artisan caste or descended from a former slave family had rights to cultivate land, but local nobles had reserved the better plots surrounding the villages. Among the Wolof, most cultivators pay annual tribute to such nobles or, in certain areas, to a marabout, in exchange for what used to be a *free* customary right. Former slaves who were granted usage of some land pay tribute to their former masters in the form of labor, a portion of the crop, or in cash (Nelson et al., 1973, p. 283). These old hierarchical arrangements are most clearly visible in the old Wolof groundnut belt and among the Tukulor in Northern Senegal whose society relied more on slave agricultural labor than that of the Wolof or Serer. In the newly developed groundnut zones of Central Senegal, that is, the "Terres Neuves," Serer tenure systems tended to become more egalitarian, that it, as long as there were vacancies, but the Wolof pattern often led to an outright dominance by the marabouts (cf. Muridism and daara). In other words, leadership in the new capitalist sector and membership of the old ruling castes overlap to a considerable extent (see also C. S. Whitaker, 1970, for such "politics of tradition" in Northern Nigeria). A stratified system also exists in the most productive agricultural zone of Northern Sudan, namely the Gezira triangle between the White and Blue Nile. In this area with substantial cash cropping (cotton), former Arab slave owners rely extensively on migrant labor from Kordofan, Darfur, or further west (such as Mecca pilgrims). This has, in some instances, led to absentee landlordism, a feature that was plainly inconceivable in the traditional sub-Saharan framework.

As already indicated, Ethiopian tenure systems also deviated substantially from the principle of circulation according to subsistence needs. At the beginning of the nineteenth century, the tenure system in the central and northern highlands (Amhara, Tigre) was based on inheritable rights to land for peasants (rist) against payment of tribute and/or rendering of labor services to the nobility (gult). The Ethiopian Church possessed land of its own in addition to *gult*-rights over peasants with *rist*-rights. In the second half of the nineteenth century, that is, following the Shewa conquest of Southern Ethiopia and the Ogaden, new *gult*-rights were given to Amhara nobility, administrators, and soldiers without extending the *rist*-rights to southern populations. These populations, who had been living closer to the more egalitarian sub-Saharan system, were thereby reduced to mere tribute-paying tenants with little security of tenure (Nelson and Kaplan, 1980, pp. 22, 98–100). The relationship between the northerners and southerners continued to develop further in this direction and it is described by Markakis and Ayele (1978) as that between "master and subject, landlord and tenant, tax collector and tax payer." This situation bears a direct relationship to the Ethiopian revolution of 1974.

A new wave of deviations from sub-Saharan principles was introduced during the colonial era. A variety of situations came into existence, depending on ecology, type of crop, and type of colonial intervention. The following sample may be helpful in picturing the range of such interventions:

1. Trading companies obtained concessions and created company estates, sometimes with smallholders on them instead of wage laborers (e.g., Ghanaian rubber plantations).
2. Colonial authorities issued occupancy permits (e.g., in Northern Nigeria) thereby "legalizing" earlier situations (cf. Fulani organization of conquered land). Alternatively, they bestowed new power on chiefs or notables by allowing them to issue titles (e.g., in Senegal).
3. Long- or short-term lease holdings were introduced in areas earmarked for new agricultural development (e.g., tenant farming in the Gezira irrigation scheme).
4. European settlement was encouraged in suitable areas (cattle raising, cash cropping) on the basis of long-term leases (99 or 999 years in the Kenyan "White Highlands" for instance) or on the basis of freeholds. European settlers engaged extensively in agriculture in Kenya and Zimbabwe, but "white farms" were also created in Malawi, Mozambique, Angola, and to a lesser degree in Zaire.
5. Colonial authorities introduced consolidation schemes in areas where land use showed fragmentation of plots scattered over a wide range (e.g., the Swynnerton Plan in Kenya's Central and Nyanza provinces), which ultimately led not only to more efficient use, but also to private ownership.

Apart from such direct colonial interventions, major changes also occurred in areas where African populations themselves initiated cash cropping (see the earlier discussion for examples of arrangements associated with Senegalese groundnut farming). The indigenous cocoa farming in Ghana illustrates an alternative set of patterns. Among the Akan who inhabit the largest part of the Ghanaian cocoa belt, the matrilineal kinship system was used to divide the land for cocoa growing, thereby respecting opportunities for women. Labor, however, was often provided by wives and children so that sons gained claims on paternal plots, which weakened matrilineal control (Manoukian, 1950, p. 50; Okali, 1983, pp. 174–178). In addition to family labor, migrant labor was imported under the *abusa* or *nkotokuando* systems. Such laborers lived on the cocoa farm with their families and were paid in kind: up to a third of the crop for farm managers (abusa) and substantially less for plucking and maintenance workers (nkotokuando). A third pattern was followed by the Krobo (that is, a subgroup of the Adangbe) who operated via *huza*-companies (Kaplan, 1973, pp. 306–307). Such a company was made up of either blood relatives or unrelated individuals who pooled their resources to acquire tracts of forest in Akan territory for cocoa farming. The tracts were subsequently divided between the *huza* members in proportion to their contribution. Colonial legal reforms permitting corporate ownership were also used by local populations in an attempt to consolidate traditional rights. The Yoruba *ebi* system provides a good example of such a legal transformation. The original *ebi* was an agnatic descent group that shared a common residence and cultivated a relatively well-demarcated area of land together with wives and children. In the modern system, the *ebi* has become a legal entity before the laws of Nigeria and owns land in the full sense of the word (Bohannan, 1967, pp. 58–59).

Not only the colonial but also the postcolonial period has been characterized by a continued and even enhanced shift in the direction of more leasing and ownership as defined by Western legal concepts. In Kenya, for instance, the government of Jomo Kenyatta continued the consolidation program introduced by the Swynnerton Plan of 1954, despite vigorous Kikuyu opposition to it during the colonial period. The net outcome was definitely enhanced productivity and an increase in standards of living, but also a firm rooting of individual ownership. Since the 1960s, many African governments have passed legislation aimed at bringing "unused" or "underutilized" land under direct state control. Such measures were primarily justified by the claim that they would facilitate major agricultural projects and would control urban sprawl. These measures were also supposed to simplify legal procedures, where courts were entangled in seemingly endless land disputes (for example, in Nigeria). More often than not resistance to such state intervention arose, not only because bureaucratization did not lead to agricultural development but also because of widespread corruption. The traditional occupants' reaction, moreover, has come to be that of avoiding any sharing of land whatsoever, for fear that a stranger could claim it. Some agronomists claim that much land is still underutilized as a result.

The introduction of cash crops during the colonial period has led subsequently to the formation of producer cooperatives or state farming enterprises. Their implementation was an obvious replacement for colonial estates, and in countries with Marxist policies the road to fully fledged state enterprises has been pursued (such as in Ghana under Nkrumah, in Angola and Mozambique, in Ethiopia after the revolution of 1974). However, as many farmers also engage in small-scale cash crop production along with subsistence farming, voluntary cooperatives, often formed on a village basis, have become central institutions in countries such as the Ivory Coast and Cameroon. The Ivoirien cooperatives function essentially as autonomous entities within the framework of free enterprise, with members holding shares and electing a managerial committee and the government providing technical assistance and financial aid according to agricultural development plans (see Roberts, 1973, pp. 303–308). Cooperatives in many other countries, however, are frequently controlled more stringently by government agencies and foreign interests and can be seen as the capitalist counterparts of state enterprises.

The Tanzanian *Ujamaa* experiment holds a special place in the annals of sub-Saharan landholding and agricultural reorganization. The *Ujamaa* (or "community") principle stems from Nyerere's rejection of both private and state ownership of land and from his concern to stay as closely as possible to the traditional pattern of communal usage. An important deviation from the traditional Tanzanian pattern, however, was the emphasis on the creation of villages in territories renown for their scattered settlement. The combination of such artificial village formation, heavy-handed bureaucracy, and more stringent government controls led to the economic failure of a project that had been regarded as most promising in the beginning.

To sum up, three features seem to dominate sub-Saharan agriculture and landholding today:

1. Most of the agricultural land and most of the farmers are still engaged in subsistence agriculture, but with reduced fallowing and increased fragmentation.
2. Individual ownership has spread and has enabled an evolution towards a rural social stratification based on wealth.
3. Bureaucratically implemented schemes and government enterprises of agricultural development often have a poor record and have not managed to close the gap between food production and population growth or to generate sufficient earnings necessary to finance food imports.

The difficult transition from pure subsistence farming to enhanced market-oriented production, combined with rural population expansion, has furthermore fuelled a steady rural exodus and exponential urban growth.

A classic finding, even in countries with controls on spatial mobility, is that an urban explosion occurs in tandem with demographic growth. Rural population growth rates of 1.5 to 3.0 percent are commonly matched by urban growth rates of 4 to 8 percent, and occasionally by rates peaking above the 10 percent level for cities. The sub-Saharan experience fitted this picture of accelerated urban growth as early as the 1950s (see W. Hance, 1970, pp. 237–244 or K. Davis, 1969, pp. 164–168), but it failed to attract attention, largely because the original levels of urbanization were so low. If one considers major cities to be those with at least a quarter million inhabitants for instance, West Africa had only 2.5 percent of its population is such places in 1960. This figure was only 1.6 percent for Central Africa and not even 1.0 percent for East Africa (see table 1.5).

TABLE 1.5   Percentage of Total Population in Urban Agglomerations of 250,000+ or 500,000+, Sub-Saharan Africa 1960–2000

	250,000+			500,000+		
	1960	1980	2000	1960	1980	2000
West Africa	2.5	16.7	NA	1.6	13.1	24.0
Central Africa	1.6	20.6	NA	1.6	17.0	27.7
East Africa	0.8	10.1	NA	0.0	9.5	15.4

SOURCE: United Nations, 1982, table 9.

Since then, the steady flow of young migrants, who also transfer a substantial portion of their fertility to the urban setting, has dramatically changed that picture. According to the latest United Nations estimates, West and Central Africa have at present 15 to 20 percent of their total population in such major urban centers and East Africa is crossing the 10 percent level. For the year 2000, no estimates are provided as it is difficult to forecast how many of the numerous smaller urban units will grow above the mark of a quarter million. An extrapolation for cities of at least half a million, however, is possible. Even when urban growth rates are taken to decline with increasing city size, the United Nations expectations for 2000 are that a quarter of the total population of West and Central Africa will be living in cities of more than 500,000. The figure for East Africa is 15 percent. With current definitions of "urban" (that is, as defined by the national censuses) and hence with much lower cutoff points for the rural–urban dichotomy, "urban" populations can easily grow toward a share of 50 percent of the total population (see table 1.6 for definitions and percentages "urban" in eight WFS countries).

Even if the outcome would be less dramatic than that pictured by these UN projections, the expansion of a social stratification system based on highly differential wages, wealth, education, and on the cleavage between modern

TABLE 1.6   Percentage of Total Population in Urban Areas (Local
Definition) in Selected Sub-Saharan Countries, early 1970s to 2000

	Base Year	1980	2000
Benin: 5 towns, 1970	16	31	54
Cameroon: Urban centers as defined in 1970 census	20	35	56
Ghana: Localities with 5000+ in 1970	29	36	51
Ivory Coast: Urban centers as defined in 1975 census	33	38	55
Kenya: Localities 2000+ in 1969	10	14	26
Lesotho: Agglomeration of Maseru, 1966	2	5	11
Senegal: Region of Cap Vert + 5 provincial towns, 1976	24	25	37
Sudan: Localities of administrative/commercial importance with at least 5000, 1973	16	25	43

SOURCE: United Nations, 1982, table 1.

and "informal" sectors of the economy is bound to continue. If the development of class stratification associated with appropriation of land in the rural areas that have developed beyond subsistence economies is taken into account, then one can envisage that the traditional and more egalitarian patterns of social organization are coming to an end in many parts of the continent.

The basic changes with respect to land tenure, lineage control, and social stratification imply that the traditional props of the sub-Saharan reproductive system are vanishing, which should be reflected in a "destabilization" of the traditional fertility and marriage patterns. However, such a process is bound to be fragmentary as some elements of the older reproductive regime may be eroded much faster than others, or alternatively, prove to be fully resistant to change. Substantial regional and ethnic variations are also expected to occur, reflecting both the weight of the past and that of modern structural transformation. The exploration of such variations with respect to major ingredients of the reproductive regimes in function of traditional and current indicators of social organization is taken up in the next chapter for sixty-one ethnic groups located in countries participating in the World Fertility Survey of the late 1970s and early 1980s.

CONCLUSIONS

The African reproductive regime has often been typified as a classic example of fertility maximization, with the prime goal being the safeguarding of the survival of societies living in a harsh environment and operating a subsistence economy based almost exclusively on human labor. This maximization hypothesis draws ample support from evidence regarding the universality of marriage, the restriction of the amount of exposure time lost through union disruptions, the strong desire for large families, the major economic and social significance of children, and, as a corollary, the high resistance so far to parity-specific forms of fertility limitation.

More elaborate views, adopting a systems analysis approach, which is essentially derived from Malthus' philosophy, consider reproductive regimes in a *dual* context: fertility levels not only need to be high enough to offset the force of mortality, they also need to be low enough to prevent population growth rates from threatening long-term subsistence means. This view stresses the importance of preventive checks on fertility and sets them in an environmental, economic, social, and cultural context. At present, three variants of such system theories can be distinguished:

1. Long-term demographic and economic equilibrium models that often draw on animal population analogies and use notions such as "unconscious rationality" or "invisible hand" mechanisms to explain functional adaptation (for example, Wrigley, 1978; Dupâquier, 1972; Coale, 1984, pp. 477–479).
2. More complex, but also more explicit, evolutionary models that stress endogenous technical progress and the mechanisms that engender it in accounting for the development of more efficient production systems capable of supporting larger populations (for example, Boserup, 1965; Simon, 1976; and Lee, 1984)
3. "Modes of production" paradigms stressing factors operating at the level of social structure such as the appropriation of means of production (for example, Goody, 1976), social pattern maintenance (for example, Lesthaeghe, 1980), or institutional forms of risk devolution (for example, Cain, 1983).

The first framework outlined above deals particularly with the mechanisms that link demographic and economic variables. Most work using this approach stems from studies of relatively advanced peasant societies such as those found in historical Western Europe or the colonial United States (Wrigley and Schofield, 1980; Smith, 1984; Grigg, 1980). The theory deals consequently with societies that have the famous "nuptiality valve" as the pivot of their system of demographic autoregulation. Most societies elsewhere, however, do not have a preventive check that operates in *both* directions, that is, limits population growth and produces simultaneously a reproductive reserve that can be released following the operation of a positive check. In fact, we suspect that this two-way mechanism and its direct link to the availability of independent means of household subsistence is as idiosyncratic to Western Europe as neolocal marriage. The "elegance" of the Western European system of autoregulation, which continues to fascinate observers (cf. Dupâquier, 1984, pp. 176–179), is an exceptional feature and needs to be treated as such in any attempt at theory formation.

The sub-Saharan experience provides an example of a powerful preventive check in the form of marked child-spacing, which reduces both fertility and childhood mortality, but the system yields no possibility for accelerating population recuperation following decimation and there is no major reproductive reserve that can be released quickly given the availability of "ecological niches." The lack of such an autocorrective feedback has been found in hunting and gathering societies as well (Howell, 1986). Aside from the problem of low protein intake and its fecundity-reducing effect, it seems that the alternative model found here rests essentially on *slow* recuperation of population, which itself is instrumental in maintaining a low-technology, low-population-density subsistence economy hinging on the availability of *open space* (see Howell, 1986). Moreover, it may well be that these populations never fill their "ecological niches": the bulk of edible natural products remains unconsumed both by pygmies in the rain forest and by bushmen in the Kalahari Desert.

Sub-Saharan cultivators basically maintained this system, but have achieved higher levels of population density than hunters and gatherers. This enabled the development of urban centers and major markets and trade routes in West Africa in particular. The picture that emerged for cultivators still has the feature of open space required for fallowing as a central element, along with the characteristic of contracting and expanding tribal land occupancy (cf. Bohannan's visualization of the "rubber sheet" map of land usage). This is consistent with the occurrence of important migration waves from the sixteenth century through the nineteenth century, and the expansion and contraction of early African states (see Fage's historical atlas, 1978). All this is somewhat reminiscent of the period of Celtic, Germanic, Slav, and Altaic migrations and dislocations in Europe (fourth to sixth century A.D.). Moreover, African tribal warfare and raids associated with these dislocations and frictions also fit the model of contracting and expanding territories and furthermore add a distinctive "struggle of life" element that surely defies any idealization based on notions of some unconscious wisdom leading to harmonious adaptation to the ecosystem. Similarly slave raids organized from the Sahel and from both the west and east coasts, and penetrating as deeply into the heartland of Africa as the Lualaba-Zaire basin, have undoubtedly contributed to this low-technology and low-population-density system of subsistence.

All of this leads to the problems raised by the second framework concerning the ways in which either demographic mechanisms themselves or exogenous forces permit technological breakthroughs, which in their turn allow for higher population densities and more complex organizational patterns. In Ronald Lee's view of the population-technology interaction, sub-Saharan populations were trapped in a situation with strong preventive checks, too sparse a population, a low marginal productivity of labor resulting from climate and leached soil, and a surplus too moderate to stimulate a technical breakthrough (Lee, 1986). Incidentally, the same trapping effect could result equally well in a densely settled population not producing a surplus, or producing a surplus that is extracted and spent unproductively (wars, conspicuous consumption by elites). Asian populations such as that of China could have been locked in this second type of subsistence economy, leaving mainly the European ones to combine system characteristics that permitted the escape from the older Malthusian subsistence constraints and created the conditions for the Industrial Revolution (Lee, 1986).

From the discussions in the previous sections it seems that the sub-Saharan preventive check was impressive and that environmental conditions restricted productivity. Furthermore, the more advanced sub-Saharan societies that developed an urban-based market system (operating on the principle that the producer owns and sells any surplus) had not made technical innovations that set them apart from other cultivator societies that were much closer to a pure subsistence economy and which lived in small, scattered settlements (such as in East Africa). This is surprising since theoretically the more advanced West African societies could have benefitted from the technology of Northern Africa (for example, from the wheel) via well-established cross-Sahara trade routes. But apparently, they did not seem to have had a use for it and continued farming without wheel, plough, or draft animals. Even today, hoe-based agriculture relying solely on manpower still prevails in many parts of the continent, and modern fertilization is not practiced by the majority of subsistence farmers.

There exists a further set of reasons to account for the African system being trapped at the low-technology, low-productivity end of the spectrum in addition to those already mentioned (leached soils, strong preventive check, low population density, modest surplus, disruptions by slave trade or warfare). This set captures the main features of social organization:

1. Prior to the colonial era, land usage patterns never showed any evolutionary tendency toward individualized land tenure by farmers, which, combined with the notion that farming is required to satisfy needs and not to maximize gain, curtailed incentives (cf. Bohannan, 1967, p. 123).

2. The social stratification system, lacking the basis of individual appropriation of resources, has resisted the formation of social classes and stressed lineage or kinship group membership and solidarity instead. This implied again subordination to a gerontocracy and restricted freedom for individual enterprise, except in the trade sector where the concept of ownership of movable goods applied.

3. The strong segregation of the male and female worlds, with women involved in agricultural work and men covering most of the communal decision making, is not conducive to innovation.

4. The cosmology involving interference of ancestral spirits accompanied by a cyclical rather than a linear notion of time shapes the nature of cause-to-effect linkages and detracts from adopting new instrumental approaches.

5. The stratification system of sub-Saharan Africa did not produce marginal groups who possessed resources and who, by virtue of their marginality, engaged in innovative economic behavior on the basis of a deviant subculture.

Taking this multiplicity of factors into account, it is clear that sub-Saharan Africa has been propelled into the twentieth century with forms of social organization and levels of technology that are not comparable to those of most Asian societies. The present agricultural and demographic crises cannot be understood without due recognition of this fact.

From this overview of organizing principles in sub-Saharan societies we shall retain the following factors as being of direct relevance for the study of the reproductive regime:

1. The degree of circulation versus concentration of wealth (that is, Goody's notion of diverging devolution) and the traditional forms of social stratification;

2. The social position of women as defined in the traditional context (cf. lineage organization and the exchange of rights in women, the productive value of women in the various types of subsistence economies, the degree of female economic independence and self-reliance);

3. The role of the various religions with respect to education, social stratification, and the social position of women;

4. The development of new forms of social stratification based on recent patterns of economic development, changes in land tenure, and urbanization.

The next chapter is devoted to the empirical testing of relationships between these major organizational and cultural aspects and the various components of the reproductive regime.

ACKNOWLEDGMENTS

The author would like to thank Frank Eelens for research assistance, and Hilary Page, Allan Hill, and Etienne van de Walle for critical comments and suggestions.

BIBLIOGRAPHY

Bisilliat, J. 1983. The feminine sphere in the institutions of the Songhay–Zarma. In *Female and male in West Africa*, ed. C. Oppong. London: Allen and Unwin, 99–106.

Bohannan, P. 1967. Africa's land. In *Tribal and peasant economies*, ed. G. Dalton. Austin: University of Texas Press, 51–60.

———. 1967. The impact of money on an African subsistence economy. In *Tribal and peasant economies*, ed. G. Dalton. Austin: University of Texas Press, 123–135.

Boserup, E. 1965. *The conditions of agricultural progress*. London: Allen and Unwin.

———. 1970. *Women's role in economic development*. London: Allen and Unwin.

———. 1981. *Population and technology*. Oxford: Basil Blackwell.

Boyd, L. H., and G. R. Iversen. 1979. *Contextual analysis: Concepts and statistical techniques*. Belmont, Calif.: Wadsworth Publishing.

Cain, M. 1983. Fertility as an adjustment to risk. *Working Papers of the Center for Policy Studies*, no. 100. New York: The Population Council.

Caldwell, J. C., and P. Caldwell. 1977. The role of marital sexual abstinence in determining fertility: A study of the Yoruba of Nigeria. *Population Studies* 31(2): 193–217.

Caldwell, J. C., and H. Ware. 1977. The evolution of family planning in an African city: Ibadan, Nigeria. *Population Studies* 31(3): 487–508.

Caldwell, J. C., and P. Caldwell. 1981. Cause and sequence in the reduction of postnatal abstinence in Ibadan City, Nigeria. In: *Child-spacing in tropical Africa—Traditions and change*, ed. H. J. Page and R. Lesthaeghe. London: Academic Press, 181–199.

Clignet, R. 1970. *Many wives, many powers—Autonomy and power in polygynous families*. Evanston, Ill.: Northwestern University Press.

Coale, A. J. 1984. Fertility in prerevolutionary rural China: In defense of a reassessment. *Population and Development Review*, 10(3):471–480.

Davis, K. 1969. *World Urbanization 1950–70: Vol. I—Basic data for cities, countries and regions*. Population Monograph Series, no. 4. Berkeley: University of California, Institute of International Studies.

Dorjahn, V. 1959. The factor of polygamy in African demography. In: *Continuity and change in African cultures*, ed. M. Herskovits and W. Bascom. Chicago: University of Chicago Press.

Dupâquier, J. 1972. De l'animal à l'homme: Le mécanisme autorégulateur des populations traditionelles. *Revue de l'Institut de Sociologie de l'Université Libre de Bruxelles* 2:177–211.

Dupâquier, J. 1984. *Pour la démographie historique*. Paris: Presses Universitaires de France.

Fage, J. D. 1978. *An atlas of African history*, 2d ed. London: Edward Arnold.

Gaisie, S. K. 1981. Child-spacing patterns and fertility differentials in Ghana. In: *Child-spacing in tropical Africa—Traditions and change*, ed. H. J. Page and R. Lesthaeghe. London: Academic Press, 237–253.

Goody, E. 1973. *Contexts of kinship: An essay in the family sociology of the Gonja of northern Ghana*. Cambridge: Cambridge University Press.

Goody, J. 1976. *Production and reproduction—A comparative study of the domestic domain*. Cambridge: Cambridge University Press.

Grigg, D. B. 1980. *Population growth and agrarian change: An historical perspective*. Cambridge: Cambridge University Press.

Hance, W. 1970. *Population, migration and urbanization in Africa*. New York: Columbia University Press.

Hill, A. 1985. The recent demographic surveys in Mali and their main findings. In: *Population, health and nutrition in the Sahel*, ed. A. Hill. London: Routledge and Kegan Paul, 44–64.

Howell, N. 1986. Feedbacks and buffers in relation to scarcity and abundance: Studies of hunter-gatherer populations. In: *The state of population theory—Forward from Malthus*, ed. D. Coleman and R. Schofield. Oxford: Basil Blackwell, 156–185.

Isiugo-Abanihe, U. 1985. Child-fosterage in West Africa. *Population and Development Review* 11(1): 53–73.

Kaplan, I., et al. 1967. *Area handbook for Ghana.* Washington, D.C.: Government Printing Office.

Lee, R. D. 1986. Malthus and Boserup: A dynamic synthesis. In: *The state of population theory—Forward from Malthus*, ed. D. Coleman and R. Schofield. Oxford: Basil Blackwell, 96–130.

Lesthaeghe, R. 1980. On the social control of human reproduction. *Population and Development Review* 6(4).

———. 1984. Fertility and its proximate determinants in sub-Saharan Africa: The record of the 1960s and 70s. Paper presented at the WFS seminar on Integrating Proximate Determinants into the Analysis of Fertility Levels and Trends, London. Liège, Belgium: Ordina for the International Union for the Scientific Study of Population.

Lesthaeghe, R., P. O. Ohadike, J. Kocher, and H. J. Page. 1981. Child-spacing and fertility in sub-Saharan Africa: An overview of issues. In: *Child-spacing in tropical Africa—Traditions and change*, ed. H. J. Page and R. Lesthaeghe. London: Academic Press, 147–179.

Lesthaeghe, R., H. J. Page, and O. Adegbola. 1981. Child-spacing and fertility in Lagos. In: *Child-spacing in tropical Africa—Traditions and change*, ed. H. J. Page and R. Lesthaeghe. London: Academic Press, 147–179.

Locoh, T. 1984. *Fécondité et famille en Afrique de l'Ouest—Le Togo méridional contemporain.* Cahier de l'INED, no. 107. Paris: Presses Universitaires de France.

Manoukian, M. 1950. Western Africa, Part I: Akan and Ga-Adangme peoples. In: *Ethnographic survey of Africa*, ed. D. Forde. London: International African Institute.

———. 1950. Western Africa, Part V: Tribes of the northern territories of the Gold Coast. In: *Ethnographic survey of Africa*, ed. D. Forde. London: International African Institute.

Markalis, J., and N. Ayele. 1978. *Class and revolution in Ethiopia.* Nottingham, Eng.: Spokesman books.

McNicoll, G. 1978. Population and development: Outlines for a structuralist approach. In: *Population and development*, ed. G. Hawthorn. London: Frank Cass, 79–99.

Molnos, A. 1973. *Cultural source materials for population planning in East Africa.* 3 vols. Nairobi: Institute of African Studies, University of Nairobi Press.

Mosley, W. H., L. H. Werner, and S. Becker. 1982. The dynamics of birth-spacing and marital fertility in Kenya. *World Fertility Survey Scientific Reports*, no. 30. Voorburg, Netherlands: International Statistical Institute.

Mueller, E., and S. Kossoudji. 1981. The economic and demographic status of female headed households in rural Botswana. *Working Paper of the Population Studies Center*, no. 81–10. Ann Arbor: University of Michigan.

Murdock, G. P. 1967. Ethnographic atlas: A summary. *Ethnology* 6(2): 109–234.

———. 1967. Postpartum sex taboo. *Paideuma* 13: 143–147.

Nelson, H. D., et al. 1974. *Area handbook for the United Republic of Cameroon.* Washington, D.C.: Government Printing Office.

———. et al. 1974. *Area handbook for Senegal.* Washington, D.C.: Government Printing Office.

Nelson, H. D., and I. Kaplan. 1981. *Ethiopia: A country study,* 3d ed. Washington, D.C.: Government Printing Office.

Okali, C. 1983. Kinship and cocoa farming in Ghana. In: *Female and male in West Africa,* ed.: C. Oppong. London: Allen and Unwin, 169–178.

Oppong, C., and K. Church. 1981. A field guide to research on seven roles of women: Focussed interviews. *Population and Labour Policies Programme Working Paper,* no. 106. Geneva: International Labour Organization.

Oppong, C., ed. 1983. *Female and male in West Africa.* London: Allen and Unwin.

Page, H. J., and R. Lesthaeghe, eds. 1981. *Child-spacing in tropical Africa—Traditions and Change.* London: Academic Press.

Roberts, T. D., et al. 1973. *Area handbook for the Ivory Coast.* Washington, D.C.: Government Printing Office.

Sala-Diakanda, M. 1979. *Approche ethnique des phénomènes démographiques—Le cas du Zaire.* 2 vols. Ph.D. dissertation. Louvain-la-Neuve, Belgium: Université Catholique de Louvain, Département de Démographie.

Saucier, J.-F. 1972. Correlates of the long postpartum taboo: A cross-cultural study. *Current Anthropology* 13(2): 238–249.

Schildkrout, E. 1983. Dependence and autonomy: The economic activities of secluded Hausa women in Kano. In: *Female and male in West Africa,* ed. C. Oppong. London: Allen and Unwin.

Schoenmaeckers, R., I. H. Shah, R. Lesthaeghe, and O. Tambashe. 1981. The child-spacing tradition and the postpartum taboo in tropical Africa: Anthropological evidence. In: *Child-spacing in tropical Africa—Traditions and change,* ed. H. J. Page and R. Lesthaeghe. London: Academic Press.

Simon, J. 1976. *The economics of population growth.* Princeton: Princeton University Press.

Sinclair, J. 1976. Educational assistance, kinship and the social structure in Sierra Leone. *Africana Research Bulletin* 2(3): 30–62.

Singarimbun, M., and C. Manning. 1976. Breastfeeding, amenorrhoea and abstinence in a Javanese village: A case study of Mojolama. *Studies in Family Planning* 7(7): 175–179.

Smith, R. 1984. Pre-industrial European demographic regimes. In: *Population and societal outlook—Populations et prospectives,* ed. S. Feld and R. Lesthaeghe. Brussels: Uitgeverij Lannoo for the King Baudouin Foundation.

Turner, H. W. 1976. The approach to Africa's new religious movements. In: *Religious innovation in modern African societies,* ed. W. van Binsbergen and R. B. Buijtenhuijs. Leyden: Afrika Studiecentrum.

United Nations. 1982. Estimates and projections of urban, rural and city populations, 1950–2025: The 1980 assessment. New York: United Nations.

Ware, H. 1981. *Women, demography and development.* Canberra: Development Studies Centre, Australian National University.

Whitaker, C. S. 1970. *The politics of tradition—Continuity and change in northern Nigeria, 1946–1966*. Princeton: Princeton University Press.

Whiting, J. W. M. 1964. Effects of climate on certain cultural practices. In: *Explorations in cultural anthropology—Essay in honour of G. P. Murdock*, ed. W. H. Goodenough. New York: McGraw-Hill.

Wrigley, E. A., and R. Schofield. 1980. *The population history of England, 1541–1871*, London: Edward Arnold.

CHAPTER TWO

The Components of Sub-Saharan Reproductive Regimes and Their Social and Cultural Determinants: Empirical Evidence

Ron Lesthaeghe
Frank Eelens

INTRODUCTION

The exploration of the various social and cultural dimensions underpinning the sub-Saharan reproductive regimes, outlined in the previous chapter, requires empirical testing. The crucial variables on the dependent and independent sides of the equation need to be measured, and such measurements must be sufficiently reliable, comparable, and representative. Until recently, such an exercise was not possible.

In the past, censuses and large-scale surveys operating with census-like questions provided essentially usable data on current marital status, polygyny, and overall fertility. The surveys following the French tradition yielded ample material on the spread and incidence of polygyny, while those using the Brass (1968) questions on recent childbearing and lifetime fertility enhanced our knowledge on fertility levels. These data sources, however, contain no information concerning child-spacing variables (birth intervals, breastfeeding, lactational amenorrhea, postpartum abstinence and overall nonsusceptibility, contraception) and, furthermore, the *current* marital status concerning divorce and widowhood is of limited value, especially when remarriage occurs at a differential pace.

In fact, demographers were relatively slow in establishing systematic measurement of child-spacing and union dissolution variables. Apart from scattered information collected by anthropologists and medical doctors through informants and patients, hardly any representative material on these issues for sub-Saharan Africa could be found prior to 1970. The first major census operations only began in the last decade of the colonial period (±1950s) and much of the 1960s was spent in extracting basic demographic parameters from these through the methods of indirect estimation (cf. the

Princeton Africa project launched by F. Lorimer, A. J. Coale, and W. Brass; see Brass et al., 1968).

The first attempts at systematic data collection with respect to the spacing variables occurred towards the end of the 1960s and chiefly in the period 1970–1975. Typical examples of intensive localized surveys that probed these issues are the multi-round studies by Cantrelle and colleagues in the Sine-Saloum region of Senegal and the single-round surveys in south-west Nigeria (that is, the early Yoruba studies by Olusanya, Ohadike, Caldwell and Okediji, Morgan). In 1974–1975 the basic questionnaire for the World Fertility Survey (WFS) was constructed; it incorporated the measurement of the various spacing variables. Moreover, a special module on "Factors Other than Contraception Affecting Fertility," known as the FOTCAF-module, was also devised, not exclusively, but especially for use in sub-Saharan Africa. In our view the systemization of the measurement of intermediate fertility variables was the single most important contribution of the WFS. When, in addition, simple methods of analysis for such variables became available (for example, Bongaarts' framework) and demographers borrowed methods of life table function analysis with covariates from statisticians, a major new area of study was opened. In short, the basic framework for fertility analysis had been drawn up by Davis and Blake in 1956, but the extensive measurement of its ingredients only became available in a comparable and standardized form from the 1970s onwards.

THE DEPENDENT VARIABLES

The data used here stem from the WFS individual questionnaires administered to women aged 15–49. The use of these data sets is conditional on official clearance and we have been permitted to analyze the information for Senegal (1978), the Ivory Coast (1980–1981), Ghana (1979–1980), Benin (1981–1982), Cameroon (1978), Kenya (1977–1978), and Lesotho (1977). Three other sub-Saharan countries, namely Sudan, Nigeria, and Mauritania, also participated in the WFS, but their data were either not released in time or are not available for analysis by third parties. On the basis of available sample sizes and information contained in the Yale Human Relations File (G. P. Murdock, 1975) with respect to ethnic clusters, sixty-one ethnic groups were set up. For each of them indicators were constructed for the intermediate fertility variables and variables related to the formation and dissolution of marital unions (which include customary marriages and "mariages d'amitié"). Sample sizes for ethnic groups range from a low of 90 women in a residual Cameroon group ("Other South") to 3603 for the Sotho. The median sample size is 460 and of the sixty-one ethnic groups fifty have a sample size greater than 200. For a few indicators, such as remarriage or the proportions single between ages 15 and 19, the population at risk falls con-

TABLE 2.1 Sample Sizes for 61 Ethnic Groups as Constructed from 7 Sub-Saharan WFS Surveys

Sample Size <200 Women, 15–49 (N = 11)

Guan (GHA)	185	Manding (SEN)	167
Duala (CAM)	182	Diola, Balante (SEN)	189
Other Cameroon South	90	Other Senegal Mande	150
Widekum (CAM)	103	Yoruba (BEN)	169
Chari-Logone (CAM)	149	Nagot (BEN)	199
Choa Arabs, Hausa (CAM)	159		

Sample Size 200–499 Women 15–49 (N = 25)

Kisii (KEN)	486	Mandara, Wandala (CAM)	350
Mijikenda (KEN)	399	Peul (CAM)	472
Other Kenyan	359	Baya, Adamawa, Benue (CAM)	490
Other Ghana Akan	460	Adja (BEN)	443
Ga-Adangbe (GHA)	460	Goun (BEN)	399
Bakosi-Bakundu (CAM)	224	Other Benin South & Central	442
Ekoi, Mbembe (CAM)	226	Dendi, Dittamari (BEN)	203
Bassa (CAM)	358	Bariba (BEN)	334
Pangwe (CAM)	351	Other Benin North	373
Kaka (CAM)	258	Lagunaires (IVO)	243
Maka (CAM)	439	Agni (IVO)	455
Bamun (CAM)	264	Guere (IVO)	261
Bafia (CAM)	417	Tuburi, Gizega (CAM)	426

Sample Size 500–999 women, 15–49 (N = 17)

Kamba (KEN)	996	Poular, Fula (SEN)	910
Meru-Embu (KEN)	573	Serer (SEN)	565
Kalenjin (KEN)	593	Baoule (IVO)	982
Fante (GHA)	581	Kru (IVO)	506
Mole-Dagbani (GHA)	800	Malinke (IVO)	691
Ewe (GHA)	743	Kulango, Senufo (IVO)	639
Other Ghana North	615	Guro, Yacuba (IVO)	560
Yaounde (CAM)	880		
Bamenda (CAM)	583		

Sample Size >1000 women 15–49 (N = 8)

Kikuyu (KEN)	2109	Wolof, Lebu (SEN)	1703
Luo (KEN)	1360	Fon (BEN)	1090
Luhya (KEN)	1213	Sotho (LES)	3603
Bamileke (CAM)	1400	Twi (GHA)	2723

CAM = Cameroon; GHA = Ghana; IVO = Ivory Coast; KEN = Kenya; BEN = Benin; LES = Lesotho;
SEN = Senegal

siderably below the numbers shown in table 2.1, where the full distribution of sample sizes is given.

We shall now consider the definitions of the various demographic variables. Entry into a sexual union is measured through five indicators. The first three pertain to first marriage itself whereas the other two pertain to premarital conceptions:

1. The mean of retrospectively reported ages at first marriage for ever-married women aged 25 + (AGEMAR). This measurement omits information about a tiny portion of women above age 25 who are not yet married, but the selection bias resulting from it is negligible.
2. The median age at first marriage estimated from life tables that incorporate all available information for both married and single women of all ages (MEDMAR).
3. The proportion of women aged 15–19 who are still single (SINGLE 15).
4. The proportion of parous women with a premarital birth (NEGINT).
5. The proportion of women with marriage durations in excess of 9 months with a birth occurring during the first 9 months of marriage (CHILDIN 9).

The data themselves are presented in Appendix A.

The first two indicators, AGEMAR and MEDMAR, have the advantage of being based on information covering the entire sample or a very large portion of it, but the estimates are made less reliable by the information yielded by older respondents (30 +) who systematically *overstate* their age at first marriage in all ethnic groups. The third indicator is restricted to the age group 15–19 and is not affected by this tendency. It also measures the recent past. However, the denominator is substantially reduced and sample error is enhanced. In the data file used here, the value of SINGLE 15 had to be estimated from the regression with MEDMAR for one ethnic group (Ekoi, Mbembe) for that reason. On the whole, the information contained in the three indicators is highly consistent as can be judged from the correlation between them (see table 2.3).

The entry into a sexual union in sub-Saharan Africa does not necessarily coincide with a first marriage, and as a result two indicators are added that capture the incidence of premarital conceptions leading to a live birth. The first is the proportion of all parous women (single or married) who report a negative interval between marriage and first live birth or who report a live birth without ever being married (NEGINT). The second is the proportion of women married for at least 9 months who report a live birth within the first 9 months following marriage (CHILDIN 9). Here, we have no way of establishing the validity of these measurements, but the distribution of the values shows sufficient heterogeneity, with regional clusters relatively well-demarcated and cutting across national boundaries (for example, lowest values are consistently found in the Islamized populations of Senegal, Ivory Coast, Ghana, and Cameroon). In other words, the proportions may be underestimated throughout, but the variables still contain meaningful information for the purpose of interethnic comparison.

The remaining nuptiality variables pertain to polygyny and to marital dissolution and remarriage. The polygyny variable is simply the proportion of currently married women who report having a polygynous husband (POLYG). Dissolution is measured respectively as the proportion of ever-married women who are ever-widowed (PEVWID) or ever-divorced (PEVDIV). The remarriage variable is the proportion of ever-divorced plus ever-widowed who had contracted a new marriage by the time of the survey (REMAR). This measurement has more severe problems: first, the population at risk is only a fraction of the total sample size, and second, the measure is affected by a truncation bias. For five Cameroon ethnic groups, no value for REMAR could be obtained directly for a lack of sufficient observations ("Other South Cameroon," Bamun, Widekum, Chari-Logone, and Duala). Values were estimated through the single best predictor of remarriage, which is—reassuringly enough—the degree of polygyny, and through a check with values for neighboring ethnic groups (for example, Duala and Other South with Ekoi, Bakosi, Bakundu, Bassa; Bamun and Widekum with other Western Highland groups, and Chari-Logone with other Northern Cameroon ethnic clusters). The insertion of these five estimated values produces a maximal shift in the correlation coefficients involving the remarriage variable of 0.04 only.

The contraception aspect is introduced through three variables. The proportion of currently married women currently using contraception is the most straightforward indicator (PCON). However, "abstinence" is included among the various contraceptive methods, which caused confusion with postpartum abstinence in the Benin survey and presumably also among the Meru-Embu in Kenya. In the Benin case, this was easily remedied through a cross-classification with the postpartum abstinence variable and the proportions currently contracepting were dramatically scaled down. Among the Meru-Embu, postpartum abstinence is short and the reduction still leaves an implausible and unexplained high incidence of contraceptive usage. The second indicator (CONPREV) is an efficiency-weighted version of PCON: users of modern contraception such as hormonal methods, IUD, or other female scientific methods were given a score of 0.97, whereas users of rhythm, withdrawal, douche or condom were assigned a score of 0.60. The score for folk methods (such as charms, herbs) was set to zero, although this is probably too drastic an intervention. The Senegalese "gris-gris" for instance (often amulets with Koranic verses) obviously yield no protection as such, but women often use them as a psychological device to fend off husbands or as a psychological support during periods of abstinence. Charms may therefore indicate lowered coital frequency. The third contraception variable (KNOW1M) pertains to the knowledge of at least one method, either modern or traditional, among all women, married or not.

The lactation and postpartum variables are all obtained as prevalence/incidence (P/I) ratios and they give an estimate of the mean durations of breastfeeding (full and partial), lactational amenorrhea, postpartum abstinence, and postpartum overall nonsusceptibility (PIRBRFD through PIRNSP). They are estimated on the basis of a file with births as the units of observation rather than women and are calculated as the ratios of the total number of surviving children born in the last 24 months whose mothers are still breastfeeding, still amenorrheic, and/or still abstaining to the average monthly number of such children. This method assumes the birth stream to be stationary, a condition that is almost met if the period of observation is restricted to the last 2 years. The number of children born 24 months ago is taken as half the number reported for this duration, given the age-heaping of children on multiples of 6 months (for a general discussion of P/I ratios, see: Ferry and Smith, 1983, p. 9; Mosley et al., 1982; or Ferry and Page, 1984).

Prevalence/incidence ratios furthermore have the advantage over retrospectively reported durations for the last closed birth interval in that they are less affected by substantial recall error, by a downward selection bias typical for the last closed interval, and by the omission of parous women with one live birth only. Moreover, the comparison of these prevalence/incidence ratios with mean durations calculated according to a more involved technique, that is, based on life tables and model schedules, yielded a very high degree of consistency, with deviations of 1 month or more predominantly occurring among populations with extremely high values (above 24 months; for example, Mole-Dagbani). Note, finally, that the postpartum nonsusceptible period is defined for each *individual* as whichever is longer, the individual's lactational amenorrhea or postpartum abstinence period. The mean duration of nonsusceptibility is therefore not the longest of either the *mean* of amenorrhea or the *mean* of abstinence, but always longer than either one. This holds, even in populations with reduced abstinence durations, for it suffices to have only one woman with abstinence longer than amenorrhea for the mean duration of nonsusceptibility to exceed that of amenorrhea (cf. chapter 3 and Lesthaeghe, 1984, p. 19).

The distribution of verbally cited desired family sizes is captured by two measures. The first is simply the mean of such quotations, following a recode to 9 of values higher than 9 and of all indeterminate answers (such as "Up to God," "As many as possible") (DESFAMS). This is obviously an arbitrary solution that further lowers the validity of this measurement, but it prevents at least a major selection bias that would result from the omission of indeterminate answers. Some readers may therefore prefer the alternative measure, that is, the proportion of women who state desired family sizes of less than six children (DESLT 6), but then this indicator is not only likely to identify populations with an incipient tendency for family limitation but also tends to pick up populations with a sterility or subfecundity problem. In the latter instance, an offspring of four or five children is highly desirable as these values represent above average completed family size.

The last factor, the occurrence of a sterility or subfecundity problem, is measured by the proportion of ever-married women with a duration of at least 10 years since first marriage who have not progressed beyond two live births (PLETWOLB). Given that childlessness is a major social stigma and proportions childless being rather low in the WFS surveys, it is suspected that childless women tended either to refuse collaboration disproportionately, or that they falsely reported at least one live birth or a foster child. As a consequence, we preferred to take two children as a cutoff point, thereby also capturing early secondary sterility and the presence of subfecundity. The exposure requirement of 10 years since first marriage is on the low side: in most natural fertility populations without pathological fecundity a small percentage of women still have second births between durations 10 and 15. In this instance, however, the loss from observation of women with such durations results in further unwarranted sample reduction.

The list of indicators and definitions is given in table 2.2 for easy reference. Means and standard deviations are added. All measures have their inherent weaknesses, but we are confident that they come close enough to the maximum reliability that can be achieved given sample fragmentation by ethnic group.

TABLE 2.2   Definitions, Means and Standard Deviations of Dependant Variables

Nuptiality

AGEMAR 25	Mean of retrospectively reported age at marriage as stated by ever-married women currently aged 25+ (age selection performed to minimize selection bias). $\bar{X} = 17.7, \sigma = 1.2$.
MEDMAR	Median age at marriage, all women (life table estimate); $\bar{X} = 17.7, \sigma = 1.3$.
SINGLE 15	Percent of all women currently aged 15–19 still single. $\bar{X} = 54.3, \sigma = 18.2$.
POLYG	Percent of currently married women presently married to a polygynous husband; $\bar{X} = 37.0, \sigma = 10.4$.

First Birth

NEGINT	Percent of parous women having a negative "marriage to first birth" interval; $\bar{X} = 16.8, \sigma = 9.4$.
CHILDIN 9	Percent of women married for at least 9 months with live birth in first 9 months of marriage; $\bar{X} = 13.7, \sigma = 5.3$.

TABLE 2.2   *Continued*

Marriage Disruption

PEVDIV   Percent of ever-married women having experienced at least 1 divorce or separation; $\bar{X} = 17.9$, $\sigma = 8.2$.

PEVWID   Proportion of ever-married women having experienced at least 1 widowhood; $\bar{X} = 6.7$, $\sigma = 2.7$.

REMAR   Percent of ever-divorced or ever-widowed women having remarried, $\bar{X} = 67.7$, $\sigma = 22.0$.

Contraception

PCON   Percent of currently married women currently using efficient and less efficient forms of contraception; $\bar{X} = 4.4$, $\sigma = 3.8$.

CONPREV   Idem as PCON, but efficiency weighed: efficient methods weight = 0.97 (pill, IUD, other female scientific, sterilization); less efficient methods weight = 0.60 (rhythm, withdrawal, condom, douche); $\bar{X} = 3.8$, $\sigma = 3.6$.

KNOWIM   Percent of all women knowing at least 1 method of contraception; $\bar{X} = 54.0$, $\sigma = 28.5$.

Breastfeeding and Postpartum Nonsusceptible Period

PIRBRED   Prevalence/incidence ratio for breastfeeding (full or supplemented), calculated for all surviving births occurring in the last 24 months; $\bar{X} = 19.8$, $\sigma = 2.7$.

PIRABST   Prevalence/incidence ratio for postpartum abstinence, surviving births last 24 months; $\bar{X} = 13.0$, $\sigma = 6.6$.

PIRAMEN   Prevalence/incidence ratio for postpartum amenorrhea, surviving births last 24 months; $\bar{X} = 13.3$, $\sigma = 2.2$.

PIRNSP   Prevalence/Incidence ratio for postpartum nonsusceptibility (i.e., either amenorrheic or in postpartum abstinence), surviving births last 24 months; $\bar{X} = 16.8$, $\sigma = 3.7$.

Desired Family Size

DESFAMS   Mean of desired family size for all women; all sizes greater than 9 or indeterminate sizes are recoded to 9; $\bar{X} = 7.1$, $\sigma = 0.8$.

DESLT 6   Proportion of women with desired family sizes less than 6; $\bar{X} = 20.0$, $\sigma = 1.1$.

Subfecundity and Sterility

PLETWOLB   Proportion of women with a duration since first marriage of at least 10 years, having had two or fewer live births; $\bar{X} = 17.0$, $\sigma = 10.7$.

The correlation coefficients between the various demographic indicators themselves are presented in table 2.3. This permits a consistency check for variables with multiple indicators such as age at first union and child-spacing. After eliminating highly collinear and redundant indicators (here: AGEMAR, MEDMAR, PIRAMEM, PIRNSP), a factor analysis is per-

TABLE 2.3 Zero-Order Correlation Coefficients between Indicators of Reproductive Regime; 61 Ethnic Groups, WFS Surveys*

		AGEMAR	SINGLE 15	MEDMAR	POLYG	PROVDIV	REMAR	NEGINT	CHILDIN 9	PIRBRFD	PIRAMEN	PIRABST	PIRNSP	PLETWOLB	PCON
AGEMAR 25	Mean age first marriage (25+)	—	.72	.87	-.47	-.08	-.32	.47	.51	-.27	-.26	.29	.09	-.08	.23
SINGLE 15	Proportion single (15–19)		—	.87	-.64	-.09	-.56	.37	.48	-.42	-.44	-.19	-.31	-.41	.50
MEDMAR	Median age first marriage (all)			—	-.50	-.19	-.44	.48	.60	-.25	-.28	.13	.00	-.37	.33
POLYG	Polygynous marriage (currently married)				—	-.06	.60	-.29	-.34	.48	.50	.16	.39	.11	-.35
PROVDIV	Ever-divorced (ever-married)					—	.37	-.17	-.14	-.38	-.14	-.18	-.27	.15	.21
REMAR	Ever-remarried (ever-dissolved)						—	-.44	-.31	.34	.43	.06	.19	.18	-.10
NEGINT	Premarital birth (parous women)							—	.32	-.24	-.23	.17	.02	.27	-.10
CHILDIN 9	Birth first 9 mths (married 9 mths+)								—	-.17	-.25	.14	.02	-.50	.27
PIRBRFD	X̄ duration breast-feeding (surviving children)									—	.83	.46	.72	.02	-.38

PIRAMEN	$\bar{X}$ duration amenorrhea (surviving children)	—	.44	.73	.13	−.40
PIRABST	$\bar{X}$ duration postpartum abstinence (surviving children)		—	.89	.20	−.43
PIRNSP	$\bar{X}$ duration postpartum nonsusceptibility (surviving children)			—	.11	−.48
PLETWOLB	2 or fewer live births (married 10+ yrs)				—	−.35
PCON	Proportion currently contracepting (currently married)					—

*Senegal, Ivory Coast, Ghana, Benin, Cameroon, Kenya, Lesotho

TABLE 2.4   Factor Analysis (PA2–VARIMAX) for Reproductive Regime
Variables; 61 Ethnic Groups, WFS Surveys

Indicators	Factor Loadings		
	Factor I	Factor II	Factor III
Proportion women single 15–19	.71	.32	−.40
Remarriage	−.75	.08	.17
Premarital birth	.71	−.27	.20
Polygyny	−.67	−.35	.10
Birth in first 9 months of marriage	.45	−.07	−.47
Duration of breastfeeding	−.47	−.50	−.06
Current use of contraception	.17	.74	−.33
Divorce	−.16	.50	.23
Desire less than 6 children	.02	.71	.01
Duration postpartum abstinence	−.01	−.54	.08
Sterility & subfecundity	.00	−.08	.99
Eigenvalues:	3.55	2.31	1.53
Percent of variance accounted for by factor:	32.3	21.0	13.9
Cumulated percent of explained variance:	32.3	53.3	67.2

formed with orthogonal rotation of axes in order to identify the basic contrasting dimensions contained in eleven demographic indicators. The factor
loadings are reported in table 2.4. They represent the zero-order correlation coefficients between the indicators and the three main factors (that is,
those with an eigenvalue greater than 1.0). The factor loadings also permit
a direct identification of the three factors: factor I essentially seizes information concerning the starting pattern of reproduction and the organization of marriage, factor II captures the spacing pattern, and factor III the
sterility and subfecundity dimension.

More specifically, factor I constrasts the regime of very early marriage for
women (low proportions single 15–19), low incidence of premarital births,
high levels of polygyny, and fast remarriage to a regime with the opposite
combination. This substantiates interpretations that consider a high incidence of polygyny as functioning through an early appropriation of female
labor and fast remarriage for widows and divorcees. Early marriage, furthermore, precludes the possibility of premarital pregnancies. The latter
point is stressed further by the fact that the high polygyny, early marriage
regime also tends to have fewer births in the first 9 months of marriage.
Hence, early marriage and enhanced control over younger women are combined.

The second factor differentiates with respect to the combination of increased contraceptive use and lower desired family size coinciding with reduced spacing through lactation and abstinence. It captures the counter-

balancing effect typical for the modernization of the sub-Saharan spacing pattern. The third factor, capturing high sterility and subfecundity, correlates with lower proportions of women with births in the first 9 months of marriage, which is highly plausible given the presence of pathological conditions. Finally, early marriage shows a further correlation with the sterility factor: apparently societies with low fecundity tend to enhance their reproductive potential by drawing women into sexual unions at younger ages.

A negative finding is also worthy of comment. It has often been stated that sterility and subfecundity are strongly positively correlated with the incidence of polygyny. The example of the Zairois ethnic groups and regions provided a typical example for it (Romaniuk, 1967) and strongly supported the interpretation in terms of positive feedback leading to an upward polygyny–sterility spiral (cf. chapter 1). The present factor analysis, which is performed on an ethnic sample that falls largely outside the Central African sterility belt, suggests that the upward spiral is not universal and that, although higher sterility may lead to more polygyny, societies may also have very high polygyny rates for reasons other than widespread infecundity. Hence, the relationship is likely to be highly asymmetric when including Central Africa: sterility is a predictor of enhanced polygyny, but high levels of polygyny are not necessarily predictive of higher sterility.

Considering the sample variations that are considerable for roughly half of the ethnic groups involved in this exercise, the pattern in the correlation matrix for the dependant variables is still highly plausible. As a result, *much caution is required when interpreting specific indicator values for groups with less than 200 women*, but it is worthwhile continuing further work with the entire sample of ethnic groups.

SOCIAL AND CULTURAL INDICATORS

In the previous chapter attention was drawn to the following aspects of social organization and culture:
1. The impact of Christianity and Islam in reshaping cosmological views and in introducing different systems of domestic organization and social stratification
2. The shift from the circulation of wealth in egalitarian societies to concentration of wealth in caste- or class-stratified societies, combined with a shift from exogamy to endogamy, toward more diverging devolution of wealth, and more control over spouse selection
3. The degree of economic encapsulation of women versus more economic independence based on the principle of possession and control of own product and the maintenance of ties with the lineage of origin
4. The advancement of female education
5. The economic evolution away from subsistence activities toward wage labor induced by urbanization and cash crop oriented agriculture.

TABLE 2.5   Definitions, Means and Standard Deviations of Independent Variables

Female Education

ILLIT	Percent of all women with 0 years of schooling or Koranic schooling only; $\overline{X}$ = 65.9, σ = 21.5.
$\overline{X}$SCHOOL	Mean number of years of schooling (Koranic = 0), all women; $\overline{X}$ = 2.5, σ = 4.0.

Religion

CHRIST, MUSLIM, TRADIT	Respectively: Percentage of all women being Christian, Muslim, or adhering to traditional religions; $\overline{X}$MUSLIM = 25.2, σ = 33.8; $\overline{X}$TRADIT = 21.1, σ = 24.5; $\overline{X}$CHRIST = 53.7, σ = 37.6.

Status of Women

TRADE	Percent of all women engaged in "sales" sector (including marketing of own agricultural produce); $\overline{X}$ = 15.5, σ = 18.2.

Social Stratification

WEALTH*	Existence of traditional forms of stratification based on differential possession of wealth, traditional existence of caste stratification, and concentration (versus circulation) of wealth via preferential cousin marriage, inheritance for women, or dowry (see table 2.6); $\overline{X}$ = 1.2, σ = 1.4.
STRATTOP	Percent of women with husbands in the following categories: Professional, clerical, or employer of wage labor; $\overline{X}$ = 18.2, σ = 8.8.
STRATWAGE	Percent of women with wage-earning husbands in agriculture, manual work, household service, or unemployed (STRATWAGE = 100 − STRATTOP − STRATSELF)
STRATSELF	Percent of women with self-employed husbands without employees, i.e., small farmers, artisans, or traders; $\overline{X}$ = 54.3, σ = 17.2.

*Variable stemming from references in Murdock's Ethnographic Atlas.

The indices constructed for the measurement of these dimensions are listed in table 2.5, together with their means and standard deviations. Female education is measured by average schooling levels ($\overline{X}$SCHOOL) and the survival of illiteracy (ILLIT). The interpretation of these variables obviously goes beyond the mere aspect of education: schooling levels also reflect the penetration of two major non-African religions, regional economic development, and the position of women within the domestic domain and economy. The religious adherence is captured through a trichotomy Christian-Muslim-traditional religion. Christianity incorporates Christian syncretic churches, but the cutoff point between Christian-syncretic and traditional or neoprimal is not clear in each of the country data files. For future occasions, more precise codes need to be introduced to achieve greater precision.

The position of women is measured *inter alia* through the proxy of female engagement in the sales sector (TRADE). Here, we stumble on the greatest flaw in the WFS questionnaire as the designers not only copied the questions for men, but, more seriously, left no room for multiple answers or for combinations. This is particularly serious as female activities are typically spread over more than one sector (such as household work + agriculture; agriculture + trade...). As a consequence, female engagement in trade was inflated or suppressed depending on the local interpretation of the question. In Benin, for instance, the range across ethnic groups is enormous with a minimum of 12 percent for the Adja and a maximum of 74 percent among the Bariba. In Ghana, with a comparable situation, the range is more plausible from 24 percent among the Twi to 56 percent for the Ga-Adangbe women who are largely located in the Accra region. Finally, it is suspected that female engagement in trade in Cameroon has been underestimated as percentages do not rise above 12 percent (Bamun). Fortunately, the question of female activity discriminates between the West and East African societies and also between strongly Islamized West African ones and others. In the future, room should definitely be made for much more detailed description of the *combination* of female economic activities.

The deviation from the relatively simple and egalitarian pattern of social stratification and deviations in the direction of more diverging devolution and endogamy are measured from entries in the Murdock Ethnographic Atlas of 1967, following essentially the operationalization used by Goody (1976). It was, however, found that stratification and diverging devolution could be merged into a single variable because of the emergence of a cumulative Guttman pattern. As shown in table 2.6, most sub-Saharan societies do not have a class or caste stratification, there is no cousin marriage of any type as they strongly adhere to the exogamy rule, and there is no diverging devolution of property through women in the form of inheritance or dowry (total score = o). The first, slight deviation occurs either when differentiations are made based on wealth or when cousin marriages are tolerated among ruling groups (total score = 1). A further deviation is the occurrence of both of these features (total score = 2). The next step is the presence of *both* class and caste stratification, often accompanied by at least the tolerance of cousin marriages (total score = 2 or 3). The maximal departure from the egalitarian sub-Saharan pattern based on endogamy and lack of diverging devolution is found in societies that adopted certain Arab practices such as

TABLE 2.6 Classification of Ethnic Groups According to Complexity of Social Stratification and Concentration versus Circulation of Wealth, as Deduced from the Murdock Codes

Pattern					
Class & Caste Stratification	Cousin-Marriage	Female Inheritance	FaBrDa Marriage and/or Dowry	Total Score	Ethnic Groups
0 = No class/caste differentiation 1 = Differentiation based on wealth 2 = Wealth + caste differentiation	0 = Absent 1 = Present	0 = Absent, or minor movable only 1 = Present, movable + real property	0 = None 1 = FaBrDa or dowry		
0	0	0	0	0	Kikuyu, Meru-Embu, Kisii, Kalenjin, Mijikenda, Diola, Kru groups, southern Mande groups, Baya, Adamawa groups, Mandara groups, Bafia, Masa-Logone, Borgou groups, 2 Mole-Dagbani groups (Nankanse, Kusasi)
1	0	0	0	1	Luo, Luhya, Cameroon Western Highland groups, Pangwe, Duala, Yoruba, 1 Mole-Dagbani group (Tallensi)
0	1	0	0	1	Baule, Senufo, several North Ghana groups (e.g., Lobi-Birifor)
1	1	0	0	2	Ashante groups, Fante, Ga, Ewe, Fon, Sotho.

col. 67: 0 versus W, col. 69: 0 versus D	col. 25: N, O, R, S versus rest	col. 74, 76: C, D versus rest	col. 25: D, Q, Fa or col. 12: D		CODES IN MURDOCK FILES
2	0	0	0	2	1 Mole Dagbani group (Mossi)
2	1	0	0	3	Manding, Serer, Bambara, Soce, Malinke
2	1	1	0	4	Wolof
2	1	0	1	4	Futajalonke, Peul
2	1	1	1	5	Tukolor, Soninke, Diula, Hausa, Arab groups.

TABLE 2.7 Economic Differentiation of Ethnic Groups: Illustration for Selected Cases on the Basis of the WFS Data on Husbands' Employment Status and Sector of Employment

	Clerical, Professional, Employers of Wage Labor	All Other Wage Earners (Agriculture, Manual, Domestic Service); Unemployed	Independent Small Farmers, Traders, Artisans (without Wage Labor)
Examples of Ethnic Groups with Strong Urban Concentration			
Lagunaires (Abidjan)	35	38	27
Ga-Adangbe (Accra)	42	31	27
Duala (Douala)	41	30	29
Examples with Strong Entrepreneurial Involvement in Market Economy			
Agni (Ivory Coast)	46	25	29
Twi (Ghana)	31	28	41
Examples with Important Wage Sector			
Kamba (Kenya)	21	54	25
Baule (Ivory Coast)	28	34	38
Fante (Ghana)	24	35	41
Bassa (Cameroon)	26	47	27
Labor Exporting Economy			
Sotho (Lesotho)	3	94	3
Examples with Mixed Wage/Subsistence Economies			
Guere (Ivory Coast)	24	28	48
Fon (Benin)	19	30	51
Guan (Ghana)	18	28	54
Kalenjin (Kenya)	18	30	52
Bamileke (Cameroon)	18	32	50

Examples with Major Traditional Sectors			
Diola (Senegal)	12	25	63
Malinke (Ivory Coast)	14	22	64
Goun (Benin)	18	15	67
Kissii (Kenya)	15	25	60
Pangwe (Cameroon)	19	20	61
Examples with Dominance of Subsistence Economy			
Poular & Fula (Senegal)	12	17	71
Adja (Benin)	14	8	78
Mole-Dagbani (Ghana)	6	22	72
Mandara groups (Cameroon)	8	18	74
Adamawa, Benue, & Baya (Cameroon)	10	14	76

NOTE: Based on cross-classification of WFS questions V804 and V805.

an inheritance for women and, above all, the Fa Br Da-type of preferential parallel cousin marriage (scores 4 and 5). The entries in the Murdock atlas of course do not always correspond exactly with the ethnic groups identified in the present exercise, but often multiple entries could be found for groups belonging to the same ethnic cluster, largely on the basis of the information contained in the more recent Yale Human Relations Area Files (1975). The final result is the classification of societies in a five category ordinal variable (WEALTH).

The last set of variables pertains to current aspects of economic modernization and stratification. The WFS data contain information on the husband's economic sector of employment, on the type of payment (wage in kind or cash, self-employed), and on the presence of employees or family labor. From the cross-classification of the WFS variables, the following three categories could be created:

1. Husbands employed as professionals or clerical workers (self-employed or wage-earning) and employers of wage labor (possibly in conjunction with family labor). These groups represent employment in the modern sector (urban, administration, teaching, etc.) and local entrepreneurial groups (e.g. owners of cocoa farms or owners of small scale industries) (STRATTOP).

2. Husbands in the wage-earning sector working as manual laborers in agriculture, industry, or domestic service. The unemployed were added to this category (STRATWAGE).

3. Self-employed farmers, artisans, or traders without wage-earning employees. In this category, small scale subsistence farming is dominant, but is complemented with traditional artisanal and trading activities (STRATSELF).

The distribution over these three categories varies considerably among the ethnic groups, and a good idea of this can be obtained from the examples presented in table 2.7. A preponderance of the top stratum combined with a sizable wage sector is, for instance, found in ethnic groups with a strong urban concentration or located in the cocoa belt of Ghana and the Ivory Coast. The dominance of the agricultural or industrial wage sector is, of course, typical for the labor exporting economy of Lesotho, but also prevails in many parts of Kenya, Ghana, the Ivory Coast, or Cameroon. At the other end of the scale, populations with more than 60 percent employment in the third category have clearly maintained a major traditional sector, and those with 70 percent or more can be considered as basically having a subsistence economy. Moreover, a fair portion of the wage earners found in such societies are probably migrant laborers. Given the limited attention paid to socioeconomic variables in the WFS as a whole, we feel that male economic activities were more adequately described than the female ones, and that the cross-

TABLE 2.8 Zero-Order Correlation Coefficients between Economic, Social, and Cultural Determinants; 61 Ethnic Groups, WFS Surveys*

		ILLIT	XSCHOOL	XIAN	MUSLIM	TRADRELI	TRADE	WEALTH	STRATTOP	STRATSELF
ILLIT	Illiteracy (all)	—	−.47	−.83	.59	.45	.24	.27	−.44	.75
XSCHOOL	Average duration schooling (all)		—	.40	−.28	−.22	−.07	−.07	.30	−.46
XIAN	Proportion Christian (all)			—	−.77	−.47	−.31	−.41	.35	−.51
MUSLIM	Proportion Muslim (all)				—	−.20	.06	.62	−.31	.44
TRADRELI	Proportion traditional religions (all)					—	.40	−.22	−.10	.16
TRADE	Proportion women engaged in trade (all)						—	.06	.13	.14
WEALTH	Index class/caste stratification, diverging devolution							—	.07	.09
STRATTOP	Husband clerical, professional, employer								—	−.61
STRATSELF	Husband small farmer, artisan, trader									—

*Senegal, Ivory Coast, Benin, Ghana, Cameroon, Kenya, Lesotho tabulation of the WFS information on husbands provides measurements of higher validity. A minor drawback of our measurement, however, is that women in a polygynous union contribute data on the same husband more than once if cowives are interviewed.

The correlation coefficients between the various social and cultural indicators are reported in table 2.8 and a factor analysis was performed to bring out the basic underlying dimensions. The procedure used was PA2-factoring with VARIMAX orthogonal rotation of axes. The results are presented in table 2.9 in the form of factor loadings, that is, the correlation coefficients

TABLE 2.9   Factor Analysis (PA2–VARIMAX) for Social and Cultural Predictors; 61 Ethnic Groups, WFS Surveys

Indicators	Factor Loadings		
	Factor I	Factor II	Factor III
Self-employed farmers, artisans, traders	.84	.14	.11
Professional, clerical, employers	−.75	.07	.15
Female illiteracy	.75	.36	.47
Years of schooling for women	−.47	−.10	−.17
Muslim	.43	.81	−.05
Caste, class, diverging devolution of wealth	−.02	.77	.01
Women in trade	.00	−.09	.51
Traditional religions	.21	−.30	.82
Eigenvalues	3.08	1.68	1.29
Percent of variance accounted for by factor	38.50	21.00	16.10
Cumulated percent of variance	38.50	59.50	75.60

NOTE: Collinear variables are dropped from analysis (CHRIST, STRATWAGE); see table 2.9 bis.

between indicators and factors. Factor I describes the dimension of socioeconomic modernization: ethnic groups with positive scores are those with substantial male employment in traditional sectors or in the subsistence economy and with considerable female illiteracy. At the other extreme ethnic groups are found with substantial wage employment (especially white-collar) and with entrepreneurs (see Appendix B). Average schooling levels for women also load on this factor in the expected direction. Finally, there is an association with the proportion Muslim, predominantly through the connection between Islamization and low levels of female schooling. Factor II captures the main structural features of a more profound Islamization, such as the emergence of caste stratification, endogamy, diverging devolution of wealth, and greater male dominance in the domestic and economic domains. Factor III identifies those West African societies who have maintained their original culture, as indicated by the high proportion of adherents to traditional religions and high female activity in the commercial sector. Such

TABLE 2.9 bis   Correlation Coefficients between Omitted Collinear Indicators and Factors Identified in Table 2.9

Omitted Indicators	Factor I	Factor II	Factor III
Christian	−.57	−.58	−.54
Males in wage sector (agriculture, manual, domestic service), unemployed	−.62	−.25	−.25

societies tend, however, to have above-average female illiteracy, largely because they have not been greatly affected by further Christianization, which generally enhances female schooling. The three factors jointly account for 75 percent of the common variance of the eight indicators involved. Note that two collinear indicators were dropped from the factor analyses (CHRIST, STRATWAGE) to prevent the correlation matrix from having a zero determinant resulting in unspecified factor scores. The correlations between the omitted variables and the three factors can obviously be obtained separately (see table 2.9 bis). The proportion of husbands employed in the wage sector as manual workers is obviously strongly correlated with factor I. The proportions Christian, however, loads equally well on all three: Christianty is instrumental in reducing female illiteracy (factor I), does not lead to caste stratification or lineage endogamy (factor II), and its penetration is obviously less pervasive in societies with robust local religions (factor III).

THE LINKS

The connection between the indicators of the reproductive regime and the social and cultural determinants can be studied through a variety of procedures. Here, we have used a series of methods that are based on the Pearson correlation matrix rather than on the phi-coefficients from 2 × 2 tables (cf. Goody's analysis). This procedure allows for the full scatter of observations to emerge and produces conservative estimates of the strength of associations. The analyses include:

1. Simple overview of correlations between social and cultural determinants and of nuptiality and first birth indicators (see table 2.10) or spacing, contraception, and desired family size indicators (see table 2.11)
2. Inspection of the zero-order correlation coefficients existing between the various reproductive regime variables and the three orthogonal factors capturing the information contained in the social and cultural set (see table 2.12)
3. A canonical correlation analysis aimed at finding out which dimension of the reproductive regime and which dimensions of the sociocultural set are optimally related to each other (see table 2.13).

TABLE 2.10 Zero-Order Correlation Coefficients between Indicators of Nuptiality or Occurrence of First Birth and Economic, Social, and Cultural Determinants; 61 Ethnic Groups, WFS Surveys*

		SINGLE 15	NEGINT	CHILDIN 9	POLYG	PROVDIV	REMAR
		Proportion Women 15–19 Still Single	Proportion of Parous Women with Premarital Live Birth	Proportion of Women Married 9+ Months with Live Birth in First 9 months	Proportion of Currently Married Women in Polygynous Union	Proportion of Ever-Married Women Ever-divorced	Proportion of Ever-divorced or Ever-widowed Women having Remarried
ILLIT	Proportion women illiterate	−.78	−.37	−.30	.65	.01	.70
XSCHOOL	Mean years of schooling, women	.39	.18	.16	−.37	.09	−.37
STRAT-TOP	Proportion of husbands in clerical, professional occupation, employers	.41	−.02	.41	−.27	.47	−.07
STRAT-SELF	Proportion of husbands self-employed as small farmers, artisans, traders	−.54	.01	−.29	.51	−.20	.43
TRADE	Proportion women in trade	.04	−.24	.28	.00	.17	.35
WEALTH	Class/Caste stratification; diverging devolution	−.30	−.56	−.43	.14	.24	.31
XIAN	Proportion women Christian	.70	.53	.43	−.57	−.03	−.69
MUSLIM	Proportion women Muslim	−.57	−.39	−.58	.53	.01	.48
TRAD-RELI	Proportion women traditional religions	−.27	−.28	.15	.15	.03	.39

*Senegal, Ivory Coast, Ghana, Benin, Cameroon, Kenya, Lesotho

TABLE 2.11 Zero-Order Correlation Coefficients between Indicators of Child-spacing or Contraception and Economic, Social, and Cultural Determinants; 61 Ethnic Groups, WFS Surveys*

		PIRBRFD	PIRABST	PIRNSP	PCON	KNOWIM	DESLT 6
		Mean Duration Breastfeeding	Mean Duration Postpartum Abstinence	Mean Duration Nonsusceptible Period	Proportion Women Currently Using Contraception	Proportion Women Knowing at least 1 Method of Contraception	Proportion Women Desired Family Size <6
ILLIT	Proportion women illiterate	.58	.25	.42	−.49	−.53	−.41
XSCHOOL	Mean years schooling for women	−.47	−.18	−.30	.19	.23	.16
STRAT-TOP	Proportion of husbands in clerical, professional occupations, employers	−.66	−.25	−.46	.52	.54	.19
STRAT-SELF	Proportion of husbands self-employed as small farmers, artisans, traders	.54	.32	.47	−.48	−.64	−.46
TRADE	Proportion women in trade	.21	.41	.38	.19	−.02	.17
WEALTH	Class/Caste stratification; diverging devolution	−.04	−.26	−.18	.01	−.31	.16
XIAN	Proportion women Christian	−.53	−.15	−.35	.29	.41	.21
MUSLIM	Proportion women Muslim	.25	−.18	.03	−.22	−.49	−.16
TRAD-RELI	Proportion women traditional religions	.47	.47	.51	−.13	.05	−.09

*Senegal, Ivory Coast, Ghana, Benin, Cameroon, Kenya, Lesotho

TABLE 2.12 Zero-Order Correlations between Demographic Indicators and the Three Factors Capturing the Information Contained in the Social and Cultural Indicators (cfr. Table 2.8); 61 Ethnic Groups, WFS Surveys

	Factor I	Factor II	Factor III
	(Traditional Economic Structure, Female Illiteracy)	(Islamization, Caste/Class, Endogamy, Diverging Devolution)	(Traditional Religion, Females in Trade)
Proportion single (15–19)	−.64	−.40	−.30
Mean age at marriage (25+)	−.32	−.43	−.07
Median age at marriage (all)	−.42	−.51	−.14
Polygyny (currently married)	.57	.35	.20
Proportion ever-divorced (ever-married)	−.30	.23	.24
Proportion remarried (ever-divorced + ever-widowed)	.43	.38	.54
Premarital birth (parous)	−.03	−.48	−.42
Birth first 9 months (married 9+ months)	−.36	−.46	.19
Mean duration breastfeeding (surviving children 24 months)	.67	−.04	.32
Mean duration lactational amenorrhea (surviving children 24 months)	.68	−.01	.31
Mean duration postpartum abstinence (surviving children 24 months)	.30	−.32	.39
Mean duration postpartum nonsusceptibility period (surviving children 24 months)	.50	−.20	.39
Current use contraceptives (currently married)	−.60	−.02	−.04
Knowledge 1 method (all)	−.63	−.33	.06
Efficiency weighted contraceptive use (currently married)	−.51	−.01	.08
Average desired family size (all)	.32	.05	.10
Proportion desire <6 children (all)	−.46	.00	−.07
Proportion ≤2 children (10 years since first marriage)	.35	.12	−.21

TABLE 2.13   Canonical Correlation Analysis for Reproductive Regime Variables versus Social and Cultural Predictors; 61 Ethnic Groups in WFS surveys; Zero-Order Correlation Coefficients between Indicators and Canonical Variates

First Canonical Variate (Y1, X1): Eigenvalue = .88; Canonical correlation = .94

Best Indicators of Y1 (r ⩾ .40)		*Best Indicators of X1 (r ⩾ .40)*	
Proportion women single 15–19	.77	Female illiteracy	−.75
Polygyny	−.67	Proportion Muslim	−.72
Knowledge of contraception	.63	Self-employed farmers, artisans,	
Current use contraception	.60	traders	−.70
Births in first 9 months of marriage	.61	Clerical, professional, employers	.66
Duration breastfeeding	−.49		
Desire less than 6 children	.49		
Subfecundity and sterility	−.41		

Second Canonical Variate (Y2, X2): Eigenvalue = .82; Canonical correlation = .91

Best Predictors of Y2		*Best Predictors of X2*	
Remarriage	.67	Traditional religion	.79
Postpartum abstinence	.54	Females in trade	.76
Breastfeeding	.50	Female illiteracy	.65
Premarital birth	−.46		

Third Canonical Variate (Y3, X3): Eigenvalue = .71; Canonical correlation = .84

Best Predictors of Y3		*Best Predictors of X3*	
Breastfeeding	−.53	Clerical, professional, employers	.71
Divorce	.50		

Fourth Canonical Variate (Y4, X4): Eigenvalue = .55; Canonical correlation = .74

Best Predictors of Y4		*Best Predictors of X4*	
Premarital birth	.80	Class/caste, diverging devolution	−.81
Births in first 9 months of marriage	.45	Self-employed farmers, artisans,	
Desire less than 6 children	−.47	and traders	.42
Postpartum abstinence	.47		

NOTE: Variables in canonical correlations are SINGLE 15, POLYG, PEVDIV, REMAR, NEGINT, DESLT 6, CHILDIN 9, PIRBRFD, PIRABST, PCON, KNOWIM, PLETWOLB versus ILLIT, MUSLIM, TRADRELI, TRADE, WEALTH, STRATTOP, STRATSELF; strongly collinear variables are omitted (AGEMAR, MEDMAR, PIRAMEN, PIRNSP, XSCHOOL, XIAN, STRATWAGE) together with the widowhood variable, which stands entirely on its own (PEVWID).

The correlation coefficients of tables 2.10 and 2.11 identify the best predictors of each of the demographic variables, but a more synoptical view can be gleaned from the associations of the demographic indicators with the three orthogonal factors that summarize the information offered by the determinants (see table 2.12). The first factor that mainly measures economic development and eradication of female illiteracy (and which obviously also captures features such as urbanization and the schooling effect of Christianity) appears to be a major predictor of all crucial demographic features that are currently transforming—or beginning to transform—the reproductive regime. The strongest correlates (coefficients = 0.60 or higher) of increased socioeconomic modernization among ethnic groups are:

1. Increased proportion of young women still single
2. Lowered durations of breastfeeding and lactational amenorrhea
3. Enhanced knowledge and use of contraception.

At this point it should be stressed that ethnic variations in proportions single have always been considerable implying that it would be dangerous to interpret the current cross-sectional findings as indicators of a temporal process. For the durations of breastfeeding there were undoubtedly also variations at the start, but the cross-section does reflect an important element of differential erosion. Finally, the use of contraceptive methods other than folk methods shared a common starting point located near zero (there seem to have been variations in the usage of coitus interruptus), and current ethnic differentiation with respect to current usage must reflect the pace of a trend. However, measurement error for rare features, such as contraceptive use, is considerable.

The breaking away from a subsistence or traditional economy and high female illiteracy is furthermore associated (coefficients comprised between 0.30 and 0.60) with:

1. Higher mean or median ages at first marriage (i.e., indicators that contain information for older cohorts rather than for the most recent one only)
2. A higher incidence of divorce
3. Less polygyny (but then, we have no measurements on the incidence of emergent forms of "polygyny" such as urban concubinage)
4. A high proportion of first births reported to have occurred in the first 9 months of marriage (no association with premarital births is found, though)
5. Lowered durations of postpartum abstinence and of the overall postpartum period of nonsusceptibility
6. An increased desire for smaller family sizes (recalling, however, that "smaller" means less than six)
7. And finally with less sterility and/or subfecundity (which reflects the fact that ethnic groups at the subsistence end of the economic scale and with high proportions of female illiteracy are also considerably disadvantaged with respect to medical assistance).

The observation that the proportion single among women aged 15 to 19 is much more closely connected with the socioeconomic development factor ($r = -0.64$) than the measure of age at first marriage for all women ($r = -0.42$) and the measure for women older than 25 ($r = -0.32$) hints at the possibility that a nuptiality change may be on its way, although such a change would be a recent phenomenon. We shall examine this matter more closely when trends rather than cross-sections are discussed in chapter 4.

The second factor, representing the features of social organization associated with Islamization, is most clearly linked with the nuptiality variables tending towards (1) much lower ages at marriage and (2) much lower incidence of premarital conceptions leading to premarital or early postmarital births. Hence, Goody's chain running from more profound Islamization via caste stratification, devolving devolution, and endogamy to greater control over young females holds remarkably well, even in this sample restricted to sub-Saharan Africa. These *structural* aspects of Islamization correlate furthermore, albeit at lower levels (r comprised between 0.30 and 0.40), with shorter durations of abstinence (cf. the Islamic prescription of 40 days postpartum abstinence only) and less knowledge of contraception.

Long durations of postpartum abstinence are best predicted for societies that have high scores on the third factor, that is, those that have surviving traditional African religions and strong female independence (or large social distance between spouses, cf. Saucier) measured by women's involvement in trade. These are clearly West African features that account for the strong concentration of the anthropological references to the long postpartum taboo in this zone (Schoenmaeckers et al., 1981). Factor III not only tends to identify ethnic groups with longer than average durations of abstinence, but also those with longer breastfeeding and lactational amenorrhea. Such societies therefore easily have the most intact traditional pattern of child-spacing.

Factor III is furthermore associated with lower than average incidence of premarital births. This is surprising: one would expect ethnic groups with strong West African traditionalism to have the typical sub-Saharan pattern of high premarital fertility as identified by Goody in contrast with Eurasian populations. Moreover, this feature cannot be accounted for by earlier marriage precluding the occurrence of premarital fertility: the partial correlation coefficient between premarital fertility and factor III, controlling for proportions single aged 15 to 19, drops only slightly below the zero-order coefficient (from −0.42 to −0.34). What seems to happen is that West African populations with high scores on factor III (i.e., Ivoirien, Beninois, and Ghanaian ones) have values for premarital fertility that are intermediate between the very low ones in Islamized groups and the very high ones among several profoundly Christianized ethnic groups. Resistance of traditional religion and female involvement in trade tend to coincide with greater traditional political complexity and strong patterns of local organization (e.g., multifunctional female societies) respectively. Typical examples of these societies are the ones that have a history of state formation such as the Invoirien and Ghanaian Akan, the Dahomey and Borgu kingdoms, the Bamileke of the Cameroon Western Highlands.

Political complexity is associated with the emergence of ruling groups and in this instance their imposition was not by an Islamic conqueror. Such groups seek political alliances and tolerate cousin marriage. These more complex West African societies—a good portion of which are matrilineal or have maintained matrilineal traits—seem to have had reasons for some control over partner selection, but they did not impose the same high level of control over younger women as the one found in societies with profound Islamization of the patterns of social organization.

The highest incidence of premarital first births are, at least in this sample of societies, found in the Cameroon forest belt and in Kenya. These ethnic groups have simpler social structures and were more decentralized and scatterred (e.g., no markets, no early urban-like concentrations). This is associated with a lack of control over partner selection for political or economic reasons, which accounts for the tolerance of premarital fertility. By the same token, weak political organization may have facilitated Christianization. But as Christianity, in contrast to Islam, did not offer social and economic but only new "moral" reasons for premarital chastity, there is an astonishing but spurious statistical result: Christianity is the strongest correlate of high premarital fertility ($r = +0.53$).

The analysis of the correlation matrix can be pursued through a technique that is particularly well suited for our purpose, namely canonical correlation analysis. We shall not go into any technical detail here as good descriptions are available elsewhere (e.g., Levine, 1977). Canonical correlation essentially combines features of multiple regression analysis, in the sense that it distinguishes between dependent (y) and independent (x) variables, and of factor analysis with orthogonality, in the sense that, on either side of independent and dependent variable sets, linear combinations of variables are made so that new variables are constructed (analogous to the factors). This construction occurs in such a way that the correlation in a pair of such new canonical variables (Y_1 and X_1) is maximal. Such a pair is called a *canonical variate*. In the first step, a canonical variate is extracted which accounts for the largest amount of variance. In the next step, a second canonical variate is formed (having the pair of canonical variables Y_2 and X_2) which is orthogonal (i.e., unrelated) to the first one. The procedure continues with further definitions of orthogonal canonical variates until a predetermined threshold is reached. The best way of studying the meaning of a canonical variate consists simply of inspecting the zero-order correlation coefficients between the new canonical variables Y_1 and X_1 on the one hand and the original x and y variables on the other. This procedure is analogous to the labeling in factor analysis via the identification of the single best correlates using factor loadings.

The results of the canonical correlation analysis are presented in table 2.13. The first canonical variate contains the new canonical variables X_1 and Y_1 which correlate at the level of 0.94. The best correlates of Y_1 are precisely those aspects of the reproductive regime that correlated well with the socioeconomic development factor in table 2.12. This is no surprise as the canonical variable X_1 in this pair is best described by low female illiteracy combined with low male employment in traditional and subsistence sectors and high male involvement in wage and entrepreneurial sectors. The only distinction with factor I is that the proportion non-Muslim joins the first canonical variate on the side of X_1. On the whole, the correlation coefficients between the indicators in the demographic set and the canonical variable Y_1 are similar or higher than those between these indicators and factor I (compare tables 2.13 and 2.12). The main exceptions are due to the incorporation of the percentage non-Muslim in X_1: the incidence of premarital births correlates higher with Y_1 in table 2.13 than with factor I in table 2.12 and the reverse holds for the duration of breastfeeding. Note, however, that X_1 captures the female illiteracy aspect of Islamization: class/caste stratification, endogamy, and devolving devolution of wealth aspects determine *another* canonical variate. As a result, we shall label the first canonical variate as the modernization dimension of the reproductive regime (Y_1) and of the socioeconomic structure (X_1).

The second canonical variate produces two canonical variables X_2 and Y_2 which correlate at the level of 0.91. The best indicators of X_2 are those of factor III in table 2.9: the persistence of traditional religions and high female involvement in economic life in societies with fairly large numbers of illiterate women. The traditionalist West African societies are again identified. The correlates in the demographic set of Y_2 are: fast remarriage, longer breastfeeding and postpartum abstinence than average, and fewer premarital births.

The third canonical variate (r between Y_3 and X_3 = 0.84) captures the association between urbanity, as identified through male activities in white collar jobs, and further reductions in breastfeeding. It also loads on a high incidence of divorce. The fourth canonical variate (r between Y_4 and X_4 =0.74) first of all signals the antagonism between traditional caste/class differentiation and endogamous preferences (scores 2 and above on the WEALTH variable) and the tolerance of premarital conceptions and especially premarital births. As indicated earlier, the high incidence of premarital births is found primarily in Central and Eastern African societies with egalitarian and decentralized political structures (i.e., with scores of WEALTH of 0 or at most 1). If, furthermore, a large subsistence sector prevails in the economy, less erosion of postpartum abstinence occurs in such societies and there is no articulation of desired family sizes below six children.

The exploratory analysis of the correlation matrix and the patterning generated by the canonical analysis have brought out the respective correlates of both *traditional* differentiation among reproductive regimes and their *current* modification. Current differences with respect to age at first marriage in older cohorts, postpartum abstinence, and premarital fertility are strongly associated with traditional organizational differences based on factors such as early Islamization, the development of caste or class organization, and a preference for some endogamy, the resistance of traditional religions, or women active in trade. Ethnic differences in breastfeeding durations, use and knowledge of contraception, and proportions single among the most recent cohort respond predominantly to socioeconomic development, that is, to the growth of a wage sector and the eradication of female illiteracy.

Another illustration: the analysis performed here sheds light on the short periods of postpartum abstinence and nonsusceptibility in Kenya. This cannot be explained in terms of Kenya having particularly high levels of female education. An explanation in terms of a clear break away from a subsistence economy would be better, since the larger Kenyan groups have a fairly sizable wage sector. Yet, many West African societies have higher scores on both counts, while maintaining a much longer taboo and better child-spacing. Hence, the institutional setting offers a clue: Kenyan populations had hardly any intact survival of traditional religion (the Kikuyu and Luo were among the very first to found their own African Christian churches), they had simple gerontocratic structures often based on age grades but no major ruling groups, strong exogamy supportive of circulation of wealth, and last but not least, high degrees of female social and economic encapsulation by the husband's patriliny. In other words, they seem to have lacked almost every institutional prop identified here as capable of stemming the tide. Moreover, even if postpartum abstinence was shorter at the onset, one should remember that, once bridewealth was paid, women were left with much less protection from their own kinsmen and with much less leverage over their husbands and cognates than West African women organized in female societies generating their own incomes. Furthermore, the lack of a more complex caste or class organization supportive of endogamous tendencies also helps in accounting for the high incidence of premarital conceptions and births in Kenya. The net result is that many Kenyan populations appear to have "lax" mores with respect to both starting and spacing patterns of reproduction.

At this stage the analysis has succeeded mainly in clarifying an overall pattern. We can, however, show greater detail by considering the orders of magnitude of cross-sectional elasticities within the various clusters of ethnic groups.

FURTHER PROBES INTO THE EFFECTS OF ORGANIZATIONAL PATTERNS AND SOCIOECONOMICS DIFFERENTIATION

From the previous analysis we know that the sixty-one ethnic groups must form clusters with respect to "institutional," "organizational," or "cultural" contexts as defined by variables such as traditional caste-/class-stratification, deviations from exogamy, the position of women and their economic activity, religious tradition, and interference from Islam or Christianity. These contexts have long historical standing and it would be worthwhile to check how they continue to have an influence on each component of the reproductive regime in the face of heterogeneous socioeconomic development. Moreover, we have not identified ethnic variation with respect to the reproductive regimes and organizational patterns in any regional detail so far. For this, the sixty-one ethnic groups were compared on the basis of the four organizational and religious variables: percentage Muslim, percentage traditional religion, the combined class/caste, endogamy, and diverging devolution score, and percentage women in trade (see table 2.14). Seven clusters are identified.

Group A consists mainly of populations experiencing profound Islamization, both in terms of percentages Muslim as well as in terms of the presence of substantial deviations from the egalitarian patterning based on circulation of wealth and exogamy. They have low to moderate proportions in trade, although one has to keep in mind here that some of the variation is not real but stems from country-specific interpretations of the WFS question. Most Senegalese groups fall into this cluster together with the more thoroughly Islamized societies of Northern Ivory Coast and Cameroon (e.g., Malinke, Peul, Choa Arabs, Cameroon Hausa).

Group B contains populations with either the combination "Muslim-traditional religion" or "Muslim-Christian," hardly any evidence of the

TABLE 2.14   Construction of Ethnic Clusters on the Basis of Religious and Organizational Characteristics; Ethnic Groups from WFS surveys

	% Muslim	% Traditional Religion	Caste/Class Diverging Devolution Score	% Women in Trade
Group A				
1. Wolof, Lebu (SEN)	100	0	4	8
2. Poular, Fula (SEN)	99	1	5	9
3. Manding (SEN)	98	2	3	3
4. Serer (SEN)	91	8	3	5
5. Senegal Mande groups (SEN)	100	0	4	4
59. Malinke (IVO)	98	2	3	37
41. Cam. Peul (CAM)	98	0	5	7
43. Choa Arabs, Hausa (CAM)	94	0	5	5
$\bar{X} =$	97	2	3&5*	10
$\sigma =$	3	3	3–5**	11

TABLE 2.14   Continued

	% Muslim	% Traditional Religion	Caste/Class Diverging De- volution Score	% Women in Trade
Group B				
39. Chari-Logone (CAM)	34	27	0	6
40. Mandara, Wandala (CAM)	38	51	0	2
38. Tuburi, Gizega (CAM)	18	50	1	4
5. Diola (SEN)	66	0	0	4
52. Baya, Adamawa, Benue (CAM)	35	4	0	7
35. Bamun (CAM)	77	2	1	12
50. Mijikenda (KEN)	47	34	0	1
X̄ =	45	24	0	5
σ =	20	22	0–1	4
Group C				
10. Mole-Dagbani (GHA)	31	56	1	32
14. Other Ghana North (GHA)	39	40	1	33
17. Yoruba (BEN)	57	13	1	59
19. Nagot (BEN)	36	12	1	34
21. Dendi, Dittamari (BEN)	49	46	0	42
22. Bariba (BEN)	34	62	0	74
23. Other Benin North (BEN)	43	49	0	48
60. Kulango, Senufo (IVO)	38	47	1	18
X̄ =	41	41	1	43
σ =	9	19	0–1	18
Group D				
15. Adja (BEN)	0	88	2	12
16. Fon (BEN)	1	64	2	41
18. Goun (BEN)	6	41	1	57
20. Other South & Central Benin (BEN)	4	67	1	30
56. Baule (IVO)	3	71	1	13
58. Guere (IVO)	2	71	0	7

TABLE 2.14   *Continued*

	% Muslim	% Traditional Religion	Caste/Class Diverging Devolution Score	% Women in Trade
61. Guro, Yacuba (IVO)	9	81	0	13
57. Kru (IVO)	1	31	0	13
X̄ =	3	64	0&1	23
σ =	3	19	0–2	18
Group E				
7. Fante (GHA)	7	9	2	36
8. Twi (GHA)	3	12	2	24
9. Other Gh. Akan (GHA)	3	20	2	24
11. Ewe (GHA)	1	32	2	37
12. Ga-Adangbe (GHA)	4	17	2	56
13. Guan (GHA)	18	29	2	41
54. Lagunaires (IVO)	10	6	2	24
55. Agni (IVO)	2	16	2	8
X̄ =	6	18	2	31
σ =	5	9	2	14
Group F				
24. Bakosi, Bakundu (CAM)	0	5	1	1
25. Ekoi, Mbembe (CAM)	1	4	1	5
26. Duala (CAM)	1	1	1	8
27. Bassa (CAM)	0	2	1	6
28. Pangwe (CAM)	1	1	0	1
29. Kaka (CAM)	2	1	0	1
30. Maka (CAM)	0	2	0	1
31. Yaounde (CAM)	0	2	0	4
32. Other Cam. South (CAM)	3	29	0	1
33. Bamenda (CAM)	3	6	1	3
34. Bamileke (CAM)	1	12	1	7
36. Bafia (CAM)	2	1	0	4
37. Widekum (CAM)	0	4	1	2
X̄ =	1	5	1	3
σ =	1	9	0–1	3

TABLE 2.14   Continued

	% Muslim	% Traditional Religion	Caste/Class Diverging Devolution Score	% Women in Trade
Group G				
44. Kikuyu (KEN)	1	3	0	1
45. Luo (KEN)	1	1	1	1
46. Luhya (KEN)	5	1	1	2
47. Kamba (KEN)	1	5	0	2
48. Kisii (KEN)	0	3	0	0
49. Meru, Embu (KEN)	1	1	0	1
51. Kalenjin (KEN)	1	8	0	0
52. Other Kenyan (KEN)	17	17	0	0
53. Sotho (LES)	0	18	2	4
$\overline{X}$ =	3	6	0	1
σ =	5	7	0–2	1

NOTE: *Mode rather than mean
**Range rather than standard deviation

early adoption of class or caste stratification, and the absence of diverging devolution of wealth or preferential cousin marriage. They also have low to moderate proportions of women engaged in trade. Such societies are predominantly found in Northern Cameroon where the people were conquered by Islamic rulers, without however becoming thoroughly Islamized. We have added the Diola from Senegal and the Mijikenda of Kenya to this group because of the religious mix with a non-Islamic component. The decision to incorporate the Mijikenda was of course a difficult one, but they are so distinct from the other Kenyan groups in terms of high proportions Muslim and adhering to traditional religion that an objective application of the criteria had to be applied here as well. If data for other East African Muslim populations such as those of Tanzania had been available, a special group would have been formed.

Group C contains West African populations with characteristics relatively similar to Group B in terms of religious mix and adherence to egalitarian and exogamous settings. They have, however, very substantial proportions of women actively involved in trade. If the latter variable is affected by differential measurement error, groups B and C would come closer to each other in terms of organizational pattern. Group C is typically located in Northern Ghana and Benin (e.g., Mole-Dagbani, Bariba).

Group D contains predominantly all the West African populations that have retained a strong adherence to traditional religion, complemented by some Christianity rather than Islam. This group is at a midpoint between the previous one (C) and the next one (E). Some societies such as the Guere, Kru, Guro, and Yacuba of the Ivory Coast and the Goun of Benin have low scores on the variable WEALTH, while the Adja and Fon of Benin have scores identical to the Southern Ghanaian ones (WEALTH score = 2) to which they are related (cf. Fon and Ewe). Nevertheless, adherence to traditional religion is overwhelming, hence the clustering in a special group.

Group E brings together the populations of Southern Ghana and related populations across the Ivoirien border. In all of them Christianity is dominant. Moreover, this group is highly homogeneous with respect to the deviation from the egalitarian setup in the sense that they had a more complex stratification with a ruling class and often a tolerance of cousin marriage. Last but not least, all the matrilineal societies related to the Akan group are present in group E, and many of them have extensive child-fostering. The degree of female involvement in trade is moderate to high.

Group F contains the societies of Southern Cameroon and the Cameroon Western Highlands. The former are typically societies without centralized authority and hence no marked tradition of caste or class stratification. In fact, populations such as the Pangwe are typical for the egalitarian and undifferentiated organization of many forest populations of Central Africa. Those in the Western Highlands, and especially the Bamileke, deviate from this principle, without however reaching the complexity of the Akan. Furthermore, all of them are Christianized, predominantly in Catholic or Presbyterian churches. Only the Bamileke and a few scattered minorities have maintained traditional religious allegiance above the 10 percent level. For the Bamileke—who are consequently the most deviant case in this group— this is not surprising given that strength of organization and maintenance of traditional religion are often associated.

Group G, finally, is made up of the Kenyan populations with the exception of the Muslim Mijikenda. They are Christianized, without complex forms of social organization, are typically exogamous, and have very few women active in trade, reflecting the high degree of female economic encapsulation in the husband's household. The problem with this group is that it is far more heterogeneous than it appears from the criteria used here and the contrast with West Africa. Obviously, if more East African ethnic groups would have been available in the WFS samples, a new and possibly entirely different grouping system would have been worked out for them. The heterogeneity is heightened by the addition of the Sotho to this group.

Admittedly, nothing is more difficult than forming ethnic clusters, and choices are always to some extent arbitrary. The grouping here is no exception. We have, however, followed as systematically as possible a few relevant criteria and their measurements as offered by the relatively highly comparable data from the WFS (with the exception of women in trade in some West

TABLE 2.15 Means and Standard Deviations of Major Characteristics for 7 Ethnic Clusters, WFS-data

		% Muslim	% Traditional Religion	Caste/Class Diverging Devolution	% Women in Trade	Socioeconomic Development Score	% Single 15–19	% Polygynous	% Ever-Divorced	% Remarried	$\bar{X}$ Duration Breastfeeding	$\bar{X}$ Duration Postpartum Abstinence	$\bar{X}$ Duration Nonsusceptibility	% Current Use Contraception	% Knowing 1 Method	% Desired Family Size <6	% ≤2 Live Births 10+ yrs of Marriage	% Premarital Birth	% Birth in First 9 Months Marriage
Group A Wolof, Lebu, Poular, Senegal Fula, Manding, Serer, Senegal Mande, Malinke, Cameroon Peul, Choa Arabs, Cameroon Hausa (N=8)	$\bar{X}$ =	97	2	3&5	10	-.57	33	46	20	86	20	7	15	3.3	28	17	21	7	7
	σ =	3	3	3–5	11	.48	13	9	7	5	1	7	3	4.1	25	6	16	4	4
Group B Chari-Logone, Mandara, Tuburi & Gizega, Diola, Adamawa groups, Bamun, Mijikenda (N=7)	$\bar{X}$ =	45	24	0	5	-1.00	36	45	16	79	21	12	17	1.8	28	19	29	18	9
	σ =	20	22	0–1	4	.38	17	4	4	18	2	6	2	2.6	26	5	10	9	4
Group C Mole-Dagbani, Other Ghana north, Benin Yoruba, Nagot, Dendi-Dit-tamari, Bariba, Other Benin north, Kulango, Senufo (N=8)	$\bar{X}$ =	41	41	1	43	-.68	48	42	15	82	23	21	22	2.9	46	16	16	15	15
	σ =	9	19	0–1	18	.42	17	7	6	7	2	3	3	1.8	19	8	6	5	5

Group D
Adja, Fon, Goun, Other Benin south, Guéré, Guro & Yacuba, Kru (N = 8)

$\bar{X} =$	3	64	0&1	23	-.01	53	37	19	82	20	17	19	4.2	61	16	12	13	17
$\sigma =$	3	19	0–2	18	.68	11	7	9	9	2	3	2	2.6	33	6	4	5	3

Group E
Fante, Twi, Other Ghana Akan, Ewe, Ga-Adangbe, Guan, Lagunaires, Agni (N = 8)

$\bar{X} =$	6	18	2	31	1.16	66	32	30	73	18	10	15	9.3	79	37	13	10	15
$\sigma =$	5	9	2	14	.73	12	5	6	4	2	2	2	5.2	7	14	3	3	3

Group F
Bakosi, Bakundu, Ekoi, Mbembe, Duala, Bassa, Pangwe, Kaka, Maka, Yaunde, Other Cameroon south, Bamenda, Bamileke, Bafia Widekum (N = 13)

$\bar{X} =$	1	5	1	3	.13	62	34	13	47	19	16	17	2.9	48	13	21	27	14
$\sigma =$	1	8	0–1	3	.89	10	11	7	19	3	5	4	2.3	18	8	11	9	3

Group G
Kikuyu, Luo, Luhya, Kamba, Kisii, Meru-Embu, Kalenjin, Other Kenya, Sotho (N = 9)

$\bar{X} =$	3	6	0	1	.69	73	27	10	43	19	6	14	6.3	85	26	10	21	17
$\sigma =$	5	7	0–2	1	.59	12	12	5	21	2	5	2	3.2	8	10	5	9	5

NOTE: Values for class/caste stratification and diverging devolution score are modes and ranges respectively.

African regions) and the Murdock Ethnographic Atlas. We are well aware of the shortcomings, especially those affecting the East African cluster. With these caveats in mind, we shall now turn to some statistical work.

The ideal format for the analysis involving sixty-one individual ethnic groups and seven organizational or cultural contexts would be provided by the technique of multilevel or contextual analysis. This technique is based on the confrontation of within-cluster intercepts and slopes a_k and b_k with the cluster's locations on the x variable, that is, $\bar{x}_k$. With only seven to thirteen ethnic groups per cluster and with enhanced relative importance of measurement error within more homogeneous clusters, not forgetting the problems typical of cluster G, estimated within-cluster slopes are not sufficiently reliable to set into motion the techniques proposed by, *inter alia*, Boyd and Iversen (1979) involving a centering procedure based on such slopes. The Bayesian approach as advocated by Mason, Wong, and Entwistle (1982) is of not much help either as we have no feasible a priori information or theory to shape the within-cluster slopes in a particular way. We could of course not resist calculating these within-cluster slopes, but a pattern could not be detected. Hence, we have to fall back on the classic default option, namely the assumption that within-cluster slopes b_k are identical to the overall slope b as exhibited in the full set of ethnic group data points. This brings us back to simpler statistical procedures such as analysis of variance and multiple classification analysis (MCA) assuming no interaction between the factor "cultural context" and the covariate "socioeconomic development score." Note, however, that we have calculated the analysis of variance results using the design in which the socioeconomic development scores were introduced first. This is the *conservative* way of estimating the contribution of cultural setting membership. If the a priori minimized contribution of the latter variable still weighs up to the maximized contribution of the former, then we have a sound reason for stating that the cultural context matters. The analysis of variance and the MCA results are presented in tables 2.16 and 2.17 (see also table 2.15 for the unadjusted means of the various demographic characteristics by cultural context).

The analysis of variance results corroborate, not unexpectedly, the findings of the previous section by showing that the cultural context effects are very strong for one set of components of the reproductive regime (the second group of variables in table 2.16) but that they cannot be given as much credit for another set (the first group of variables). In addition to these results, further information can be gleaned from the various plots presented in figure 2.1. Here we have shown the location of the seven cluster centers $(\bar{y}, \bar{x})$, together with an indication of within-cluster heterogeneity, both with respect to x and y. The vertical and horizontal lines correspond respectively to plus or minus $1\sigma_y$ and $1\sigma_x$. Moreover, the seven within-cluster correlation coefficients r_k are reported in order to bring out the direction of within-cluster

TABLE 2.16   Proportion of Variance of Reproductive Regime Components Explained by Socioeconomic Development Score and Membership of Institutional/Cultural Cluster; Analysis of Variance Results for 61 Ethnic Groups, WFS Surveys

Component of Reproductive Regime	Proportion of Variance Explained By:		
	Socioeconomic Development Score	Cluster Membership	R
Duration postpartum amenorrhea	45.5	13.0	.77
Duration breastfeeding	45.3	10.8	.75
Percent single, women 15–19	41.0	19.8	.78
Knowledge at least 1 method of contraception	39.5	16.8	.75
Current use contraception	35.4	10.9	.68
Polygyny	32.5	12.4	.67
Duration postpartum nonsusceptibility	30.5	25.1	.75
Occurrence of premarital birth	0.0	51.9	.72
Duration postpartum abstinence	8.9	50.1	.77
Percent ever-widowed	1.0	49.4	.71
Percent remarried	18.2	47.1	.81
Percent ever-divorced	9.0	38.6	.69
Median age at first marriage, all women	17.2	37.6	.74
Birth first 9 months of marriage	12.6	37.6	.70
Mean age at first marriage, women 25+	10.1	33.1	.66
Percent desired family size <6	21.6	27.9	.70
Percent ≤2 live births 10+ yrs marriage	12.0	21.7	.58
Average desired family size	10.2	16.9	.52

NOTE: Analysis of variance design with socioeconomic development score introduced prior to cluster membership.

slopes and the degree of association. Finally, the MCA results in table 2.17 show the relative position of each cluster as measured against overall means, under the assumption that all clusters would have equal average development scores and equal within-cluster slopes. In other words, they indicate how much difference is left between the cultural settings, once socioeconomic development scores are under control. We shall now inspect the results for each component of the reproductive regime.

The child-spacing variables are treated first. Breastfeeding and postpartum amenorrhea for mothers of surviving children born in the last 2 years show very little variation between cultural settings once the socioeconomic development score is controlled for. Moreover, as we can see from figure 2.1, panel A, the cluster means $(\bar{y}_k, \bar{x}_k)$ tend to fall on a common downward slope, and in addition, all within-cluster slopes are *consistently* negative (cf. signs of

TABLE 2.17 Average Vales of Demographic Parameters in the Form of Deviations from the Grand Mean for 7 Institutional/Cultural Clusters after Adjustment for Differences in Socioeconomic Development Scores (MCA results); 61 Ethnic Groups, WFS Surveys

	Nuptiality & First Birth							Spacing				Contraception		Desired Family Size		Sterility & Subfecundity	Identification of Cluster Pattern			
	Percent single, 15–19	Median age at marriage, all	Polygyny	Percent ever-divorced	Percent remarried	Percent with premarital birth, parous women	Percent birth first 9 months of marriage	Duration breastfeeding, surviving children	Duration postpartum amenorrhea, surviving children	Duration postpartum abstinence, surviving children	Duration nonsusceptible period, surviving children	Percent knowledge at least 1 method	Current use contraception, currently married women	Percent desiring family size <6	Average desired family size	Percent ≤2 live births, 10+ years marriage	Average percent Muslim	Average percent traditional religion	Class/Caste; diverging devolution score	Average percent women in trade
Grand Mean:	54	17.7	37	18	68	17	14	20	13	13	17	54	4	20	7.2	17				
Adjusted Deviations																				
Group A	−17	−1.8	7	4	14	−10	−7	−1	−1	−7	−3	−20	0	−1	0.2	4	97	2	3 to 5	10
Group B	−11	−1.1	4	1	5	0	−5	0	−1	−3	−2	−16	−1	−1	0.0	12	45	4	0 & 1	5
Group C	−2	.4	2	−1	10	−2	2	2	1	7	3	−1	0	−3	0.2	−1	41	41	0 & 1	43
Group D	−1	.2	0	1	14	−4	3	3	0	4	2	7	0	−4	0.3	−5	3	64	0 to 2	23
Group E	3	.3	−1	9	13	−6	1	0	2	−1	0	13	3	13	−1.9	−5	6	18	2	31
Group F	7	.8	−2	−2	−20	10	1	−1	−1	3	1	−7	−2	−7	0.3	4	1	5	0 & 1	3
Group G	14	.6	−7	−9	−20	4	3	0	0	−5	−2	24	1	5	−0.1	−7	3	6	0 & 1	1

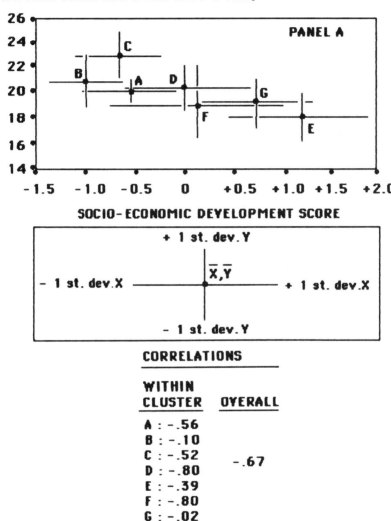

FIGURE: 2.1. Location of Ethnic Clusters with Respect to Various Components of the Reproductive Regime (Y) and the Socioeconomic Development Score (X); Overall and within Cluster Correlations (r_{XY})

FIGURE 2.1, PANEL A: Y = Duration of Breastfeeding in Months within-cluster correlation coefficients). With the present data set, that is, not being able to differentiate more precisely between the magnitudes of within-cluster slopes, all we can say is that socioeconomic development erodes breastfeeding and amenorrhea durations in a consistent way and that there seem to be few institutional and cultural elements among the ones introduced here that decelerate or accelerate this process.

Exactly the opposite holds true with respect to the other component of child-spacing, namely postpartum abstinence. Here organizational cluster membership explains five times as much of the variance than socioeconomic development scores, despite the use of an analysis of variance design that suppresses the impact of the organizational or cultural setting. The clusters are furthermore widely scattered (figure 2.1, panel B) and the adjusted deviations from the grand mean in the MCA table remain impressive. Postpartum abstinence is highly reduced in the profoundly Islamized and Kenyan societies; it is still very high in West African societies where traditional religions combined with a moderate to high participation of women in the market economy have been maintained. Nevertheless, within-cluster slopes tend to be negative (Group G, our problem case, is the exception), meaning that postpartum abstinence is reduced according to socioeconomic development in each setting, but that the relative position of the various clusters is being maintained at very different levels.

The two patterns for lactation and postpartum abstinence respectively are fused in order to explain overall postpartum nonsusceptibility. In table 2.16, socioeconomic development scores and cultural context membership have been given comparable explanatory power. In other words, ethnic groups with high development scores, but belonging to different organizational settings, are less differentiated with respect to the length of the postpartum nonsusceptible period—in addition to having lower levels—than societies with low scores on the development dimension. This feature, which is a logical consequence of the joint action of the two previous ones, is shown in panel C of figure 2.1. The difference in dynamics for breastfeeding/amenorrhea and for postpartum abstinence leads to an additional phenomenon. Societies who have the strong cultural props of long postpartum abstinence are at present also at the top with regard to duration of lactation (see group C in panels A and B). But, given the relatively moderate overall slope of breastfeeding (the lowest group mean is still 18 months for surviving children) and the high dispersion of the groups for abstinence (the range of group means stretches down from 21 months to 6 months only), very highly differentiated degrees of dissociation between lactation and postpartum abstinence durations have come into existence. Further within-cluster specifications of this differential dissociation are, however, impossible. Given the relatively volatile nature of the magnitudes of within-cluster slopes (not their signs), this data set does not allow us to compare such within-cluster slopes for breastfeeding with

**DURATION POSTPARTUM ABSTINENCE
IN MONTHS (SURVIVING CHILDREN
BORN LAST 2 YEARS)**

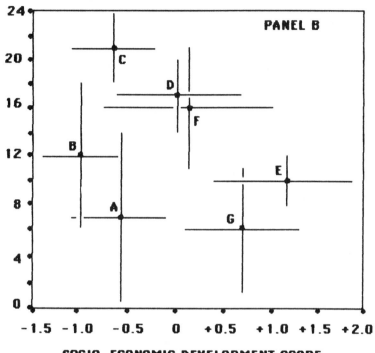

SOCIO-ECONOMIC DEVELOPMENT SCORE

CORRELATIONS

WITHIN CLUSTER	OVERALL
A : -.10	
B : -.25	
C : -.74	
D : -.08	-.30
E : -.29	
F : -.65	
G : +.38	

FIGURE 2.1, PANEL B: Y = Duration Postpartum Abstinence in Months

DURATION OF OVERALL POSTPARTUM NON-SUSCEPTIBLE PERIOD IN MONTHS (SURVIVING CHILDREN BORN LAST 2 YRS)

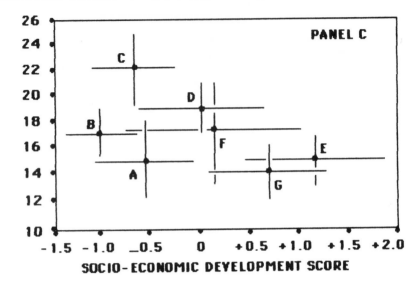

SOCIO-ECONOMIC DEVELOPMENT SCORE

CORRELATIONS

WITHIN CLUSTER	OVERALL
A : -.28	
B : +.17	
C : -.00	
D : -.15	-.50
E : -.53	
F : -.73	
G : +.21	

FIGURE 2.1, PANEL C : Y = Duration of Overall Postpartum Nonsusceptible Period in Months

those for abstinence. The addition of one ethnic group or a change in ethnic cluster membership for one data point, for instance, could considerably alter the magnitudes of these respective slopes.

Current contraceptive use and knowledge of at least one method of con-

**PER CENT CURRENT USE OF
CONTRACEPTION
(CURRENTLY MARRIED WOMEN
AGED 15-49)**

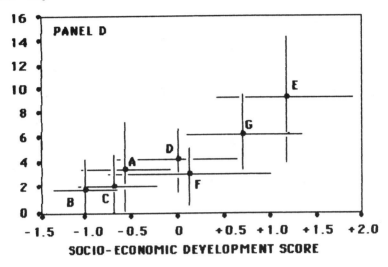

SOCIO-ECONOMIC DEVELOPMENT SCORE

CORRELATIONS

WITHIN
CLUSTER   OVERALL

A : +.41
B : +.25
C : +.65   +.60
D : +.09
E : +.49
F : +.52
G : +.13

FIGURE 2.1, PANEL D: Y = Percent of Currently Married Women, 15–49, Currently Using Contraception

traception follows the pattern of breastfeeding: here too, organizational or cultural setting membership effects have only a moderate resistance to the control for socioeconomic development scores (see tables 2.16 and 2.17). This is explained by the fact that the contextual averages are located on an upward slope (panels D and E in figure 2.1) and that within-context slopes are systematically positive as well. Note that there is again a problem with the direction of the within-cluster slope for the East African group (G),

**PER CENT KNOWING AT LEAST
ONE METHOD OF CONTRACEPTION
(ALL WOMEN AGED 15-49)**

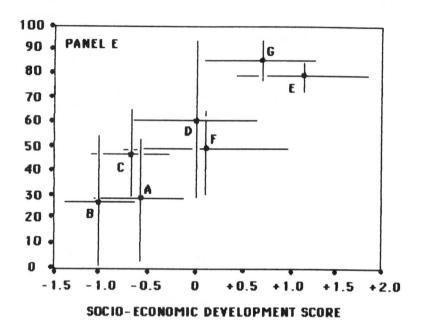

SOCIO-ECONOMIC DEVELOPMENT SCORE

CORRELATIONS

WITHIN
CLUSTER   OVERALL

A : +.11
B : +.57
C : +.00
D : +.46   +.63
E : +.47
F : +.61
G : -.36

FIGURE 2.1, PANEL E: Y = Percent of All Women, 15–49, Knowing at Least One
Method of Contraception

which underlines once more that some other unidentified factors are operating within this group. The remainder of the contextual effects, as exhibited by the MCA results for current use and knowledge of contraception, hints at the fact that the combination of high socioeconomic development scores and an institutional setting permitting high female social and economic inde-

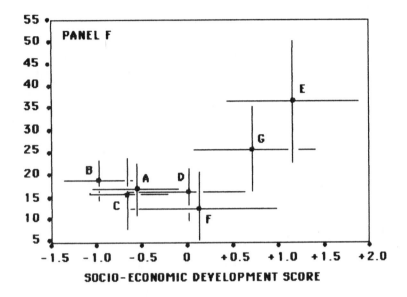

PER CENT STATING DESIRED
FAMILY SIZE LESS THAN
6 CHILDREN (ALL WOMEN
AGED 15-49)

SOCIO-ECONOMIC DEVELOPMENT SCORE

CORRELATIONS

WITHIN
CLUSTER   OVERALL

A : +.62
B : -.69
C : +.71
D : +.34   +.46
E : +.00
F : -.09
G : +.79

FIGURE 2.1, PANEL F : Y = Percent of All Women, 15–49, Stating Desired Family Sizes of Less Than 6 Children

pendence is conducive to enhanced contraceptive use. Such combinations are typical for southeastern Ivory Coast and southern Ghana. Finally, the observation that, even then, the cluster average for current contraceptive use among currently married women is barely 10 percent is worthy of consideration.

Of the two measures of desired family size, the proportion not wishing to go beyond six children shows the clearest pattern (see panel F in figure 2.1).

The location of the cluster means for this variable stays systematically below the 20 percent level for societies with low to moderate scores on the socioeconomic development scale. Note, that with 10 to 15 percent of women not progressing beyond two children after 10 years since first marriage, such a level of 20 percent not "wanting" to move beyond six is really indicative of no desire for any manifest family limitation whatsoever. Hence, only for the two clusters with the highest score on the socioeconomic development dimension is there a takeoff toward higher proportions. After the control for the wage sector and female literacy dimension, only one cluster stands out in the MCA: it comprises again the ethnic groups of southeastern Ivory Coast and southern Ghana which had well above average levels of contraceptive use and no major infecundity problem. Hence, we can safely accept that we are dealing here with the only cluster of societies in which there has been a real takeoff in modern contraceptive behavior with genuine intentions for preventing a further decline of the older spacing pattern (they already have relatively short durations of postpartum abstinence) or for some family limitation at parities below six.

We shall now turn to the nuptiality and reproductive starting pattern indicators. With the exception of the proportion single among women aged 15 to 19 and the percentage of married women in a polygynous union, all other nuptiality and reproductive starting pattern variables are predominantly associated with cultural cluster membership, even when the analysis of variance design used here artificially reduces its explanatory power. The dominance of the contextual effect is particularly striking for premarital fertility, which is not linked at all to socioeconomic development scores, either across or within contexts (see panel G in figure 2.1 and table 2.16). Consequently, the organizational variables picked by Goody are endowed with remarkable predictive power. The weight of socioeconomic development scores is also unimpressive when it comes to account for births occurring in marriage, but stemming from premarital conceptions. Here, there is no differentiation across cultural contexts, except for clusters A and B which have a major Islamic component and low proportions of such births. This further substantiates Goody's prediction that the adoption of Islam results in more control over young women. As soon as traditional religion emerges as the chief complement to Islam, the effect of the latter disappears (cf. cluster C, which is in line with the others in panel H of figure 2.1).

The effects of cultural setting membership and of socioeconomic development scores on age at first marriage are highly dependent on the age groups considered. We have already pointed out this feature when the correlation coefficients were considered between indicators SINGLE 15, MEDMAR and AGEMAR 25 with the socioeconomic development dimension. If data for older women are taken (i.e., 25 +), cultural setting effects dominate. If the youngest cohort is considered (i.e., women aged 15–19) via the proportion

**PER CENT OF PAROUS WOMEN
WITH PREMARITAL BIRTH**

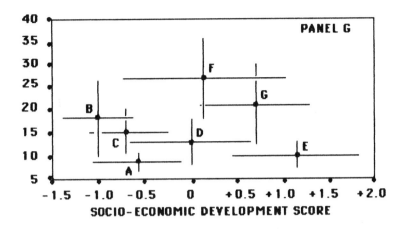

FIGURE 2.1, PANEL G : Y = Percent of Parous Women, 15–49, with Premarital Birth

still single, the socioeconomic development dimension dominates. This dominance is not only evident through the patterning of cluster means on an upward slope (panel I), but also through the prevalence of positive within-cluster slopes. The only two explanations that can be offered for this duality are either that substantially differential reporting error for retrospectively reported ages at marriage is associated with cluster membership (older women pull up their ages at first marriage), or that genuine change is taking place with respect to cohort marriage behavior. For the latter hypothesis to hold, such change must have been both *recent* and *substantial*. We shall come back to this issue when trends are discussed in a later chapter.

So far, the findings of this empirical testing have fit our theoretical expec-

PER CENT OF MARRIED WOMEN WITH BIRTH IN FIRST 9 MONTHS OF MARRIAGE (WOMEN MARRIED AT LEAST 9 MONTHS, AGED 15-49)

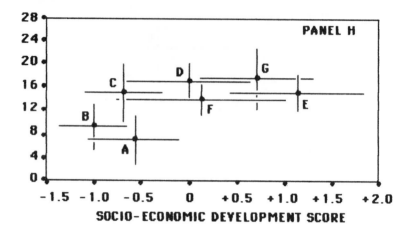

CORRELATIONS

WITHIN
CLUSTER   OVERALL

A : -.06
B : +.75
C : +.06
D : -.34   +.36
E : +.50
F : +.13
G : -.23

FIGURE 2.1, PANEL H : Y = Percent of Women, 15–49, Married for at Least 9 Months with Birth During the First 9 months of Marriage

tations rather better than we had expected. A real puzzle emerges, however, when it comes to dealing with polygyny. We had expected polygyny to respond mainly to the cultural context, but, as the earlier analyses had shown, it is the socioeconomic development score that explains most of the variation. Inspection of the location of the various contextual clusters, as shown in panel J, reveals that the cluster means fall indeed on a downward slope with respect to socioeconomic development, which partially accounts for the overall negative association. This cross-sectional finding is supportive of the

PER CENT SINGLE WOMEN
IN AGE GROUP 15-19

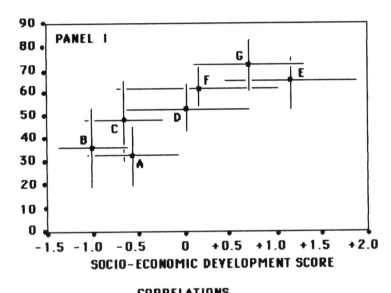

FIGURE 2.1, PANEL I : Y = Percent Women Single in Age Group 15–19

thesis that socioeconomic modernization would weaken the institution of polygyny, either directly or indirectly by pushing up the age at first marriage for women. However, within-cluster slopes have contradictory signs: three are positive, three are negative, and one is virtually zero. Moreover, as we shall see shortly, the incidence of divorce tends to rise within clusters with increasing scores on socioeconomic development, thereby fueling polygyny to a moderate extent. Hence, the within-cluster dynamics seem to be rather complicated, and it may very well be that, despite the *overall* downward slope (which has a Muslim versus non-Muslim component as well) within-cluster

**PER CENT IN POLYGYNOUS UNION
(CURRENTLY MARRIED WOMEN,
AGED 15-49)**

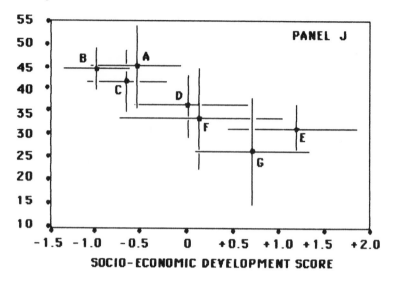

FIGURE 2.1, PANEL J : Y = Percent of Currently Married Women, 15–49, in Polygynous Unions

dynamics are genuinely different. Obviously, trend data are again needed to crack the problem.

The results for the percentages ever-divorced and remarried are shown in panels K and L. Here, very substantial contextual patterning occurs, as also reflected in the outcomes of the analysis of variance and MCA. Cluster means on percentages ever-divorced are located in the 10 to 20 percent band, except for the E cluster, which contains all the matrilineal societies of the Ivory Coast and Ghana. In this cluster, the incidence of divorce is much

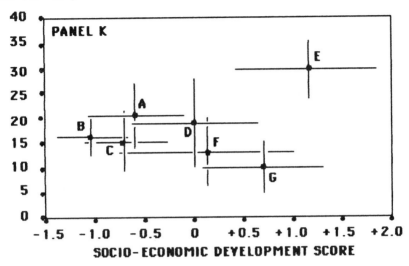

PER CENT EVER DIVORCED
(EVER MARRIED WOMEN,
AGED 15-49)

SOCIO-ECONOMIC DEVELOPMENT SCORE

CORRELATIONS

WITHIN
CLUSTER   OVERALL

A : +.28
B : -.26
C : +.10
D : +.81   +.30
E : -.38
F : +.34
G : +.25

FIGURE 2.1, PANEL K: Y = Percent of Ever-Married Women, 15–49, Ever-Divorced

higher (30 percent on average). Matrilinearity does seem to be associated with high divorce, although all groups in cluster E have levels above 20 percent: typically matrilineally organized ethnic groups such as the "Other Akan" (41 percent), Fante (32), Agni (32), and Twi (27) are at the high end, societies with a mixture such as the Lagunaires (27) or the Ga-Adangbe (28) are in the middle, and those with predominance of patrilineal traits such as the Ewe (25) or without corporate lineages such as the Guan (23) are at the lower end. Other matrilineal societies not incorporated in this cluster, such

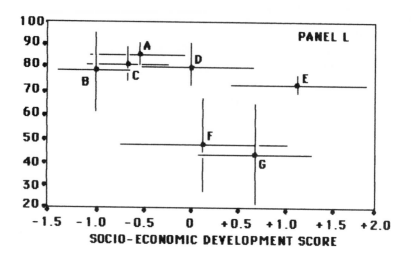

**PER CENT REMARRIED
(WOMEN WITH DISRUPTED
FIRST UNION, AGED 15-49)**

CORRELATIONS

**WITHIN
CLUSTER   OVERALL**

A : -.32
B : -.57
C : -.76   -.43
D : -.44
E : +.43
F : -.43
G : -.06

FIGURE 2.1, PANEL L: Y = Percent of Women, 15–49, with Disrupted First Union
Already Remarried

as the neighboring Baule of the Ivory Coast, have equally marked proportions
ever-divorced (32). The within-cluster slope for group E (negative) is equally
out of line with the slopes in most of the other clusters (positive). The same
holds for the within-cluster slopes with respect to remarriage: it is positive in
group E and negative in all the others. Hence, the overall picture seems to be
increasing divorce with socioeconomic development levels but decreasing
speed of remarriage, except for cluster E where the reverse holds. However, it
should be pointed out that the indices used here are affected by truncation
and that a closer inspection of the age pattern is required.

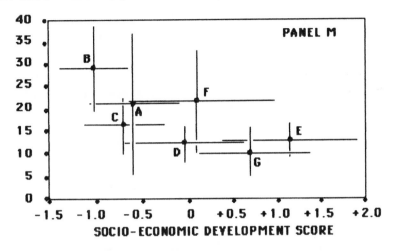

FIGURE 2.1, PANEL M : Y = Percent of Women with Durations of Marriage of at Least 10 Years Having 2 or fewer Children

The last issue to be treated is that of sterility and subfecundity. The plot of the clusters and the within-cluster correlation coefficients are given in panel M. The overall slope tends to be negative and the same holds for several within-cluster slopes. However, our sample only captures the Cameroon segment of the wide Central African sterility belt (pulling up the means for clusters A, B, and F) and misses other important locations such as those in East Africa outside Kenya (e.g., Tanzania). We have the impression that the overall tendency is indeed towards lower sterility levels as subsistence economies are drawn into contact with the outside world, thereby gaining better access to antibiotics. On the other hand, we should not rule out the existence of the opposite trend in large cities and especially those that have a high incidence of prostitution, fueled, *inter alia*, through immigration of childless women from other areas. Once more, trend data would elucidate at least part of the problem.

CONCLUSIONS

First of all it should be stressed that the results presented here do not stem from a representative sample of all sub-Saharan societies and that the West African information far outweighs the rest. The advantage has been a relatively detailed unfolding of the various reproductive patterns and their correlates specific to this region (i.e., from Senegal to Cameroon). The disadvantage, of course, emerges clearly when dealing with the eastern and southern African groups (cluster G), which seem to have their own system of internal differentiation with respect to variables such as premarital conception, age at first union and polygyny, postpartum abstinence (compare Kenya with Lesotho), and subfecundity. These internal variations are not adequately accounted for.

A second caveat pertains to the characterization of the position of women. Ideally, this position should be studied through the use of *several* dimensions, which are furthermore not always overlapping (see M. K. Whyte, 1978). Here, we explicitly measured a central variable, namely the possibility of independent income generation for women and its correlate, the existence of segregated household budgets. The other features pertaining to female roles and positions are only brought out indirectly, that is, through the clustering of the original sixty-one ethnic groups, and their association with variables such as matrilineal organization (cluster E), depth of Islamization (cluster A), or the lack of more complex traditional polity and its associate, the relative absence of multifunctional female associations (cluster G). Obviously, there is ample room left for further theory formulation and testing.

The findings of this chapter illustrate the fact that the various components of the reproductive regime exhibit different patterns of association with socioeconomic development and aspects of social organization. The three variables that show consistent within- and across-cluster effects of female schooling and the growth of the wage sector are (1) the duration of breastfeeding and postpartum amenorrhea, (2) the use of contraception other than abstinence, and (3) the indicator of female age at first marriage (proportions single 15–19). The relationship between these three variables and the degree of socioeconomic development not only holds at the aggregate level of analysis, as shown in this chapter for ethnic groups, but has repeatedly been documented in analyses performed with individual-level data (e.g., Adegbola and Page for Lagos, 1981; Mosley et al. for Kenya, 1982; Ferry and Page for Kenya, 1984; Gaisie for Ghana, 1985; Abbas and Kalule-Sabiti for Northern

Sudan, 1985; Mpiti and Kalule-Sabiti for Lesotho, 1985). These micro-level analyses, using female education as a proxy for socioeconomic development, show a typically sub-Saharan feature: socioeconomic development erodes child-spacing through reduced breastfeeding and, at best, just barely succeeds in reestablishing an equilibrium via increased contraception. In many instances, a positive relationship emerges between marital fertility levels and schooling, and it is only the introduction of the effect of later marriage for the more educated women that redresses the balance. The analysis of ethnic differences in this chapter reproduced these features.

The "multiple phase"-theory of fertility transition recognizes the initial balancing, typical of the preparatory stage of the transition, of the three major components of reproduction (marriage, contraceptive use, breastfeeding and amenorrhea). It also describes individual variation within a given society and accounts for the present interethnic variation. At both levels of analysis, differences with respect to the "component mix," reflecting the impact of socioeconomic development, are larger than differences with respect to overall fertility levels in societies that are not afflicted by a major sterility problem. Apart from a few exceptions, the unfolding of differential levels of fertility, typical of a genuine fertility transition, has not emerged yet. Speculation suggests that this second phase could not be reached before the end of this century in the majority of sub-Saharan populations because of the counteractive effects of shortened breastfeeding and increased contraception. Bongaarts et al. (1984) provide illustrative calculations on the subject: in table 2.18 estimates of the prevalence of contraception required by the year 2000 for bringing about marital fertility reductions of up to 30 percent are given, assuming (1) a postpartum nonsusceptible period stabilized at 16 months and (2) nonsusceptibility was reduced from 16 to 8 months. In the unlikely event of unaltered nonsusceptibility, contraceptive prevalence (i.e., percentage of current users among married women) would have to be approximately 26 percent to bring about a modest marital fertility reduction of 20 per-

TABLE 2.18   Estimates of Levels of Contraceptive Prevalence Needed To Achieve Specified Reductions in Marital Fertility by the Year 2000

Percent Reduction in Marital Fertility by Year 2000	*Required Percentage Contraceptive Users by Year 2000*	
	If Nonsusceptible Period Remains at 18 months	If Nonsusceptible Period Declines to 8 Months
0	5	29
10	15	37
20	26	45
30	36	53

SOURCE: Bongaarts, Frank, and Lesthaeghe, 1984.

cent. In the much more likely event of a reduction of nonsusceptibility to 8 months, contraceptive prevalence would need to increase to 46 percent to produce the same fall in marital fertility. Considering that contraceptive prevalence of 20 percent is presently achieved in hardly any populations (e.g., Ga-Adangbe in and around Accra and several other urban populations with more than primary schooling), large fertility differentials between individuals within a given society *and* between ethnic groups themselves are indeed unlikely to emerge within the next decade.

The effects of ethnicity and social organization have some influence on this socioeconomically induced pattern. Only two such effects with respect to contraception and female age at marriage are worth mentioning. The first pertains to the possible contraceptive increasing effect of belonging to the West African group of populations with high female levels of schooling, female economic independence, and largely matrilineal organization (i.e., group E in Ghana and the Ivory Coast). The effect of ethnic cluster, as distinct from the effect of the high socioeconomic development score, is not as marked when contraceptive prevalence itself is considered (table 2.17 shows a modest positive residual for contraceptive prevalence in group E after controlling for socioeconomic development scores), but it emerges more forcefully in the form of a substantial positive residual for knowledge of contraception and preference for smaller family sizes. Hence, independently of socioeconomic development levels, the Akan and related groups exhibit a greater readiness for contraceptive use and family limitation than others.

The second ethnic-specific effect illustrates the lowered age at marriage effected by Islamization (see large negative residuals for proportions women 15–19 single in table 2.17 for ethnic clusters A and B). Such societies, conforming with Goody's thesis, exercise strong social controls over women, not only by marrying them off at young ages, which reduces premarital conceptions, but also by maintaining a high speed of remarriage and concomitantly high levels of polygyny. The maximized use of the reproductive age span seen in these two clusters is contributed to not only by the low levels of female literacy but also by other arrangements that affect the social position of women.

The most powerful effect of ethnic cluster-membership or social organization characteristics on fertility is seen in operation through the length of postpartum abstinence. The cluster means for this variable have a wide range of 16 months, whereas the corresponding range for breastfeeding is only 6 months, and that of current contraceptive use is 20 percentage points. The impact of this heterogeneity in durations of the postpartum taboo on fertility must therefore be considerable. Islamized societies of clusters A and B, East African societies of group G, and the matrilineal societies of Ghana and the Ivory Coast of group E have average durations of postpartum abstinence that are 6 to 12 months shorter than those of the other West African societies.

The persistence of traditional religion, combined with more female economic self-reliance, patrilinearity, and absence of caste organization or diverging devolution of property through women are associated with the survival of a long postpartum taboo.

As indicated, the demographic significance of the postpartum taboo must be stressed in the context of a fertility transition. Societies with a long, upheld taboo are more likely to experience high or even rising fertility levels if the taboo is weakened than societies that practice short durations of abstinence. The reason for this is the mechanism shown in table 2.18: starting from long durations of postpartum abstinence, a reduction implies a rapid decline of the overall nonsusceptible period and the consequent need for a large increase in contraceptive prevalence to maintain current fertility levels. By contrast, societies with eroded postpartum abstinence are, at least at present, at a relative advantage in converting a given increase in contraceptive use into a net fertility reduction. Patrilineal and non-Islamized West African societies have, by virtue of their long postpartum abstinence periods, reduced the size of the initial fertility increase in the past, but they may experience this increase at present or in the near future and witness a postponement of the overall fertility decline. Obviously, Islamized societies and societies with strong adherence to traditional religions are at a major disadvantage with respect to adopting contraception and delaying the age at marriage for women by virtue of low female literacy, so that the onset of a genuine fertility transition is likely to be confined to the more developed and Christianized parts of West and East Africa. The former have the advantage of greater female economic and social independence, the latter that of having progressed beyond the decline in postpartum abstinence and nonsusceptibility. Assuming similar developments in these two regions with regard to female schooling and growth of the modern wage sectors in the economy, it is for the future record to show which of these two features, greater female social independence or prior reduction in postpartum nonsusceptibility, will be decisive in bringing about the first cases of a sustained fertility decline.

BIBLIOGRAPHY

Abbas, I., and I. Kalule-Sabiti. 1985. The proximate determinants of fertility in north Sudan. *World Fertility Survey Scientific Reports*, no. 73. Voorburg, Netherlands: International Statistical Institute.

Adegbola, O., and H. J. Page. 1981. Nuptiality and fertility in Lagos. In: *Nuptiality and fertility*, ed. L. Ruzicka. Liège, Belgium: Ordina for the International Union for the Scientific Study of Population.

Akinkunmi, J. O. 1984. Sexual abstinence, breast-feeding and fertility: A study of eastern Nigeria. M. A. thesis. Legon: University of Ghana, Regional Institute for Population Studies.

Bertrand, J. T., W. E. Bertrand, and M. Malonga. 1983. The use of traditional and modern methods of fertility control in Kinshasa, Zaire. *Population Studies* 37(1): 129–136.

Bongaarts, J., O. Frank, and R. Lesthaeghe. 1984. The proximate determinants of fertility in sub-Saharan Africa. *Population and Development Review* 10(3): 511–537.

Brass, W., et al. 1968. *The demography of tropical Africa.* Princeton: Princeton University Press.

Boyd, L. H., and G. R. Iversen. 1979. *Contextual analysis: Concepts and statistical techniques.* Belmont, Calif.: Wadsworth.

Carael, M. 1981. Child-spacing, ecology and nutrition in the Kivu province of Zaire. In: *Child-spacing in tropical Africa—Traditions and change,* ed. H. J. Page and R. Lesthaeghe. London: Academic Press, 275–286.

Davis, K., and J. Blake. 1956. Social structure and fertility: An analytic framework. *Economic Development and cultural change* 4(4): 211–235.

Ferry, B. 1981. The Senegalese surveys. In: *Child-spacing in tropical Africa—Traditions and change,* ed. H. J. Page and R. Lesthaeghe. London: Academic Press, 265–285.

Ferry, B., and D. P. Smith. 1983. Breast-feeding differentials. *World Fertility Survey Comparative Studies,* no. 23. Voorburg: International Statistical Institute.

Ferry, B., and H. J. Page. 1984. The proximate determinants of fertility and their effect on fertility patterns: An illustrative analysis applied to Kenya. *World Fertility Survey Scientific Reports,* no. 71. Voorburg: International Statistical Institute.

Gaisie, S. K. 1984. The proximate determinants of fertility in Ghana. *World Fertility Survey Scientific Reports,* no. 53. Voorburg: International Statistical Institute.

Goody, J. 1976. *Production and reproduction—A comparative study of the domestic domain.* Cambridge: Cambridge University Press.

Hennart, P. 1983. *Allaitement maternel en situation nutritionelle critique: Adaptations et limites.* Zaire: CEMUBAC—Université Libre de Bruxelles and IRS-Lwiro.

Henin, R. A., D. Ewbank, and H. Hogan, eds. n.d. *The demography of Tanzania: An analysis of the 1973 National Demographic Survey of Tanzania.* Dar Es Salaam, Tanzania: Bureau of Statistics and BRALUP.

Henin, R. A., A. Korten, and L. Werner. 1982. Evaluation of birth histories: A case study of Kenya. *World Fertility Survey Scientific Reports,* no. 36. Voorburg: International Statistical Institute.

Hill, A., S. Randall, and O. Sullivan. 1982. The mortality and fertility of farmers and pastoralists in central Mali, 1950–81. *Centre for Population Research paper,* no. 84-2. London School of Hygiene and Tropical Medicine.

Lesthaeghe, R. 1984. *Fertility and its proximate determinants in sub-Saharan Africa: The record of the 1960s and 70s.* Liège, Belgium: International Union for the Scientific Study of Population, Committee on the Comparative Analysis of Fertility and Family Planning.

Levine, M. S. 1977. *Canonical analysis and factor comparison.* London: Sage Publications, University Series on Quantitative Applications in the Social Sciences, no. 07-006.

Locoh, T., and G. Adaba. 1981. Child-spacing in Togo: the Southeast Togo Survey EFSE. In: *Child-spacing in tropical Africa—Traditions and Change,* ed. H. J. Page and R. Lesthaeghe. London: Academic Press, 255–264.

Mason, W., G. Y. Wong, and B. Entwistle. 1982. The multilevel linear model: A better way to do contextual analysis. *Working paper of the Population Studies Center*, no. 82-36. Ann Arbor: University of Michigan.

Mosley, W. H., L. H. Werner, and S. Becker. 1982. The dynamics of birth-spacing and marital fertility in Kenya. *World Fertility Survey Scientific Reports*, no. 30. Voorburg: International Statistical Institute.

Mpiti, A. M., and I. Kalule-Sabiti. 1985. The proximate determinants of fertility in Lesotho. *World Fertility Survey Scientific Reports*, no. 78. Voorburg: International Statistical Institute.

Murdock, G. P. 1975. *Outline of world cultures.* 5th ed. New Haven: Human Relations Area Files.

Page, H. J., and R. Lesthaeghe. 1981. *Child-spacing in tropical Africa—Traditions and change.* London: Academic Press. (especially chaps. 3 and 7 by P. Caldwell and J. C. Caldwell [Ibadan]; chap. 8 by Bracher and Santow [Ibadan]; chap. 6 by O. Adegbola, H. J. Page, and R. Lesthaeghe [Lagos]; and chap. 9 by I. Orubuloye [Ekiti and Ibadan villages]).

Pison, G. 1982. *Dynamique d'une population traditionelle—Les Peuls Bandé du Sénégal Oriental.* Cahier de l'INED no. 99. Paris: Presses Universitaires de France.

Randall, S. C. 1984. A comparative demographic study of three Sahelian populations: Marriage and child-care as intermediate determinants of fertility and mortality. Ph.D. dissertation. London School of Hygiene and Tropical Medicine.

République du Burundi. 1974. *Enquete démographique 1970–71.* 2 vols. Bujumbura: Ministère du Plan.

République du Zaire, SICAI, and Département de démographie. 1977–78. *Etude démographique de l'ouest du Zaire (EDOZA).* Louvain-la-Neuve, Belgium: Université Catholique de Louvain, Département de Démographie.

Romaniuk, A. 1967. *La fécondité des populations congolaises.* Paris: Mouton.

Sala-Diakanda, M. 1979. Approche ethnique des phénomènes démographiques—Le cas du Zaire. 2 vols. Ph.D. dissertation. Louvain-la-Neuve: Université Catholique de Louvain, Département de Démographie.

Schoenmaeckers, R., I. H. Shah. R. Lesthaeghe, and O. Tambashe. 1981. The child-spacing tradition and the postpartum taboo in tropical Africa: Anthropological evidence. In: *Child-spacing in tropical Africa—Traditions and change,* ed. H. J. Page and R. Lesthaeghe. London: Academic Press, 25–71.

Tabutin, D. 1979. Tendances et niveau de fécondité au Zaire. Paper presented at the Colloquium on the Demography of Africa. Abidjan, Ivory Coast.

Tambashe, O. 1984. "Niveaux et corrélats de la fécondité à Kinshasa. Ph.D. dissertation." Brussels: Vrije Universiteit, Interuniversity Programme in Demography.

Vimard, P. 1980. *Nuptialité et fécondité sur le Plateau de Dayes, sud-est Togo—Principaux résultats.* Lomé, Togo: Office de la Recherche Scientifique et Technique d'Outre Mer.

Weiss, E. M. 1981. *The Calabar rural MCH-FP project: Final report.* New York: The Population Council and the Ministry of Health, Government of Nigeria.

Whyte, M. K. 1978. *The status of women in preindustrial societies.* Princeton: Princeton University Press.

CHAPTER THREE

Regional Variation in Components of Child-Spacing: The Role of Women's Education

Ron Lesthaeghe
Camille Vanderhoeft
Samuel Gaisie
Ghislaine Delaine

INTRODUCTION

In this chapter, our primary aim is the assessment of the effect of female education on each of the fertility components separately as well as on their overall balance with respect to child-spacing.The chapter differs from the previous one on a number of points. First of all, only the postpartum variables (lactation, lactational amenorrhea, postpartum abstinence) and contraception are considered. The other components of fertility, namely abortion and coital frequency, are omitted for lack of reliable data, and the problem of sterility is considered in chapter 4. Second, we shall pay attention to the *balance* between the fertility-increasing potential of shorter lactation or abstinence and the fertility-lowering effect of contraception. This involves a more technical section in which we evaluate the joint effect of declining lactational amenorrhea and postpartum abstinence.

The data used in this chapter are again those of the World Fertility Survey. The units of analysis are no longer ethnic groups but a set of thirty-three larger regions. This shift was necessary to obtain larger sample sizes. The spacing variables and their net effect are studied according to individual female education and age within regions. These micro-level effects are subsequently compared across regions in terms of a set of macro-level or contextual characteristics of the regions themselves. In other words, the spacing differentials associated with female education in each region are related to aggregate regional characteristics. Such multi-level analyses are performed separately for three broad age groups. The subject of the chapter is closely related to the notion of the two-phase fertility transition, which we shall now consider.

Ever since the pre-WFS surveys of the 1960s and 1970s started measuring the components of child-spacing, there has been a growing body of evidence showing the importance of the postpartum variables (that is, lactational amenorrhea and postpartum abstinence, which together constitute the overall period of postpartum nonsusceptibility) in explaining both fertility trends and differentials (see for instance Henin, 1968; Ohadike, 1968; Olusanya, 1969; Morgan, 1975; Caldwell and Caldwell, 1977; Romaniuk, 1980; Page and Lesthaeghe, 1981; Mosley, Werner, and Becker, 1982). Examples of tracing back fertility differentials to variations in postpartum nonsusceptibility and contraception are found in studies that attempted to explain regional contrasts (such as Gaisie's account of regional differentials in Ghana, 1981), higher fertility among the educated than among the illiterate women (for example, Adegbola, Page, and Lesthaeghe, 1981), or higher fertility in urban than in rural settings (Tabutin et al., 1981). These intermediate fertility variables are also likely to be major components of fertility increases associated with the settlement of nomads (such as, Henin, 1968).

These studies inspired the notion of a two-phase fertility transition (Lesthaeghe et al., 1981). During the first phase, any fertility-lowering effect gained from the small increments in contraceptive use is neutralized or even outpaced by the fertility-increasing effect of shortened periods of postpartum nonsusceptibility. Only during the second phase is contraceptive prevalence rising fast enough to counteract any further decline in lactational amenorrhea and/or postpartum abstinence. The initial phase, frequently characterized by a fertility bulge, corresponds essentially to a situation with continued high demand for children combined with a rise in supply (that is, rising levels of natural fertility). In this period, fertility of the educated and/or of urban women can be higher than that of the illiterate and/or rural women. Fertility levels also tend to rise with socioeconomic development. The second phase of the transition comes into existence when demand for children falls and when supply reaches a new plateau (Kocher, 1973). Only during this second phase are the "classic" fertility differentials restored.

As suggested earlier, rises in supply are not solely produced by declining periods of nonsusceptibility. The determinants of fecundity have played a role as well. This is especially true for Central African areas, which experienced high levels of infecundity prior to the 1970s (see Brass et al., 1968; Tabutin et al., 1981; Frank, 1983). In these areas increases in fecundity have been associated with reductions in the incidence of venereal disease.

The data from the WFS round of surveys provide additional opportunities for studying the balance between contraception and postpartum variables. Largely as a result of the size of the project, cross-cultural and interregional comparisons can now be made involving populations that show major variation in social organization and economic setting. In addition, intraregional analyses of individual differentials are still feasible. Consequently, individual and contextual variables can now be combined into a multilevel analysis.

More specifically, as a result of the WFS the following questions can be addressed:

1. Are the regional levels of contraceptive use-effectiveness and the regional average durations of postpartum nonsusceptibility a function of regional background characteristics? This is the typical "ecological" or aggregate view.

2. Are the regional values of contraception and postpartum nonsusceptibility for *specific subgroups of women* a function of regional background characteristics? A subgroup of women can, for instance, be specified by a particular level of education, age group, and so forth (for example, only women 25–34, illiterate, are considered). We are still dealing with ecological correlations, but controls have been built in with respect to important *individual* characteristics. The regression results can be compared for the various subgroups across regions, which yield information that is not available in the traditional "ecological" setup.

3. Are the *differences* between values for *two contrasted subgroups* within each region (for example, between illiterate women, 25–34, and women 25–34 with 5+ years of schooling) a function of regional background characteristics? The magnitude of a shift associated with an increase in *individual* education within each region is related, *across regions*, to aggregate socioeconomic and cultural traits. This corresponds to a classic question in contextual analysis: are slopes of individual level variables in each context a function of contextual characteristics? The interaction effects are of particular importance here: the shifts in direction of within-region slopes or differentials with changing characteristics of contexts (such as regional socioeconomic development) are the features required for testing the two-phase nature of the transition. Moreover, the comparison of within-region slopes across all regions may indicate how far the transition has evolved morphologically and which contextual variables produce accelerating or decelerating effects.

The types of analysis proposed so far presuppose that the values of the various dependent variables for *each subgroup within each region* can be calculated with sufficient accuracy. This is especially crucial for the third type of analysis as the dependent variable is the difference between two such values. This means not only that sufficiently large sample sizes must be used, but also that the estimation techniques make an optimal use of these samples.

MEASUREMENT OF DEPENDENT VARIABLES BY REGION AND SUBGROUP

The individual-level variables considered in all subsequent analyses have been restricted to just two: age and education. Their combination has repeatedly captured an impressive proportion of the basic dimension of individual modernization, not only in sub-Saharan Africa, but in most developing countries. Age or cohort locates the individual in history, and in times of change such a location is essential. Education is a key variable for economic stratification since it is a major determinant of standard of living, income, or sector of employment. It is furthermore a crucial component of "Weltanschauung" and determines tastes, a reorientation of priorities, and adoption of other lifestyles (such as "Westernization"). Three age groups are retained (15–24, 25–34, 35+) and combined with three education levels (no schooling or Koranic only, 1–4 years, 5+ years of formal schooling), producing a matrix with nine cells. Information for all nine cells is only available in a limited number of regions: many areas do not have a sufficiently long tradition of female education so that there is often a shortage of educated women in the older age groups. A few regions have information for only three cells as a result of the total lack of schooling for women.

The estimation of mean durations of the postpartum variables and use of contraception for nine possible age-education subgroups by region requires a sufficiently large sample. To ensure this, regions were often grouped. Grouping was not only performed on the basis of geographical proximity, but also of cultural affinity. The ethnic variables employed in chapter 2 and the location of tribes were of some consequent use in setting up larger regions with a maximum degree of cultural homogeneity. Socioeconomic characteristics were also taken into account: large urban units and their hinterland were kept as separate units of analysis. The original fifty-one regions identified in the eight WFS countries were condensed into thirty-three regions. The modal sample size categories are 750–999 and more than 1500 ever-married women (eight regions each); and five regions contain less than 500 ever-married women (Khartoum, Cotonou, Ivory Coast urban savannah, Nairobi, Volta). The estimation of the duration of the postpartum variables (breastfeeding, lactational amenorrhea, abstinence, and overall nonsusceptibility) was based on samples of surviving children born in the last 3 years rather than on the retrospectively reported durations for the last closed interval (often strongly biased downward) or the information for the current open birth interval (biased upward). Table 3.1 shows the thirty-three new regions and the sample sizes for ever-married women and their surviving children born in the last 36 months. Sample sizes for children are smaller than those for ever-married women: in thirteen regions such sample sizes drop below 500 with a minimum of 239. Of the remaining twenty regions, fourteen have sample sizes between 500 and 1000, and six have samples in excess of 1000. It must be noted that only children of ever-married women were taken into account to achieve comparability with the data for Northern Sudan and Lesotho, where only ever-married women were interviewed.

The mean durations of the four postpartum variables were estimated

TABLE 3.1 New Regions and Sample Sizes of Ever-Married Women 15–49 and Their Surviving Children Born in the Last 36 Months; 8 WFS Countries

	Ever-Married Women (N)	Surviving Children (N)
Senegal		
Cap Vert & Thiès	959	668
Central	143	855
Fleuve & Oriental	595	366
Casamance	505	288
Ivory Coast		
Abidjan	900	582
Forest, Urban	610	377
Savannah, Urban	384	245
Forest, Rural	2091	1270
Savannah, Rural	985	661
Ghana		
Greater Accra & East	1310	784
West & Central	775	460
Volta	478	305
Ashanti & Brong-Ahafo	1540	944
North & Upper	840	452
Benin		
Atacora & Borgou	1039	693
Central & South	2185	1484
Cotonou	353	239

	Ever-Married Women (N)	Surviving Children (N)
Cameroon		
Central-South & East	1379	1000
Littoral & Southwest	928	480
North	2558	836
Northwest & West	1657	797
Yaounde & Douala	671	622
Northern Sudan		
Khartoum	326	331
North & East	594	459
Central	775	527
Kordofan & Darfur	912	596
Kenya		
Nairobi	299	371
Central & Eastern	1892	1525
Coast	600	349
Rift Valley	1164	990
Western & Nyanza	2349	1552
Lesotho		
Lowlands	1483	822
Foothills, ORV, Mountains	1903	1073

separately by region, but jointly for the various age-education groups within each region. Children who were already weaned or whose mothers were no longer amenorrheic or abstaining following that child's birth were coded as 1; the others were coded as 0. In the jargon of failure time models, a designation as code 1 means a "failure," or in this instance, a transition from the initial state (breastfed, amenorrheic, abstaining, nonsusceptible) to a new postpartum state (weaned, menstruating, sexually active, exposed to conception). The data now take the following form:

$$(d_{tz}, n_{tz}, t, z)$$

meaning that there are n_{tz} grouped observations (children) with current age t in completed months and characterized by two covariates (here the mothers' age and education categories). The number having undergone the "failure" or the transition is d_{tz}.

If $F(.\,;z)$ is the distribution of failure time t for observations with covariates z, then d_{tz}/n_{tz} is a raw estimate of $F(t+0.5\,;z)$, that is, the probability that an item with covariates z has "failed" at or before exact age $t+0.5$. $F(.\,;z)$ should be a monotonically increasing sequence in t in the absence of sampling fluctuations. The raw estimates d_{tz}/n_{tz} do not provide such a smoothly increasing set of values. Therefore, a model will be useful only if it provides estimates $\hat{F}(t\,;z)$ of $F(t\,;z)$, such that a monotonically increasing sequence in t is established.

At first, work started with the following set of parametric models:

$$F(t; z) = \Phi^{-1} \left(\theta\,(z).h_o\,(t; \delta, \alpha) + \beta(z) \right) \qquad \text{(eq. 3.1)}$$

where

$h_o\,(.\,;\,\delta,\,\alpha)$ is a monotonically increasing function of t with two parameters δ and α;

$\Phi^{-1}\,(.)$ is a cumulative distribution function depending on two parameters m_1 and m_2;

$\theta(.)$ and $\beta(.)$ are parameter functions of the covariates z (age and education), with $\theta(.) > 0$.

The explicit formulae for h_o and Φ^{-1} are:

$$\begin{aligned} h_o\,(t; \delta, \alpha) &= ((t+\alpha)^\delta - 1)/\delta \qquad \text{for } \delta \neq 0,\ t > -\alpha \\ &= \log\,(t+\alpha) \qquad \text{for } \delta = 0,\ t > -\alpha \end{aligned}$$
(or a nonparametric function—cf. logit model)

$$\Phi^{-1}(w) = \int_{-\infty}^{\omega} f_w(u)\,du$$

in which $f_w\,(.)$ is the probability density function of the generalized exponential F distribution. Equation 3.1 can now be written as:

$$\Phi(F(t; z)) = \theta(z).h_o (t; \delta, \alpha) + \beta(z) \qquad \text{(eq. 3.2)}$$

For fixed parameters m_1, m_2, δ, and α the model is for any fixed covariate z a generalized linear model, with linear parameters $\theta(z)$ and $\beta(z)$. Joint estimation of the parameters $\theta(z)$ and $\beta(z)$ for different subsamples z is possible with the GLIM3 package if the parameter functions $\theta(.)$ and $\beta(.)$ are linear functions of the covariates z, that is, if $\theta(z) = \theta_1 z_1 + \ldots \theta_k z_k$ and $\beta(z) = \beta_1 z_1 + \ldots + \beta_k z_k$. For such parameter functions eq. 3.2 becomes:

$$\Phi(F(t; z)) = \theta. z \, h_o (t; \delta, \alpha) + \beta. z \qquad \text{(eq. 3.3)}$$

So far, eq. 3.3 still covers a broad range of models and the following specifications were tested:

1. The *probit model* in which Φ^{-1} in eq. 3.1 is the cumulative standard normal distribution (Finney, 1952).
2. The *logit model* in which Φ^{-1} is the cumulative logistic distribution function (Ashton, 1972). The logit model has been used by Lesthaeghe and Page (1981) to link observed schedules of breastfeeding and amenorrhea to a common standard schedule.
3. *Exponential gamma models* where Φ^{-1} is a cumulative exponential gamma distribution function, used for instance by Ginsberg (1973) to model amenorrhea; in this instance h_o (t) is simply t.
4. *The Weibull model* where Φ is the complementary log-log transformation and h_o is the logarithm of time (here: of the child's age). This model is a special gamma model, which has the properties of both the proportional hazards and accelerated failure time models if $\theta(z)$ does not depend on z. In fact, Kalbfleish and Prentice (1980) show that it is the only model for which these two classes of models coincide.

These various possibilities were tested out with data for Nairobi, Lesotho lowlands, Abidjan, and Khartoum, both on the breastfeeding and the abstinence schedules. Various parameter values for m_1, m_2 and δ, α were also tried. The conclusions were that:

1. There is no evidence that one particular model is better interregionally or for a particular set of data (i.e., breastfeeding, abstinence).
2. If Φ is the complementary log-log transformation, the results are best when $\delta = 0$, that is, better when $h_o (t) = \log t$, than with $\delta = 0.5$ or 1.0.
3. If $\delta = 0$, the complementary log-log transformation is the most suitable candidate for Φ.
4. At a 5 percent significance level, the Weibull model is not significantly different from the "best" model in most analyses.
5. It was found that $\theta.z$ could be simplified to θ for each region.

As a consequence, we opted systematically for the application of a Weibull model with two parameters:

$$\log \left[-\log \left(1 - F(t; z) \right) \right] = \theta. \log t + \beta. z \qquad \text{(eq. 3.4)}$$

The values of θ and $\beta.z$ differ between regions, so that we have a simple *proportional hazards model* (or accelerated failure time model) to estimate mean durations of the postpartum variables in the 3 × 3 "education-age" matrix for each region separately. Finally, it should be noted that eq. 3.4 should only be used for events that are universal. The weaning of children is such an event, but the ultimate proportion resuming menstruation or sex is not necessarily unity. A modification for nonuniversality can be introduced as

$$\log \left[-\log \left(1 - (F(t; z)/C(z)) \right) \right] = \theta. \log t + \beta. z \qquad \text{(eq. 3.5)}$$

with $C(z)$ being the proportion ultimately experiencing the event. Such $C(z)$ parameters were estimated for seven national data files with z being the age of the mother. The mean durations with $C = 1$ and $C = C(z)$ were compared. It turned out that $C(z)$ could be fairly volatile (and even greater than 1.0), and as a consequence C was uniformly set equal to unity.

The last problem pertains to the selection of an appropriate model capturing the effects of the covariates age and education. Here, use was made of a forward selection procedure leading to an additive or a multiplicative model. The forward selection procedure is described in figure 3.1, and the results are reported by country for breastfeeding, abstinence, and overall nonsusceptibility in table 3.2. The model with interaction between age and education ($E * A$) fits the data better than the additive model in three of the thirty-three regions for breastfeeding and in four of the twenty-nine regions for postpar-

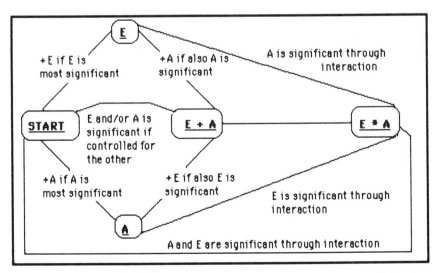

FIGURE 3.1. Forward Selection Procedure of Model Specifying Age and Education Effects on Spacing Variables.

TABLE 3.2   Outcomes of the Forward Selection Procedure in Regions with Respect to the Significance of Covariates Age and Education

	No Covariates Significant	Education only	Age only	Education + Age	Education * Age
Breastfeeding					
Kenya (5 regions)	0	0	1	2	2
Ghana (5 regions)	0	5	0	0	0
Lesotho (2 regions)	0	1	1	0	0
Cameroon (5 regions)	0	4	0	1	0
Benin (3 regions)	2	1	0	0	0
Ivory Coast (5 regions)	0	2	2	0	1
North Sudan (4 regions)	2	0	0	2	0
Senegal (4 regions)	0	2	1	1	0
33 regions	4	15	5	6	3
Abstinence					
Kenya (5 regions)	1	0	2	2	0
Ghana (5 regions)	1	2	1	0	1
Lesotho (2 regions)	1	0	1	0	0
Cameroon (5 regions)	0	3	2	0	0
Benin (3 regions)	2	0	1	0	0
Ivory Coast (5 regions)	0	1	2	0	2
North Sudan (4 regions)	3	0	0	0	1
Senegal (4 regions)			No information		
29 regions	8	6	9	2	4
Nonsusceptible period					
Kenya (5 regions)	1	0	1	2	1
Ghana (5 regions)	1	2	0	1	1
Lesotho (2 regions)	0	1	1	0	0
Cameroon (5 regions)	0	4	1	0	0
Benin (3 regions)	1	0	2	0	0
Ivory Coast (5 regions)	0	1	1	1	2
North Sudan (4 regions)	0	4	0	0	0
Senegal (4 regions)			No information		
29 regions	3	11	7	4	4

NOTE: Significance is tested at 10 percent level and based on the log-likelihood ratio chi-squared statistic.

tum abstinence and overall postpartum nonsusceptibility. Differences in mean durations of these postpartum variables in the nine education-age cells of these regions as estimated from the $(E * A)$ and the $(E + A)$ models respectively were also compared. It turned out that the bulk of differences in excess of 1 month were produced for cells with thirty or fewer observations. In other words, interaction effects tended to be induced by outliers that were often the result of small sample size. As a consequence, we systematically opted for an estimation procedure based on a simple additive model $(E + A)$ in all regions and for dropping information inferred from age or education *marginals* with thirty or fewer observations. This implies that estimates can still be obtained for *cells* with thirty or fewer observations, provided that the surrounding cells contain enough cases and that joint estimation with an additive model is indeed appropriate. The mean duration values of the various postpartum variables are given in Appendix C for the regions and the age-education categories. Note that the information for literate women aged 35+ has been dropped: this subgroup contained too few women in most regions. Finally, the mean durations of postpartum amenorrhea for the Senegalese regions are estimated on the basis of the mean durations of breastfeeding and the Bongaarts equation (1981):

$$\bar{X}amen = 1.753 \exp (0.1396 \ \bar{X}brfd - 0.001872 \ \bar{X}brfd^2) \quad \text{(eq. 3.6)}$$

An alternative, and much simpler, way of estimating the mean durations of the postpartum variables consists of calculating the prevalence-incidence ratios or stationarity means. This is a classic method encountered in numerous epidemiological applications. It is assumed that the phenomenon studied shows no marked trend during the observation period (in this case 3 years) and that the birth stream is constant (stationarity hypothesis). The mean is simply the ratio of the total number of persons observed in the initial state (in this case: still breastfed, mother still amenorrheic, etc.) to the number of persons entering this initial state per unit of time (the monthly number of births). As age-heaping occurs on children's ages that are multiples of 6 months, it is advisable to subtract half the number of births reported for the last month when this is a multiple of 6 (for example, if the last month is 24 or 36) prior to the calculation of the average monthly birth stream. Eelens and Donné (1985) computed such stationarity means for the original regions in the sub-Saharan WFS countries, and it is of interest to compare their results with the Vanderhoeft estimates based on the accelerated failure time model described above. The results of the comparison is presented in Appendix D. As can be seen there, the results of the two estimation procedures match each other very closely. For forty-one regions, differences in excess of 1 month in the duration of breastfeeding were encountered in only five regions; there was only one such case of disagreement out of the thirty-six regions for abstinence and overall nonsusceptibility. Stationarity means are consequently seen to be reliable. They are also easy to calculate when samples contain at least 500 observations (spread, in this case, over a 24-month observation period). When intraregion differentials are used, sample sizes drop, so that the stationarity hypothesis required for the prevalence-incidence ratios is rapidly violated. Instead, information on the temporal pattern of the postpartum variables must be borrowed from a larger population (for example, the entire region) or from a standard time schedule. In other words, a baseline hazard function had to be imposed on the age-education subgroups within a region, and the use of the stationarity means, which could not accomodate such an operation, had to be dropped.

The estimates of contraceptive use-efficiency were obtained for the same age-education groups within the thirty-three regions for currently married women only. The estimates are proportions of current users weighted by a fixed schedule of method efficiency. Inaccuracy with respect to contraceptive effectiveness is not a major source of error in estimating overall contraceptive use-effectiveness: current use in sub-Saharan Africa covers rarely more than 20 percent of currently married women. More significant for the results was the decision to eliminate abstinence from the list of contraceptive methods. This was done as a result of the very substantial overlap with *postpartum* abstinence. In most countries and in most translations of the questionnaire, the distinction between postpartum and other periods of abstinence was sufficiently clear, resulting in few mentions of abstinence as a current contraceptive method, but in some instances totally unrealistic figures of contraceptive use resulted from confusion with the postpartum taboo. This was particularly so for all the questionnaires in Benin and for those administered to the Meru-Embu ethnic group in Kenya.

The efficiency weighted percentages of current use among currently married women are also given in Appendix C. Estimates for literate women above age 35 are again omitted owing to the small sample sizes in many regions.

THE COMPONENTS OF THE OVERALL POSTPARTUM NONSUSCEPTIBLE PERIOD (NSP)

For any woman, the period of postpartum nonsusceptibility is simply the longest duration of either her period of lactational amenorrhea or her period of postpartum abstinence. For a population, the average duration of postpartum nonsusceptibility is *not* equal to the longest of either the mean duration of amenorrhea or the mean for abstinence, but larger than both. If in a given population most women have abstinence periods exceeding those of amenorrhea, the mean duration of abstinence would obviously be longer than the mean for amenorrhea. Yet, as soon as there is at least one woman for whom amenorrhea exceeds abstinence, the mean duration of abstinence would be an underestimate of the mean duration of postpartum nonsusceptibility: the former fails to take account of the extra nonsusceptibility period for that woman. The argument obviously holds in situations where mean amenorrhea durations exceed abstinence durations. Hence,

$$\bar{X}nsp = (\bar{X}amen \text{ or } \bar{X}abst) + E$$

where $(\bar{X}amen \text{ or } \bar{X}abst)$ is the longest of the two means and E an extra bonus value of nonsusceptibility. A simple way of establishing the *net* contribution of postpartum abstinence to postpartum nonsusceptibility in a population consists of relating the difference between the mean duration of the overall nonsusceptible period (calculated from the individual's experience) and the mean duration of lactational amenorrhea (i.e., $Xnsp - \bar{X}amen$) to the difference between the mean duration of postpartum abstinence and that of lactational amenorrhea (i.e., $\bar{X}abst - \bar{X}amen$). The former difference measures the part of the overall nonsusceptible period that is not due to lactational amenorrhea and must therefore be the *net* contribution of postpartum abstinence (that is, the "abstinence bonus"). The relationship between $(\bar{X}nsp - \bar{X}amen)$ and $(\bar{X}abst - \bar{X}amen)$ has been plotted in figure 3.2. Panel 1 of this figure contains the observations computed from the stationarity means for the original forty-seven regions in the WFS countries used so far (Eelens and Donné, 1985). Panel 2 contains the values based on the Vanderhoeft accelerated failure time model (AFT) for twenty-eight grouped regions. Country codes are also shown in figure 3.2 so that one can readily see where the net contribution of postpartum abstinence to overall nonsusceptibility is considerable and where it is negligible. Several curves were fitted through these two data sets and the results are shown in table 3.3. It emerges that:

1. The function of the form $Y = A \exp (\lambda X + \gamma X^2)$ produces the best fit in both instances.
2. The parameter estimates are hardly different depending on the use of the stationarity means or the AFT-means.

The net abstinence bonus can hence be computed from:

$$(\bar{X}nsp - \bar{X}amen) = 2.79 \exp (0.1684(\bar{X}abst - \bar{X}amen) \\ - 0.003157 (\bar{X}abst - \bar{X}amen)^2) \qquad \text{(eq. 3.7)}$$

This function implies that the abstinence bonus is of the order of 2.8 months when mean durations of abstinence and amenorrhea are identical, irrespective of their length. The net abstinence bonus drops to less than 1 month if average lactational amenorrhea exceeds the average duration of postpartum abstinence by 6 months (even if the postpartum taboo would still be of the order of, say, 12 months!). Populations with little or no abstinence bonus are typically those of Northern Sudan, Kenya, and most of Ghana. At the other end, the bonus increases to 6–12 months in several West African populations

$$Y=2.7899*EXP(.1684*X-.003157*X*X)$$

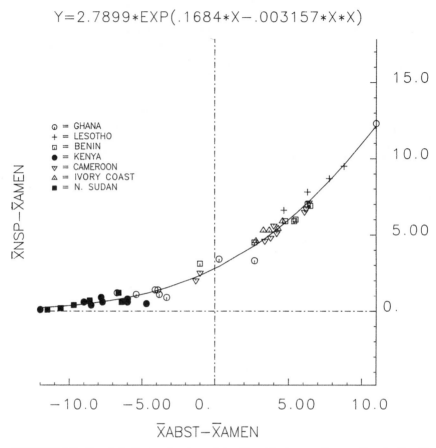

FIGURE 3.2. Panel 1: Determination of the Net Abstinence Bonus, Results for 47 Regions Using Stationarity Means

located in the Ivory Coast, Northern Ghana, Benin, Cameroon, and also in Lesotho.

Table 3.3 and panel 3 of figure 3.2 also show the results for the 224 age-education groups. If the mean durations for the three postpartum variables are sufficiently well estimated by the AFT-model described in the previous section, the differences between these means should be reliable as well and the link between $(\bar{X}nsp - \bar{X}amen)$ and $(\bar{X}abst - \bar{X}amen)$ should follow the specification of eq. 3.7. This holds true to a remarkable extent, which is reassuring for all future work that will be based on these age-education specific measures.

Finally, data on lactational amenorrhea and postpartum abstinence were

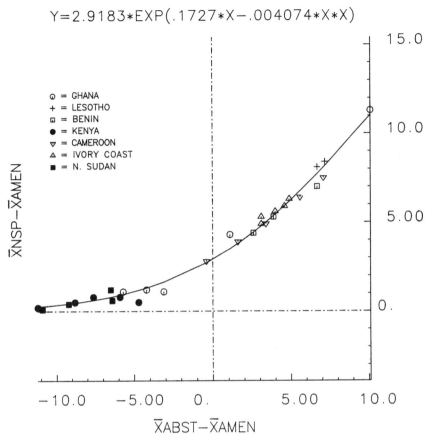

$$Y=2.9183*EXP(.1727*X-.004074*X*X)$$

FIGURE 3.2. Panel 2: Determination of the Net Abstinence Bonus, Results for 28 Regions Using AFT Means

not collected in the Senegalese survey. However, lactational amenorrhea averages could be inferred from the breastfeeding data through the Bongaarts equation (see eq. 3.6). Postpartum abstinence information is, fortunately, available from other surveys conducted in Western and Central Senegal. Their results are reported in table 3.4 and indicate that abstinence durations lie between the Koranic prescription of 40 days and 6 months. Since average durations of lactational amenorrhea in the WFS are of the order of 13 to 17 months, the difference ($\bar{X}abst - \bar{X}amen$) is more extreme than −7.0 months, so that the abstinence bonus is at most 1 month. The average lengths of overall nonsusceptibility in the Senegalese regions were therefore taken as the Bongaarts estimate of lactational amenorrhea plus 1 month.

TABLE 3.3   Estimation of the Abstinence Bonus $(\bar{X}nsp\text{-}\bar{X}amen)$ on the Basis of the Relative Lengths of Abstinence and Lactational Amenorrhea $(\bar{X}abst\text{-}\bar{X}amen)$

Function Fitted	Results with Stationarity Means (47 Regions)	Results with AFT Means (28 Grouped Regions)	Results with AFT Means (224 Age-Education Groups in Regions)
$Y = A + BX + CX^2$	$A = 2.854$ $B = 0.5108$ $C = 0.02658$ Scaled Deviance $= 7.35$ DF $= 45$	$A = 2.997$ $B = 0.5255$ $C = 0.02580$ Scaled Deviance $= 3.18$ DF $= 26$	$A = 3.029$ $B = 0.5098$ $C = 0.02280$ Scaled Deviance $= 95.9$ DF $= 222$
$Y = A.e^{\lambda X}$	$A = 2.8634$ $\lambda = 0.1394$ Scaled Deviance $= 10.92$ DF $= 46$	$A = 2.9654$ $\lambda = 0.1389$ Scaled Deviance $= 7.01$ DF $= 27$	$A = 2.9654$ $\lambda = 0.1305$ Scaled Deviance $= 151.6$ DF $= 223$
$Y = A \exp (\lambda X + \gamma X^2)$	$A = 2.7899$ $\lambda = 0.1684$ $\gamma = -.003157$ Scaled Deviance $= 6.54$ DF $= 45$	$A = 2.9183$ $\lambda = 0.1727$ $\gamma = -.004074$ Scaled Deviance $= 3.33$ DF $= 26$	$A = 2.8950$ $\lambda = 0.1759$ $\gamma = -.004810$ Scaled Deviance $= 96.4$ DF $= 222$

TABLE 3.4   Estimated Mean Durations of Postpartum Abstinence in Senegal; Western and Central Regions

Area of Ethnic Group	Mean Duration Postpartum Abstinence
Dakar-Pikine, 1968–1969	2.8 months
Khombole, 1968–1969	2.4
Thienaba, 1968–1969	2.3
Saloum region, 1963–1968	
• Wolof	2.3
• Fulani	4.6
• Serer	2.3
• Tukulor	5.8
Sine-Saloum region, 1982	5.0
• Wolof	4.2
• Serer	5.2
• Fulani	6.3

SOURCE: Delaine, 1976; Cantrelle and Ferry, 1979; Cantrelle et al., 1981; Anderson et al., 1984.

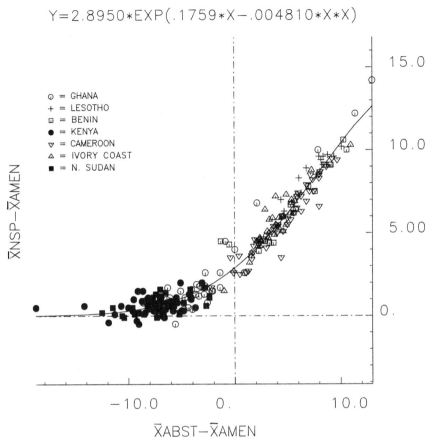

FIGURE 3.2. Panel 3: Determination of the Net Abstinence Bonus, Results for 224 Age-Education Groups in Regions Using AFT Means

EFFECTS OF SOCIOECONOMIC AND CULTURAL VARIABLES ON REGIONAL PATTERNS OF CHILD-SPACING FOR DIFFERENT AGE AND EDUCATION SUBGROUPS

The present analysis follows to some extent the analysis performed in chapter 2 for ethnic groups. A major difference stems from the fact that some aspects of social organization can no longer be quantified (for example, diverging devolution of property and traditional caste/class stratification) as regions usually contain several ethnic groups. This loss of information is alleviated by the finding in chapter 2 that diverging devolution of property and the existence of a traditional caste/class stratification mainly affected the nuptiality and premarital fertility variables rather than the child-spacing ones.

An advantage of the regional over the ethnic data file is that some controls for individual characteristics are possible in the former (that is, control for age-education group membership).
The independent variables retained in the present analyses are:

1. An index at the regional level of socioeconomic development, which is the principle component extracted from the following four indicators:
   • percentage of all women 15–49 illiterate
   • the average duration of female schooling (all women 15–49)
   • the percentage of husbands of women 15–49 employed in clerical or professional jobs or employers of wage labor
   • the percentage of husbands of women 15–49 who are self-employed without wage labor as farmers, traders, or artisans.

   The results of the principle component analysis are displayed in table 3.5, which shows that 73 percent of the common variance is covered by the first component. It measures essentially the expansion of female schooling and the growth of a wage sector in the economy (variable: DEV.SCORE). The values of the variables used for the computation of this principle component are given in Appendix E.
2. The percentages of females 15–49 in each region reporting themselves as Muslim or as followers of traditional religions (variables ISLAM and TRAD.RELIG.)
3. The percentage of women 15–49 in each region engaged in trade (variable: TRADE). Note that the caveats formulated in chapter 2 with respect to this variable are still valid.

TABLE 3.5   Construction of Socioeconomic Development Score for 33 Regions via Principle Component Analysis; WFS Countries

Indicator	$\bar{X}$	σ	Correlation with Principle Component
Percent women illiterate	62.4	25.5	−.92
Average duration of schooling for women	2.4	1.8	+.95
Percent husbands in clerical, professional jobs or employers of wage-earning employees	20.2	10.7	+.60
Percent husbands as self-employed farmers, artisans, or traders (without wage-earning employees)	44.5	22.3	−.90
Percent of common variance explained by principle component			72.8 percent

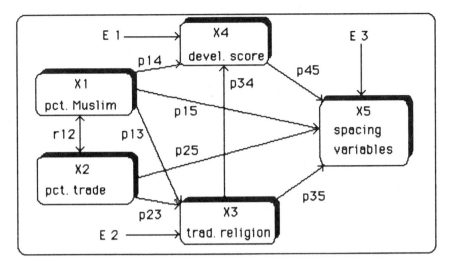

$$r12 = -0.23 \quad p13 = -0.19 \quad p14 = -0.67 \quad E\ 1 = 0.70$$
$$p23 = +0.49 \quad p34 = -0.52 \quad E\ 2 = 0.72$$

FIGURE 3.3. Path Model Linking Regional Characteristics to Spacing Variables

The relationships between these independent variables have been given a causal structure (see figure 3.3). The causal ordering starts with the percentage of Muslims and the percentage of women engaged in trade, that is, two historically rooted variables of major cultural and organizational significance. The percentage following traditional religions is seen as dependent on these two, despite the fact that adherence to traditional religion constitutes a "primal" condition. The reason for its location further down the causal ordering is that traditional religions have been under such severe pressure from both Islam and Christianity and that, at least at present, they can be thought of as a residue. Resistance of traditional religion to the non-African religions has been supported by the prior existence of more complex forms of social organization and the functions fulfilled by traditional religion with respect to pattern maintenance of the social structures. In the generally more complex societies of West Africa, the presence of female secret societies, female title-taking societies and work parties, female mutual assistance associations, and professional organizations of market women and traders (not to mention overlapping membership) testify to the strength and degree of interdependence of traditional religion and economy. In the path diagram of figure 3.3 the tradition of economic self-reliance for women, captured by the proxy variable "women in trade" is seen as one of the elements that have sustained the survival of traditional religion.

The socioeconomic development score is made dependent on the two religion variables, largely because both Islam and traditional religion, in contrast to Christianity, have not been associated with the development of female education. Of course, the level of socioeconomic development and most notably the growth of a modern wage economy are also contingent on numerous other factors, but these exert their influence through an unspecified (or latent) variable E_1. Note, furthermore, that there is no direct influence from the percentage of women in trade on the regional development score. This link was dropped on the basis of negligible zero order and beta coefficients. As a result, the model is over-identified.

With the present model the effect of Islam can be broken down into:

1. A direct effect p_{15} on the spacing variable considered
2. An indirect effect via traditional religion, that is, $p_{13}.\ p_{35}$
3. An indirect effect via traditional religion and development score, that is, $p_{23}.\ p_{34}.\ p_{45}$.

Also the effect of women in trade consists of three components:

1. The direct effect p_{25}
2. The indirect effect via traditional religion $p_{23}.\ p_{35}$
3. The indirect effect via traditional religion and development score, that is, $p_{23}.\ p_{34}.\ p_{45}$.

Traditional religion affects the spacing variables through its direct effect p_{35} and via its indirect effect on development scores, that is, $p_{34}.\ p_{45}$. The level of socioeconomic development of a region has a direct effect only, namely p_{45}.

All of these effects are measured through path coefficients that are simply the standardized regression (or beta) coefficients in a set of multiple regressions. The effect of the latent variables is also the classic $\sqrt{1 - R^2}$ in which R is the multiple regression coefficient. The causal structure of figure 3.3 has been quantified with the regional values of breastfeeding, postpartum abstinence, overall postpartum nonsusceptibility, and contraceptive use-effectiveness as the ultimate dependent variables. Moreover, this is done for regional values calculated on the basis of information for different subgroups of women (once for all women, once for illiterate women in each of the three age groups, once for women with 1–4 years of schooling in the two youngest age groups, and once for women with 5+ years of schooling, also aged below 35). This yields a total of eight quantified models for each of the four spacing variables.

In all thirty-two models the path coefficients connecting the background variables (that is, X_1 through X_4) are estimated with the full sample of thirty-three regions. Path coefficients involving direct effects leading to the spacing variable (that is, X_5) may be estimated on a smaller sample of regions as some lack the more educated subgroups. The information is presented in a series of tables, all containing the measurement of the direct effect, the combined indirect effects, and the total effect (that is, direct + all indirect effects).

The latter is furthermore compared to the zero-order correlation coefficient between each predictor and the ultimate dependent variable. The total effect should yield a good approximation of the zero-order coefficient, and any discrepancy between them stems from the fact that the model is over-identified and that direct effects may be estimated on the basis of a reduced sample. On the whole, however, the correspondence between total effects and zero-order coefficients is convincing, both in terms of sign and orders of magnitude.

The results for regional variation in breastfeeding are reported in table 3.6. The following conclusions can be drawn:

1. For all women taken together and for illiterate women irrespective of age, traditional religion has a strong positive effect on the regional breastfeeding duration. This positive effect operates both directly and indirectly (that is, via the feature that regions with strong adherence to traditional religion have less female education and hence a lower socioeconomic development score). This indirect effect is positive because lower levels of socioeconomic development produce a moderate effect in the direction of longer breastfeeding.

2. The percentage Islam has a small negative direct effect on the breastfeeding average for the region, but this direct effect is almost entirely neutralized by the positive indirect effect. Islamized regions also have lower than average levels of female schooling, a feature that supports longer lactation.

3. A similar trade off between direct and indirect effects occurs for the percentage of women in trade. The direct effect is negative, but the indirect effect via traditional religion is positive and usually stronger. The overall effect of female self-reliance is therefore often positive, but modest.

4. Considering the four predictors together, only traditional religion, with an overall positive effect, and the socioeconomic development score, with a negative effect, stand out as major determinants of regional variation in breastfeeding among illiterate women of all ages.

5. However, as soon as the regional average durations of lactation are considered for the better educated subgroups, the positive effect of traditional religion and the negative effect of socioeconomic development are weakened. Also, the multiple correlation coefficients decrease. On the other hand, the effect of an Islamic environment is strengthened, in the sense that a negative effect on breastfeeding is produced. Educated women in Islamic societies are a strongly selected group (probably more strongly selected than their counterparts in non-Islamic societies with overall higher levels of female education), which contributes regional values for durations of breastfeeding that are shorter than the regional values calculated for identical education-age groups elsewhere.

TABLE 3.6 Quantification of Path Model Explaining Regional Variation in Breastfeeding

	Direct Effect	All Indirect Effects	Total Effect	Zero-Order Correlation
All Women: $\bar{X}$ = 19.6 mos. $\quad \sigma$ = 3.5 mos. $\quad R$ = .79 $\quad$ E3 = .61 $\quad$ N = 33				
% Muslim	+.00	+.02	+.02	−.00
% Traditional Religion	+.75	+.15	+.90	+.67
% Women in Trade	−.30	+.44	+.14	+.08
Development Score	−.28	—	−.28	−.54
Illiterate Women 35–49: $\bar{X}$ = 21.5 $\quad \sigma$ = 3.7 $\quad R$ = .74 $\quad$ E3 = .67 $\quad$ N = 32				
% Muslim	−.05	+.04	−.01	−.02
% Traditional Religion	+.66	+.16	+.82	+.60
% Women in Trade	−.32	+.40	+.08	+.03
Development Score	−.30	—	−.30	−.51
Illiterate Women 25–34: $\bar{X}$ = 20.2 $\quad \sigma$ = 3.2 $\quad R$ = .79 $\quad$ E3 = .61 $\quad$ N = 32				
% Muslim	−.21	+.18	−.03	−.07
% Traditional Religion	+.55	+.25	+.80	+.65
% Women in Trade	−.22	+.39	+.17	+.09
Development Score	−.49	—	−.49	−.57
Illiterate Women 15–24: $\bar{X}$ = 20.6 $\quad \sigma$ = 3.9 $\quad R$ = .75 $\quad$ E3 = .66 $\quad$ N = 32				
% Muslim	−.22	+.12	−.10	−.11
% Traditional Religion	+.57	+.21	+.78	+.61
% Women in Trade	−.29	+.38	+.09	+.04
Development Score	−.41	—	−.41	−.50
Women 1–4 Yrs of Schooling, 25–34: $\bar{X}$ = 18.4 $\quad \sigma$ = 2.3 $\quad R$ = .53 $\quad$ E3 = .85 $\quad$ N = 27				
% Muslim	−.35	−.05	−.40	−.35
% Traditional Religion	+.40	+.02	+.42	+.29
% Women in Trade	−.40	+.21	−.19	−.11
Development Score	−.04	—	−.04	−.01
Women 1–4 Yrs of Schooling, 15–24: $\bar{X}$ = 18.6 $\quad \sigma$ = 2.6 $\quad R$ = .42 $\quad$ E3 = .91 $\quad$ N = 27				
% Muslim	−.19	+.01	−.18	−.17
% Traditional Religion	+.36	+.07	+.43	+.32
% Women in Trade	−.26	+.21	−.05	−.03
Development Score	−.13	—	−.13	−.17
Women 5+ Yrs of Schooling, 25–34: $\bar{X}$ = 15.9 $\quad \sigma$ = 2.4 $\quad R$ = .55 $\quad$ E3 = .83 $\quad$ N = 23				
% Muslim	−.21	−.21	−.42	−.37
% Traditional Religion	+.55	−.10	+.45	+.31
% Women in Trade	−.45	+.22	−.23	−.09
Development Score	+.19	—	+.19	+.09
Women 5+ Yrs of Schooling, 15–24: $\bar{X}$ = 16.3 $\quad \sigma$ = 2.4 $\quad R$ = .61 $\quad$ E3 = .79 $\quad$ N = 23				
% Muslim	−.30	−.16	−.46	−.39
% Traditional Religion	+.53	−.06	+.47	+.29
% Women in Trade	−.53	+.23	−.30	−.17
Development Score	+.11	—	+.11	+.06

The results for postpartum abstinence are summarized in table 3.7. Firstly, regional variation is much larger for durations of the postpartum taboo than for the durations of lactation: standard deviations for abstinence are of the order of 6 to 8 months as compared to 2 to 4 months for breastfeeding. The conclusions with respect to the predictors are:

1. The level of socioeconomic development in the regions has a negative effect on abstinence, irrespective of the age-education subgroup considered. This result is in line with findings within ethnic clusters in the previous chapter. However, the impact of the regional level of development weakens when subgroups with 5+ years of schooling are considered.

2. Equally consistent is that adherence to traditional religion as a regional characteristic is positively associated with a more intact postpartum taboo. In fact, traditional religion has a marked positive direct effect and on top of this also a clearly positive indirect effect for all age-education groups (operating via lower socioeconomic development and lower female education). This is in line with the across-ethnic cluster comparison in chapter 2.

3. In contrast with the results for breastfeeding, the Islamic nature of the region contributes substantially to the lowering of postpartum abstinence durations. The negative direct effect is no longer neutralized by a positive indirect effect (as was found for breastfeeding) when abstinence is considered. This holds again for all age-education groups. Hence, the eroding effect of Islam on the long postpartum taboo is no longer kept in check by lower female education as was still true for lactation.

4. The variable concerning women in trade has a small positive direct effect on abstinence plus a larger positive indirect effect (resulting from the association with traditional religion). The net outcome is an overall positive effect, which, in absolute value, is of a comparable magnitude of those of Islam or socioeconomic development score. This positive effect weakens, however, for the subgroups with 5+ years of schooling as a result of a change in sign of the direct effect.

5. On the whole, the most striking fact for these analyses with postpartum abstinence is that the Islamic character of the region now assumes a major role that is diametrically opposed to that of traditional religion. Also noteworthy is the confirmation of the weakened effect of the local development level on the regional pattern of postpartum abstinence among the better educated.

When lactational amenorrhea (with results that closely resemble those for breastfeeding) and postpartum abstinence are combined into overall postpartum nonsusceptibility, many of the above observations can be maintained

TABLE 3.7   Quantification of Path Model Explaining Regional Variation in
Postpartum Abstinence

	Direct Effect	All Indirect Effects	Total Effect	Zero-Order Correlation
All Women: X̄ = 12.1 σ = 7.2 R = .80 E3 = .60 N = 29				
% Muslim	−.46	+.25	−.21	−.31
% Traditional Religion	+.34	+.28	+.62	+.71
% Women in Trade	+.11	+.31	+.42	+.36
Development Score	−.54	—	−.54	−.40
Illiterate Women 35+: X̄ = 14.1 σ = 8.3 R = .80 E3 = .60 N = 28				
% Muslim	−.52	+.31	−.21	−.31
% Traditional Religion	+.27	+.32	+.59	+.68
% Women in Trade	+.13	+.28	+.41	+.35
Development Score	−.62	—	−.62	−.42
Illiterate Women 25–34: X̄ = 12.3 σ = 7.3 R = .79 E3 = .61 N = 28				
% Muslim	−.50	+.30	−.20	−.31
% Traditional Religion	+.23	+.31	+.54	+.67
% Women in Trade	+.21	+.26	+.47	+.40
Development Score	−.60	—	−.60	−.39
Illiterate Women 15–24: X̄ = 12.3 σ = 7.4 R = .74 E3 = .67 N = 28				
% Muslim	−.49	+.28	−.21	−.31
% Traditional Religion	+.19	+.29	+.48	+.63
% Women in Trade	+.22	+.23	+.45	+.39
Development Score	−.56	—	−.56	−.35
Women with 1–4 Yrs of Schooling, 25–34: X̄ = 10.3 σ = 6.7 R = .71 E3 = .72 N = 24				
% Muslim	−.59	+.26	−.33	−.41
% Traditional Religion	+.15	+.26	+.41	+.57
% Women in Trade	+.15	+.20	+.35	+.33
Development Score	−.50	—	−.50	−.24
Women with 1–4 Yrs of Schooling, 15–24: X̄ = 10.6 σ = 7.1 R = .66 E3 = .75 N = 24				
% Muslim	−.52	+.21	−.31	−.39
% Traditional Religion	+.17	+.22	+.39	+.55
% Women in Trade	+.17	+.19	+.36	+.35
Development Score	−.42	—	−.42	−.20
Women with 5+ Yrs of Schooling, 25–34: X̄ = 8.9 σ = 5.8 R = .60 E3 = .80 N = 23				
% Muslim	−.42	+.03	−.39	−.41
% Traditional Religion	+.38	+.09	+.47	+.50
% Women in Trade	−.10	+.24	+.14	+.18
Development Score	−.18	—	−.18	−.09
Women with 5+ Yrs of Schooling, 15–24: X̄ = 9.0 σ = 5.8 R = .58 E3 = .81 N = 23				
% Muslim	−.44	+.03	−.41	−.44
% Traditional Religion	+.33	+.08	+.41	+.46
% Women in Trade	−.10	+.20	+.10	+.17
Development Score	−.16	—	−.16	−.04

TABLE 3.8 Quantification of Path Model Explaining Regional Variation in Length of the Overall Postpartum Nonsusceptible Period

	Direct Effect	All Indirect Effects	Total Effect	Zero-Order Correlation
All Women: $\bar{X} = 16.2$ $\sigma = 4.3$ $R = .79$ $E3 = .61$ $N = 33$				
% Muslim	−.33	+.16	−.17	−.21
% Traditional Religion	+.50	+.24	+.74	+.70
% Women in Trade	−.08	+.37	+.29	+.23
Development Score	−.47	—	−.47	−.47
Illiterate Women 35–49: $\bar{X} = 18.5$ $\sigma = 5.3$ $R = .79$ $E3 = .61$ $N = 32$				
% Muslim	−.44	+.17	−.27	−.32
% Traditional Religion	+.45	+.24	+.69	+.70
% Women in Trade	−.06	+.34	+.28	+.25
Development Score	−.46	—	−.46	−.38
Illiterate Women 25–34: $\bar{X} = 16.6$ $\sigma = 4.0$ $R = .77$ $E3 = .64$ $N = 32$				
% Muslim	−.33	+.23	−.10	−.17
% Traditional Religion	+.43	+.28	+.71	+.66
% Women in Trade	−.08	+.35	+.27	+.19
Development Score	−.53	—	−.53	−.51
Illiterate Women 15–24: $\bar{X} = 16.3$ $\sigma = 4.5$ $R = .70$ $E3 = .71$ $N = 32$				
% Muslim	−.34	+.19	−.15	−.20
% Traditional Religion	+.36	+.24	+.60	+.61
% Women in Trade	+.01	+.30	+.31	+.25
Development Score	−.47	—	−.47	−.41
Women with 1–4 Yrs of Schooling, 25–34: $\bar{X} = 14.09$ $\sigma = 3.4$ $R = .71$ $E3 = .70$ N = 27				
% Muslim	−.65	+.21	−.44	−.49
% Traditional Religion	+.19	+.23	+.42	+.54
% Women in Trade	+.04	+.20	+.24	+.26
Development Score	−.44	—	−.44	−.16
Women with 1–4 Yrs of Schooling, 15–24: $\bar{X} = 14.4$ $\sigma = 3.9$ $R = .60$ $E3 = .80$ N = 27				
% Muslim	−.51	+.18	−.33	−.38
% Traditional Religion	+.14	+.20	+.34	+.48
% Women in Trade	+.11	+.17	+.28	+.28
Development Score	−.38	—	−.38	−.15
Women with 5+ Yrs of Schooling, 25–34: $\bar{X} = 12.8$ $\sigma = 3.5$ $R = .69$ $E3 = .72$ N = 23				
% Muslim	−.66	+.13	−.53	−.53
% Traditional Religion	+.25	+.17	+.42	+.46
% Women in Trade	−.16	+.20	+.04	+.10
Development Score	−.32	—	−.32	−.07
Women with 5+ Yrs of Schooling, 15–24: $\bar{X} = 12.3$ $\sigma = 4.0$ $R = .65$ $E3 = .76$ N-23				
% Muslim	−.58	+.07	−.51	−.52
% Traditional Religion	+.29	+.12	+.41	+.47
% Women in Trade	−.12	+.20	+.08	+.16
Development Score	−.23	—	−.23	−.03

(see table 3.8). As the results for the nonsusceptible period will be contrasted with those for contraceptive use-effectiveness, we have also plotted the effects in figure 3.4 for the age group 25–34. These results can be taken as typical for the other age groups as well. The conclusions with respect to postpartum nonsusceptibility are:

1. The impact of the religions remains important. Regions with considerable adherence to traditional religions have positive direct and positive

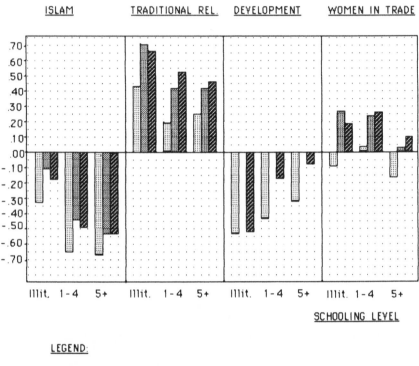

FIGURE 3.4. Direct and Total Effects of Regional Characteristics on the Length of the Postpartum Nonsusceptible Period for Women Aged 25–34 with Various Levels of Education

indirect effects (again via lower female schooling). The impact of traditional religion as a local feature is strongest for illiterate women and diminishes slightly when educated subgroups are considered (see figure 3.4). The impact of Islam is negative, despite positive indirect effects operating via lower education. The Islamic environment has furthermore a stronger negative impact on the length of postpartum nonsusceptibility when better educated women considered (see figure 3.4). In all of this, the results obtained for postpartum abstinence have left a dominant trace.

2. The impact of the regional level of development is negative throughout, but its size strongly diminishes in better educated subgroups.

3. The effect of women in trade on regional levels of postpartum nonsusceptibility is positive but small. This stems from the finding that its direct effects on breastfeeding and on abstinence respectively went in opposite directions for most age-education subgroups.

A similar analysis is also performed for contraceptive use-effectiveness. The results are presented in table 3.9 and in figure 3.5 for the age group 25–34 only. The main features are:

1. By far the largest influence on contraceptive use-effectiveness for all age-education subgroups is that exerted by the socioeconomic development score of the region (see figure 3.5). As expected, the effect is positive.

2. The effect of the two religious denominations is much smaller, and total effects are often negative. This result is not produced so much by the direct effect (that of Islam is positive in most instances) as by the indirect impact operating through lower female education and lower development scores. These indirect effects are negative throughout and either neutralize a positive direct effect or reinforce a small negative one.

3. The effect of women in trade is equally modest and signs are rather volatile. Zero-order correlations are close to zero or have a slight tendency to being positive.

Before concluding this section, attention should again be directed to the declining impact of the regions' levels of socioeconomic development on the three postpartum variables when considering the more educated subgroups. This phenomenon is rather striking as can be seen from the zero-order correlations reported in table 3.10. There is, however, the possibility that it is produced by the selection procedure in which the least developed regions (often Islamized or located in Benin) are eliminated from the analysis for subgroups with more education, simply because not enough educated women could be found in such regions. The phenomenon is all the

TABLE 3.9   Quantification of Path Model Explaining Regional Variation in Contraceptive Use-Effectiveness (Current Use, Currently Married Women)

	Direct Effect	All Indirect Effects	Total Effect	Zero-Order Correlation
All Women: $\bar{X} = 3.8\%$ $\sigma = 3.7\%$ $R = 0.80$ $E3 = 0.60$ $N = 33$				
% Muslim	+.30	−.60	−.30	−.25
% Traditional Religion	+.21	−.51	−.30	−.25
% Women in Trade	−.11	−.15	−.26	+.01
Development Score	+.99	—	+.99	+.76
Illiterate Women 35–49: $\bar{X} = 2.0$ $\sigma = 2.5$ $R = .70$ $E3 = .71$ $N = 33$				
% Muslim	+.10	−.52	−.42	−.37
% Traditional Religion	+.27	−.43	−.16	−.11
% Women in Trade	−.17	−.08	−.25	+.02
Development Score	+.82	—	+.82	+.67
Illiterate Women 25–34: $\bar{X} = 1.9$ $\sigma = 1.9$ $R = .47$ $E3 = .88$ $N = 33$				
% Muslim	+.09	−.29	−.20	−.22
% Traditional Religion	+.06	−.25	−.19	−.03
% Women in Trade	+.16	+.15	+.31	+.21
Development Score	+.49	—	+.49	+.43
Illiterate Women 15–24: $\bar{X} = 0.9$ $\sigma = 1.4$ $R = .39$ $E3 = .92$ $N = 33$				
% Muslim	+.00	−.28	−.28	−.24
% Traditional Religion	+.17	−.22	−.05	−.03
% Women in Trade	−.12	−.03	−.15	−.00
Development Score	+.43	—	+.43	+.37
Women with 1–4 Yrs of Schooling, 25–34: $\bar{X} = 6.4$ $\sigma = 8.0$ $R = .56$ $E3 = .82$ $N = 33$				
% Muslim	+.57	−.41	+.16	+.18
% Traditional Religion	+.11	−.36	−.25	−.27
% Women in Trade	−.00	−.13	−.13	−.02
Development Score	+.69	—	+.69	+.36
Women with 1–4 Yrs of Schooling, 15–24: $\bar{X} = 2.9$ $\sigma = 3.8$ $R = .45$ $E3 = .89$ $N = 33$				
% Muslim	+.48	−.39	+.09	+.12
% Traditional Religion	+.22	−.32	−.10	−.16
% Women in Trade	−.09	−.05	−.14	−.04
Development Score	+.61	—	+.61	+.29
Women with 5+ Yrs of Schooling, 25–34: $\bar{X} = 10.7$ $\sigma = 6.9$ $R = .53$ $E3 = .84$ $N = 23$				
% Muslim	+.28	−.21	+.07	+.04
% Traditional Religion	−.19	−.23	−.42	−.23
% Women in Trade	+.33	−.20	+.13	+.19
Development Score	+.44	—	+.44	+.37
Women with 5+ Yrs of Schooling, 15–24: $\bar{X} = 4.2$ $\sigma = 3.0$ $R = .69$ $E3 = .72$ $N = 25$				
% Muslim	−.08	−.18	−.26	−.29
% Traditional Religion	−.36	−.23	−.59	−.27
% Women in Trade	+.37	−.29	+.08	+.23
Development Score	+.44	—	+.44	+.62

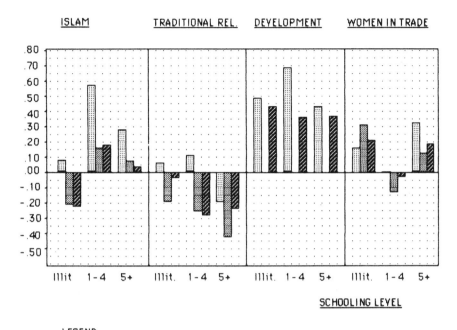

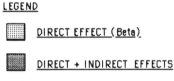

FIGURE 3.5. Direct and Total Effects of Regional Characteristics on the Percentage Use-Effectiveness of Contraception for Women Aged 25–34 with Various Levels of Education

more striking, because it does not appear to exist for contraceptive use-effectiveness: the correlation for women with 5+ years of education is not lower than for the other groups, despite the dropping out of eight and ten regions respectively. The way to find out whether sample size reduction is responsible for the change in impact of regional development scores consists of running the correlations again for the subset of regions that have full information for all age-education subgroups. The results of this operation are shown in table 3.11. The outcome is that the declining sequence in the correlation coefficients with increasing individual schooling, as shown in table

TABLE 3.10 Zero-Order Correlations between Development Score and the Spacing Variables for the Age-Education Subgroups (N = Number of Regions Involved)

Age-Education Subgroup	With Breast-feeding		With Absti-nence*		With Non-suscep-tible Period		With Contra-ception	
	r	N	r	N	r	N	r	N
Illiterate, 15–24	−.50	32	−.35	28	−.41	32	+.37	33
Illiterate, 25–34	−.57	32	−.39	28	−.50	32	+.43	33
Illiterate, 35+	−.51	32	−.42	28	−.38	32	+.67	33
1–4 yrs, 15–24	−.17	27	−.20	24	−.15	27	+.29	33
1–4 yrs, 25–34	−.01	27	−.24	24	−.16	27	+.36	33
5+ yrs, 15–24	+.06	23	−.04	23	−.03	23	+.62	25
5+ yrs, 25–34	+.10	23	−.09	23	−.07	23	+.37	23
All Women	−.54	33	−.40	29	−.47	33	+.76	33

*No data for Senegalese regions.

TABLE 3.11 Zero-Order Correlations between Development Score and the Spacing Variables for Regions that have Information for all Age-Education Subgroups

Age-Education Subgroup	With Breast-feeding	With Absti-nence*	With Non-suscep-tible Period	With Contra-ception
	N = 19	N = 19	N = 19	N = 23
Illiterate, 15–24	−.40	−.14	−.33	+.40
Illiterate, 25–34	−.39	−.17	−.42	+.52
Illiterate, 35+	−.26	−.22	−.32	+.73
1–4 yrs, 15–24	−.26	−.16	−.19	+.63
1–4 yrs, 25–34	−.19	−.20	−.27	+.54
5+ yrs, 15–24	−.17	−.17	−.18	+.58
5+ yrs, 25–34	−.08	−.19	−.17	+.37
All Women	−.49	−.25	−.48	+.86

3.10, is attenuated when sample size is fixed, but that socioeconomic development levels of regions are still more strongly associated with regional patterns of breastfeeding and of nonsusceptibility among illiterate than among literate women. Furthermore, the weakening of the link is especially clear for women with 5 or more years of schooling. For abstinence, however, the originally declining sequence is not maintained, as all correlation coefficients drop, whereas the patterns for contraception remain unchanged. Hence, sample size reduction and selectivity were responsible for exaggerating the difference in the associations with the background variables between the various education categories, but they are not responsible for generating a completely fallacious pattern.

ARE EDUCATIONAL EFFECTS WITHIN REGIONS RELATED TO CONTEXTUAL VARIABLES?

So far we have treated the spacing variables separately for each of the age-education subgroups. Comparisons between these groups were only performed at the level of the regression results. Another way of approaching this consists of making the comparisons first and only subsequently seeking to predict the magnitude of the within-region age-education contrasts (see Appendix F) on the basis of the various background variables. This approach is followed for the *difference* in length of the nonsusceptible period between:

1. Illiterate women 35+ and illiterate women 15–24
2. Illiterate women 25–34 and women of the same age but with 1–4 years of schooling
3. Illiterate women 25–34 and women of the same age but with 5+ years of education
4. Illiterate women 15–24 and women 15–24 with 1–4 years of schooling
5. Illiterate women 15–24 and women 15–24 with 5+ years of education.

The first contrast considers the current age effect among illiterate women, whereas the remaining four contrasts measure the impact of individual schooling on the length of the nonsusceptible period. The regression of these *differences* in nonsusceptibility produced by individual characteristics (age or education) with regional characteristics merely consists of measuring the interaction effect between individual and contextual characteristics. This was, however, not done in one step. It had been noted that large differences in nonsusceptibility between age or education groups could only emerge in regions where the most traditional women still had long periods of nonsusceptibility and obviously not in regions where the length of the nonsusceptible period was shorter to start with. Hence, a measure of *relative* difference was required. To achieve this, the difference in nonsusceptibility between the two contrasted groups was related first to the length of the nonsusceptible period (NSP) of the most conservative group in the pair. The residuals, E, from this regression were taken as measures of relative difference and these were regressed on the regional background variables in the next step. For example, in figure 3.6 the difference in nonsusceptibility between older and younger

Y = nsp (Illit,35-49)
  - nsp (Illit,15-24)

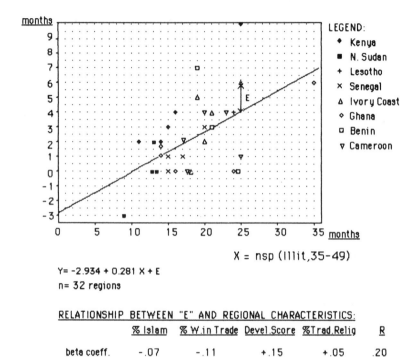

X = nsp (Illit,35-49)

Y= -2.934 + 0.281 X + E
n= 32 regions

RELATIONSHIP BETWEEN "E" AND REGIONAL CHARACTERISTICS:

	% Islam	% W.in Trade	Devel.Score	%Trad.Relig	R
beta coeff.	-.07	-.11	+.15	+.05	.20
zero order	-.14	-.05	+.17	-.03	

FIGURE 3.6. Definition of a Relative Measure of Decline in Postparum Nonsusceptibility Associated with Age (E) and Relationship with Regional Characteristics

illiterate women in the various regions was plotted against the values for the older group. The best fitting linear relationship was established and the values of E are simply the distance of each data point to the regression line. Hence, E measures whether the contrast in nonsusceptibility between these two age groups is larger or smaller than what one would expect on the basis of the length of the nonsusceptible period for the most conservative, that is, the oldest, group. From the subsequent regression of E with four regional (that is, contextual) characteristics, also shown in figure 3.6, it appears that only 4 percent of the variance of E is accounted for. Consequently, the regional level of development, its Islamic character, its history of economic self-reliance for women, or its adherence to traditional religion all fail to specify the pattern any further.

This picture changes when education groups are contrasted rather than

y = nsp (Illit,25-34)
   -nsp (1-4 yrs,25-34)

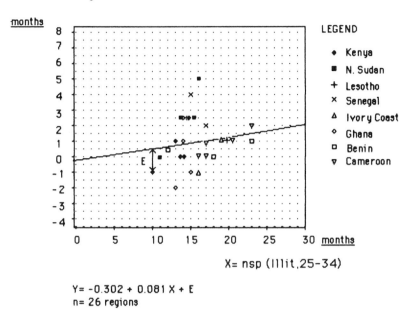

X= nsp (Illit,25-34)

Y= -0.302 + 0.081 X + E
n= 26 regions

RELATIONSHIP BETWEEN "E" AND REGIONAL CHARACTERISTICS:

	%Islam	%W. in Trade	Devel. Score	%Trad. Relig.	R
beta coeff.	+.60	-.25	-.05	-.05	.75
zero order	+.70	-.42	-.36	-.34	

FIGURE 3.7. Definition of a Relative Measure of Decline in Postpartum Nonsusceptibility Associated with Education (E) and Relationship with Regional Characteristics

age groups of illiterate women. An example is given in figure 3.7 for women 25–34 and the effect of 1–4 years of schooling versus none or Koranic schooling only. In this instance there appears to be a good deal of additional structure ($R = 0.75$ and $R^2 = 0.56$): the Islamic character of the region enlarges the contrast in nonsusceptibility between illiterate women and women with some schooling, whereas all the other contextual variables reduce it. The positive effect of percentage Muslim remains dominant when three more educational contrasts with respect to nonsusceptibility are made, as shown in table 3.12. Clearly, female education in Islamic areas greatly reduces the

TABLE 3.12 Contextual Effects on the Relative Difference (E) in Postpartum Nonsusceptibility (nsp) between Educational Groups

Educational Contrast*	Beta (top) and Zero-Order Correlation Coefficients (bottom)					
	% Islam	% Woman in Trade	Development Score	% Traditional Religion	R	N
Women 25–34						
nsp (illit.) − nsp (1–4 yrs)**	+.60	−.25	−.05	−.05	.75	26
	+.70	−.42	−.36	−.34		
nsp (illit.) − nsp (5+ yrs)	+.62	+.05	−.05	−.04	.65	22
	+.65	−.12	−.36	−.17		
Women 15–24						
nsp (illit.) − nsp (1–4 yrs)	+.56	−.30	−.10	+.16	.70	26
	+.63	−.35	−.46	−.14		
nsp (illit.) − nsp (5+ yrs)	+.87	−.14	+.32	+.25	.70	22
	+.66	−.18	−.22	−.18		

*The regressions are in order of appearance of the 4 contrasts:

$Y = -0.302 + 0.081\,X + E$

$Y = 2.838 + 0.029\,X + E$

$Y = 0.245 + 0.063\,X + E$

$Y = 1.675 + 0.112\,X + E$

where Y is the difference in nonsusceptibility (nsp) between the education subgroups, and X the nsp-value for the illiterate group. The regression results in the table pertain to the residuals E.

**See also Figure 3.7.

period of postpartum nonsusceptibility in comparison to the other regions. A strong selection effect is likely to have contributed to this result: educated women in Muslim areas are rarer and therefore more atypical than elsewhere.

The other three contextual variables tend to produce modest negative effects, as already shown in figure 3.7. The effect of women in trade and of adherence to traditional religions captures the typical West African feature of better preserved traditions of child-spacing and especially postpartum abstinence. Considering that the periods of postpartum nonsusceptibility for illiterate women are still very long in less Islamized West African populations and that there is consequently ample room for a marked decline associated with female education, it is indeed remarkable to find that postpartum nonsusceptibility among educated women tends to be relatively close to that of illiterate women. Hence, individual schooling reduces the length of the nonsusceptible period, but has less of an effect in societies with an extant tradition of female self-reliance and a West African organizational pattern in general.

The effect of the regional level of development on the relative decline in postpartum nonsusceptibility associated with education is also of interest. It might have been expected that the education gap with respect to postpartum nonsusceptibility would be widest in the most developed regions. But, this is clearly refuted by the regression results. Instead it is found that illiterate women reduce breastfeeding and abstinence when living in the more developed regions to a striking degree. The unstandardized regression coefficients from the earlier analysis treating the education groups separately are of relevance here, and they are reported in table 3.13 for a shift in development score of one unit (also $\cong 1\sigma$): illiterate women reduce their nonsusceptible period on average with 2.0 to 2.5 months, whereas women with full primary education (5+ years) reduce it with only about 1 month when development scores of the region of residence increase by one unit. The net result is that the relative gap between education groups with respect to the

TABLE 3.13   Reduction in Postpartum Nonsusceptible Period among Age-Education Groups Associated with a Shift in Regional Development Score of 1 Unit

Age Group	Illiterate Women		1–4 Yrs of Schooling		5+ Yrs of Schooling	
	$\bar{X}$	Reduction	$\bar{X}$	Reduction	$\bar{X}$	Reduction
35+	18.5 mos.	−2.5 mos.	—	—	—	—
25–34	16.6	−2.1	14.9	−1.5	12.8	−1.1
15–24	16.3	−2.1	14.4	−1.5	12.3	−0.9

length of postpartum nonsusceptibility tends to *shrink* when the respective means are lowered as a consequence of higher regional levels of development.

POSTPARTUM NONSUSCEPTIBILITY AND CONTRACEPTION: THE BALANCE

Mean durations of postpartum nonsusceptibility and efficiency weighted proportions currently using contraception among currently married women can be converted to a comparable metric using the Bongaarts indices (Bongaarts and Potter, 1983). The index of postpartum nonsusceptibility C_i measures what proportion of total fecundity would remain after allowing for the sole effect of postpartum nonsusceptibility. The total fecundity rate TF measures the average number of children that would be born to women who are exposed during their entire fertile age range (15–49) in the absence of contraception and any prolongation of the postpartum nonsusceptible period beyond a minimum of 1.5 months. If $C_i = 0.60$, the total fecundity rate TF would be reduced by 40 percent, and the remaining 60 percent constitutes the total natural fertility rate TN. Hence,

$$TN = TF \times C_i \qquad \text{(eq. 3.8)}$$

The values of TF are usually comprised between 13.5 and 16.5 children, but lower values can be encountered in populations with pathological fetal wastage, subfecundity or sterility, or with reduced coital frequency. The measure C_i is defined as:

$$C_i = 20.0/18.5 + \text{NSP} \qquad \text{(eq. 3.9)}$$

If no breastfeeding or postpartum abstinence is practiced, the birth interval equals about 18.5 months for waiting time to conception, time loss associated with some fetal loss and gestation, plus 1.5 months of postpartum amenorrhea. The index C_i is then a simple ratio between such a minimum birth interval and an interval prolonged by an extra period of postpartum nonsusceptibility. For instance, if the total duration of postpartum nonsusceptibility equals 18 months, there is an extra prolongation of 16.5 months and $C_i = 20/36.5 = 0.55$. If the total fecundity rate $TF = 15$ children, then the total natural fertility rate $TN = 15 \times 0.55 = 8.25$ children: the total fecundity rate is almost reduced to half by the impact of extra child-spacing produced by lactational amenorrhea and/or abstinence. The values for C_i are given in Appendixes G and H, for the various age-education groups. The lowest value of $C_i = 0.43$ for the northern and upper regions in Ghana, meaning that postpartum nonsusceptibility reduces the TF by more than half, whereas the highest values of C_i of about 0.80 are found in Nairobi, Khartoum, and the North and Eastern regions of Sudan, implying that the total fecundity rate is merely reduced by 20 percent. The range of regional values in age and education groups encountered in the WFS countries is hence enormous.

The index of contraception C_c is obtained as

$$C_c = 1 - (1.08 \times u \times e) \qquad \text{(eq. 3.10)}$$

where u is the proportion of users among women currently in a sexual union and e the method-specific effectiveness. The parameters u and e are already combined in our measure of contraceptive use-effectiveness used so far. The coefficient 1.08 represents an adjustment for the fact that some couples do not use contraception if they know or believe that they are sterile. The index C_c indicates which portion of the total natural fertility rate TN is realized after allowing for the fertility reducing capacity of contraception. The outcome of $TN \times C_i C_c$ should represent the total marital fertility rate $TMFR$. Hence,

$$TMFR = TF \times C_i \times C_c \qquad \text{(eq. 3.11)}$$

where the product $C_i \times C_c$ measures the combined effect of postpartum non-susceptibility and contraception. The *lower* the value of $C_i C_c$ is, the *more* the TF is reduced, and the *lower* the value of the $TMFR$ for a given TF will be. The values of C_c and of the product $C_i C_c$ are also given in Appendixes G and H.

Given that one possesses a measure of the combined effect of nonsusceptibility and contraception, differences between educational groups can be established as

$$\Delta(\text{illit, literate}) = C_i C_c \text{ (illiterate)} - C_i C_c \text{ (literate)} \qquad \text{(eq. 3.12)}$$

A *positive* value of Δ indicates that the product $C_i C_c$ for the literate group is *lowest* and hence that *more* child-spacing occurs among them as a result of postpartum nonsusceptibility and contraception. In other words, for identical values of TF, the value of the $TMFR$ would be lowest among the literate group. *Negative* values of Δ imply that *less* spacing is associated with female education.

The values of Δ are also reported in Appendixes G and H. Moreover, a count has been made of the regions where female education is associated with more versus less overall spacing. The results of these counts are presented for women 25–34 in figure 3.8 showing the contrast between illiterate women and women with 1–4 years of schooling, and in figure 3.9 for illiterate women and women with 5+ years of education. Partial primary education produces more spacing ($\Delta(0, 1-4) \geq +0.020$) in eight out of twenty-six regions for which the comparison could be made, and full primary education ($\Delta(0, 5+) \geq +0.020$) in only four of the eighteen regions. The reason why so few regions have better overall spacing being associated with full primary education is that such schooling reduces postpartum nonsusceptibility by a considerable amount, therefore requiring contraceptive use-effectiveness to rise

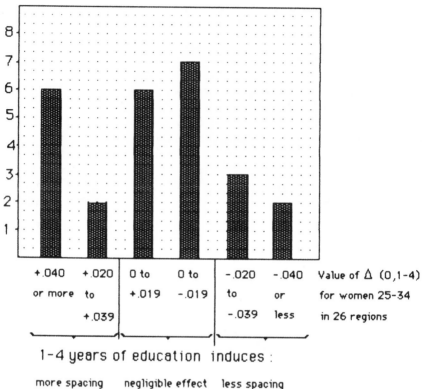

FIGURE 3.8. Number and Identification of Regions with an Increase or Decrease in Overall Child-Spacing; Effect of Partial Primary Education

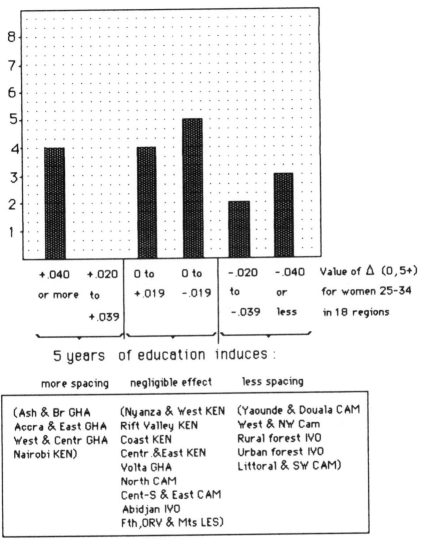

FIGURE 3.9. Number and Identification of Regions with an Increase or Decrease in Overall Child-Spacing; Effect of Full Primary Education or More

to levels in the vicinity of 20 percent before the balance is restored. Of these four regions, three are located in Ghana and the fourth is Nairobi. In other major urban areas such as Cap Vert and Thiès, Khartoum, Abidjan, Douala, and Yaounde, contraceptive use-effectiveness among women with full primary education is not high enough to compensate for their shorter durations of postpartum nonsusceptibility. Partial primary education often reduces postpartum nonsusceptibility by a smaller amount and lower levels of contraceptive use-effectiveness are needed to restore the balance. As a consequence Δ(o, $1-4$) is also larger than $+$o.o2o in an additional number of regions, such as the Rift Valley, Cotonou, Khartoum, and the Central Region of Northern Sudan (that is, Gezira and the Two Niles). Among women $15-19$ education virtually always reduces overall spacing: young women start with reduced periods of nonsusceptibility but not with enhanced contraception. The value of Δ(o, $5+$) for such women exceeds $+$o.o2o only in one of the nineteen regions studied, namely in Greater Accra and the adjacent Eastern Region.

The magnitude of the effect on overall spacing induced by individual education can also be related to our set of contextual variables. The dependent variables are Δ(o, $1-4$) and Δ(o, $5+$) for women $15-19$ and $25-34$ respectively. The results are presented in figures 3.10 and 3.11 and in table 3.14 in the form of overall effects (zero-order correlation coefficients) and direct effects (beta-coefficients). The most striking feature is that the socioeconomic development score of the region proves to be the most dominant determinant of the value of Δ. Moreover, the relationship is positive. Hence, declining durations of postpartum nonsusceptibility associated with increments in individual female education are compensated to a larger extent by rising contraceptive use-effectiveness in regions with higher scores on socioeconomic development than in regions with lower scores. Female economic self-reliance (see percent women in trade) and Christianity (that is, the complement of Islam and traditional religion) act in the same direction as socioeconomic development, but the effects are usually more modest. Much of this stems from the fact that postpartum nonsusceptibility for literate women, and especially for women with full primary education, was less differentiated according to regional development levels than contraceptive use-effectiveness (see figures 3.4 and 3.5). In other words, relatively similar reductions in postpartum nonsusceptibility induced by individual schooling in the various regions are confronted with regionally more diversified rises in contraceptive use-effectiveness. Hence, factors responsible for regional heterogeneity in education related increases in contraception also emerge when explaining education related differentials in overall spacing. To sum up, the inverse relationship between individual education and overall spacing, that is, a typical feature during the first phase of the transition, weakens with advancing regional development. At present, however, this inverse relationship has yielded to the opposite pattern (women with full primary education having better spacing than illiterate women) in very few regions. These are Southern Ghana and Nairobi. The pattern reversal can be taken as an indicator of the shift toward the second phase of the transition.

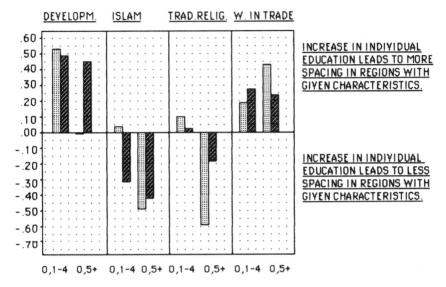

FIGURE 3.10. Effects of Regional Characteristics on the Change in Overall Child-Spacing Produced by Partial and Full Primary Education Respectively; Results for Women Aged 15–24

CONCLUSIONS

The analysis strategy used in this chapter is largely based on relating levels or differentials by age and education in the various components of child-spacing to contextual characteristics of thirty-three regions. Once again, it should be borne in mind that these regions are not representative of the whole of sub-Saharan Africa and that the sample is weighted in favor of West Africa. The most relevant findings were the following:

1. Individual schooling reduces breastfeeding and abstinence and enhances contraceptive use-effectiveness virtually in every region.

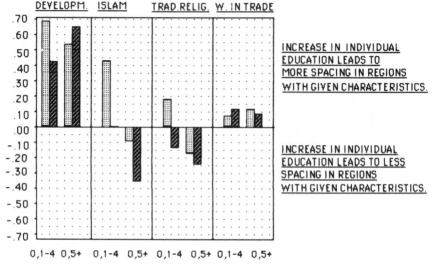

FIGURE 3.11. Effects of Regional Characteristics on the Change in Overall Child-Spacing Produced by Partial and Full Primary Education Respectively; Results for Women Aged 25–34

However, the magnitude of these shifts varies considerably for each of these spacing variables depending on contextual characteristics of the regions.

2. The continued existence of traditional religion in an area supports traditional methods of spacing, that is, prolonged breastfeeding and the long postpartum taboo, but has a negative overall effect on contraception largely because traditional religion is associated with low female education and low socioeconomic development scores.

3. The Islamic character of an area strongly reduces postpartum nonsusceptibility, mainly as a result of eroding the postpartum taboo. Part of this negative influence is, however, alleviated by the indirect effect operating via low overall female schooling, which is supportive of pro-

TABLE 3.14   Relationship between Education-Induced Effect on Child-Spacing (Δ) and Contextual Variables in WFS Regions

	Women Aged 15–24			
	$\Delta = C_i C_c(\text{illit}) - C_i C_c(1\text{–}4 \text{ yrs})$		$\Delta = C_i C_c(\text{illit}) - C_i C_c(5+ \text{ yrs})$	
	r	β	r	β
% Muslim	−.31	+.04	−.42	−.49
% Traditional Religion	+.02	+.10	−.18	−.56
% Women in Trade	+.27	+.19	+.24	+.43
Development Score	+.49	+.53	+.45	−.01
R		.55		.63
N		26		19

	Women Aged 25–34			
	$\Delta = C_i C_c(\text{illit}) - C_i C_c(1\text{–}4 \text{ yrs})$		$\Delta = C_i C_c(\text{illit}) - C_i C_c(5+ \text{ yrs})$	
	r	β	r	β
% Muslim	.00	+.43	−.35	−.09
% Traditional Religion	−.13	+.18	−.24	−.17
% Women in Trade	+.12	+.07	+.09	+.12
Development Score	+.42	+.69	+.65	+.54
R		.53		.66
N		26		18

longed breastfeeding and lactational amenorrhea. The Islamic nature of a region furthermore exerts a negative effect on contraceptive use-effectiveness, but again, this operates entirely through the low level of female education. In the balance, the single most important contribution to child-spacing in such areas is made by the long duration of lactational amenorrhea, but if the new generations of women were to receive education beyond Koranic schooling and follow the ways of those who are currently making up the group of literate women, chances are that also lactational amenorrhea would shrink and that child-spacing would collapse. This shows how important it will be for these areas to combine future efforts in female education with efforts in the domain of family planning.

4. Christianity is less supportive of traditional forms of spacing than traditional religion but less erosive with respect to the postpartum taboo than Islam. However, Christianity has a negative effect on overall postpartum nonsusceptibility as a result of its indirect effect operating via increased overall levels of female education. By the same token, Christianity is positively related to contraceptive use-efficiency.

5. The tradition of female economic self-reliance has a modest but overall positive effect on postpartum nonsusceptibility thanks to its positive effect on the length of postpartum abstinence. Its effect on contraception is neutral, except for the better educated women for whom it is positive. In the balance, female economic self-reliance is supportive of slightly better overall child-spacing for illiterate women (effect via long abstinence) and for women with full primary education (effect via contraception).

6. The effect of the regional development level on the postpartum variables is negative, but the religious variables have a stronger predictive power. By contrast, its effect on contraceptive use-effectiveness dominates the effects of all other contextual variables by a very substantial amount.

7. The age effect, only measured for illiterate women, cannot be predicted adequately by the four contextual variables. The only pattern found in the data is that the age differential is greatest where overall spacing is longest for the oldest group.

8. The effect of *individual* female education, measured for the youngest and the middle age groups, is largely determined by the regional levels of development. The other contextual variables have additional effects in such a way that:

   • overall child-spacing *declines most* with increased individual schooling in regions that have low development scores, high proportions Muslim or traditional religion, and no female economic-self reliance.

   • overall child-spacing *declines less* with individual schooling in areas that have higher development scores, higher proportions Christian, and, furthermore, a tradition of greater female independence. In such areas, the education gap with respect to overall child-spacing is gradually being closed via increased use of contraception.

   • overall child-spacing *improves* with individual education in a few regions only; they are characterized by the highest overall levels of female education, but are not necessarily urban.

The main conclusion to be drawn from this analysis is that female education is of paramount importance for the future of the demographic transition in sub-Saharan Africa. It operates both as an individual and as a contextual variable. At the onset, educated women are a select few and they start off with much less child-spacing than the illiterate women, who still benefit from the traditionally long postpartum nonsusceptible period. As more women are educated, thereby increasing the contextual level of education, illiterate women also reduce lactation and abstinence, and a fertility increase emerges in the area. During the third stage, however, when contextual levels of education have reached an average of 4 to 6 years (that is, when the majority of women have had some primary schooling), contraceptive use rises, the better educated women fully correct for lowered postpartum nonsusceptibility, a positive spacing-education differential emerges and fertility may start its decline. *The pace of this scenario is, however, strongly influenced by cultural and organizational settings,* summarized in this chapter by way of a few additional and admittedly crude contextual variables.

ACKNOWLEDGMENTS

The work by Gaisie and Delaine was made possible thanks to financial support from USAID through the Population Council's International Awards Program (agreements CP84.12A and CP82.39A). Vanderhoeft's contribution was financed by a grant from the National Bank of Belgium. Frank Eelens and Luc Donné provided additional analysis assistance.

BIBLIOGRAPHY

Adegbola, O., H. J. Page, and R. Lesthaeghe. 1981. Child-spacing and fertility in Lagos. In: *Child-spacing in tropical Africa—Traditions and Change*, ed. H. J. Page and R. Lesthaeghe. London: Academic Press, 147–180.

Anderson, J. E., H. I. Goldberg, F. M'Bodgi, and A. Abdel-Aziz. 1984. Postpartum practices and child-spacing in Senegal and Jordan. Paper presented at the Annual Meetings of the Population Associations of America, Minneapolis, Minn.

Ashton, W. D. 1972. *The logit transformation.* London: Griffin.

Bongaarts, J., and R. Potter. 1983. *Fertility, biology and behaviour.* London: Academic Press.

Brass, W., et al. 1968. *The demography of tropical Africa.* Princeton: Princeton University Press.

Caldwell, J. C., and P. Caldwell. 1977. The role of marital sexual abstinence in determining fertility: A study of the Yoruba in Nigeria. *Population Studies* 31(2): 193–217.

Cantrelle, P., and B. Ferry. 1979. Approche de la fécondité naturelle dans les populations contemporaines. In: *Natural fertility—Fécondité naturelle,* ed. H. Leridon and J. Menken. Liège, Belgium: Ordina for the International Union for the Scientific Study of Population.

Cantrelle, P., H. Leridon, and P. Livenais. 1981. Fécondité, allaitement et mortalité infantile: Différences inter-ethnique dans une même région (Sine-Saloum). Paris: ORSTOM (mimeo).

Delaine, G. 1976. Observation des variables intermédiaires dans le cadre de la fécondité naturelle—Etude d'allaitement. Mémoire de DEA. Paris: Université de Paris, Institute de démographie.

Eelens, F., and L. Donné. 1985. The proximate determinants of fertility in sub-

Saharan Africa: A factbook based on the results of the World Fertility Survey. *Working Paper of the Interuniversity Programme in Demography*, no. 85–3. Brussels: Vrije Universiteit.

Ferry, B. 1977. Etude de la fécondité à Dakar (Sénegal)—Objectifs, méthodologie et résultats. Dakar, Senegal: ORSTOM (mimeo).

Finney, D. J. 1971. *Probit analysis*. 3d ed. Cambridge: Cambridge University Press.

Frank, O. 1983. Infertility in sub-Saharan Africa. *Working Paper of the Center for Policies Studies*, no. 97. New York: The Population Council.

Gaisie, S. K. 1981. Child-spacing patterns and fertility differentials in Ghana. In: *Child-spacing in tropical Africa—Traditions and change*, ed. H. J. Page and R. Lesthaeghe. London: Academic Press, 237–253.

Ginsberg, R. B. 1973. The effect of lactation on the length of the postpartum anovulatory period: An application of a bivariate stochastic model. *Theoretical Population Biology* 4: 276–299.

Henin, R. A. 1968. Fertility differentials in the Sudan, with reference to the nomadic and settled population. *Population Studies* 22(1): 147–164.

Kalbfleisch, J. D., and R. L. Prentice. 1980. *The statistical analysis of failure time data*. New York: Wiley.

Kocher, J. E. 1973. *Rural development, income distribution and fertility decline*. New York: the Population Council.

Lesthaeghe, R., and H. J. Page. 1980. The postpartum non-susceptible period: Development and application of model schedules. *Population Studies* 34(1): 143–169.

Morgan, R. W. 1975. Fertility levels and fertility change. In: *Population growth and socio-economic development in West Africa*, ed. J. C. Caldwell. New York: Columbia University Press, 187–235.

Mosley, W. H., L. H. Werner, and S. Becker, 1982. The dynamics of birth-spacing and marital fertility in Kenya. *World Fertility Survey Scientific Reports*, no. 30. Voorburg: International Statistical Institute.

Ohadike, P. 1986. A demographic note on marriage, family and family growth in Lagos, Nigeria. In: *The population of tropical Africa*, ed. J. C. Caldwell and C. Okonjo. London: Longmans, Green and Co, 379–392.

Olusanya, P. O. 1969. Modernization and the level of fertility in western Nigeria. In: *Proceedings of the International Population Conference (London)*. Liège: International Union for the Scientific Study of Population.

Romaniuk, A. 1980. Increase in natural fertility during the early stages of modernization—Evidence from an African case study: Zaire. *Population Studies* 34(2): 293–310.

Tabutin, D., M. Sala-Diakanda, Ngondo A Pitshandenge, and E. Vilquin. 1983. Fertility and child-spacing in western Zaire. In: *Child-spacing in tropical Africa—Traditions and change*, ed. H. J. Page and R. Lesthaeghe. London: Academic Press, 287–302.

Vanderhoeft, C. 1983. A unified approach to models for analysis of zero-one data with applications to intermediate fertility variables. *Working Paper of the Interuniversity Programme in Demography*, no. 1983–5. Brussels: Vrije Universiteit.

CHAPTER FOUR

A Comparative Study of the Levels and the Differentials of Sterility in Cameroon, Kenya, and Sudan

Ulla Larsen

Children are the cloth of the body.
Without children you are naked.
Yoruba saying (Nigeria)

Numerous populations in sub-Saharan Africa experience very low fertility (Page and Coale, 1972). Effective intentional practices to lower reproduction are uncommon in Africa and most populations approximate natural fertility. The occurence of infertility is a major problem for individuals, since most Africans desire large families (at least six children). Low fertility also indicates serious health problems, because low fertility is strongly linked to sexually transmitted diseases, such as gonorrhea. If the prevalence and incidence of sterility were better understood, more effective campaigns to reduce sterility could be carried out. However, if the levels of sterility were reduced, fertility and the population growth rate would most likely increase rapidly, thereby causing other problems. Thus, the prevalence of sterility in certain areas of sub-Saharan Africa and the effective prevention or treatment of sterility are complex issues.

Sterility is defined as the inability of a noncontracepting, nonlactating, sexually active woman to have a live birth. Primary sterility is defined biologically as never developing the capacity to reproduce, whereas secondary sterility refers to the termination of previously possessed reproductive ability. In practice, sterility is difficult to measure. Celibate women are never at risk of having a child or of testing their reproductive capacity. Therefore, in establishing operational definitions, only noncelibate women are considered. Those who have never had a live birth are usually considered to have primary sterility, while secondary sterility is measured among women who are unable to have a live birth subsequent to an earlier live birth.

Studies of sterility in Africa have been hampered by the fact that no method of measuring the levels of sterility by age from incomplete birth histories has been available until now (Larsen, 1985). In addition, until recently demographic data for sub-Saharan Africa have been both scarce and of poor quality. In the last decade several sources have become available; surveys, carried out by several African countries in collaboration with the World Fertility Surveys (WFS), provide a particularly rich body of information. The present study is based on WFS data from Cameroon, Kenya,[1] and Sudan.[2] These three countries were selected because they represent many of the variations in reproductive characteristics in sub-Saharan Africa, such as difference in age at first marriage and duration of postpartum abstinence (Lesthaeghe, 1984b). Total fertility is relatively low in Cameroon and Sudan, and relatively high in Kenya; Sudan is the only country for which the WFS included questions about female circumcision.

In this chapter, the discussion begins with a description of the geographic distribution of subfertility in sub-Saharan Africa. Next, theoretical models of sterility are established, previous research on differentials in subfertility is reviewed, and the covariates of sterility to be examined in this study are defined. Subsequently, age-specific sterility rates and the levels of primary sterility are estimated for all women and for selected subgroups. Finally, in order to examine the effects of several covariates simultaneously on the prevalence or incidence of sterility at different time points or across cohorts, a hazards models analysis is conducted.

SUBFERTILITY IN SUB-SAHARAN AFRICA

Sterility is strongly associated with low levels of fertility. Therefore, a map of the geographic variations in the levels of fertility for peoples of Africa south of the Sahara provides a good indication of the prevalence of sterility. Page and Coale (1972) estimated total fertility rates for all the populations in sub-Saharan Africa for which data were available (figure 4.1). Their study shows that the low fertility areas are concentrated in Central Africa and include, among other countries, Cameroon, Central African Republic, the western part of Sudan, Congo, and Gabon. Recently, this distribution pattern of subfertility has been confirmed by Frank (1983a, 1983b), who mapped the proportion childless among women aged 45–49.

MODELS OF STERILITY

A couple's inability to have a live birth may be due to impairment of the reproductive system of the wife, the husband, or both. In general, female factors are thought to cause sterility in 50 to 70 percent of all sterile couples (Sherris and Fox, 1983). However, the contribution of female factors might be overestimated, since sterility investigations traditionally have concentrated on women rather than men.

Female sterility is primarily due to one or more of the following reasons: (1) ovaries may fail to produce a viable egg, preventing the possibility of

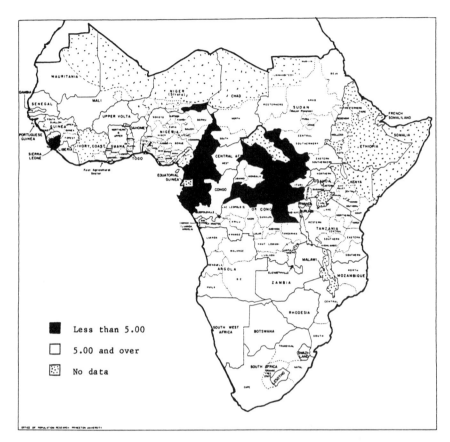

FIGURE 4.1. Total Fertility Rates for Selected Areas or Peoples of Africa South of the Sahara (Source: Page and Coale, 1972)

conception; (2) fallopian tubes may be blocked, distorted, or infected, preventing normal movement of the egg or sperm in the tubes; (3) the uterus may be distorted or the uterine lining (endometrium) inadequate or infected, preventing implantation or survival of the embryo; (4) the cervix may be malformed, infected, or secrete abnormal mucus, preventing sperm from reaching the upper reproductive tract; and (5) systemic infection or hormonal imbalance may result in fetal death (figure 4.2).

Sterility is most frequently caused by a pelvic inflammatory disease (PID), which originates in the cervix and can ascend to the upper reproductive tract and block the fallopian tubes. PID can also lead to fluid filled swellings, adhesions, scarring, and other permanent damage of the fallopian tubes. Permanent sterility is more likely to occur if the infection is severe, if treatment is delayed, or if a woman has had multiple episodes of PID. An

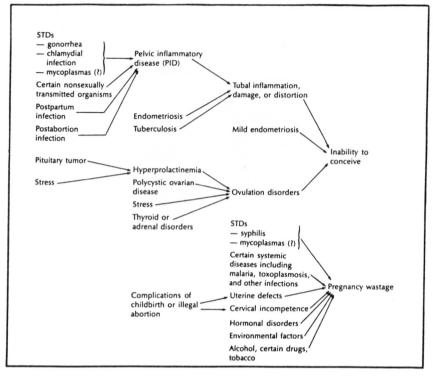

FIGURE 4.2. Relationships of Selected Direct and Indirect Causes of Female Infertility (Source: Sherris and Fox, 1983)

estimated 60 percent of women with PID become sterile if they are not treated with antibiotics (Sherris and Fox, 1983). The most common source of PID is a sexually transmitted disease, such as gonorrhea and chlamydia. However, the risk of PID is also fairly high when childbirth or abortion is carried out under unhygienic conditions, because microorganisms ascend more easily through a dilated cervix.

Sterility can result from the inability to carry a pregnancy to term as well as the inability to conceive. Pregnancy wastage often results from causes that cannot be prevented, such as abnormalities of the fetus and problems with the uterus or cervix. Other causes are preventable and they include sexually transmitted diseases, such as syphilis, and certain systemic diseases, such as malaria. The risk of pregnancy wastage is high for women with syphilis because this disease can infect the fetus, causing intrauterine death. Malaria can result in pregnancy wastage because malarial infection of the placenta impairs fetal nutrition and increases the risk of spontaneous abortion.

Female circumcision has been indicated as increasing the risk of sterility, but evidence is lacking. It is hypothesized that circumcision predisposes women to infections leading to sterility because scarring and closure of the external genitalia prevent proper drainage of urine and menstrual blood. Also, circumcised women often experience pain during sexual intercourse and difficulties at childbirth. All of these problems may lead to primary sterility. In addition, the risk of secondary sterility may be increased because at each delivery most circumcised women have to be cut to allow delivery of the fetus and the incision is subsequently stitched. This procedure frequently causes infections and subsequent sexual intercourse is often more difficult, even impossible in some cases. It should be noted that there are different types of female circumcision. The most common is a Pharaonic circumcision, which is a removal of the clitoris, the labia minora, the labia majora, and a closing of the vagina to only a small opening to allow elimination of urine and menstrual blood. Less common is a Sunna circumcision, where only the prepuce of the clitoris is removed. Other types are also performed which vary in degree between a Sunna and a Pharaonic circumcision. It is generally agreed that a Pharaonic circumcision may especially enhance the risk of sterility (Aziz, 1980; People, 1979; Shandall, 1967).

Male sterility is usually due to blockage of sperm ducts, or disorders in sperm production resulting in poor semen quality, that is, semen that contains too few sperm and/or abnormal sperm (figure 4.3). A less common cause is a sexual malfunction that prevents ejaculation of semen. Genital

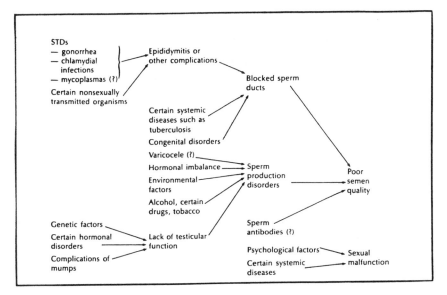

FIGURE 4.3. Relationships of Selected Direct and Indirect Causes of Male Infertility (Source: Sherris and Fox, 1983)

infections cause poor semen quality and sterility by creating inflammation or blockage in the upper reproductive tract. The infection is usually due to sexually transmitted diseases, such as gonorrhea and chlamydia, but it can also be caused by urogenital tuberculosis and other diseases (Sherris and Fox, 1983).

THE COVARIATES OF STERILITY

Empirical analyses of sterility in sub-Saharan Africa are complicated by the fact that data about the major factors directly related to sterility are usually not available. Therefore, most previous research on sterility in sub-Saharan Africa has used indirect evidence of sterility, and variables related only indirectly to sterility, as does this study. The variables included are selected on theoretical grounds and on the basis of the literature on factors related to subfertility. Clearly these factors must be related to be health problems described in the previous section, although our analysis cannot delineate these relationships because of the lack of available data.

The major limitations of the WFS surveys as a source of information about sterility are as follows. First, the WFS surveys provide only data about women's reproductive histories; hence, sterility of a couple is ascribed always to the woman. Second, no data are available about women's medical histories, for example, whether a woman has had a venereal disease or whether she has had medical treatment. Third, the WFS surveys collected no information about location of childbirth and about who assisted with the delivery (midwifery) for Kenya or Sudan. In Cameroon, midwifery information is provided only for the last pregnancy. Finally, the WFS surveys asked questions about female circumcision only in Sudan.

As a consequence of the lack of data about medical history, midwifery, and female circumcision, proxies are used for health information. One further problem with these data must be noted. There is evidence indicating that the prevalence of venereal diseases leading to sterility has decreased since knowledge about the effects of antibiotics became available around 1950 (Tabutin, 1982). Infections following a childbirth or an abortion can also be cured with penicillin, and midwifery is likely to have improved in the last few decades. Furthermore, in Sudan the ratio of Sunna to Pharaonic circumcisions has increased slightly, suggesting that complications leading to sterility from female circumcision may have decreased (Shandall, 1967). Thus, it is possible that place of the delivery, type of attendant at the birth, and circumcision have different relations to sterility in different cohorts, that the levels of sterility by age have declined in recent decades, and that the prevalence of sterility may vary across cohorts.

The WFS surveys generally provide information about socioeconomic variables only at the time of survey, so that we are forced to limit the analysis to a time period during which it is reasonable to assume that the covariates do not change. Due to this restriction, two models are established: model 1 of sterility status (sterile or fecund) 5 years before survey (we need at least 5 years of exposure to determine sterility status) includes socioeconomic variables; model 2 of sterility status at different points in time or by cohorts excludes most of these variables. In model 1 it is assumed that the single observation made on a covariate (such as education) at the time of the survey holds for the previous 5 years. This assumption should not bias the results substantially because none of the socioeconomic variables analyzed change much in 5 years. For instance, in the societies studied, few married women move or start to go to school and most husbands do not change their work statuses. However, it is not valid to assume that all covariates are constant from entry into first marriage until survey; for example some women divorce and other women acquire cowives. Therefore, model 2, which looks at women at 5-year age intervals over their entire married lifetime, is restricted to either constant covariates or to time-varying covariates for which data at different points in time are available.

Both models include the following as covariates: region, religion, residence (urban or rural), education, type of circumcision, number of times married, use of contraception, and age. Model 1 adds the covariates: husband's education, husband's work status, and marital status (monogamous versus polygamous unions and wife order). Model 2 includes the basic set of covariates plus time period and cohort. The justification for inclusion of these variables is described below.

Geographic variations in sterility can provide clues to the presence of environmental variations (such as prevalence of venereal diseases) related to sterility, and to cultural patterns that affect sexual practices (such as more sexual partners). Subfertility has been found to vary greatly from region to region in all three countries. For instance, the percent childless is higher in the North, Center-South and East regions than in the West regions of Cameroon (Santow and Bioumla, 1984; Nasah, Azefor, and Ondoa, 1974). Furthermore, previous research shows that geographic boundaries of subfertility are often ethnic boundaries (Caldwell and Caldwell, 1983; Retel-Laurentin, 1974; Romaniuk, 1968). For example, the Mijikendas and the Kikuyus are neighboring tribes in Kenya and the former group has much lower fertility than the latter (Kenya Fertility Survey 1977–1978, 1980). Lesthaeghe (1985) and Retel-Laurentin (1974) noted that in subfertile societies, marital mobility is high and tribal customs permit wider sexual contacts, while ethnic groups that practice strict marriage laws have higher fertility.

Region is used as a proxy for venereal diseases and the sexual practices associated with its frequency. It would be preferable to use ethnicity instead of region, but no data are available about ethnic groups in Sudan. There are also too many distinct ethnic groups in Cameroon (thirty-four) and Kenya (forty-three) to examine the levels of sterility across ethnic groups. In a previous study of Cameroon and Kenya, ethnic groups located in the same area were combined and it was found that the differentials in sterility by ethnicity are very similar to the variations across region (Larsen, 1985). It is problematic, however, to use region in model 2, due to the fact that some women migrate after first marriage. More specifically, if some women move from a region with low sterility to a region with high sterility, then the estimated effects for the latter region at survey will be biased downwards, indicating lower sterility than is the case, because some women actually spent a part of their life in a more healthy environment. Likewise, migration in the opposite direction will cause the effects estimates for the low sterility region to be biased upwards, masking the explanatory power of region.

Romaniuk (1968) pointed out that low fertility areas often are close to waterways, such as lakes, rivers, and the sea, and that subfertility seems to follow the Arab slave routes. In accordance with this finding Romaniuk observed that Muslims suffer more from subfertility than non-Muslims. Today, it is uncertain whether the Arab slave traders spread venereal diseases, thus causing sterility, or whether the prevalence of sterility in these areas is predominantly due to cultural practices among Muslims. For instance, female circumcision is more frequently practiced among Muslims than non-Muslims, although female circumcision is not an ordinance from Islam (Shandall, 1967). Religion is included for Cameroon and Kenya, but not for Sudan, where only 38 women are non-Muslim in a sample of 3115 women (the WFS survey is restricted to northern Sudan). On the other hand, the effects of type of female circumcision are analyzed only for Sudan (no data about female circumcision are available for Cameroon and Kenya). The differentials between women with a Pharaonic circumcision and other women and examined (as few as 112 women (3.6 percent of the women surveyed) were not circumcised, so the differentials between never circumcised and circumcised women cannot be analyzed).

Urban or rural residence is hypothesized to be linked to the prevalence of venereal diseases and different practices of midwifery. In general, prostitution is more common in cities; hence, exposure to venereal diseases and subsequent sterility is likely to be higher in urban than in rural areas, even though medical treatment is more readily accessible in urban areas. Conversely, secondary sterility due to infections from a previous childbirth or abortion is probably greater for women who live in rural areas where more births are delivered at home under poor sanitary conditions by a family member or an untrained midwife. Previous research shows that the pattern of low fertility by residence is not systematic; subfertility is more widespread in rural than in urban areas in Central Africa, while the Yorubas in Nigeria experience very little difference in fertility by residence, and fertility is higher in rural than urban Ghana (Caldwell and Caldwell, 1983). In order to determine the impact of residence on sterility and to test the hypothesis that barren women tend to migrate from rural to urban areas to hide their childlessness (Frank, 1983*b*), the differentials in sterility by residence and whether a woman has migrated since her childhood (moved from a rural to an urban area), are analyzed.

Education of the wife and of her husband and husband's work status are used as indicators of socioeconomic status. Education is assumed to be linked to lower sterility because educated people are better informed. As a consequence, they are more likely to seek treatment for a venereal disease, and they are probably better able to avoid an infection leading to sterility, for example, by being more aware of the importance of hygienic conditions at childbirth. Education is also generally associated with higher income, and educated people can therefore better afford medical treatment and sanitary facilities. Information about education is available only at survey. It is assumed that women did not continue their education after they married, so this variable is included in both models. Education of the husband and his work status are included only in model 1 because some women divorce and do not have the same husband from the time of their first marriage until the survey. It is hypothesized that the employers (men who employ one or more people) have the highest income and are the best informed, that men who are self-employed (for example, in agriculture or trade) are more traditional and poorer, while the employees are a heterogeneous group.

In many African societies it is considered the husband's right to have offspring, and childlessness or subfertility is usually blamed on the wife. It is common practice to dissolve subfertile unions; consequently, as a group, divorced women have lower fertility. However, most divorced women remarry shortly thereafter and often become higher order wives in polygamous unions. Not surprisingly, polygamous unions generally have lower fertility than monogamous unions (Frank, 1983*b*; Henin, 1981). A study of Cameroon and Ghana shows that the proportion of women with no live birth at any expected duration of marriage is lower for women of rank 1 in polygamous unions compared to women in monogamous unions, while women of rank 2 and rank 3+ in polygamous unions have the highest proportion of childlessness (Lesthaeghe, 1984*a*). For other regions, subfertility might be higher in polygamous than monogamous unions because a man adds a new wife to a subfertile union to achieve higher parity (Henin, 1981).

To test whether women married more than once have higher sterility, the covariate, number of times married, is included in both model 1 and model 2. In model 2, number of times married may, of course, change with age but the marital history of each woman in the WFS surveys provides this information. The effects of marital status are examined only in model 1 because the dates cowives entered polygamous unions are not available. It is, therefore, assumed that marital status did not change in the 5 years preceding the survey. Marital status is grouped differently in the three countries analyzed because the individual WFS questionnaires varied; for example, the survey for Sudan provides no data about wife order in polygamous unions.

In order to measure the effects of contraception on sterility, it would be ideal to know the ages at which each woman starts and stops using contraception. However, the WFS surveys only provide data about whether a woman has ever used and whether she is currently using contraceptives at survey. Women who have used efficient methods of contraception during a long period have lower fertility and are very likely falsely to be classified as sterile. Many women in the societies studied do not contracept efficiently, and it is hypothesized that contraception only decreases fecundity slightly. In contrast, some methods of contraception (such as the condom and diaphragm) protect against venereal diseases and subsequent sterility. In addition, women who have used contraception tend to have more education and are probably more inclined to seek treatment for venereal diseases and to have trained assistance at childbirth, two factors that protect against sterility. Information about the ever use of contraception is employed in the present study, because it covers both past and current users. We are forced to assume that women who report that they have used contraception were contracepting throughout their entire married life, although most of these women probably contracepted only in certain periods. Consequently, the direct effects of contraception on fecundity are measured very poorly, while the indirect effects of being better informed probably vary less with time.

In Cameroon, information about midwifery (location at delivery and assistance of delivery) is available for the last pregnancy, as mentioned previously. However, it is problematic to interpret the effects of midwifery on sterility in analyses of individual women. For instance, women who delivered their last birth in a hospital or who were assisted by a doctor may have higher sterility than other women, due to the fact that these women experienced complications at their last delivery and therefore received special medical care. Otherwise, we would assume that women who delivered their last birth in a hospital or were assisted by a doctor are less likely to be sterile than women who delivered at home or were assisted by an untrained midwife. Furthermore, since data about midwifery are available only about the last pregnancy; it is not possible to determine the effects of midwifery on sterility throughout a woman's reproductive life, since we would be forced to make the false assumption that midwifery had been the same for all births. Due to these shortcomings, the present study examines the effects of midwifery on sterility only at the group level.

There are three major dependent variables: levels of primary sterility, incidence of secondary sterility, and prevalence of sterility (both primary and secondary). These variables are measured both at the group and at the individual level. For example, the prevalence of sterility by age group in a population or one of its subgroups is estimated at the group level without assigning an age at sterility to *individual* women in that group. At the individual level, each woman must be assigned a sterility status at each age. Since the second procedure is far more subject to error, both are used in different circumstances. Depending on the question to be addressed, the age range of women included in a particular analysis varies. For estimates of levels of primary sterility, only women married before age 20 are considered. (It becomes very difficult to distinguish between biological primary sterility and early secondary sterility in populations where menarche precedes the initiation of sexual relations by a relatively long time.) At the group level, age-specific prevalence rates of sterility are estimated by standard 5-year age intervals for women in the age range from 20–45. Sterility below age 20 is not examined in these analyses because of the complications caused by adolescent subfecundity. For women above age 45 the ability to have a live birth decreases sharply and biological aging is the predominant cause of sterility. At the later ages of the reproductive span, it also becomes more difficult to distinguish sterile from fecund women, a problem that is especially pronounced in studies of individual women (Larsen, 1985). Therefore, at the individual level, the analysis of the covariates of the incidence of sterility is limited to the age range from 20–40, while the covariates of the prevalence of sterility are analyzed for the age interval 20–45.

Finally, in order to determine a woman's status (sterile or fecund) at any age, at least 5 subsequent years of exposure are needed (the methods of measuring sterility are described below). Consequently, the closest to interview we can determine current sterility status is 5 years before survey, as utilized in model 1. In model 2 each woman's status is determined 5 years before survey, 10 years before survey, and so forth. The oldest women entered first marriage so long ago that we can determine their status 25 years before survey. As an alternative variable to time period, the link between different cohorts and sterility may be analyzed. In model 2 the cohorts examined are women born in the following periods: before 1933, 1933–1937, 1938–1942, 1943–1947, and 1948 and later.

Methods of Measuring Sterility

Primary sterility is measured among women who married below age 20 by the proportion childless after at least 7 years of marriage (Larsen, 1985; Vincent, 1950). Age-specific prevalence rates of sterility are estimated by a measure originally proposed by Louis Henry (1965, 1961) and termed "the proportion subsequently infertile." This method substitutes the number of infertile couples at a given age for the number of sterile couples at that age, where a couple is defined as being infertile if it has no live birth at that age or later (at least the next 5 years, if incomplete birth histories are used). The proportion sterile is then estimated as the number of infertile couples at a given age divided by all couples at that age. The relation between the estimated proportion sterile at a given age and the age at which this proportion sterile is attained was determined in a simulation study where the exact age at sterility of each woman as well as the exact proportion sterile at each age is known (Larsen, 1985).

An individual woman's status (sterile or fecund) at particular ages is determined on the basis of the length of the open birth interval. Women whose last live birth occurred less than 5 years before censoring are assigned the status of fecund when last observed; otherwise an age at onset of sterility is assigned. The age assigned is determined by the age at the last live birth (or marriage, if childless), but it is generally not equal to the age at the last reproductive event; the latter age usually precedes the actual age at onset of sterility. The correspondence between an individual woman's age at the last reproductive event and the age at onset of sterility has been determined in a simulation study (Larsen, 1985).

The introduced group and individual measures of sterility are robust to interpopulation variations in reproductive characteristics (age at marriage, the age pattern of sterility, and so forth) and to sampling variation in samples of at least 500 women. The primary sterility estimate requires a sample of at least 1000 women. Finally, individual assignments of ages at onset of sterility are quite sensitive and specific, although the accuracy declines with age (Larsen, 1985).

THE LEVELS OF STERILITY IN CAMEROON, KENYA, AND SUDAN

This section examines the prevalence of primary sterility and the levels of sterility by age for all women in a population and for selected subgroups. In order to carry out this analysis we need to define the sample of women who have been exposed to childbirth.

Only women in the age range from 15 to 50 who have been in one union for at least 5 years are considered. The required 5-year period of exposure might introduce a bias, because subfertile unions are frequently dissolved and even though divorced women usually remarry, they may not have been in a union 5 years or longer at censoring. The period of exposure is assumed to begin at first marriage, but there is evidence indicating that women are often sexually active prior to marriage (see Lesthaeghe, 1984a). This bias has little effect on the results, since the group measures of sterility and the assignment of individual ages at onset of sterility are quite robust to misassignment of age at first marriage (initiation of sexual relationships) (Larsen, 1985). Exposure ends at the time of survey, if the first marriage is intact, or at the dissolution of first marriage. In the latter case, the woman reenters the analysis at entry into second marriage, and so forth.

The study of sterility is complicated by the fact that not all women in the married state are sexually active. Some women practice postpartum abstinence, while other women have terminated all sexual activity, or are temporarily contracepting. Fortunately, the group and individual measures of sterility are not sensitive to variation in the period of postpartum abstinence (Larsen, 1985). The effects of terminal abstinence are also negligible, but only because it is rarely practiced. Only 2 percent (seventy-two women) in Cameroon and 1 percent (forty-eight women) in Kenya report terminal abstinence. No information is available about this question for Sudan.

Most people in Cameroon, Kenya, and Sudan want large families. Nevertheless, as many as 13 percent (564 women) in Cameroon, 32 percent (1306 women) in Kenya, and 24 percent (476 women) in Sudan report having used contraception. Consequently, the estimates of sterility may be biased, because fecund women who have contracepted efficiently over a long period of time might be falsely classified as sterile. Hence, to determine the effects of contraception on sterility, the levels of sterility by age are estimated separately for all women and for women who have never used contraception. Contraception appears to have almost no effect on the levels of sterility in these countries (table 4.1). In Sudan, only above age 35 is there slightly higher sterility for all women compared to women who have never used contraception. In Cameroon and Kenya women who have never used contraception have slightly higher age-specific rates of sterility than all women. These differences are small, so all women are included in the subsequent analysis.

The levels of sterility by age are highest in Cameroon, intermediate in

TABLE 4.1   The Proportion Subsequently Infertile Estimated for All Women and Women Who Have Never Used Contraception for Cameroon, Kenya, and Sudan and for All Women Married at Age 15–19 in England

	Proportion Subsequently Infertile						
	Cameroon		*Kenya*		*Sudan*		*England 1550–1849**
Age Group	All Women	Never Users	All Women	Never Users	All Women	Never Users	Women Married at Age 15–19
20–24	.17	.18	.05	.07	.09	.09	.07
25–29	.26	.27	.08	.10	.14	.14	.13
30–34	.38	.39	.14	.16	.27	.27	.23
35–39	.51	.52	.26	.28	.46	.44	.35
40–44	.69	.69	.52	.55	.74	.71	.58
Sample Size	4468	3212	4037	2731	2228	1859	—

*Estimates for England 1550–1849 are from Trussell and Wilson, 1984.

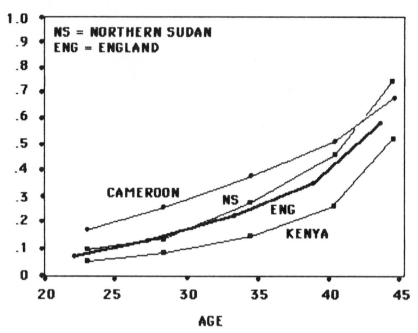

FIGURE 4.4. Age-Specific Sterility Rates in Three African Countries Compared to Those in Prenineteenth-Century England

Sudan, and lowest in Kenya for all ages below age 40 (figure 4.4). The age structure of the estimates is similar to that of a natural fertility population sample derived from reconstitutions of English families from 1550 to 1850 (Trussell and Wilson, 1985). The proportion sterile is systematically lower in Kenya than in England and systematically higher in Cameroon, while the proportion sterile in Sudan rises more steeply with age than in any of the other three populations. The levels of primary sterility for all women follow the same pattern as the age-specific rates of sterility (table 4.2). It is possible, however, that the estimates of primary sterility are too low because childlessness is probably underreported. There is also evidence of age misreporting

TABLE 4.2   The Proportion Childless among Women Married before Age 20 Estimated for Cameroon, Kenya, and Sudan

	Cameroon	Kenya	Sudan
All Women	.11	.02	.04
Sample Size	3518	3135	1826

and time misplacements of births and the impact of these reporting errors will be discussed later in this paper.

As a first step in the analysis of covariates of the prevalence of sterility, the samples of all women in Cameroon, Kenya, and Sudan were divided into subgroups defined by a single demographic or socioeconomic characteristic and the levels of sterility within groups was estimated. Variables had to be considered singly to maintain adequate sample sizes within each group. The characteristics analyzed include region, religion, residence, education, husband's education, husband's work status, type of circumcision, number of times married, marital status, location at delivery of last pregnancy, assistance of delivery of last pregnancy, and cohort.

The within-group differentials in sterility by demographic and socioeconomic factors are quite consistent across Cameroon, Kenya, and Sudan (tables 4.3 and 4.4). These observed differentials in sterility within a group may not be due to an association between the examined variable and sterility. Instead, they may be confounded by the effects of other covariates associated with sterility. For instance, uneducated women and women in certain regions appear to have higher sterility than educated women and women in other regions. However, it is possible that educated women live in regions with low sterility and that the apparent differentials by education are due to differences by region. In order to measure differentials in sterility within a variable and across variables it is necessary to estimate the effects of those variables hypothesized to be associated with sterility simultaneously. The requisite analysis cannot be carried out at the group level because of the sample size questions already described. Therefore, an individual level analysis was carried out to determine the effects of each variable simultaneously with several other variables hypothesized to be associated with sterility.[3]

Methods

In order to analyze simultaneously the effects of several demographic and socioeconomic factors on sterility at different points in time or by cohort, a hazards model approach is used. In general, a hazard or risk is the conditional probability of the occurrence of an event (dying, becoming sterile, and so forth) at a given age, provided that one has survived to that age without the event occurring. For example, assume that time can take only positive values ($t = 1, 2, 3, \ldots$) and that we observe a total of n independent individuals ($i = 1, \ldots, n$) beginning at time $t = 1$[4]. Then the discrete-time hazard rate is defined as

$$P_{it} = Pr(T_i = t \mid T_i \geq t, x_{it})$$

where T is a variable giving the time of event occurrence, and x_{it} is a vector of explanatory variables, which may take on different values at different discrete times.

TABLE 4.3 The Levels of Sterility by Age and by Demographic and Socioeconomic Factors Estimated by the Proportion Subsequently Infertile for Cameroon, Kenya, and Sudan

Proportion Subsequently Infertile

Region[1]

Variable: Age Group	Cameroon									Kenya							Sudan			
	CS	E	Li	N	NW	W	SW	Ya	Do	Na	Ce	Co	Ny	RV	W	E	Kh	N&E	Ce	K&D
20–24	.22	.19	.11	.25	.07	.08	.07	.14	.14	.04	.04	.10	.07	.03	.05	.05	.07	.07	.06	.12
25–29	.32	.28	.16	.38	.13	.13	.14	.22	.23	.06	.05	.15	.09	.07	.10	.07	.13	.11	.12	.18
30–34	.44	.37	.26	.54	.21	.21	.31	.37	.34	.30	.08	.24	.15	.11	.14	.11	.27	.21	.24	.34
35–39	.58	.50	.42	.65	.33	.31	.46	.59	.47	.57	.14	.46	.31	.25	.30	.18	.52	.50	.42	.43
40–44	.79	.66	.57	.75	.51	.52	.56	.94	.73	.87	.34	.63	.57	.47	.54	.50	.88	.77	.69	.66
Sample size	643	594	319	1143	473	414	205	252	383	222	640	313	919	780	494	644	428	540	575	685

Religion

Age Group	Cameroon			Kenya	
	Christian	Muslim	Other	Christian	Muslim
20–24	.13	.32	.12	.05	.14
25–29	.21	.46	.15	.07	.16
30–34	.33	.59	.27	.13	.22
35–39	.47	.70	.34	.25	.42
40–44	.65	.86	.49	.52	.54
Sample size	3156	810	491	3585	177

Residence[2]

Age Group	Cameroon				Kenya				Sudan			
	Rural	Urban	Rural to Urban	Urban to Rural	Rural	Urban	Rural to Urban	Urban to Rural	Rural	Urban	Rural to Urban	Urban to Rural
20–24	.17	.21	.17	.23	.05	.18	.08	.06	.09	.08	.06	.08
25–29	.25	.33	.28	.32	.08	.22	.13	.06	.14	.15	.06	.16
30–34	.37	.46	.35	.45	.12	.46	.30	.19	.26	.30	.18	.34
35–39	.50	.57	.44	.53	.24	.63	.55	.39	.40	.56	.51	.56
40–44	.67	.79	.56	.89	.50	.74	.91	.73	.69	.80	.87	.72
Sample size	3210	498	464	178	3316	88	499	134	1103	793	162	168

Education[3]

	No Schooling	Primary	Secondary & Higher	No Schooling	Primary	Secondary & Higher	No Schooling	Primary & Higher
20–24	.18	.14	.11	.06	.04	.01	.09	.05
25–29	.26	.24	.17	.10	.05	.07	.14	.12
30–34	.39	.34	.43	.15	.08	.41	.28	.34
35–39	.51	.50	.63	.28	.18	.62	.44	.76
40–44	.68	.79	.84	.51	.53	.67	.72	1.00
Sample size	3310	972	184	2369	1551	112	1817	530

Husband's Education

	No Schooling	Primary	Secondary & Higher	No Schooling	Primary	Secondary & Higher	No Schooling	Incomplete Primary	Primary & Higher
20–24	.18	.14	.15	.06	.05	.04	.10	.06	.05
25–29	.27	.23	.26	.10	.07	.06	.15	.12	.14
30–34	.40	.33	.38	.15	.12	.17	.28	.23	.28
35–39	.51	.49	.54	.29	.22	.32	.44	.49	.64
40–44	.67	.71	.85	.53	.50	.62	.71	.77	.90
Sample size	2471	1487	474	1343	2174	419	1368	530	330

Husband's work status

	Employer	Self-Employed	Employee	Employer	Self-Employed	Employee	Employer	Self-Employed	Employee
20–24	.19	.18	.14	.04	.07	.05	.09	.11	.06
25–29	.32	.26	.23	.04	.10	.07	.14	.16	.12
30–34	.37	.39	.33	.11	.15	.13	.26	.27	.28
35–39	.45	.51	.50	.23	.26	.27	.50	.44	.47
40–44	.59	.69	.74	.54	.53	.51	.86	.70	.74
Sample size	252	2856	1334	358	1540	2128	372	803	1053

Type of circumcision

	Pharaonic	Other
20–24	.09	.07
25–29	.14	.14
30–34	.27	.26
35–39	.46	.45
40–44	.74	.74
Sample size	1749	434

TABLE 4.3 Continued

Proportion Subsequently Infertile

Times in union

Variable	Age Group	Cameroon 1	Cameroon 2+	Kenya 1	Kenya 2+	Sudan 1	Sudan 2+
Times in union	20–24	.15	.36	.05	.14	.07	.21
	25–29	.23	.47	.08	.15	.12	.26
	30–34	.35	.59	.13	.24	.25	.41
	35–39	.46	.72	.23	.46	.43	.64
	40–44	.63	.86	.52	.51	.70	.92
Sample size		4062	406	3930	~107	2143	85

Marital status[+]

Cameroon

Age Group	Monogamous	Polygynous	1	2	3
20–24	.16	.18	.16	.20	.17
25–29	.24	.26	.23	.31	.25
30–34	.38	.37	.34	.43	.37
35–39	.52	.49	.46	.58	.46
40–44	.69	.67	.61	.83	.63
Sample size	2224	1634	750	617	267

Kenya

Age Group	Monogamous	Polygynous	1	2	3	4
20–24	.04	.08	.08	.07	.09	.11
25–29	.05	.13	.13	.09	.19	.16
30–34	.09	.20	.20	.16	.21	.25
35–39	.22	.31	.32	.29	.25	.38
40–44	.49	.58	.67	.51	.48	.60
Sample size	2591	1611	404	422	80	255

Sudan

Age Group	Monogamous	Polygynous
20–24	.07	.14
25–29	.12	.20
30–34	.25	.34
35–39	.44	.54
40–44	.70	.86
Sample size	1731	497

Location of delivery, last pregnancy (Cameroon)

Age Group	Home	Dispensary	Hospital
20–24	.13	.05	.06
25–29	.24	.11	.14
30–34	.39	.20	.25
35–39	.50	.33	.37
40–44	.67	.47	.62
Sample size	1669	626	1302

Assistance at delivery, last pregnancy	Family Member	Midwife, Nurse	Doctor	Other
20–24	.13	.05	.09	.11
25–29	.25	.11	.21	.17
30–34	.40	.21	.35	.31
35–39	.52	.32	.47	.37
40–44	.70	.53	.52	.55
Sample size	1559	1800	141	128

Cohorts	Born Before 1941	Born 1941–1955	Born Before 1941	Born 1941–1955	Born Before 1941	Born 1941–1955
20–24	.20	.15	.04	.06	.10	.08
25–29	.27	.23	.07	.10	.16	.12
30–34	.38	.35	.13	.15	.28	.18
35–39	.51	—	.26	—	.46	—
40–44	.69	—	.52	—	.74	—
Sample size	1907	2418	1549	2460	619	1459

1. **Cameroon:** CS = Center-South; E = East; Li = Littoral; N = North; NW = Northwest; W = West; SW = Southwest; Ya = Yaounde; Do = Douala. **Kenya:** Na = Nairobi; Ce = Central; C = Coast; Ny = Nyanza; RV = Rift Valley; W = Western; E = Eastern. **Sudan:** Kh = Khartoum; N&E = Northern & Eastern; Ce = Central; K&D = Kordofan & Darfur.

2. Rural = childhood residence and residence at survey are rural.
   Urban = childhood residence and residence at survey are urban.
   Rural to Urban = childhood residence is rural and residence at survey is urban.
   Urban to Rural = childhood residence is urban and residence at survey is rural.

3. Different grouping in the questionnaire for Sudan (no schooling, primary and higher).

4. **Cameroon:** 1 Polygamous, rank 1; 2 Polygamous, rank 2; 3 Polygamous, rank 3+. **Kenya:** 1 Polygamous 2 wives, rank 1; 2 Polygamous 2 wives, rank 2; 3 Polygamous 3+ wives, rank 1; 4 Polygamous 3+ wives, rank 2+.

TABLE 4.4   The proportion childless among women married below age 20 estimated by different demographic and socioeconomic characteristics for Cameroon, Kenya and Sudan

Variable/Category	Proportion childless		
	Cameroon	Kenya	Sudan
Region[1]			
1	.13*	.01**	.04**
2	.12**	.02*	.04*
3	.05**	.04*	.04
4	.17	.03	.04
5	.03*	.01	—
6	.04*	.02*	—
7	.02**	.01*	—
8	.05**	—	—
9	.04**	—	—
Religion			
Christian	.07	.02	—
Muslim	.20	.05**	—
Other	.09		
Residence[2]			
Rural	.11	.02	.04
Urban	.13*	.03**	.04
Rural to urban	.09*	.04*	.06**
Urban to rural	.09**	.03**	.02**
Education[3]			
No schooling	.12	.03	.04
Primary	.05	.01	.03*
Secondary and higher	.06**	.00**	
Husband's Education[5]			
No schooling	.13	.02	.04
Primary	.07	.02	.04
Secondary and Higher	.06*	.02*	.02*
Husband's Work Status			
Employer	.15*	.02*	.04*
Self-employed	.11	.03	.05
Employee	.07	.02	.03
Type of Circumcision			
Pharaonic	—	—	.04
Other	—	—	.04*
Times Married			
1	.09	.02	.04
2+	.26*	.07**	.07**
Marital Status[4]			
Monogamous	.10	.01	.03
Polygamous	.12	.04	.07*

TABLE 4.4   *Continued*

Variable/Category	*Proportion childless*		
	Cameroon	*Kenya*	*Sudan*
1	.09	.03*	—
2	.14	.04*	—
3	.13**	.08**	—
4	—	.03**	—
Cohorts			
Born before 1941	.13	.02	.05*
Born 1941–1955	.09	.02	.03

* Fewer than 500 cases
** Fewer than 250 cases
1. **Cameroon**; 1 Center-South; 2 East; 3 Littoral; 4 North; 5 Northwest; 6 West; 7 Southwest; 8 Yaounde; 9 Douala. **Kenya**: 1 Nairobi; 2 Central; 3 Coast; 4 Nyanza; 5 Rift Valley; 6 Western; 7 Eastern. **Sudan**: 1 Khartoum; 2 Northern & Eastern; 3 Central; 4 Kordofan & Darfur.
2–4. See footnotes 2, 3, 4 to table 4.3.
5. Different grouping in the questionnaire for Sudan (no schooling, incomplete primary, primary and higher).

In the present study the logistic regression function is used to specify how the hazard rate depends on time and the explanatory variables. The explanatory variables for individuals i are in the form of a vector $x_{it} = (x_{i1t}, x_{i2t}, \ldots, x_{ijt})$, where there are j variables. Here, the value for an individual on a specific characteristic variable can vary over time. Then the logistic regression function for individual i at time t is

$$P_{it} = 1/(1 + \exp(-a - b'x_{it})).$$

In logit form, this becomes

$$\log(P_{it}/(1 - P_{it})) = a + b'x_{it}$$

where a is a constant and b' is the vector of regression coefficients associated with the risk factors x_{it}. When the risk factors x_{it} are restricted to be categorical variables, the regression coefficients can be used to determine the odds of the occurrence of the event under study, where the odds are defined as the ratio of the probability the event occurs to the probability it does not occur. In this case, all the x_{ijt} are dummy variables where x_{ijt} equals 1 if individual i is in the category represented by the jth variable and is zero otherwise. The predicted odds of an event occurring for individual i in interval t are $\exp(a + b'x_{it})$.

The ratio of two odds is called the relative odds. Hence, the odds at a given time for individual i relative to the odds for individual i' are $\exp(a + b'x_{it} - a - b'x_{i't})$. In general, it is of interest to determine the relative odds when all factors but one are the same for the two groups of people. For example, if there is a three-category variable represented by two dummy variables x_{i1t} and x_{i2t}, and individual i has $x_{i1t} = 1$ and $x_{i2t} = 0$, whereas individual i' has $x_{i'1t} = 0$ and $x_{i'2t} = 1$, then the relative odds (RO) are exp $(b_1 - b_2)$. Thus, for a given variable, if RO is greater than 1, then the odds of an event are higher for individual i who is in category 1 relative to individual i' who is in category 2; if RO is less than or equal to 1, those in category 1 have lower than or the same odds of an event as those in category 2 when the categories on all other variables are exactly the same.

In practice, this procedure treats each discrete age interval for each individual as a separate observation or unit of analysis. For each of these observations in the incidence analysis, the dependent variable is coded 1 if an event occurred to that individual in that age interval; otherwise it is coded 0. Thus, if an individual experienced an event at age interval 5, at least five different observations could be created. For the fifth observation the dependent variable would be coded 1. For the other four observations, the dependent variable would be coded 0. In the prevalence analysis, the dependent variable is coded 1 if an event occurred in that age interval or in a previous age interval; otherwise it is coded 0.

The explanatory variables for each of these new observations would be assigned whatever values they had at that particular unit of age. When prevalence rates (such as, the probability of being sterile) are estimated, all individuals exit the analysis at censoring, whereas when incidence rates (for example, the probability of becoming sterile) are estimated, individuals exit the analysis either at censoring or at the time of the event, whichever comes first. These observations are pooled and the models are estimated by a maximum likelihood procedure.[5]

A backward stepwise procedure was used to determine the model that fits the data best. The idea behind this procedure is that we have one model (the unrestricted model) and a second model (the restricted model), which is a subset of the unrestricted model. A restricted model is established when some parameters are constrained either to equal some given value (for example, $b_0 = 0$) or to be related in a specific way to other parameters (such as, $b_1 = 2b_2$). The maximized log-likelihood in the restricted model is less than or equal to the maximized log-likelihood in the unrestricted model, since the maximum likelihood estimates in the restricted model are possible values of the parameters in the unrestricted model. Consequently, if the restrictions are valid, the value of the restricted log-likelihood function should be almost as large as that of the unrestricted model. If W_R is the log-likelihood of the restricted model, and W_U is the log-likelihood of the unrestricted model, each evaluated at their respective maximum likelihood estimates, then $-2(W_R - W_U)$ is distributed asymptotically as a χ^2 variate with degrees of freedom equal to the difference in the number of free parameters in the two models. If the χ^2 statistic is not significantly different from zero, the restricted model is accepted as fitting the data nearly as well as the unrestricted model. Thus, the backward stepwise procedure first fits the model to all the covariates analyzed, and then eliminates covariates one-by-one on the basis of minimum loss in the likelihood value.

In the present study only the effects of age and the effects of each covariate (main effects) are estimated, while the effects of any interactions are not examined. Hence, it is implicitly assumed that there is no interaction between age and any of the covariates so that the model is a proportional hazards model. In such a model, there is a constant underlying hazard function and the effect of a covariate is to raise or lower this hazard function by the same proportional amount at every age. This restriction appears to be a reasonable one because the factors that cause sterility are most likely independent of age, with the exception of biological aging. For instance, PID has the same damaging effect on all women's reproductive systems and primary sterility due to female circumcision occurs before menarche. It is very easy to assess the quantitative impact of one variable relative to another in a main effects model by analyzing relative odds, while it becomes more complicated when interactions are also included (Trussell and Hammerslough, 1983; Allison, 1982; Cox, 1972).

The Covariates of Sterility in Cameroon, Kenya, and Sudan

The effects on sterility of several covariates that are analyzed simultaneously (multivariate models), as well as the effects of age interval and each covariate considered separately (univariate models) are estimated in this section.[6] The prevalence of sterility is defined as the proportion of sterile women at a given age (referred to as proportion being sterile), while the incidence of sterility refers to the proportion of women who became sterile during the last 5 years (referred to as proportion becoming sterile). First, the results of the analysis of the prevalence and incidence of sterility 5 years before the survey are reported. Second, the prevalence and incidence of sterility at different points in time or across cohorts are addressed.

In the analysis of sterility 5 years before survey the covariates examined are the variables defined in model 1. The differentials in the prevalence and incidence of sterility follow the same pattern in the three countries examined (table 4.5). In general, most variables are significant in the univariate models of the prevalence of sterility, while fewer variables contribute significantly to the fit in the multivariate models (table 4.6). For instance, educated women have lower prevalence of sterility than uneducated women in the univariate models for Cameroon and Kenya, while education is not significant in the multivariate models. This implies that the factors associated with lower sterility are overrepresented among educated women, and, when the effects of these other variables are controlled, the apparent beneficial aspects of education are reduced.

Several of the variables included in the analysis have a significant effect on

TABLE 4.5*a*   Relative Odds[†] of Sterility 5 Years before Survey: Prevalence and Incidence Estimated from Univariate and Multivariate Models for Cameroon

Variable/Category	Relative Odds		Relative Odds	
	Prevalence of Sterility		Incidence of Sterility	
	Univariate	Multivariate	Univariate	Multivariate
	Cameroon			
Age				
20–24	1.00	1.00	1.00	1.00
25–29	1.37	1.38	2.01	2.08
30–34	2.51	2.68	2.73	2.83
35–39	4.14	4.34	3.75	4.20
40–44	5.11	5.61	—	—
Region				
Center-South	1.29*	1.16*	.66*	.26
East	1.01*	.83*	.71*	.29
Littoral	.72*	.63*	.59*	.26
North	1.96	1.12*	1.02*	.42*
Northwest	.56	.46	.44	.19
West	.50	.36	.39	.16
Southwest	.76*	.65*	.81*	.31
Yaounde	1.00	1.00	1.00	1.00
Douala	.84*	.77*	.83*	.72*
Religion				NS
Christian	1.00	1.00	1.00	
Muslim	2.71	1.94	1.54	
Other	1.10*	.91*	1.03*	
Residence**		NS	NS	
Rural	1.00			1.00
Urban	1.13*			.62*
Rural to urban	.75*			.32
Urban to rural	1.45*			1.74*
Education		NS	NS	NS
No schooling	1.00			
Primary	.67			
Secondary and higher	.74*			
Husband's Education		NS	NS	NS
No schooling	1.00			
Primary	.69			
Secondary and higher	.74*			
Husband's Work Status	NS		NS	NS
Employer		1.00		
Self-employed		.91*		
Employee		.68		
Times Married				NS
1	1.00	1.00	1.00	
2+	2.16	1.78	1.53	

TABLE 4.5a   *Continued*

Variable/Category	Relative Odds		Relative Odds	
	Prevalence of Sterility		Incidence of Sterility	
	Univariate	Multivariate	Univariate	Multivariate
		Cameroon		
Marital Status		NS		NS
Monogamous	1.00		1.00	
Polygamous rank 1	1.03*		.68	
Polygamous rank 2	1.04*		.91*	
Polygamous rank 3+	.91*		.65*	
Ever Used Contraception			NS	NS
No	1.00	1.00		
Yes	.64	.66		

†All odds are calculated relative to a reference category indicated by having odds = 1.00.
*Not significantly different from the reference category at the 5% level using a two-tailed test.
**Rural = childhood residence and residence at survey are rural.
  Urban = childhood residence and residence at survey are urban.
  Rural to urban = childhood residence is rural and residence at survey is urban.
  Urban to rural = childhood residence is urban and residence at survey is rural.
NS Nonsignificant variable at the 5% level.
—Not used category.

TABLE 4.5b   Relative Odds† of Sterility 5 Years before Survey: Prevalence and Incidence Estimated from Univariate and Multivariate Models for Kenya

Variable/Category	Relative Odds		Relative Odds	
	Prevalence of Sterility		Incidence of Sterility	
	Univariate	Multivariate	Univariate	Multivariate
		Kenya		
Age				
20–24	1.00	1.00	1.00	1.00
25–29	1.91	1.97	1.73	1.72
30–34	2.98	2.88	2.15	2.16
35–39	4.16	3.97	2.42	2.42
40–44	7.88	7.42	—	—
Region				
Nairobi	1.00	1.00	1.00	1.00
Central	.26	.26	.25	.24
Coast	.88*	.62*	.35	.30
Nyanza	.69*	.53	.54*	.51*
Rift Valley	.37	.35	.33	.33
Western	.63*	.43	.50*	.42
Eastern	.40	.33	.39	.35
Religion		NS	NS	NS
Christian	1.00			

TABLE 4.5b   Continued

Variable/Category	Relative Odds		Relative Odds	
	Prevalence of Sterility		Incidence of Sterility	
	Univariate	Multivariate	Univariate	Multivariate
		Kenya		
Muslim	2.05			
Other	1.01*			
Residence**		NS	NS	NS
Rural	1.00			
Urban	1.73*			
Rural to urban	1.77			
Urban to rural	1.58*			
Education		NS	NS	NS
No schooling	1.00			
Primary	.66			
Secondary and higher	.83*			
Husband's Education		NS		NS
No schooling	1.00		1.00	
Primary	.69		.65	
Secondary and higher	.82*		.96*	
Husband's Work Status	NS	NS	NS	NS
Employer				
Self-employed				
Employee				
Times Married				
1	1.00	1.00	1.00	1.00
2+	2.56	2.46	2.67	2.70
Marital Status			NS	NS
Monogamous	1.00	1.00		
Polygamous 2 wives rank 1	2.10	1.96		
Polygamous 2 wives rank 2	1.34*	1.19*		
Polygamous 3+ wives rank 1	2.29	2.05		
Polygamous 3+ wives rank 2+	1.87	1.49		
Ever Used Contraception			NS	NS
No	1.00	1.00		
Yes	.59	.69		

†All odds are calculated relative to a reference category indicated by having odds = 1.00.
* Not significantly different from the reference category at the 5% level using a two-tailed test.
** Rural = childhood residence and residence at survey are rural.
   Urban = childhood residence and residence at survey are urban.
   Rural to urban = childhood residence is rural and residence at survey is urban.
   Urban to rural = childhood residence is urban and residence at survey is rural.
NS Nonsignificant variable at the 5% level.
—Not used category.

TABLE 4.5c   Relative Odds† of Sterility 5 Years before Survey: Prevalence and Incidence Estimated from Univariate and Multivariate Models for Sudan

Variable/Category	Relative Odds		Relative Odds	
	Prevalence of Sterility		Incidence of Sterility	
	Univariate	Multivariate	Univariate	Multivariate
	Sudan			
Age				
20–24	1.00	1.00	1.00	1.00
25–29	2.08	2.06	1.33*	1.33*
30–34	2.74	2.58	.91*	.88*
35–39	7.71	7.25	3.32	3.18
40–44	11.23	10.65	—	—
Region				
Khartoum	1.00	1.00	1.00	1.00
Northern & Eastern	.64	.62	.47	.48
Central	.51	.49	.42	.44
Kordofan & Darfur	.93*	.79*	.79*	.78*
Residence**	NS	NS	NS	NS
Rural				
Urban				
Rural to urban				
Urban to rural				
Education	NS	NS	NS	NS
No schooling				
Incomplete primary				
Primary and higher				
Husband's Education	NS	NS	NS	NS
No schooling				
Incomplete primary				
Secondary and higher				
Husband's Work Status	NS	NS	NS	NS
Employer				
Self-employed				
Employee				
Type of Circumcision	NS	NS	NS	
Pharaonic				1.77*
Other				1.00*
Times Married				
1	1.00	1.00	1.00	1.00
2+	2.12	1.95	1.84	1.70
Marital Status			NS	NS
Monogamous	1.00	1.00		
Polygamous	1.71	1.57		

TABLE 4.5c   *Continued*

Variable/Category	Relative Odds		Relative Odds	
	Prevalence of Sterility		Incidence of Sterility	
	Univariate	Multivariate	Univariate	Multivariate
Ever Used Contranception No Yes	NS	NS	NS	NS

˙All odds are calculated relative to a reference category indicated by having odds = 1.00.
*Not significantly different from the reference category at the 5% level using a two-tailed test.
**Rural = childhood residence and residence at survey are rural.
Urban = childhood residence and residence at survey are urban.
Rural to urban = childhood residence is rural and residence at survey is urban.
Urban to rural = childhood residence is urban and residence at survey is rural.
NS Nonsignificant variable at the 5% level.
—Not used category.

the prevalence of sterility, while relatively few are associated with the incidence of sterility. This may result from the fact that incidence is measured less precisely than prevalence of sterility and measurement errors might obscure the effects on estimates of incidence (Larsen, 1985). Also, sample sizes decrease more sharply with age when the incidence of sterility is analyzed, and small sample sizes may permit fewer variables to reach statistical significance. Finally, certain factors may affect the ability to have another live birth at only certain ages, and these effects are not captured by a model without interaction terms.

The results from the analysis of individual women support the findings obtained at the group level. For instance, the prevalence of sterility relative to the age interval 20–24 rises fastest in Sudan, more moderately in Kenya, and slowest in Cameroon in both the univariate and multivariate models 5 years before survey. This pattern was expected, because the age-specific rates of sterility are substantially higher in Cameroon compared to Sudan at ages 20–24 and about the same at ages 40–45 (in fact higher in Sudan). It should also be noted that the multivariate odds of becoming sterile increase moderately up to age 35 and then more rapidly in all three countries. Thus, this analysis provides further evidence that biological aging affects the ability to reproduce most substantially above age 35. There is no evidence of a rapid rise as early as age 30, as some researchers have suggested (Federation CECOS, et al., 1982; DeCherney and Beikowitz, 1982).

The covariates examined in the analysis of sterility by time period or cohort are defined in model 2. The description of the effects of these covariates on sterility is restricted to the results from the multivariate models (table 4.7). The findings in the models that include time period are similar to those

TABLE 4.6 Significant/Nonsignificant Covariates of Sterility 5 Years before Survey: Prevalence and Incidence Estimated from Univariate (U) and Multivariate (M) Models for Cameroon, Kenya, and Sudan

Variable	Cameroon Significance — Prevalence of Sterility U	M	Incidence of Sterility U	M	Kenya Significance — Prevalence of Sterility U	M	Incidence of Sterility U	M	Sudan Significance — Prevalence of Sterility U	M	Incidence of Sterility U	M
Age	S	S	S	S	S	S	S	S	S	S	S	S
Region	S	S	S	S	S	S	S	S	S	S	S	S
Religion	S	S	S	NS	S	NS	NS	NS	NS	—	—	—
Residence	S	NS	NS	S	S	NS	NS	NS	NS	NS	NS	NS
Education	S	NS	NS	NS	S	NS	NS	NS	NS	NS	NS	NS
Husband's education	S	NS	NS	NS	S	NS	S	NS	NS	NS	NS	NS
Husband's work status	NS	S	NS	NS	NS	NS	NS	NS	NS	NS	NS	NS
Type of circumcision	—	—	—	—	—	—	—	—	NS	NS	NS	S
Time married	S	S	S	NS	S	S	S	S	S	S	S	S
Marital status	S	NS	S	NS	S	S	NS	NS	S	S	NS	NS
Ever used contraception	S	S	NS	NS	S	S	NS	NS	NS	NS	NS	NS

S Significant variable at the 5% level.
NS Nonsignificant variable at the 5% level.
— Not used category.

TABLE 4.7a Relative Odds† of Sterility by Time Period or Cohort: Prevalence and Incidence Estimated from Multivariate Models for Cameroon

Variable/Category	Relative Odds		Relative Odds	
	Models with Time Period		Models with Cohort	
	Prevalence of Sterility	Incidence of Sterility	Prevalence of Sterility	Incidence of Sterility
	Cameroon			
Age				
20–24	1.00	1.00	1.00	1.00
25–29	1.90	2.27	1.46	1.23
30–34	3.17	2.54	2.25	1.64
35–39	5.30	3.59	2.96	1.95
40–44	7.48	—	9.00	—
Cohort				NS
Born before 1933			1.17*	
Born 1933–1937			.97*	
Born 1938–1942			.99*	
Born 1943–1947			.76*	
Born 1948+			1.00	
Time Period/Years	NS	NS		
Before 1978 Survey				
5				
10				
15				
20				
25				
Region				
Center-South	1.38*	.83*	1.69	1.05*
East	.92*	.59	1.17*	.74*
Littoral	.55	.49	.59	.50
North	.87*	.62	.94*	.64*
Northwest	.37	.39	.41	.45
West	.28	.29	.29	.28
Southwest	.47	.44	.56	.53
Yaounde	1.00	1.00	1.00	1.00
Douala	.68	.76*	.85*	.86*
Religion				
Christian	1.00	1.00	1.00	1.00
Muslim	2.25	1.73	2.81	2.40
Other	.80	.87*	.81*	1.02*
Residence**		NS		NS
Rural	1.00		1.00	
Urban	1.26		1.35	
Rural to urban	1.03*		1.14*	
Urban to rural	1.31		1.55	
Education	NS	NS	NS	NS
No schooling				

TABLE 4.7a *Continued*

Variable/Category	*Relative Odds*		*Relative Odds*	
	Models with Time Period		Models with Cohort	
	Prevalence of Sterility	Incidence of Sterility	Prevalence of Sterility	Incidence of Sterility
	Cameroon			
Primary				
Secondary and higher				
Times in union				
1	1.00	1.00	1.00	1.00
2+	2.07	1.86	2.09	1.73
Ever used contraception[†]				
No	1.00	1.00	1.00	1.00
Yes	.46	.73	.44	.65

[†] All odds are calculated relative to a reference category indicated by having odds = 1.00.
* Not significantly different from the reference category at the 5% level using a two-tailed test.
** Rural = childhood residence and residence at survey are rural.
  Urban = childhood residence and residence at survey are urban.
  Rural to urban = childhood residence is rural and residence at survey is urban.
  Urban to rural = childhood residence is urban and residence at survey is rural.
[†] Status at survey.
NS Nonsignificant variable at the 5% level.
— Not used category.

TABLE 4.7b   Relative Odds[†] of Sterility by Time Period or Cohort: Prevalence and Incidence Estimated from Multivariate Models for Kenya

Variable/Category	*Relative Odds*		*Relative Odds*	
	Models with Time Period		Models with Cohort	
	Prevalence of Sterility	Incidence of Sterility	Prevalence of Sterility	Incidence of Sterility
	Kenya			
Age				
20–24	1.00	1.00	1.00	1.00
25–29	2.10	1.94	1.34	.89*
30–34	2.86	2.02	2.01	1.20*
35–39	4.26	2.67	3.78	2.66
40–44	7.45	—	20.66	—
Cohort			NS	NS
Born before 1933				
Born 1933–1937				
Born 1938–1942				
Born 1943–1947				
Born 1948+				
Time Period/Years				
Before 1977–1978 Survey				
5	1.00	1.00		
10	.73	1.02*		

TABLE 4.7*b*   *Continued*

Variable/Category	Relative Odds		Relative Odds	
	Models with Time Period		Models with Cohort	
	Prevalence of Sterility	Incidence of Sterility	Prevalence of Sterility	Incidence of Sterility
	Kenya			
15	.54	.54		
20	.61	.67		
25	.55	.65*		
Region				
Nairobi	1.00	1.00	1.00	1.00
Central	.71*	.30	.67*	.23
Coast	1.21*	.59*	1.44*	.65*
Nyanza	1.19*	.51	1.02*	.36
Rift Valley	.79*	.42	.91*	.38
Western	1.06*	.48	1.11*	.42
Eastern	.78*	.37	.76*	.28
Religion	NS	NS	NS	NS
Christian				
Muslim				
Other				
Residence**		NS		NS
Rural	1.00		1.00	
Urban	3.35		3.43	
Rural to urban	1.75		1.63	
Urban to rural	1.78		1.98	
Education				
No schooling	1.00	1.00	1.00	1.00
Primary	.58	.74	.51	.59
Secondary and higher	.86*	1.16*	1.41*	1.56*
Times in union				
1	1.00	1.00	1.00	1.00
2+	2.17	2.44	2.11	1.98
Ever used contraception[†]				
No	1.00	1.00	1.00	1.00
Yes	.56	.68	.53	.73

[†]   All odds are calculated relative to a reference category indicated by having odds = 1.00.

*   Not significantly different from the reference category at the 5% level using a two-tailed test.

** Rural = childhood residence and residence at survey are rural.

      Urban = childhood residence and residence at survey are urban.

      Rural to urban = childhood residence is rural and residence at survey is urban.

      Urban to rural = childhood residence is urban and residence at survey is rural.

[†]   Status at survey.

NS Nonsignificant variable at the 5% level.

— Not used category.

TABLE 4.7c   Relative Odds† of Sterility by Time Period or Cohort:
Prevalence and Incidence Estimated from Multivariate Models for Sudan

Variable/Category	*Relative Odds*		*Relative Odds*	
	Models with Time Period		Models with Cohort	
	Prevalence of Sterility	Incidence of Sterility	Prevalence of Sterility	Incidence of Sterility
		Sudan		
Age				
20–24	1.00	1.00	1.00	1.00
25–29	2.24	1.09*	1.45	.94*
30–34	3.55	1.19*	2.64	1.99
35–39	7.18	2.15	4.43	2.82
40–44	13.87	—	25.80	—
Cohort				NS
Born before 1933			1.26*	
Born 1933–1937			.85*	
Born 1938–1942			.92*	
Born 1943–1947			.68*	
Born 1948+			1.00	
Time Period/Years				
Before 1979 Survey	NS	NS		
5				
10				
15				
20				
25				
Region				
Khartoum	1.00	1.00	1.00	NS
Northern & Eastern	.83*	.67	1.02*	
Central	.79*	.59	.96*	
Kordofan & Darfur	1.35*	.95*	1.69	
Residence**		NS		
Rural	1.00		1.00	1.00
Urban	1.35		1.37	1.40
Rural to urban	.77*		.63*	.80*
Urban to rural	1.18*		1.19*	1.47*
Education	NS	NS	NS	NS
No schooling				
Incomplete primary				
Primary and higher				
Type of circumcision	NS	NS	NS	NS
Pharaonic				
Other				

TABLE 4.7c　Continued

Variable/Category	Relative Odds		Relative Odds	
	Models with Time Period		Models with Cohort	
	Prevalence of Sterility	Incidence of Sterility	Prevalence of Sterility	Incidence of Sterility
		Sudan		
Times in union				
1	1.00	1.00	1.00	1.00
2+	2.12	1.91	2.44	2.19
Ever used contraception[†]	NS	NS	NS	NS
No				
Yes				

[†]　All odds are calculated relative to a reference category indicated by having odds = 1.00.
*　Not significantly different from the reference category at the 5% level using a two-tailed test.
**　Rural = childhood residence and residence at survey are rural.
　Urban = childhood residence and residence at survey are urban.
　Rural to urban = childhood residence is rural and residence at survey is urban.
　Urban to rural = childhood residence is urban and residence at survey is rural.
[†]　Status at survey.
NS　Nonsignificant variable at the 5% level.
—　Not used category.

in the models that include cohort (table 4.8). Furthermore, the variables found to be significant in these models are generally also significant in the models of sterility 5 years before survey. This pattern suggests that sterility is relatively invariant across cohorts and during recent decades. In line with this finding the variations across cohorts are not significant in any of the three countries.[7] Time period, however, is significant in the models for Kenya, where the multivariate odds of being sterile are significantly lower 10, 15, 20, and 25 years before survey relative to 5 years before survey (0.73, 0.54, 0.61, and 0.55 vs. 1.00), while the probability of becoming sterile is significantly lower only 15 and 20 relative to 5 years before survey (0.54 and 0.66 vs. 1.00). It should be noted that the major difference between the covariates included in the analysis 5 years before survey and those in the models incorporating time period or cohort is that the former contains marital status (monogamous vs. polygamous unions).

Discussion

The levels of sterility by age for all women are highest in Cameroon, moderate in Sudan, and lowest in Kenya. The estimated age-specific rates of sterility may be lower than the true rates because in each of these countries, there is evidence of a tendency to misreport births as occurring closer to the time of survey than they did in actuality: that is, if date at last birth is mis-

TABLE 4.8 Significant/Nonsignificant Covariates of Sterility by Time Period or Cohort: Prevalence (P) and Incidence (I) Estimated from Multivariate Models for Cameroon, Kenya, and Sudan

Variable	Cameroon — Significance				Kenya — Significance				Sudan — Significance			
	Time Period		Cohort		Time Period		Cohort		Time Period		Cohort	
	P	I	P	I	P	I	P	I	P	I	P	I
Age	S	S	S	S	S	S	S	S	S	S	S	S
Cohort	—	NS	S	NS	—	—	NS	NS	—	—	S	NS
Time Period	NS	S	—	—	S	S	—	—	NS	S	—	—
Region	S	S	S	S	NS	S	S	NS	S	S	S	NS
Religion	S	S	NS	NS	S	NS	NS	NS	—	—	—	—
Residence	S	NS	S	NS	S	S	S	S	S	NS	S	S
Education	NS	NS	NS	NS	—	—	—	—	NS	NS	NS	NS
Type of circumcision	—	—	—	—	—	—	—	—	S	S	S	NS
Time in union	S	S	S	S	S	S	S	S	S	S	S	S
Ever used contraception	S	S	S	S	S	S	S	S	NS	NS	NS	NS

S Significant variable at the 5% level.
NS Nonsignificant variable at the 5% level.
— Not used category.

placed in the direction of the date at survey, then the proportion subsequently infertile at a given age is underestimated and, at the individual level, age at
onset of sterility is assigned later than the true age of sterility. Furthermore,
some women might have overstated their age, which has the same effect on
the estimated levels of sterility as does the time misplacement of the date of
the last birth (Santow and Bioumla, 1984; Rizgalla, 1984; Henin, Korten,
and Werner, 1982).

Primary sterility follows the same pattern as overall sterility, being highest
in Cameroon, moderate in Sudan, and as low in Kenya as in well-docu-
mented natural fertility populations. However, it seems likely that primary
sterility is underestimated, due to poor quality of data on childlessness.
In sub-Saharan Africa, having children is very highly valued and barren
women tend to hide their childlessness. For instance, childless women may
avoid being interviewed, report "Don't know" to questions about children
ever born, or fail to distinguish between bearing and rearing children. The
evaluations of the WFS data for Cameroon, Kenya, and Sudan find evidence
of too few nulliparous women among the older cohorts. This problem is especially pronounced for Cameroon (Santow and Bioumla, 1984; Rizgalla, 1984;
Henin, Korten, and Werner, 1982).

The relative variations in sterility across cohorts are not significantly
different in either of the three countries analyzed.[8] This result was somewhat unexpected, because the age-specific rates of sterility are slightly
higher for women born before 1941 compared to women born in the period
1941–1955 in Cameroon and Sudan, while the younger cohort has higher
sterility in Kenya. It is possible that women born before 1941 in Cameroon and
Sudan more frequently have the characteristics that are related to sterility, and
when the effects of these characteristics are controlled, these cohort differences
disappear. Also, some of the variations across cohorts found at the group level
are caused by sampling error.

Time period has a significant effect on the prevalence and incidence of
sterility only in Kenya, where it appears that sterility has increased in recent
decades. The findings that sterility did not change during the last decades in
Cameroon and Sudan, and that it increased in Kenya, were also unexpected.
As discussed previously, it was hypothesized that the availability of penicillin
had reduced the prevalence and incidence of PID leading to sterility and that
Pharaonic circumcision was practiced less in recent years. Time misplacements of birth dates towards the time at survey are more severe among older
women and are worse when last births occurred a long time before survey
(Santow and Bioumla, 1984; Rizgalla, 1984; Henin, Korten, and Werner,
1982). Therefore, it is conceivable that the estimated cohort and time period
effects reflect the mistiming of reported births in these data sets. More specifically, if some women, who had their last child say in the period 20–24 years
before survey, reported their last reproductive event to have occurred in the

period 15-19 years before survey, then the estimated levels of sterility in the more recent time period are too high relative to the more remote period. Furthermore, this type of deficiency in the WFS data also biases estimates of fertility, for example, misplacements of birth dates towards the time of survey can provide too-high estimates of fertility in recent years and exaggerate the increase in fertility during the last decades. Thus, drawbacks of the survey data could in part explain the paradox that age-specific rates of fertility have been increasing simultaneously with an increase (or no change) in the levels of sterility. The rise in fertility may also be due to changes in other reproductive characteristics, such as shorter periods of postpartum abstinence.

In Kenya, if the time-period estimates are valid, the incidence of sterility was significantly lower 15 and 20 relative to 5 years before survey; otherwise there is no significant difference in the multivariate odds of becoming sterile by time period. This finding suggests that the incidence of sterility was low in the period 1952-1953 to 1962-1963. The penicillin campaigns in Kenya, for example, in the Rift Valley, were carried out in the 1950s and it is possible that the effects of reduced PID from the use of penicillin caused a lower incidence of sterility in this period (Caldwell and Caldwell, 1983). Women of all ages were treated with penicillin and consequently these campaigns had a time-period effect, rather than a cohort effect. Large-scale penicillin campaigns have not been carried out since the early 1960s and it is possible that untreated PID leading to sterility is again becoming more prevalent in Kenya. This statement is based on the observation that traditional moral codes are being relaxed in Kenya and, as a consequence, prostitution, which is generally strongly linked to the spread of venereal diseases, is more common today than in the past.

The prevalence of sterility in Kenya rose gradually during the period studied, with the exception of the period about 15 years before survey. However, the levels of sterility at survey are relatively low in Kenya compared to Cameroon and Sudan, as well as to the English historical population. Subfertility and probably also sterility have historically been more prevalent in Central and West Africa than in East Africa (Page and Coale, 1972). Therefore, evidence of declining sterility in the former areas, for example, in Zaire (Tabutin, 1982), may not apply to East Africa. Furthermore, the findings indicating a striking decline in sterility during recent decades in Zaire (Tabutin, 1982) are based on information about childlessness. However, fewer women may stay barren, even though a large proportion of women have secondary sterility at an early age. It would be interesting to extend the analysis by Tabutin to include estimates of the proportion subsequently infertile by age to determine the trend in the age structure of sterility.

Regional differentials in sterility are pronounced, and the capitals—and in general urban residence—are associated with higher sterility. This pattern suggests that venereal diseases are more prevalent in the cities, possibly due to the more widespread practice of prostitution. There is no support for the hypothesis that infertile women migrate to the cities. Environmental differences and variations in sexual practices, other than prostitution, might also influence the prevalence and incidence of sterility. For instance, the regions with low sterility in Cameroon, Kenya, and Sudan are those characterized by better economic prosperity, for example, the Central Region in Sudan and the Central Region in Kenya.

The quality of the WFS data for Cameroon varies by region and therefore the estimates of regional differentials in sterility might be biased. The data for the North Region are particularly poor and the estimates of primary sterility and age-specific rates of sterility in the North Region may be underestimated (for example, there is evidence of omission of childless women and a shift of birth dates towards the date of interview (Santow and Bioumla, 1984). Also, the effects of living in the North relative to the reference region (Yaounde) on both the incidence and prevalence of sterility are probably biased downward, reducing the explanatory power of the region variable.

Sterility often follows ethnic as well as regional boundaries, indicating that cultural practices within ethnic groups affect the risk of sterility. For example, in the West Region in Cameroon, 98 percent of the women in the WFS sample belong to the Bamileke and Bamoun tribes with strict marriage laws and little allowance for promiscuity. Sterility is low in the West Region relative to Yaounde in both the models of the prevalence and incidence of sterility. In contrast, there is generally no significant difference between the prevalence of sterility in the Center-South Region and in Yaounde. Several different ethnic groups live in the Center-South Region and exogamy and promiscuity are common practices among these tribes. Thus, the prevalence of sterility might be associated with cultural practices regarding marriage.

There is also evidence suggesting that religious practices influence the age at onset of sterility, since Muslims have consistently higher sterility than Christians. Most Muslims, in both Kenya and Cameroon, live in the areas that were invaded by the Arab slave traders, where venereal diseases are known to have been introduced, and so many individuals may consequently be susceptible to early sterility. Female circumcision is more widely practiced among Muslims and religion may operate as a proxy for female circumcision, a covariate that is not controlled in Cameroon and Kenya. This hypothesis is supported by the fact that Muslims have substantially higher primary sterility than Christians (0.20 vs. 0.07 in Cameroon) and female circumcision is hypothesized to affect primary sterility most. Also, in the models with cohort or time period, religion is significant both when the incidence (secondary sterility) and prevalence (primary and secondary sterility) of sterility are estimated for Cameroon. It is not significant in any of the multivariate models for Kenya, where there are relatively few Muslims and female circumcision is also practiced among non-Muslims.

In Sudan, the effect of type of female circumcision (Pharaonic vs. other types of circumcision and never circumcised) on sterility was not significant, except in the model of the incidence of sterility 5 years before survey. This finding may be real, even though it is hard to believe that the mutilation, subsequent infections, and other complications from circumcision do not affect the ability to have a live birth. The large majority of women in Sudan were circumcised and had a Pharaonic circumcision. Therefore, the present analysis should be extended to a population in which a larger proportion of women were not circumcised, in order to allow an analysis of the differentials between women with a Pharaonic circumcision, other types of circumcision, and no circumcision.

Women who are uneducated and women whose husbands are uneducated generally have higher sterility below age 30, while women who have or whose husbands have secondary and higher education suffer more from sterility at the older ages when only differences in this single variable are considered. This pattern does not hold when the effects of other covariates are controlled. Education and husband's education are not significant in the multivariate models for Cameroon and Sudan. Thus, the apparent differentials in sterility by education found at the group level are due to the effects of other variables, such as residence. In Kenya, education is significant in the models including time period or cohort and women with no schooling have higher sterility. However, it is not conclusive that socioeconomic status is linked to lower sterility in Kenya because husbands' work statuses have no impact on sterility.

In Cameroon, women who delivered their last pregnancy at home have much higher age-specific rates of sterility than women who delivered in dispensaries (local clinics), which suggests that sanitation and proper care at childbirth affect the ability to have further children. Women who delivered in hospitals have intermediate rates of sterility. These elevated levels of sterility for women who delivered in hospitals compared to dispensaries may be caused by the fact that some women who experienced complications at the last childbirth may be more likely to go to the hospital for special care. Variations in sterility according to the nature of assistance with the last delivery reveal a similar pattern. Sterility is more prevalent among women who were assisted at the last delivery by a family member, as opposed to a midwife or nurse. Finally, the few women who had assistance from a doctor have high age-specific rates of sterility relative to those who were assisted by a nurse or midwife.

The number of times a woman has married is strongly related to age-specific rates of sterility, as well as to the levels of primary sterility. Sterility is more prevalent among women married more than once, probably because childless or subfertile unions are more likely to be dissolved.

The effects of type of marriage (monogamous or polygamous) are more diverse. Marital status has a significant effect on the prevalence of sterility 5 years before survey in the multivariate models for Kenya and Sudan, but not for Cameroon. (In Cameroon, the effects of number of times married and marital status may be confounded because women in polygamous unions are more likely to have been married more than once.) In Kenya and Sudan, sterility is more prevalent among women in polygamous unions.

In Kenya, in unions with two wives, sterility is more prevalent among women of rank 1, while women of rank 2 do not have significantly different sterility from women in monogamous unions. This result can be interpreted as indicating that husbands in subfertile unions are prone to take another wife. In unions with three or more wives, all women, regardless of rank, have significantly higher sterility than women in monogamous unions, with wives of rank 1 having the highest levels. This finding supports each of the following three hypotheses: (1) husbands in subfertile unions are prone to take another wife; (2) they may also divorce a subfertile wife, who may then be likely to remarry and to be a higher order wife in a polygamous union; (3) women in polygamous unions might spread infections and subsequent sterility to their cowives. However, from our data, it is not possible to distinguish among these hypotheses.

The differences in the levels of sterility between women who have used contraception and nonusers are only significant for Cameroon and Kenya. In both countries, women who ever used contraception have a lower prevalence of sterility than women who never used, while no significant difference was found in the incidence of sterility. (Since the effects of efficient use of contraception to terminate childbearing would be indistinguishable from sterility, it appears that contraceptive use was not sufficient to end childbearing at earlier ages than nonusers.) The lower sterility of contraceptive users may partly be due to the protection against venereal diseases provided by methods like the condom and diaphragm. The negative relationships could also be due to sterile or subfecund women being less likely to adopt contraception. Furthermore, women who use contraception are often selected for higher socioeconomic status. Therefore, contracepting women are probably more informed about health issues, can better afford medical treatment, and are less likely to become sterile from PID.

CONCLUSIONS

The levels of sterility found within either Cameroon or Sudan are surprisingly invariant across cohorts and over recent decades, and in Kenya sterility increased in the 1960s and 1970s. With the available data, it is not possible, however, to explain these unexpected features. Also, it has not been determined why sterility is so prevalent in Cameroon relative to Kenya, although venereal diseases seem the most plausible cause. In each of the three countries examined, fertility has increased in recent years and this pattern was assumed to be linked in part to a decline in sterility and in part to more complete reporting of recent births. However, we could find *no* evidence of a decline in sterility. To determine whether sterility actually has remained unchanged, or even increased in Kenya, further studies based on other data sets would be worthwhile.

The detrimental influence of venereal diseases on fecundity was hypothesized to have been reduced by the use of penicillin. Unfortunately, the WFS surveys do not provide information on medical history so that the link between venereal diseases and sterility cannot be addressed directly. To do so, we would need to know the incidence of venereal diseases, how frequently they were treated with penicillin, and how effective penicillin is in preventing venereal disease–induced sterility. This last point is particularly relevant in light of reports of penicillin resistance in Cameroon. Syphilis and malaria are diseases known to cause pregnancy wastage. A further avenue of research even without medical data might be to use the WFS surveys for Cameroon and Kenya, where complete pregnancy histories were obtained (not just live birth histories), to assess the impact of pregnancy wastage on sterility. These data would still present problems, however, since reports of non–live-birth pregnancies are notoriously inaccurate.

In this chapter, type of female circumcision has been singled out as a factor that may increase the risk of primary sterility and secondary sterility at an early age. The effects of female circumcision on the ability to reproduce should be analyzed further in one of the East African countries where female circumcision is widely practiced but not universal, as it is in available data sets from Sudan. Unfortunately, questions about female circumcision were not asked in the WFS survey for Kenya, where the practice is frequent but not universal.

The effects of midwifery on subsequent sterility were addressed in this study, but also need further research. The WFS survey for Cameroon provides information about location of delivery and assistance at childbirth, but only for the last pregnancy. In order to ascertain the impact of midwifery on the ability to have another live birth, information about all childbirths must be available, since we cannot assume that all previous births were delivered under the same circumstances.

The analysis of Cameroon, Kenya, and Sudan confirms that WFS surveys are a useful source for a comparative study of the levels and the differentials of sterility in sub-Saharan Africa. Unfortunately, time misplacements of births and age misreporting often distort African WFS surveys, and care must be taken in the interpretation of the results from studies based on these data. Before further research in undertaken, it might be fruitful to examine whether the population and individual measures of sterility employed herein are robust to such distortions of the data as are detected in some of the African WFS surveys. This type of analysis could be carried out by a simulation of common patterns of misresponse. It is quite possible that we could modify the present techniques, if necessary, to allow for certain types of deficient data. Finally, in African countries where two or more surveys have been carried out in recent years, it may be possible to evaluate the consistency of the data and thus determine trends in sterility with greater precision.

Those variables most strongly related to sterility were found to be region and residence: sterility was higher in urban than rural areas. Women who have been married more than once and women in polygamous unions experience more sterility than women who remain in first marriages and women who have no cowives. Contraception has only a minor effect on sterility with ever-users having lower sterility in Cameroon and Kenya. Muslims have generally higher sterility than Christians. Education of the woman or her husband and husband's work status have almost no impact on sterility.

It is of interest to examine here some of the policy implications of our findings. If we assume that sterility at an early age is predominantly due to disease and, in particular, to venereal diseases, then these results indicate wide geographic variation in the diseases and thus provide information for targeting campaigns against venereal diseases to the most affected districts. These campaigns might have two components: education (on the causes and treatment of venereal diseases) and medical care (perhaps through single-round penicillin campaigns or establishment of permanent treatment centers).

It is worthwhile to speculate also on the extent to which sterility has reduced fertility in Cameroon and Sudan in comparison to Kenya, and, conversely, to speculatle on the rise in fertility to be expected if the age-specific prevalence of sterility could be reduced to the Kenyan levels. To do so, let us assume that the low levels of sterility in Kenya in the 1970s measured from the WFS data were prevailing in Cameroon and Sudan, and the fertility to those individuals who were not sterile remained unchanged. In this case, the total fertility rate in the age interval 20–45 would increase from 5.5 to 7.3 in Cameroon and from 5.3 to 6.9 in Sudan. In other words, if sterility were reduced in these countries we would expect a substantial increase (of about 30 percent) in the total number of children born to each woman and an even more rapid population growth than these regions are experiencing. Thus sterility seems, at least in sizable areas of Africa, to be an important check on fertility and one that must be taken into account in planning or predicting furture change in these areas.

In general, it is important that this analysis of Cameroon, Kenya, and

Sudan be extended to more sub-Saharan countries in order to assess the magnitude and geographic distribution of sterility and to assess the potential scope of interventions aimed at reducing sterility. As a final note, it is advisable that attempts to reduce sterility be made in the context of integrated family planning services so that successful efforts to combat infertility do not result in an unexpected increase in population growth.

ACKNOWLEDGMENTS

An earlier version of this paper was presented at the session on "African Demography—Macro Approaches" at the Annual Meeting of the Population Association of America, Boston, March, 1985. I would like to thank Jane Menken, James Trussell, Barbara Vaughan, and Chris Wilson for their suggestions and contributions in the preparation of this manuscript.

NOTES

1. The Kenyan survey covers primarily the western and southern regions. It does not include the northern parts of the Rift Valley or the eastern and northeastern regions.

2. Sudan is divided into eighteen provinces, twelve of which comprise the northern part of the country which was covered by this survey.

3. In the subsequent analysis the term "effects" is used to indicate an association between sterility and a covariate, although it does not imply anything about a causal relationship.

4. Time could also be a continuous variable, but the present study uses a discrete-time method.

5. A maximum likelihood procedure that takes weighting into account was used (see the MLOGIT Procedure developed by Salford Systems for use with SAS).

6. Note that a model involving a categorical covariate has one fewer variables than the number of categories.

7. The effects of cohort are significant in the models of the prevalence of sterility in Cameroon and Sudan, but the odds of being in any category relative to the reference category (born 1948+) are not significantly different for any of the cohorts examined.

8. See note 7.

BIBLIOGRAPHY

Aziz, F. 1980. Gynecologic and obstetric complications of female circumcision. *International Journal of Gynaecology and Obstetrics* 17: 560–563.

Allison, P. D. 1982. Discrete-time methods for the analysis of event histories. In *Sociological methodology, 1982*, ed. S. Leinhardt. Washington, D.C.: Jossey-Bass.

Caldwell, J. C., and P. Caldwell. 1983. The demographic evidence for the incidence and course of abnormally low fertility in tropical Africa. *World Health Statistics Quarterly* 36: 2–34.

Cox, D. R. 1972. Regression models and life tables (with discussion). *Journal of the Royal Statistical Society, Series B* 34: 187–220.

DeCherney, A., and G. Beikowitz. 1982. Female fecundity and age. *The New England Journal of Medicine* 307: 424–426.

Enquête nationale sur la fécondité du Cameroun 1978. Rapport principal. 1983. Huddersfield, Eng.: H. Charlesworth and Co. Ltd.

Federation CECOS, D. Schwartz, and M. J. Mayaux. 1982. Female fecundity as a function of age. *The New England Journal of Medicine* 307: 404–406.

Female circumcision. 1979. *People* 6: 24–30.

Frank, O. 1983*a*. Infertility in sub-Saharan Africa: Estimates and implications. *Population and Development Review* 9: 137–145.

————. 1983*b*. Infertility in Sub-Saharan Africa. *Working Papers of the Center for Policy Studies*, no. 97. New York: The Population Council.

Henin, R. A., A. Korten, and L. H. Werner. 1982. *Evaluation of birth histories: A case study of Kenya.* Voorburg, Netherlands: International Statistical Institute. (World Fertility Survey Scientific Report no. 36).

Henin, R. A. 1981. Fertility, infertility and sub-fertility in eastern Africa. In *International Population Conference, Manila, 1981.* Liège: Ordina Editions, 667–607.

Infertility in Africa. 1978. *People* 5: 23–34.

Henry, L. 1965. French statistical work in natural fertility. In *Public Health and Population Change*, ed. M. Sheps and J. C. Ridley. Pittsburg: University of Pittsburg Press, 333–350.

Henry, L. 1961. Some data on natural fertility. *Eugenics Quarterly* 8: 81–91.

Kenya fertility survey 1977–1978: First report. 1980. Nairobi: Central Bureau of Statistics.

Larsen, U. M. 1985. "Measures of sterility: A comparative study of the levels and the differentials of sterility in Cameroon, Kenya and Sudan." Ph. D. dissertation. Princeton: Princeton University.

Lesthaeghe, R. 1984*a*. *Fertility and its proximate determinants in sub-Saharan Africa: The record of the 1960's and 70's.* Liège, Belgium: International Union for the Scientific Study of Population, Committee on the Comparative Analysis of Fertility and Family Planning.

Lesthaeghe, R. 1984*b*. *On the adaptation of sub-Saharan systems of reproduction.* Liège, Belgium: International Union for the Scientific Study of Population, Committee on the Comparative Analysis of Fertility and Family Planning.

Lunganga, K. 1983. Pathological factors associated with infertility: The case of Upper Volta, 1971. In *Studies in African and Asian demography: CDC annual seminar, 1982.* Cairo, Egypt: Cairo Demographic Centre: 259–285.

Nasah, B. T. 1979. Aetiology of infertility in Cameroon. *Nigerian Medical Journal* 9: 601–605.

Nasah, B. T., M. A. N. Azefor, and B. N. Ondoa. 1974. Clinical and pathological conditions affecting fertility in Cameroon. In *Sub-fertility and infertility in Africa,* ed. B. K. Adadevoh. Ibadan, Nigeria: The Caxton Press, 75–78.

Page, H. J., and A. J. Coale. 1972. Fertility and child mortality south of the Sahara. In *Population growth and economic development in Africa*, ed. S. H. Ominde and C. N. Ejiogu. London: Heinemann, 51–67.

Retel-Laurentin, A., and C. Armagnac. 1983. Changes in foetal and child mortality in

Upper Volta (1969–77): Effects of medical treatment in a low fertility area. Unpublished manuscript.

Retel-Laurentin, A. 1974. Sub-fertility in black Africa—The case of the Nzakara in Central African Republic. In *Sub-fertility and infertility in Africa,* ed. B. K. Adadevoh. Ibadan: The Caxton Press, 69–80.

Rizgalla, M. 1984. *Evaluation of the Sudan fertility survey 1978–79.* Voorburg, Netherlands: International Statistical Institute.

Romaniuk, A. 1968. Infertility in tropical Africa. In *The population of tropical Africa,* ed. J. C. Caldwell and C. Okonjo. London: Longmans, 214–224.

Santow, G., and A. Bioumla. 1984. *An evaluation of the Cameroon fertility survey 1978.* Voorburg: International Statistical Institute.

Shandall, A. 1967. Circumcision and infibulation of females. *Sudan Medical Journal* 5: 178–212.

Sherris, J. D., and G. Fox. 1983. Infertility and sexually transmitted diseases: A public health challenge. *Population Reports, Series L: Issues in World Health* 4: L113–151.

The Sudan fertility survey 1979: Principle report. 1982. Khartoum, Sudan: Department of Statistics.

Tabutin, D. 1982. Evolution régionale de la fécondité dans l'ouest du Zaire. *Population* 37: 29–50.

Trussell, J., and C. Hammerslough. 1983. A hazards-model analysis of the covariates of infant and child mortality in Sri Lanka. *Demography* 20: 1–27.

Trussell, J., and C. Wilson. 1985. Sterility in a population with natural fertility. *Population Studies* 39: 269–287.

Vincent, P. 1950. La stérilité physiologique des populations. *Population* 5: 45–64.

CHAPTER FIVE

The Demography of Polygyny in Sub-Saharan Africa

Noreen Goldman
Anne Pebley

INTRODUCTION

A common feature of African marriage customs is polygyny, a form of nuptiality in which some husbands have more than one wife. Although polygyny is not unknown in other populations, its incidence today is rarely as high as in sub-Saharan Africa. For example, between 1 and 7 percent of married men in North African and Middle Eastern Moslem countries are in polygynous marriages (Huzayyin, 1976; Torki, 1976; Issa and Eid, 1976; Momeni, 1975; Tabutin, 1979), and less than 10 percent of nineteenth-century American Mormon men were polygynists (Smith and Kunz, 1976). By contrast, between 12 and 38 percent of married African men are reported in polygynous marriages (van de Walle, 1968; van de Walle and Kekevole, 1984).

Because the sex ratio below age 50 is about unity in African populations that do not experience heavy migration, and because virtually all African men marry, there has been considerable speculation about the demographic and social arrangements that permit high levels of polygyny. Examination of the age distributions by sex in a stable population, shown in figure 5.1, indicates that a surplus of women relative to men can be readily generated by a difference in the ages at which men and women first marry. If, on average, women marry at age 20 and men at age 28, the surplus of eligible women, shown in the shaded area to the left of the graph, will be substantial. A small surplus of women, shown in the shaded sliver on the right of the graph, is also generated at older ages by differences in the longevity of women and men.

Another commonly cited explanation for the frequency of polygyny is that widows usually remarry, often to an already-married kinsman of their deceased husband (Murdock, 1959; Caldwell, 1976; McDonald, 1985). For example, Caldwell (1976) has suggested that while polygyny is socially per-

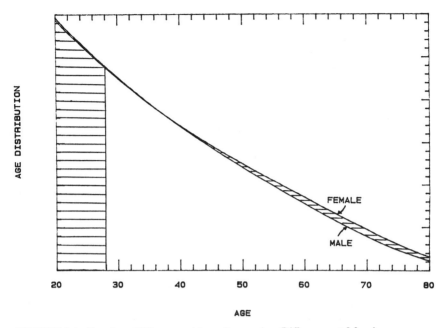

FIGURE 5.1. Surplus of Women with an 8-year Age Difference at Marriage

NOTE: This figure is based on male and female stable age distributions with a rate of increase of 0.02 and Coale and Demeny West model life tables, level 13 ($e_0 = 50$ for women, 47.1 for men).

missible in Bangladesh and while the age differences at marriage for men and women are as large as in sub-Saharan Africa, polygyny may be uncommon in Bangladesh because widows do not traditionally remarry. By contrast, McDonald (1985) reports that in Senegal, 91 percent of all women who stated that they had been widowed in their first marriages were remarried within 5 years, and among those who remarried, 75 percent were in polygynous unions.

The effects of both age differences at marriage and the extent of widow remarriage in producing a surplus of potential wives are likely to vary with the rate of growth experienced by a population. In the case of age differences, the slope of the age distribution curve is steeper with a higher growth rate and flatter with a lower growth rate. Thus, on the one hand, when men marry at older ages than women, we would expect that the surplus of women would be larger with higher growth rates. The extent of widow remarriage, on the other hand, may have a greater effect at lower rates of growth when older women comprise a larger portion of the female population. While most African countries are now experiencing moderate or high rates of population growth, growth rates were certainly considerably lower before World War II because of higher mortality rates. Growth rates are also likely to drop to lower levels again in the future, this time through declines in fertility.

In this chapter, we investigate the contributions of age differences between spouses at first marriage and widow remarriage in permitting high levels of polygyny. We also examine the ways in which these associations change with different demographic regimes, in order to determine whether probable declines in future growth rates are likely to make polygyny more difficult to maintain at current levels. Our objective, however, is solely to describe the demographic conditions that *allow* polygyny to occur. We make no attempt to argue either that polygyny exists because African societies value universal marriage of women, or that large age differences and universal marriage exist to support polygyny.

METHODS

Measurement of Polygyny

The frequency of polygyny can be measured in several ways. Van de Walle (1968) proposed three measures: m, the ratio of currently married women to currently married men; p, the proportion of husbands who have more than one wife; and w, the number of wives per polygynist. These measures are interrelated in the following way:

$$m = 1 + p(w - 1).\qquad\text{(eq. 5.1)}$$

Since, by definition, more women are involved in polygynous marriages than men, we might consider another measure of the frequency of polygyny: the proportion of all married women who are in polygynous marriages, which we call f, where:

$$f = \frac{pw}{m} = \frac{pw}{1 + p(w - 1)}\qquad\text{(eq. 5.2)}$$

We use census data from Cameroon and Senegal, collected in 1976, to illustrate the relations among these measures.[1] The data are shown in table 5.1.

Senegal clearly has a higher frequency of polygyny than Cameroon. More than half of all wives and almost a third of all husbands are involved in polygynous marriages. Though these proportions are smaller in Cameroon, the index w, which van de Walle terms the intensity of polygyny, indicates that men who participate in polygynous marriages have roughly the same number of wives in both countries. In fact, van de Walle's calculations from data collected in the 1950s and 1960s in a wide range of African countries indicates that the average number of wives per polygynist is usually less than 2.5. Contrary to the western stereotype of polygynists with large harems, the vast majority (71 percent in Cameroon, for example) are married to only two women.

TABLE 5.1   Measures of Polygyny from 1976 Census Data for Cameroon and Senegal

	Cameroon	Senegal
Ratio of currently married women to currently married men (m)	1.30	1.50
Percent of married men who have two or more wives (p)	23.6%	31.3%
Mean number of wives per polygynist (w)		
• Calculated from p and m	2.3	2.6
• Reported	2.5	NA
Percent of married women in polygynous marriages (f) (calculated from p and m)	45.8%	54.3%
Ratio of ever-married women to ever-married men	1.41	1.62

NA = not available.
SOURCES: Cameroon, Bureau Central du Recensement. 1976. *Recensement général de la population et de l'habitat d'avril 1976*, vol. 2, tome 2; and Senegal, Bureau National du Recensement. 1976. *Principaux résultats du recensement général de la population d'avril 1976*, tables 6 and 7 and p. 11.

To assess the effects of changes in demographic parameters on the surplus of women available for marriage, we use a different index: the ratio of women above the female age at first marriage to men above the male age at first marriage . The advantage of this measure is that it reflects the *potential* for polygyny in the population rather than the current marriage practices of the population. In practice, since marriage of both men and women is virtually universal in African societies, as shown later, this index of potential is essentially equivalent to the ratio of ever-married women to ever-married men. The last row in table 5.1 shows the ever-married ratio for Cameroon and Senegal in 1976. The differences between these ratios and the ratios of currently married women to currently married men shown at the top of table 5.1 are due to widowhood, divorce, and separation. In the next section, we describe the assumptions and procedures which we use to calculate our index of polygyny.

Stable Population Model

The number of men and women at each age in a population closed to migration is completely determined by its history of fertility and mortality rates. Sub-Saharan African countries appear to have experienced declines in mortality since World War II, but little fertility change over the past few decades. To the extent that fertility has declined, such changes appear to be very recent and would only affect the population at the youngest ages. Since our focus in this paper is on adults who were all born at least 15 to 20 years ago, an assumption of constant fertility seems adequate for describing the age distributions of these populations. Previous research indicates that the age distributions resulting from mortality declines usually differ only slightly from those generated by the assumption of constant mortality at current levels (Coale and Demeny, 1967). For these reasons, we rely on a stable population model, one in which fertility and mortality are assumed to have been constant over a long period of time, for most of our calculations.

The advantage of stable models is that the effect of various demographic parameters on the surplus of women can be readily assessed by a comparison of two or more stable populations. Such findings can be interpreted as either comparisons among different stable populations (with varying characteristics) or as assessments of the effects of long-term changes within a given population once it has reachieved stability at the new levels of the parameters. An obvious limitation of the stable model is that short-term period effects that result from demographic changes are ignored. Since demographers have recently become concerned with the effects of mortality decline on the availability of women for marriage (see, for example, Preston and Strong, 1986), we examine the short-term effects of mortality decline on our measure of the surplus of women in a later section.

In a stable population, the number of persons at a given age x can be represented by $Be^{-rx}l_x$, where l_x is the underlying life table, r is the rate of population growth, and B is the number of births. In words, the number of people at a given age, x, is determined by the original size of the cohort at birth times the probability that members of the cohort survive from birth to age x. Although the effect of fertility on the age distribution is not apparent from this expression, fertility is the major determinant of the rate of growth r.[2] Fertility affects the relative size of birth cohorts and hence the slope of the age distribution. For example, high levels of fertility result in large rates of growth and invariably lead to young (steep) age distributions. The consequences of the mortality level are more difficult to assess because there are two kinds of effects: mortality partly determines the rate of growth (and hence the relative sizes of birth cohorts) and, in addition, mortality affects the proportions surviving to each age. These effects can counteract each other: for example, reductions in mortality usually raise the rate of growth— producing a younger age distribution—and simultaneously increase the proportions surviving to each age—producing an older age distribution (Coale, 1972).

If we assume that the female and male stable populations have a common growth rate, r, but separate life tables, l_x^f and l_x^m, respectively, the number of females and males at age x can be expressed as:

$$\text{Number of females} = B^f e^{-rx} l_x^f \qquad \text{(eq. 5.3)}$$

$$\text{Number of males} = B^m e^{-rx} l_x^m, \qquad \text{(eq. 5.4)}$$

where B^f and B^m are the number of female and male births, respectively. The ratio of $B^m h/B^f$, which we call S, is simply the sex ratio at birth.[3]

If we also assume that women first marry at age a_f and men at age a_m, the ratio of the number of ever-married women to the number of ever-married men, which we call Z, can be defined as:

$$Z = \frac{\text{\# ever-married women}}{\text{\# ever-married men}} = \frac{\int_{a_f}^{\omega} e^{-rx} \, l_x^f \, dx}{S \int_{a_m}^{\omega} e^{-rx} \, l_x^m \, dx}, \qquad \text{(eq. 5.5)}$$

where ω is the oldest age of life.

In real populations, women as well as men marry over a range of ages rather than at a single age. In order to assess the effect of a distribution of ages at marriage rather than a single age for each sex, we compared calculations of Z in which ages at marriage are fixed for each sex (eq. 5.5) with calculations in which a distribution, or schedule, of ages at marriage is employed for each sex. To incorporate schedules of age at marriage in Z, we let $g^f(x)$ and $g^m(x)$ represent the first marriage frequencies for each sex. Then $G^f(x)$ and $G^m(x)$, where

$$G^f(x) = \int_0^x g^f(y) \, dy$$

and

$$G^m(x) = \int_0^x g^m(y) \, dy,$$

denote the proportions of women and men who marry by age x. The ratio Z can be redefined to incorporate $G(x)$ in the following way:

$$Z = \frac{\text{\# ever-married women}}{\text{\# ever-married men}} = \frac{\int_0^{\omega} e^{-rx} \, l_x^f \, G^f(x) \, dx}{S \int_0^{\omega} e^{-rx} \, l_x^m \, G^m(x) \, dx} \qquad \text{(eq. 5.6)}$$

In eq. 5.6 the number of ever-married persons at each age is expressed as the product of the total number of that age and the proportion of persons married prior to that age. Our calculations made using eq. 5.6 are based on a Coale-McNeil curve of first marriage frequencies in which the rate of first marriages $g(x)$ for each sex is expressed as a double exponential curve with three parameters: the mean age at marriage, the standard deviation of age at marriage, and the proportion that eventually marries (Coale and McNeil, 1972; Rodriguez and Trussell, 1980).[4] The comparison of our calculations, under a wide variety of conditions, reveals that the values of Z based on eq. 5.6 barely differ from those based on eq. 5.5 which a_f and a_m take on the mean values of $g^f(x)$ and $g^m(x)$, respectively. For example, evaluation of eq. 5.6 with mean ages at first marriage for women and men of 20 and 25, a standard

TABLE 5.2   Parameters of Age at Marriage, Reported Ratios of
Ever-Married Women to Men, and Estimated Ratios, WFS Data

	Cameroon (1978)	Senegal (1978)	Sudan (1979)
Mean Age at Marriage*			
Female (a_f)	18.9	17.9	21.0
Male (a_m)	26.8	28.4	27.8
Age difference ($a_m - a_f$)	7.9	10.5	6.8
Percents Ever-Married			
Women aged 50–54	98.1	99.5	98.7
Men aged 50–54	94.2	98.0	97.8
Ratios			
$\dfrac{\text{Ever-married women}}{\text{Ever-married men}}$	1.52	1.61	1.35
$\dfrac{\text{All women aged } a_f +}{\text{All men aged } a_f +}$	1.51	1.64	1.32
Estimate of Z according to eq. 5.3**	1.47	1.71	1.39

*Estimated by fitting a first marriage schedule to reported proportions ever-married by age for each sex (Coale, 1971; Rodriguez and Trussell, 1980); distributions of age and marital status are derived from the household survey in each country.
**The calculations are based on the above values of a_f and a_m (with linear interpolation to accommodate nonintegral ages), estimated total fertility rates of 6.3, 7.1, and 6.0 for Senegal, Cameroon, and Sudan, respectively (based on the period 0–4 years before each World Fertility Survey) and Coale and Demeny West model life tables, level 9 for Senegal and level 13 for Cameroon and Sudan. All of the calculations incorporate a sex ratio at birth (S) of 1.03 males per female.

deviation of 4.6 for each sex, and proportions of one eventually marrying for each sex, yields a ratio Z of 1.247.[5] Evaluation of eq. 5.5, with values of a_f and a_m equal to 20 and 25, yields a value for Z of 1.248.

Further indication that use of fixed ages at marriage in lieu of age distributions would not alter our results is given by data presented later from three African fertility surveys. These estimates, shown in table 5.2, indicate that reported numbers of ever-married women per ever-married men, from survey data in Cameroon, Senegal, and Sudan, are almost equal to the ratios of the number of women (of all marital statuses) above the mean age at first marriage for females to the number of men (of all marital statuses) above the mean age at first marriage for males. Since we conclude that allowance for variance in age at marriage does not alter the value of the ratio Z, all future calculations are based on fixed ages a_f and a_m.

Implicit in the use of Z as a measure of the potential for polygyny is the assumption that all persons above the age at first marriage are either married or eligible for remarriage. Since part of our objective is to determine the extent to which widow remarriage contributes to the surplus of women in the population, we use a modified version of Z, which we call Z', in which no widows remarry. To construct Z', we assume that the mortality experience of women is independent of that of men, that is, that spouses have independent risks of dying and that mortality is independent of marital status, assumptions that are undoubtedly false (see, for example, Goldman and Lord, 1983), but which are sufficient for purposes of our model. We include in the numerator of Z' only women whose husbands are still alive, that is, we multiply the number of ever-married women at each age by the life table probability that the husband survived to the time they reached that age, given the age difference between spouses:

$$Z' = \frac{\begin{array}{c}\text{\# of ever-married women}\\\text{who have never been}\\\text{widowed}\end{array}}{\text{\# of ever-married men}} = \frac{\displaystyle\int_{a_f}^{\omega} e^{-rx}\, l_x^f\left(\frac{l_{x+a_m-a_f}^m}{l_{a_m}^m}\right)}{S\displaystyle\int_{a_m}^{\omega} e^{-rx}\, l_x^m\, dx} \cdot \quad \text{(eq. 5.7)}$$

The ratio Z' could be further modified, by inclusion of the term

$$\left(\frac{l_x^f + a_f - a_m}{l_{a_f}^f}\right)$$

in the denominator, to describe a situation in which neither widows nor widowers are considered marriageable. Since the definition of a widower is problematic in polygynous populations, and, in any case, social prohibitions against widower remarriage are virtually non-existent, we do not consider this latter case.

Since almost everyone ultimately marries in sub-Saharan countries, we have not introduced a factor (denoted by C in the Coale-McNeil marriage model) which signifies that only a fraction of persons of marriageable age would ultimately marry. The ratio C^f/C^m would enter the expression for Z simply as a multiplicative factor and its effects can, therefore, be assessed readily.

In all of our calculations, numerical values for Z or Z' are obtained by evaluating equations 5.5, 5.6, and 5.7 with a single-year summation. For example, in eq. 5.5, Z is evaluated as

$$Z = \frac{\displaystyle\sum_{x=a_f}^{\omega-1} e^{-r(x+0.5)}\, L_x^f}{S\displaystyle\sum_{x=a_m}^{\omega-1} e^{-r(x+0.5)}\, L_x^m} \cdot \quad \text{(eq. 5.8)}$$

Single-year values of person-years lived (L_x^f and L_x^m) are obtained by linear interpolation of values presented in the Coale and Demeny model life tables

(Coale and Demeny, 1983).[6] When we alter levels fertility or mortality, we calculate the population growth rate (rate of natural increase) from a life table and fertility schedule, and then substitute it into the appropriate equation for Z.

RESULT

Indices of Polygyny in Cameroon, Senegal, and Sudan

To determine whether the results of our model adequately describe the demographic determinants of polygyny in African populations, we compare them with data from two countries and part of a third which participated in the World Fertility Survey. These countries, Cameroon, Senegal, and Northern Sudan, were chosen because their data sets were available to us and because they included questions on marital status of men and women in their household questionnaires. Each of the three countries conducted a household survey in which the sex, age, and marital status of each household member were listed. Subsequently, an extensive fertility questionnaire, including a complete marital history, was administered to all women between ages 15 and 49 who were listed on the household schedule. Most of the data for our calculations come from published tabulations derived from the household survey (République Unie du Cameroun, 1978; République du Sénégal, 1981; Democratic Republic of the Sudan, 1982).

Since one of the main objectives of the household survey was to identify women who were eligible for the individual interview, men may have been less completely enumerated in the household survey than women. Selective omission of men would bias upward the ratios calculated from these data. To determine whether such underreporting occurred, we calculated the sex ratios for persons under age 45 in each household sample. In the absence of error (and sex-selective migration), the sex ratio for the age range from 0 to 45 should be very close to 1. In fact, for each of the three countries, there were 0.95 men per woman (or 1.05 women per man), a value that suggests only a modest undercount of males and a slight inflation of our ratios.

Our calculations for individual countries depend on the accuracy of WFS data on age, age at marriage, and marital status. Serious age-heaping is apparent in the age distributions in all three countries, but it should have little effect on our ratios since they involve the cumulation of numbers of men and women above a certain age. We believe that information on whether a person has ever been married or is currently married is likely to be reasonably well reported. On the other hand, dating of marriages and reports of marriage dissolution are much less likely to be accurate.

In table 5.2, we compare ratios of women to men above their respective mean ages at first marriage from WFS data for Cameroon, Senegal, and Sudan with the corresponding estimates from our model. The first part of the table presents the nuptiality parameters required for calculation of these ratios. Figures in the first two rows show the mean ages of marriage for men and women calculated from a first marriage schedule fitted to reported proportions ever married by sex from the household survey. All three populations have sizable differences in the mean ages of men and women at first marriage. The difference for Senegal is by far the largest, with men, on average, being 10.5 years older at first marriage than women. The data in table 5.2 also indicate that virtually all men and women eventually marry in each of the three countries: the percentages of women and men aged 50–54 who have ever been married are at least 98 percent, with the exception of men in Cameroon (94 percent).

Two indices reflecting the potential for polygyny based entirely on reports of age and marital status in each household survey are shown in table 5.2. The first ratio relates ever-married women to ever-married men[7] and the second is a ratio of all women over the mean female age at first marriage to all men over the mean male age at first marriage. The two ratios are very close for each country, reflecting the fact that marriage is almost universal for both men and women. The comparison provides further confirmation that using the mean age at marriage rather than an age-at-marriage distribution for subsequent calculations does not affect our findings. The third ratio in table 5.2 is the estimate of Z calculated from eq. 5.5 using parameters based on actual values for each population. We used model life tables (Coale and Demeny, 1983, West family) at level 13 ($e_0 = 50.0$ for females and 47.1 for males) for Cameroon and Sudan and at level 9 ($e_0 = 40.0$ for females and 37.3 for males) for Senegal; these values are based on recent estimates of life expectancies for these countries (Population Reference Bureau, 1985). Age specific fertility rates were calculated from the individual data for the 5-year period before each survey and yielded estimated total fertility rates of 6.3, 7.1, and 6.0 for Cameroon, Senegal, and Sudan respectively (République Unie du Cameroun, 1983; République du Sénégal, 1981; Democratic Republic of the Sudan, 1982). A sex ratio at birth of 1.03 was used for all calculations. Despite probable errors in reports of age and marital status and in our choices of population parameters, and violations of the assumption of stability, the estimates of Z are consistent with those from the WFS data, for each country. These comparisons suggest that our stable population model approximates the steepness of the adult age distribution and hence the ever-married ratio in each of the three populations.

In the next section, we use this model to explore in detail the effects of changes in each of the demographic parameters on the ratios of women to men (Z). An alternative way to evaluate our findings would be to consider changes in the *surplus* of women relative to men, which can be measured by $Z - 1$. For the sake of consistency, all of our results are presented in terms of Z, rather than $Z - 1$, although a case could be made for each approach. Had we chosen to use a measure of surplus, the observed changes (in percentage terms) would clearly have been much greater.

For most of the discussion below, we assess the effects of varying fertility and mortality regimes by a comparison among different stable populations. Although we sometimes refer to "changes" in fertility or mortality, these changes should be interpreted as either eventual long-term changes (when a given population has reachieved stability), or as variations among different stable populations. These distinctions are particularly important in the case of fertility, since even drastic declines in fertility will have no effect on the ratio for a period of about 20 years following the change. Short-term effects of mortality change are considered in a separate section.

The Effect of Age Differences at Marriage

An examination of the age distribution in figure 5.1 makes it apparent that age difference at marriage has a major impact on the potential surplus of wives. For example, consider two populations in which all women first marry at the same age (a_f) and in which men first marry at an older age (a_m) than women. Since all women between ages a_f and a_m are married whereas no men of comparable age are, the population with the larger age difference at marriage must have the higher ratio. The extent to which a given age difference produces a surplus (or deficit) of females is a function of the steepness of the age distribution. For example, it appears from figure 5.1 that changes in demographic rates which would bring about a younger population (for example, increases in fertility), would give more weight to the portion of the age distribution between the female and male ages at marriage and would increase the size of the surplus for a given age difference.

Calculations based on a wide range of schedules of fertility and mortality indicate that, unlike age differences, the absolute ages at marriage have almost no effect on the ratio. For example, changes in the ages at marriage from 20 and 25 for females and males to 17 and 22, respectively, alter the ratio by only one percent.[8] For this reason, throughout the analysis, we fix the female age at marriage at 20 and let the male age at marriage vary according to the required age difference, unless otherwise specified.

Figure 5.2 shows the ratios which result from selected age differences at marriage with the same schedule of mortality but a wide range of fertility conditions. Since the impact of changes in fertility changes on the ratio can only be determined by first evaluating the effect of the fertility changes on the rate of growth (and hence on the age distribution), figure 5.2 depicts the ratios under different rates of growth, r, rather than under varying schedules of fertility. Clearly, fertility differences that have no effect on the rate of growth (such as a higher mean age of childbearing and a counteracting difference in the level of fertility) do not affect the ratio of marriageable persons.

Not surprisingly, the results indicate that, at any given growth rate, the

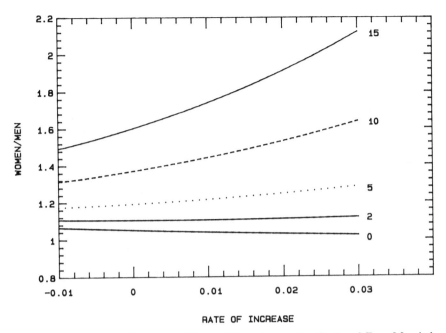

RATE OF INCREASE

FIGURE 5.2. The Effect of the Rate of Increase on the Ratio of Ever-Married Women to Ever-Married Men at Selected Age Differences at Marriage (Male Minus Female Age at Marriage, in Years)

NOTE: These calculations are based on Coale and Demeny West model life tables, level 13 ($e_0 = 50$ for women, 47.1 for men), and an age at marriage of 20 for women.

ratio increases markedly as the age difference between spouses increases. For example, with a 2-percent growth rate, an age difference of 5 years produces a ratio of 1.22 whereas a 10-year difference results in a ratio of 1.50. Note that even when men and women marry at the same ages, there is a modest surplus of females, in spite of a sex ratio at birth of 1.03 males per female. This results from the fact that the underlying mortality schedules incorporate a higher life expectancy for females (by almost 3 years) than for males.

The effect of different growth rates on the surplus of women is shown for selected age differences at marriage ranging from 0 to 15 years, with men marrying at older ages than women. When men's age at marriage exceeds that of women by more than 2 or 3 years, the size of the female surplus is larger at higher rates of growth, as expected. The curves for larger age differences have increasingly steep slopes, which indicate the progressively larger effects of changes in the growth rate on the ratio Z. For small age differences, however, the situation is reversed: the surplus of women is slightly *lower* at higher rates of growth. This unanticipated result is a consequence of commonly observed sex differences in life expectancy which produce a male population of marriageable age which is *younger* on average than the female population of marriageable age. In Appendix I, these relationships are derived mathematically.

Effect of Differences in Fertility and Mortality

While many African populations are currently experiencing very high population growth rates, it is likely that growth rates in the past were much lower. Furthermore, growth rates are also likely to decline in the future with socioeconomic development. How much would a decline in the growth rate affect a society's ability to maintain a high frequency of polygyny? At a rate of growth of 3 percent, an age-at-marriage difference of 8 years results in a ratio of 1.5 ever-married women per ever-married man, which is quite similar to ratios currently observed in some African populations. A reduction in the growth rate to 2 percent, due to a decline in fertility, at a constant age difference at marriage, would eventually result in a relatively modest decrease of 5 percent in the ratio. Thus, unless accompanied by a reduction in the age difference at marriage (or other social changes), a decline in the growth rate poses little threat to the surplus of potential wives for polygynous marriages.

While the effect of changes in fertility as reflected in changes in the growth rate in figure 5.2 have a noticeable though modest effect on Z, changes in mortality rates have virtually no effect, at least within the range of life expectancy common to most African countries (40 to 60 years). For example, if ages at marriages for women and men are 20 and 25, respectively, and fertility is held constant, an increase in life expectancy from 40 to 50 years would reduce the ratio only from 1.29 to 1.28. If life expectancy were increased further to 60 years, the ratio would remain at 1.28.[9] The reason is that, in effect, the tendency of decreases in mortality rates to produce older male and female populations is counteracted by an increase in the rate of growth (also resulting from the same decrease in mortality rates), which makes the population younger. The net effect on the age distribution is very small for ages above 20.

The different effects of changes in fertility and mortality rates can be seen in figure 5.3. The top two curves depict the age distributions of two populations with the same fertility schedule: the solid line is that of a population with a life expectancy of 40 (and a growth rate of 0.021) and the dashed line is that of a population with a life expectancy of 60 (but a growth rate of 0.033). The similarity of the two distributions at adult ages contrasts with the third curve on each graph in figure 5.3.[10] This curve shows that a much younger age distribution would result from the higher rate of growth ($r = 0.033$) which would occur at the low life expectancy (40) but at a *higher level of fertility*. These results follow from well-known findings of stable

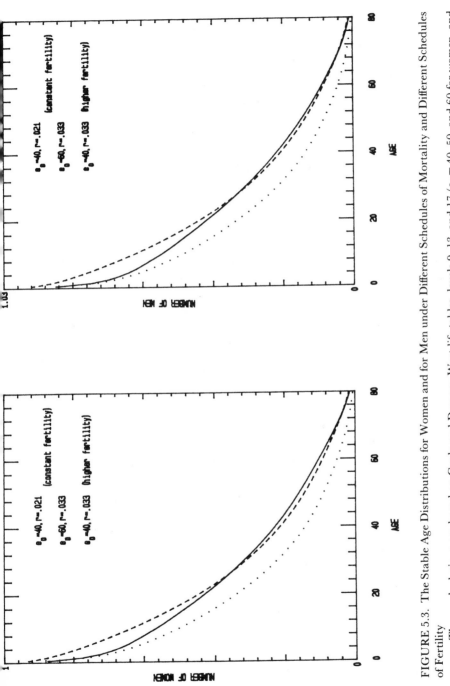

FIGURE 5.3. The Stable Age Distributions for Women and for Men under Different Schedules of Mortality and Different Schedules of Fertility

NOTE: These calculations are based on Coale and Demeny West life tables, levels 9, 13, and 17 ($e_0 = 40$, 50, and 60 for women, and 37.3, 47.1, and 56.5 for men) and a Coale-Trussell model fertility schedule (GRR = 3 or TFR = 6.1, mean age of childbearing = 29 years).

population theory about the greater (and more clear-cut) effect of changes in fertility relative to changes in mortality on the age distribution of a population.

Period Effects Resulting from Mortality Change

The results described above indicate that mortality changes have no significant long-term effect on the ever-married ratio. Nevertheless, it is plausible that these changes would have a noticeable impact on the ratio during the period of change and shortly thereafter. For example, Preston and Strong (1986) have suggested that recent mortality declines in many developing countries have resulted in a sizable surplus of women of marriageable age. In particular, if age differences at first marriage were large, female cohorts of marriageable age would be subject to reduced mortality rates much sooner than their male counterparts.

In order to examine the short-term effects of mortality decline, we replace our stable population model with a population projection that incorporates changing mortality and fixed fertility rates.[11] The calculation starts with a stable population age distribution that is then projected annually. Mortality rates for each year, within an assumed 20-year period of change, are calculated by linear interpolation between specified beginning and final life tables. After year 20, mortality rates are assumed to remain fixed at the new lower level for the remainder of the projection period (75 years) . In order to obtain upper-bound estimates of such mortality effects, we have chosen a large age difference at first marriage: ages of 20 and 30 for women and men respectively.

In figure 5.4a we show the resulting ratios for three projections of mortality decline for a 75-year period. Recall that the mortality change takes place entirely during the first 20 years. In the first two projections, we consider a moderate and a large mortality decline respectively. Both projections are based on model life tables (Coale and Demeny, West) for the beginning and final schedules. The first projection, which is based on a rise in life expectancy from 40 to 50 years over a 20-year period, is characterized by very little variation in the ever-married ratio Z. Not surprisingly, the second projection, which incorporates an improvement in life expectancy from 40 to 60 years over a 20-year period, shows greater variation in Z, but still a rather modest short-term change in the ratio considering the large magnitude of the mortality change. Moreover, both these projections suggest that the short-term effects lead to a reduction rather than an increase in the ever-married ratio. As shown earlier, the long-term effects of both of these changes on Z is virtually zero.

Our results appear to be inconsistent with those from an earlier study by Preston and Strong (1986) who argue that some types of mortality change bring about significant changes in the marriage market. In fact, the two sets

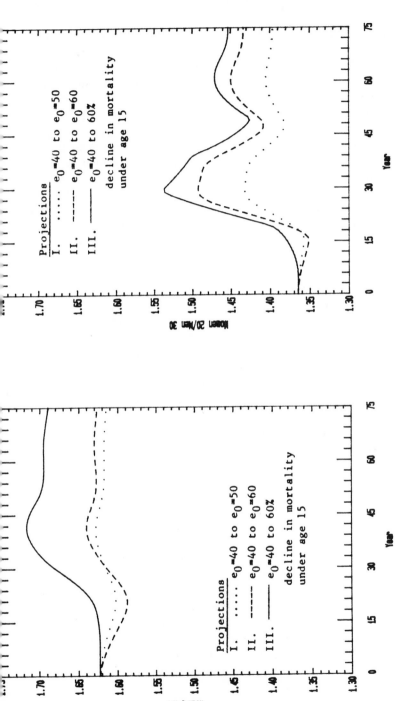

FIGURE 5.4. The Ratio of Ever-Married Women to Ever-Married Men and the Ratio of Women Aged 20 to Men Aged 30 under Three Projections of a 20-year Mortality Decline

NOTE: These calculations are based on Coale and Demeny West model life tables, a Coale-Trussell model fertility schedule (GRR = 3 or TFR = 6.1, mean age of childrearing = 29 years), and ages at marriage of 20 and 30 for women and men respectively.

of results can be reconciled if we take into account the nature and magnitude of the mortality declines considered by Preston and Strong. Among their projections, the one that generates a significant surplus of marriageable females is a decline restricted to the young ages. In addition, the magnitude of the decline incorporated in their examples is enormous: for example, an absolute decline in the infant mortality rate of 100 per 1000 and a 35 percent increase in the probability of surviving to age 15.

Using our projection model described above, we have experimented with similar patterns of mortality decline. The third projection shown in figure 5.4a is essentially a replication of the latter example used by Preston and Strong. We begin with a life expectancy of 40 years and assume that death rates for each single-year age group under 15 decline by 60 percent over a 20-year period; in the resulting life table, the probability of surviving to age 15 is 35 percent higher than in the original life table (and life expectancy at birth is about 10 years higher for each sex). The resulting trajectory of Z indicates a modest rise in the ratio, with a maximum rise of 5.5 percent and an eventual rise of 3.9 percent. Of course, such a drastic improvement in infant and child mortality (which, according to values of $l(15)$, is associated with an increase from $e_0 = 40$ to $e_0 = 65$) is extremely unlikely to occur without substantial reductions in adult mortality. The fact that such patterns of mortality decline have a noticeable impact on the ratio is not surprising since the type of demographic change incorporated in the third projection is virtually equivalent to an increase in fertility. Our previous results have demonstrated that changes in fertility (which operate through the rate of growth) bring about modest long-term changes in the ever-married ratio.

It is important to recognize that these findings do not suggest that typical patterns of mortality decline have no impact on the marriage market. In particular, if we focus on the cohorts of prime marriageable age, it is clear, as Preston and Strong (1986) argue, that reductions in mortality can produce a substantial surplus of women at these ages. Figure 5.4b shows the ratio of women age 20 to men age 30 for the same three projections described earlier. The results indicate that, even with a moderate decline (projection 1), a significant surplus of marriageable women is created during the period that follows the decline. Not surprisingly, the surplus is considerably larger for the latter two projections. Although measures of this type may be useful for explaining phenomena such as the "marriage squeeze," such measures are less appropriate than Z or similar indices for assessing the potential for polygyny, in part because of the wide dispersion of ages of both husbands and wives in polygynous systems. These illustrations make it clear that, both in the short-term and in the long-term, realistic patterns of mortality reduction have little impact on the potential for polygyny. As we will see later, the exception to this finding is a situation in which widows do not remarry.

Widow Remarriage

Until this point, our calculations have been based on the assumption that all men and women above their respective ages at marriage are eligible for marriage. In order to determine how much widowhood contributes to the surplus of potential wives, we need to compare these figures with calculations in which no widows remarry (that is, widows are ineligible for marriage). In table 5.3, we compare the effects of age differences between spouses, growth rates, and mortality on polygyny under two conditions: (1) all widows are eligible for remarriage, as in preceding examples, and (2) widows do not remarry. The comparison in the first panel of table 5.3 shows that even when there is no age difference between men and women at first marriage, widow remarriage makes a substantial difference to the ratio of ever-married women to men. If men and women marry at the same ages and widows do not remarry, there would be a *surplus of men relative to women* with a

TABLE 5.3   The Effect of Eliminating Widow Remarriage on the Ratio of Ever-Married Women to Ever-Married Men, by Selected Values of Age Difference at Marriage, Rate of Increase, and Life Expectancy

	Widows Remarry (Z)	Widows Do Not Remarry (Z')	Percent Difference
*Age Difference at Marriage**			
0	1.02	0.85	16.7
2	1.12	0.92	17.9
5	1.28	1.03	19.5
10	1.61	1.24	23.0
15	2.07	1.50	27.5
*Rate of Increase**			
.00	1.19	0.84	29.4
.01	1.22	0.90	26.2
.02	1.25	0.97	22.4
.03	1.29	1.04	19.4
Life Expectancy For Females†			
40	1.29	0.96	25.6
50	1.28	1.03	19.5
60	1.28	1.09	14.8
70	1.28	1.14	10.9

*Calculations are based on a fixed fertility schedule (Coale and Trussell model fertility schedule, GRR = 3, mean age of childbearing = 29 years).

**Calculations are based on a Coale and Demeny West model life table, level 13, and ages at marriage of 20 and 25 for women and men respectively.

†Calculations are based on a fixed fertility schedule (see footnote *), ages at marriage of 20 and 25 for women and men respectively, and Coale and Demeny West model life tables, levels 9, 13, 17, and 21.

ratio of 0.85. If widows are allowed to remarry under these circumstances, the ratio would increase to just over 1. The effect of widow remarriage on the ratio increases as the age difference widens: larger age differences increase the number of widows at each age since women who marry much older men are more apt to outlive their spouses. For example, at an age difference of 10 years, widow remarriage would increase the ratio dramatically from 1.24 to 1.61 women per men.

The second panel shows the differences in the ratio that would occur at different rates of growth. Widow remarriage has the greatest impact when the growth rate is lowest. This effect is due to differences in the age distributions: populations with low rates of growth have a higher proportion of people at older ages, and widows, therefore, constitute a greater percentage of the population.

The figures in the third panel of table 5.3 indicate that, as previously shown, when all widows remarry, mortality has virtually no effect on the ratio. However, if widows do not remarry, the ratio is substantially lower at lower expectations of life simply because widowhood is more common. Thus, our conclusion that mortality has little effect on the ratio must be qualified: reductions in mortality will increase surplus of potential wives in societies that prohibit or restrict widow remarriage.

Comparison of the Effects of Demographic Parameters

The results of changes in the age difference at marriage, the growth rate, and widow remarriage are summarized in table 5.4. The objective of these comparisons is to determine how large a change in each of these parameters, taken one at a time, would be required to bring about a 10 percent reduction in the ratio for several stable populations. For a population at a high rate of growth (0.03) and a large age difference (8 years), a reduction of the age difference to just under 6 years would reduce Z by 10 percent. The same

TABLE 5.4   Changes in Demographic Parameters,* Taken One at a Time, Needed To Bring about a 10 Percent Reduction in Z

Age Difference at Marriage**	Rate of Increase	Z	Age Difference at Marriage**	Rate of Increase	% Widows Not Eligible for Remarriage
8	.03	1.49	5.8	.01	47
8	.01	1.35	4.9	−.029	35
3	.03	1.17	0.7	—†	6
3	.01	1.14	−0.4	—†	41

*For all calculations, female age at marriage equals 20 years and the life table is described by a Coale and Demeny West model life table, level 13, for males and females (e_0 = 50 and 47.1 respectively).
**Male age at marriage minus female age at marriage.
†Under these conditions, it is impossible to obtain Z < 1.12 for any rate of increase.

reduction in Z would be achieved by the substantial reduction in the growth rate to a value of 0.01 or by a situation in which only about half of widows were eligible for remarriage. For populations with a smaller age difference at marriage of 3 years, reductions in Z on the order of 10 percent could only be achieved by a further lowering of the age difference at marriage (with females marrying at older ages than males in some cases) or with restrictions on widow remarriage, but they could *not* be achieved by changes in the rate of growth. As was shown in figure 5.2 and in appendix, the effect of changes in the growth rate on Z is either small or negative when age differences at marriage are small. The values in table 5.4 also indicate that, in order to achieve a 10 percent reduction in Z, the restriction on widow remarriage need not be as large in populations with small rates of growth or with large age differences because of the greater prevalence of widows in these populations.

  In summary, our results indicate that the most important determinants of the ratio of ever-married women to men are the age difference at marriage and the inclusion of widows as potential marriage partners. At large age differences, changes in fertility have a modest influence on the ratio, but at age differences under 2 or 3 years there is no notable effect on Z. Substantial changes in mortality, at least within the range of life expectancy examined here, barely alter the ratio, as long as widows are eligible for remarriage.

CONCLUSIONS

The above comparisons suggest that the high ratios of marriageable women to men observed and estimated for Cameroon, Senegal, and Sudan are in large part due to substantial age differences at marriage which range between 7 and $10\frac{1}{2}$ years. Further calculations not presented here indicate that differences in the ratios *among* the three countries are due to variations in these age differences at marriage. For example, the reason that Senegal has the largest of the ratios (an observed ratio of 1.6 and an estimated one of 1.7) is almost entirely because its age difference at marriage exceeds those of Cameroon and Sudan by about 3 to 4 years; only a small part of the difference is due to Senegal's higher total fertility rate. The previous section indicated that virtually none of the disparities could be due to variations in life expectancy.

  It is also apparent that the high prevalence of polygyny made possible by these ratios would not exist if widows could not remarry. The values of Z' in table 5.5 shown together with those of Z, based on estimated demographic parameters for the three countries, indicate that the ever-married ratio would be reduced by one-quarter, on average, if widows could not remarry. In absolute terms, the difference between values of Z and Z' is largest in Senegal, a not unexpected result since Senegal has the largest age difference at marriage and the lowest life expectancy, conditions that are conducive to a high prevalence of widowhood.

TABLE 5.5   Selected Indices of Polygyny and Measures of
Widow Remarriage

	Cameroon	Senegal	Sudan
Estimate of Z according to eq. 5.3*	1.47	1.71	1.39
Estimate of Z' according to eq. 5.5*	1.17	1.25	1.09
$\dfrac{\text{Ever-married women}}{\text{Ever-married men}}$**	1.52	1.61	1.35
$\dfrac{\text{Currently married women}}{\text{Currently married men}}$**	1.33	1.51	1.17
Estimated percent of ever-widowed women who are currently married†	30	68	27
Estimated percent of currently married women who were previously widowed†	9	23	7

* These estimates are calculated as described in table 5.2, footnote **.
** These ratios are calculated from WFS household survey data for each country.
† Female age distributions by current marital status from the household survey and model life tables were used to estimate the percent of ever-married women at each age who had ever been widowed. These calculations are based on the assumptions of constant mortality for men and fixed ages at marriage for men and women (see table 5.2, footnote **).

Throughout this chapter, we have used observed and estimated ratios that reflect the *potential* for rather than the *prevalence* of polygyny. An index of the prevalence of polygyny in each population—the ratio of currently married women to currently married men at the time of the survey—is shown in the second panel of table 5.5. The fact that this currently married ratio is fairly close in size to the ever-married ratio suggests that women whose marriages have ended tend to remarry quickly. The comparison also suggests that the remarriage rates for widows are likely to be higher in Senegal than in the other two countries.

The extent to which widow remarriage contributes to the high prevalence of polygyny at any one point in time in each country can be examined more directly. If reports of marriage dissolution and remarriage in the WFS individual surveys had been accurate, we could have tabulated the number of currently married women who reported being widowed at some time in the past. Examination of the accuracy of reports of marriage dissolution in the three surveys, however, indicated that widowhood was reported much less frequently than it must have occurred.[12] One possible explanation for this pattern is the practice of levirate marriage in which a widow is often automatically inherited by her husband's brother. The woman herself may consider marriage to her brother-in-law as a continuation of her first marriage, rather than as widowhood and a subsequent remarriage. An additional problem with data in the individual survey is that they are restricted to women under age 49.

Because reports of widowhood in each survey are not adequate for our purposes, we have used a different approach for estimating the contributions of widows to the surplus of married women in each country. Based on the assumption of constant mortality at current levels and on fixed ages at marriage for women and men (as given in table 5.2), we estimated the percent of ever-married women at each age who had ever been widowed and compared these values to the numbers currently widowed as reported in the household surveys.[13] Although the measures derived from this calculation are subject to considerable uncertainty, they illustrate the relative importance of widow remarriage in the three countries.

The results are shown in the last panel of table 5.5. The next-to-last row shows the estimated percentage of ever-widowed women who are currently married, an indicator of the extent of widow remarriage. The difference between Senegal and the other two countries is striking. Almost 70 percent of Senegalese women who have ever been widowed are married at the time of the survey compared to less than a third in Cameroon and Sudan.

The figures in the last row in table 5.5 measure the contribution of former widows to the surplus of currently married women. Again, the pattern of remarriage in Senegal is markedly different from those in Cameroon and Sudan: an estimated 23 percent of currently married women were formerly widowed in Senegal compared to less than 10 percent in the other two countries.

The ratios in table 5.5 indicate that both the potential for, and the prevalence of, polygyny are greatest in Senegal. As noted earlier, the greater surplus of ever-married women (or of women of marriageable age) is due almost entirely to larger age differences at marriage in Senegal than in Cameroon or Sudan. The greater surplus of currently married women results not only from these age differences, but also from the greater prevalence of remarriage in Senegal.

Many countries in sub-Saharan Africa are currently experiencing high rates of population growth, due to high fertility rates and moderate declines in mortality. In the next two decades, these countries are likely to experience at least moderate reductions in growth rates as fertility rates begin to decline more rapidly than mortality rates. Our analysis shows that although these demographic changes may have a noticeable effect on the potential for polygyny, they are unlikely to have a large impact on the ability of African societies to maintain high levels of polygyny. Instead, our results indicate that the two major factors permitting high levels of polygyny in these societies are primarily social: the differences in age at marriage between men and women and the extent of widow remarriage.

ACKNOWLEDGMENTS

This research was supported by grant #AGR CP48.07A from USAID and the Population Council Program on the Determinants of Fertility in Developing Countries; grant #R01 HD11720 from NICHD; and the Andrew W. Mellon Foundation. The authors would like to thank Ansley Coale and Graham Lord for their advice throughout the course of this project, Donna Sulak for producing the figures, and Gilles Pison and Etienne van de Walle for suggestions that significantly improved this paper.

NOTES

1. In subsequent analyses, we use data from the World Fertility Survey (WFS) in each of the three countries. However, since these surveys do not contain information on the number of wives per husband and are administered only to women aged 15 to 59, we use data from the censuses (conducted 2 years before the WFS surveys) to make the comparisons above. Comparable census data were not available for Sudan.

2. The rate of natural increase is the solution of the characteristic equation $1 = \int_0^\omega e^{-rx} l(x)m(x)dx$, where $m(x)$ is the female birth rate at age x, and $l(x)$ is the female life table.

3. All of the calculations in this paper are based on a sex ratio at birth of 1.03.

4. The original $g(x)$ curve of first marriage frequencies (Coale and McNeil, 1972) is based on the following three parameters: a_0, the starting age at marriage; k, the pace at which marriages occur relative to a standard; and C, the proportion which eventually marries. The $g(x)$ curve can be reexpressed as a function of more meaningful parameters (Rodriguez and Trussell, 1980): μ, the mean age at first marriage: σ, the standard deviation of age at first marriage, and C, the proportion which eventually marries. In our calculations, the values of $G(x)$ are obtained from $g(x)$ by the trapezoidal rule of numerical integration.

5. These parameters are equivalent to values of a_0 of 12.1 and 17.1, for women and men, $k = 0.7$ and $C = 1$ for both sexes. The calculations are based on a rate of growth of 2 percent and Coale and Demeny West model life tables, level 13 ($e_0 = 50$ for women, 47.1 for men). Changes in the rate of increase and the life table have no notable effect on the above comparison.

6. Several recent studies suggest that the age pattern of mortality in African populations may deviate substantially from standard model life tables, particularly in infancy and childhood (see, for example, Blacker and Hill, 1985). To assess the effects of restricting our mortality estimates to the collection of Coale-Demeny model life tables, we substituted mortality schedules calculated by Pison and Langaney (1985), based on data from the Bandafassi of Western Senegal. At a similar value of life expectancy, these life tables incorporate higher infant and child mortality rates and lower adult rates than do the model schedules; in addition, they are based on almost identical life expectancies for males and females, rather than sex differences in life expectancy of about 2 to 3 years which characterize comparable model life tables. In

order to hold life expectancy fixed in our calculations, we used the Brass logit procedure (see, for example, Brass, 1971) and the reported Bandafassi schedule as a standard to generate new life tables with life expectancies of about 40 years. The resulting
calculations indicate that, given male and female life expectancies implied by the
Coale and Demeny schedules (e_0 of 40.0 and 37.7 years for females and males respectively), the ratio Z is virtually unaffected by the use of the Bandafassi mortality pattern. However, mortality schedules that imply the same life expectancies for males
and females are associated with substantially lower Z values than are the Coale and
Demeny model schedules.

7. The WFS ratios for Senegal and Cameroon shown in table 5.2 can be compared with those from the 1976 censuses, which are shown in table 5.1. The ratio from
the Senegal census is the same as that from WFS data, while the ratio from the
Cameroon census of 1.41 is somewhat lower than the WFS ratio.

8. We do not take into account the effects of changing female (and possibly male)
ages at marriage on fertility rates.

9. This calculation is based on a model fertility schedule (Coale and Trussell,
1974) with a gross reproduction rate of 3 (or a total fertility rate of 6.1) and Coale and
Demeny West model life tables of levels 9, 13, and 17, which are based on life expectancies of 40.0, 50.0, and 60.0 years, respectively, for women, and corresponding life
expectancies of 37.3, 47.1, and 56.5 years for men.

10. In fact, the mean ages of marriageable women in the first two distributions are
almost identical: 38.9 and 38.5 for the lower and higher life expectancies, respectively.
By contrast, the mean age for the third distribution is 36.6.

11. As in earlier calculations, we use a Coale-Trussell model fertility schedule
with GRR equal to 3 (TFR equal to 6.1) and a mean age of childbearing of 29 years.

12. This conclusion is based on a series of comparisons of reported proportions
ever-widowed by successive durations of marriage (based on a life table calculation in
which divorce is treated as a censoring) with the corresponding estimated proportions
from a model life table under the assumption that current ages at marriage and levels
of mortality prevailed for the past 20 years. These comparisons indicate that union
dissolutions brought about by the death of husband were underreported by at least 50
percent: for example, by 20 years of marriage, the reported proportions of women
ever-widowed from their first marriages were 12, 16, and 9 percent in Cameroon,
Senegal, and Sudan while the expected proportions were 18, 26, and 19 percent respectively.

13. Divorced women were excluded from the calculation.

BIBLIOGRAPHY

Blacker, J., and A. Hill. 1985. Age patterns of mortality in Africa: An examination of
    recent evidence. In *International Population Conference 1985*, Florence, Italy; Liège,
    Belgium: Ordina for the International Union for the Scientific Study of Popula-
    tion.

Brass, W. 1971. On the scale of mortality. In: *Biological aspects of demography*. London:
    Taylor and Francis.

Caldwell, J. C. 1976. Marriage, the family and fertility in sub-Saharan Africa, with special reference to research programmes in Ghana and Nigeria. In: *Family and marriage in some African and Asiatic countries*, ed. S. A. Huzayyin and G. T. Acsadi. Cairo: Cairo Demographic Centre.

Coale, A. J. 1971. Age patterns of marriage. *Population Studies* 25: 193–214.

———. 1972. *The growth and structure of human populations: A mathematical investigation.* Princeton: Princeton University Press.

Coale, A. J., and P. Demeny. 1967. *Methods of estimating basic demographic measures from incomplete data: Manual IV.* Population Studies, no. 42. New York: United Nations.

Coale, A. J., and D. R. McNeil. 1972. Distribution by age of the frequency of first marriage in a female cohort. *Journal of the American Statistical Association*, 67: 743–749.

Coale, A. J., and J. Trussell. 1974. Model fertility schedules: Variations in the age structure of childbearing in human populations. *Population Index* 40: 185–258.

Democratic Republic of the Sudan, Ministry of National Planning. 1982. *The Sudan fertility survey 1979: Principal report.* Khartoum: Department of Statistics.

Goldman, N., and G. Lord. 1983. Sex differences in life cycle measures of widowhood. *Demography* 20(2): 177–195.

Huzayyin, S. A. 1976. Marriage and remarriage in Islam. In: *Family and marriage in some African and Asiatic countries*, ed. S. A. Huzayyin and G. I. Acsadi. Cairo: Cairo Demographic Centre.

Issa, S. A., and I. Eid. 1976. Nuptiality and divorce in the East Bank of Jordan, 1968–1975. In: *Family and marriage in some African and Asiatic countries*, ed. S. A. Hyzayyin and G. T. Acsadi. Cairo: Cairo Demographic Centre.

McDonald, P. 1985. Social organization and nuptiality in developing societies. In: *Reproductive change in developing countries*, ed. J. Cleland and J. Hobcraft. Oxford: Oxford University Press.

Murdock, G. P. 1959. *Africa: Its peoples and their culture history.* New York: McGraw-Hill.

Momeni, D. A. 1975. Polygyny in Iran. *Journal of Marriage and the Family* 37(2): 453–456.

Pison, G., and A. Langaney. 1985. The level and age pattern of mortality in Bandafassi (eastern Senegal): Results from a small-scale and intensive multi-round survey. *Population Studies* 39(3): 387–405.

Population Reference Bureau. 1985. *1985 World population data sheet.* Washington D.C.

Preston, S. H., and M. A. Strong. 1986. Effects of mortality declines on marriage patterns in developing countries. Chap. 9 in *Consequences of mortality trends and differentials.* New York: United Nations.

République du Sénégal. 1978. *Principaux résultats du recensement de la population d'avril 1976.* Dakar: Bureau National du Recensement.

———. 1981. *Enquête Sénégalaise sur la fécondité: Rapport national d'analyse.* Dakar: Direction de la Statistique.

République Unie du Cameroun. 1978. *Recensement général de la population et de l'habitat d'avril 1976.* Yaoundé: Bureau Central du Recensement.

———. 1983. *Enquête nationale sur la fécondité du Cameroun: Rapport principal.* Yaoundé: Direction de la Statistique et de la Comptabilité Nationale.

Rodriguez, G., and J. Trussell. 1980. Maximum likelihood estimation of the parameters of Coale's model nuptiality schedule from survey data. *World Fertility Survey Technical Bulletin*, no. 7/Tech 1261. London: World Fertility Survey.

Smith, J., and P. R. Kunz. 1976. Polygyny and fertility in nineteenth century America. *Population Studies* 30(3): 465–480.

Tabutin, D. 1979. Nuptiality and fertility in the Maghreb. In: *Nuptiality and Fertility*, ed. L. Ruzicka. Liège: Ordina for the International Union for the Scientific Study of Population.

Torki, F. G. 1976. Trends and differentials in age at marriage in Kuwait, 1965–1975. In: *Family and marrige in some African and Asiatic countries*, ed. S. A. Huzayyin and G. Acsadi. Cairo: Cairo Demographic Centre.

van de Walle, E. 1968. Marriage in African censuses and inquiries. In: *The demography of tropical Africa*, ed. W. Brass et al. Princeton: Princeton University Press.

van de Walle, E., and J. Kekovole. 1984. The recent evolution of African marriage and polygyny. Paper presented at the annual meeting of the Population Association of America, Minneapolis, Minn.

CHAPTER SIX

The Nuptiality Regimes in Sub-Saharan Africa

Ron Lesthaeghe
Georgia Kaufmann
Dominique Meekers

THE ISSUES

In most comparative studies of nuptiality it has been usual to characterize sub-Saharan patterns of marriage as "early and universal." This categorical generalization was shown to be inadequate in the now classic study of van de Walle (1968), which used the then somewhat underweight body of available census and survey data to rigorously examine this accepted opinion. The pioneering work of van de Walle has been taken up and expanded in this chapter.

Although the starting pattern of procreation is not the most significant Malthusian preventive check on population growth in sub-Saharan Africa, it is still worth noting the range of the mean age at first marriage for women, which was found to vary between 15 and 21 years. Such a discrepancy in the average ages of entry into a first sexual union between African populations must have some implications. Interestingly, the Northwest European marriage pattern, first described by Hajnal (1965), of late age at marriage with neolocal, nuclear household formation, exhibits a similar range for mean ages at first marriage among historical European populations. At the very least, the presence of a similar variation in sub-Saharan Africa requires an explanation and it is surprising that there is such a paucity of systematic statistical analysis addressing this problem. At present, most African countries have been covered by at least one census or large-scale survey, and hence it is due time to reopen the African nuptiality file on ethnic and regional variation.

The suspicion that women's ages at first marriage are rising, thereby shortening the overall reproductive age span, provided the second reason for revisiting the subject. The connection between socioeconomic development

NUPTIALITY REGIMES   *239*

or a rise in female literacy and the postponement of marriage with the concomitant increase in the age at first birth has been described for many Third
World societies (see Casterline and Trussell, 1980; McCarthy, 1982; Mc-
Donald, 1985). The strength and regularity of this positive association in
developing countries everywhere is such that the absence of a link is cause to
suspect the quality of the data. International evidence, furthermore, indicates that modest rises in female schooling, leading to partial or full primary
education only, produces a delay of female entry into regular sexual unions.
This trend is not a mere symptom of the practical difficulties of attending
school over age 13 while fulfilling a wife's marital duties in the husband's
household, but it is the result of changes generated before reaching a marriageable age.

As predicted, it was found that the pattern of rising age at marriage
associated with increased levels of female education and literacy was true for
sub-Saharan Africa as well. Taking data from several countries, mostly
World Fertility Survey participants, it was found for women below 25 that
the median age at first marriage rises from 1 year in Benin to over 3 years in
Cameroon, Nigeria, and Senegal, as one moves from illiteracy to full primary
education (5 to 7 years of schooling). This result, shown in table 6.1, is not
produced by a cohort effect underlying both the rise in age at marriage and
the rise of literacy, since the data are derived only from the two youngest age
groups.

Since the African cross-sectional pattern by education fits the worldwide
experience, and given the increase in female literacy since the 1960s, there is
reason for expecting an incipient trend towards overall later female marriage.
If this proves to be true, sub-Saharan populations will respond to certain

TABLE 6.1   Median Ages at First Marriage for African Women Aged 15–24
by Education, 1973–1982

	Education			
	Illiterate or Koranic Only	1–4 Years	5–7 Years	8+ Years
Benin, 1981	18.0	18.8	19.0	—
Cameroon, 1978	15.6	16.9	18.1	20.9
Ghana, 1979	17.3	17.4	18.2	19.4
Ivory Coast, 1980	16.8	16.8	17.9	19.9
Kenya, 1978	17.1	18.1	19.4	22.2
Nigeria, 1982	15.1	17.0	18.8	23.8
Senegal, 1978	15.9	17.8	19.7	21.9
Tanzania, 1973	16.9	17.2	18.0	20.9

NOTE: Medians for Tanzania are for women 25–29.
SOURCE: Eelens and Donné, 1985; Adegbola, personal communication; Henin et al., n.d.

elements of socioeconomic development, first by a change in nuptiality. This would not constitute an exceptional sequence of events: numerous populations in Latin America and Asia are known to have followed a similar path. In other words, a nuptiality transition has often been a prelude to a subsequent marital fertility transition, and the hypothesis can be advanced that sub-Saharan reproductive regimes have reached this starting point in their adaptation to new conditions. Additional evidence supporting such an outcome has been produced by the analysis of the WFS-data for ethnic groups. From chapter 2 it will be recalled that the spatial distribution of the nuptiality indicator for the youngest age group was very similar to that of literacy and of emerging social stratification by class and was no longer related to the geographic pattern of traditional elements of social organization. By contrast, Goody's variables concerning devolution (inheritance, caste, endogamy) were more successful in predicting the ethnic variation in the age at first marriage for the older women. Obviously, cross-sectional evidence is never an adequate substitute for well-measured trends, but it wets the appetite for further inquiry.

The third reason for returning to the issue of nuptiality is the claim that increased Westernization would lead to a restructuring of the sub-Saharan marriage regimes. In this sense, Westernization is taken to mean the adoption and penetration of Western ideals of conjugal closeness which are spread through the mass media, school textbooks, and Christian doctrine and teaching. Two features of the African nuptiality regime are often suggested to be the most affected by these cultural changes: first of all, increased preference for and tolerance of free partner choice, and second, a weakening in the practice of polygyny.

The hypothesis proposing a shift towards free partner choice is supported by a substantial body of anthropological and sociological research (cf. Dries, 1985, for a bibliography and discussion). Caldwell (1980) has argued that the connection between primary education and changing reproductive behavior can at least be partially accounted for by the spread of Western ideals on partner choice through education and socialization. Indeed, in many parts of Africa literacy is a byproduct of Christian penetration, with its concomitant ideology favoring conjugal closeness. Once a population is literate it is much more open to Western thinking, strongly promoting futher "individualization of marriage."

The literature also draws attention to the disruptive influence of migration, urbanization, and early industrialization (for example, mining) on the traditional social system. The outcome is the possibility of social change, as in new ways of choosing partners in a sexual union. But the weakening of lineage control is perhaps more general. The unilineal system is based on corporate property ownership (land and cattle) and economic interdependence of lineage members. As the lineages lose control over land and economic independence emerges as a result of integration into the capitalist economy, the freedom of the young lineage members is strengthened as the control of their elders is weakened. This imbalance in social control is further exasperated by the younger members acquiring new skills and abilities (Lesthaeghe, 1980).

The empirical literature describing the evolution of free partner choice not only links it with urban areas, but also testifies to the ambiguity accompanying the change. Even when the choice is individually made, parental consent is still sought so as not to sever the lifeline to the lineage network. It seems that although in the more developed areas of sub-Saharan Africa a change in ways of partner selection is taking place, this has not involved the complete disintegration of lineage control and influence. Despite losing, completely or partially, some of their major rights, kinship groups still fulfil many other duties and functions, which may prove to be crucial to survival in the current economic climate in Africa. At this juncture it is difficult to imagine individuals rejecting the supportive potential of the traditional kinship system completely.

An international study of the various forms of partner selection is beyond the scope of this chapter. The available information is limited to certain areas and the direct measurement of free versus arranged partner selection cannot be attempted through simple demographic or statistical indicators. This is not the case, however, for the second subject of inquiry: polygyny. Western sociologists (such as, Hunter, 1967; Goode, 1970; Gough, 1977) have tended to predict a decline in the incidence of polygyny as part of the universal progression towards a nuclear and conjugal family. The evolutionary notions behind this implicitly view the Western family form as more rational than others. Goode, for example, argues that (1970, p. 188):

> It [i.e. polygyny] will, without question, eventually almost completely disappear as a pattern of behaviour. The new legal codes are gradually moving towards its abolition, women will avoid it where they can, and men will not generally be able to afford it.

Not unsurprisingly, Goode was unable to specify a time horizon for this evolution, and any consequent empirical testing of the hypothesis runs the risk of being premature. There are, however, some arguments that are contrary to this evolutionary view. From the functionalist point of view, polygyny has a number of important institutional functions, and as long as there are no viable alternatives to take its place, the existence of the institution is not gravely endangered.

Polygyny, by its nature, causes a large differential marriage age between the sexes, which greatly increases the chance of widowhood for women. But, being functionally coherent, polygyny also provides an efficient remarriage net for widows and divorcées and effectively prevents widowhood for men

(Goody, 1976). Amongst the highly polygynous Konkomba of Ghana and Togo, for instance, instant betrothal is the common practice since all girls and women are already spoken for, resulting in late marriage for men and in frequent widow and fiancée inheritance (Goody, 1973). The institutional alternative to polygyny, in this sense, would be some other social welfare mechanism for the care of the single and elderly. The question remains as to whether such an alternative exists, or is in the making, in response to an initial decrement in the incidence of polygyny.

Since in the lineage system the greatest wealth is sons, polygyny is an insurance against subfecundity or a succession of daughters. Given that large areas of central Africa suffered from high levels of sterility induced by venereal disease, the tendency to increase levels of polygyny there can be seen as a response to subfecundity. In populations where knowledge of contagious diseases and medical treatment is far more disseminated, the logical response would be to curb polygynous practice. In central Africa, however, the logical response to the infecundity problem was simply to marry again. At present, the incidence of venereal disease has declined in this area, probably through the use of antibiotics. Since venereal infection is no longer a major threat, one could argue that the high polygyny levels that came into existence in the past can now be maintained without the risks. This is likely to be an attractive proposition for men over 30 in a region that is largely rural and traditional.

The second point made by Goode in the quotation above concerns the financial ability of men to support a plurality of wives. This argument goes straight to the central issue of polygyny, namely its economic basis. Boserup (1970) was among the first to systematically relate the practice of polygyny to the economic relations of production. Goody (1973, 1976) clearly demonstrates the existence of relationships between hoe-culture and polygyny, and plough-culture and monogamy. Traditionally polygyny was a response to the high productive and reproductive value of women in societies with low levels of agricultural technology and high female participation in cultivation (cf. chapter 1). In many parts of Africa women have continued to be prime economic assets, especially in the agricultural sector. In West Africa, women have a major additional involvement in trade. They continue to generate substantial independent incomes, contributing to household and child care expenses (Schwimmer, 1979). With the current practice of men migrating to the cities leaving their wives in the fields, it is difficult to envisage a radical change in this division of labor. Finally, Clignet (1975) noted how it is the newly arrived migrants who do not practice polygyny (nor would they as young men if they remained at home) and that with time and success, the more established city dwellers return to polygyny or an urban variant thereof (for example, "outside wives"). In East Africa women do more agricultural work, but the men's pastoral activity is seen as more significant. Women in these predominantly patrilineal societies are valued primarily as producers of sons. Nevertheless, the impact of a monetary income can, as expected by Goode, greatly affect the marital pattern. In Botswana as a result of adapting pastoralism to cattle trading, the relative contribution of women has seriously diminished, and women have been so excluded from the new economic system that not only has polygyny fallen, but marriage itself has gone into decline (Kuper, 1985). To sum up, polygyny can be advantageous to both sexes: men can accrue power and prestige: women gain support, solidarity with cowives, help with child care, and relief from sexual duties. It is probably a more powerful and viable institution than Goode envisaged.

Legal abolition, female education, and Christian conversion have been cited as major forces countering polygyny. In the Ivory Coast, polygyny was legally abolished in 1964, which has done nothing to stop it. Several ethnic groups in the Ivory Coast have been maintaining some of the highest levels of polygyny in Africa. The data on education do show, however, that polygyny declines with increased schooling. Whether this has to do with female choice or other structural factors is debatable: for instance, how capable is a woman with A-levels of farming? The effect of Christianity on polygyny is ambiguous. The Catholic church, in particular, has been waging war against plural marriages throughout its missionary history. The result is either a lax interpretation of official doctrine or its total disregard because of its impracticability. Syncretic churches and Islam have absorbed polygyny and have consequently fared well in terms of recruitment. Hence, the incidence of polygyny may vary substantially by religious denomination, but this should be viewed against the backdrop of selectivity of recruitment. Only in the rare instances where the Catholic church has no major competitors and has a close historical alliance with the state, as in Rwanda, is an effect to be expected.

The immediate concerns of this chapter are the verification and measurement of facts. In the light of this discussion, a realistic research agenda offers the following possibilities:

1. The construction of a nuptiality file and a polygyny file based on census and survey information
2. The study of interregional and interethnic variations for teasing out the sources of this variation
3. The measurement of trends, whenever possible.

MEASUREMENT PROBLEMS AND THE DEFINITION OF INDICATORS

The broad definition of marriage used in most censuses and surveys fits the needs of demographers since they are only interested in whether or not an individual is in a regular sexual union. Sometimes further distinctions are made between different types of unions: legal, traditional, consensual, and so forth. Occasionally census reports contain tabulations of the frequency of the different types of unions. The broad definition found in censuses is in fact a reflection of the situation in reality: different ethnic groups and religious faiths proscribe different forms of marriage. In fact, the legal codes of countries often specify different regulations for different union types. In Tanzania, for instance, Muslim and traditional marriage are presumed to be potentially polygynous, while others are not. But in fact the form of marriage can be changed by a mutal declaration of the spouses (Marriage Act of 1971), so that in practice all marriages are potentially polygynous.

Although such a broad definition of marriage covers most sexual unions, there still remains a problem in comparing the different types of unions internationally because of variations in local legislation and interpretation. A form of union often excluded is that of a visiting relationship. These "outside wives" or "deuxièmes bureaux" are commonly found in urban areas and are presumably classified as consensual unions (marriages d'amitié) or single. Whereas from the demographer's point of view these women are effectively married in that they are in a regular sexual union and often have children, from the anthropological point of view they are not. Marriage legitimates and thereby institutes social inclusion of sexuality and fertility. From this point of view "outside wives" are more akin to concubines than to women in a polygynous union since they are external and often illicit. But demographically they are of significance as an alternative mode of reproduction in societies undergoing socioeconomic change. As pointed out before, in many cases these women will be lost between the different marital status categories. Some surveys, however, and the WFS in particular, include a final question referring to the existence of any partner, which allows "single" women to admit to having a partner and being recorded as being in a union.

More serious than the problem of definitions is the undisputed tendency of the ages of women to shift across the 5-year age boundaries according to marital status. Married women younger than 15 tend to be recorded as 15–19 years old, and single women older than 20 tend to be dropped down into the same age group. Similarly, married women 15–19 may be pushed into the 20–24 category when age-heaping is particularly prevalent (rounding to 20). This practice can be severely aggravated if literacy levels are low and if the interviewer uses marital status or parity to determine a woman's age. In 1955, Romaniuk (1968) found in Zaire that there was an evident correlation between the regional index of age misreporting for women aged 10–14 and 15–19 and the estimated mean age at marriage ($r = 0.74$ and 0.48 respectively). This was attributed to age overstatement by married and postpubescent girls and to the fact that interviewers had been explicity instructed to estimate ages on the basis of marital status. Interestingly, Romaniuk also found a similar phenomenon for men, but solely for the age group 15–19, despite the lack of such instructions. It can be assumed that in practice interviewers used the same techniques for age estimation for men and women alike, but given the concentration of marriage for women in just one age group (15–19), interviewers could assign ages more easily on the basis of marital status for women than for men.

Since the degree of literacy among young women in non-Muslim areas was greatly enhanced in the 1960s and 1970s, it is plausible to assume that the quality of the age data has correspondingly improved. In sub-Saharan Africa, furthermore, the overall regional variation in the proportions of single women and men is so great that the relative error involved in interregional comparison is moderate. The quality of the age data collected after 1970 is probably more reliable, but the unevenness over time creates major problems in estimating trends. Indeed, the analysis of trends is very susceptible to bias given the differential degree of distortion of the two or three successive estimates used. The cross-sectional analyses based on spatial and ethnic patterns may, therefore, prove to be more accurate than the trend analyses.

A third problem that arises in survey data analysis is the increasing unreliability of retrospectively reported ages at first marriage with the advancing age and decreasing literacy of respondents. There is a tendency to round ages to multiples of 5, which is accompanied by an upward shift to 20 and 25. Van de Walle's golden rule is to never trust retrospectively reported ages at marriage for women who cannot specify their age or year of birth. This rule has its obvious value and the estimation of cohort changes in ages at marriage should consequently be discouraged if the information stems from such retrospectively reported figures obtained in a single survey. Despite this, cohort comparisons are often attempted, notably in WFS reports, with the resulting dubious interpretation of apparent trends.

These points can be documented for the WFS-countries. As displayed in figure 6.1, quartile and median ages at first marriage often show a U-curve. The left arm of the U is indicative of marital status–related age misstatement. If married women gave or were assigned ages that were too high, the age group 15–19 will contain too many single women. This proportion can be enhanced even more when older single women are subjected to the reverse error. Quartiles and median values for the youngest age group are considerably inflated in such circumstances. The left arm of the U-curve is very pronounced in the WFS data for Northern Sudan, but equally present in the data for Nigeria, Senegal, and Kenya. The right arm of the U tends to rise at about age 30 or 35 and results from an upward rounding of retrospectively reported ages at first marriage. In figure 6.1, the right arm is most obvious in the data for Nigeria and Cameroon. The Ghanaian data have the flattest profile and those for Lesotho (not shown here) are almost free of such distortions. Not surprisingly, the countries with large Muslim and illiterate

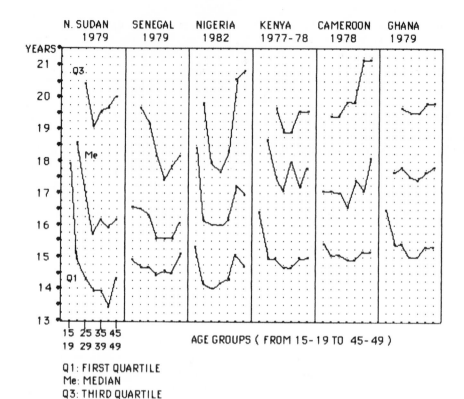

FIGURE 6.1. Quartile and Median Ages at First Marriage for Women as Reported in World Fertility Surveys for Selected Sub-Saharan Countries

populations (Senegal, Northern Sudan, Nigeria) exhibit the strongest U-pattern, whereas those with the most literate populations (Ghana and Lesotho) show relatively minor irregularities.

It is worthwhile to document these points by inspecting the heaping pattern and other indicators of data quality for a particular country. Such a check was carried out on the Kenyan WFS data, which in terms of overall quality were by no means at the poor end of the spectrum. Table 6.2 contains the relevant information. First of all it can be noted that the highest first quartile is for the age group 15–19 and the highest median for 20–24. The lowest median is found in the age group 30–34 and medians and third quartiles rise again thereafter. Hence, the U-shape seems to prevail. The cohort pattern of rounding retrospectively reported ages at marriage now warrants attention. The pattern of rounding to age 10 is highly erratic with over 30 percent of women 35–39 stating this figure, as opposed to only 3 to 8 percent for the youngest and the two oldest cohorts. Child marriage

TABLE 6.2 Quality of Estimates of Median Age at First Marriage and Indicators of Accuracy of Event Dating, Kenya WFS 1977–1978

	Age Group						
	15–19	20–24	25–29	30–34	35–39	40–44	45–49
Median age at first marriage	—	18.7	17.5	17.1	18.1	17.2	17.8
Proportion not yet married	.76	.18	.04	.01	.004	.003	.002
Proportion with retrospective reported age at marriage of:							
• 10 years	(.04)	.13	.24	.16	.32	.04	.08
• 15 years	(.15)	.17	.19	.17	.14	.10	.07
• 20 years	—	.23	.25	.17	.14	.09	.13
• 25 years	—	—	.15	.18	.25	.16	.26
Proportion self-reporting illiterate	.12	.13	.18	.14	.17	.11	.14
Proportion reporting complete date of birth	.40	.26	.18	.08	.04	.03	.02
Proportion reporting year of birth only	.21	.18	.21	.14	.11	.08	.08
Proportion of married women reporting complete date of first marriage	(.11)	.23	.25	.16	.12	.07	.07
Proportion of married women reporting year of first marriage only	(.03)	.09	.18	.16	.19	.15	.20
Proportion of parous women reporting complete date of last birth	(.09)	.22	.25	.16	.13	.08	.08
Proportion of parous women reporting year of last birth only	(.01)	.05	.11	.12	.22	.19	.30
N (all women)	1930	1505	1515	991	892	596	671

NOTE: Values in parentheses pertain to a highly selected group that had already progressed to marriage or a first birth at a young age.

undoubtedly has declined in Kenya for the more recent cohorts, but the difference between the 35–39 age group and those aboved 40 is entirely implausible. The remarkable attraction to 25 as the age at marriage for those over 30 also suggests dubious data quality. Heaping does not disappear for younger cohorts aged 20–24 and 25–29. They show heaping around a younger age (mainly 20), as expected. The age pattern of self-reported literacy, given in table 6.2, shows a distribution which, in contrast to the increasing levels of schooling, is virtually horizontal. Moreover, the proportions capable of reporting actual dates of birth, first marriage, or even of birth of the last born child (that is, the most recent event) decline with age. In sum, it is rare for more than a quarter of the women to be able to accurately fix a year to an event. In view of this, it seems prudent to follow van de Walle's advice.

Bearing these arguments in mind, it can be concluded that comparisons between regions and ethnic groups based on proportions single by age can be attempted, but that singulate mean ages at marriage for women are likely to be *too high* for populations with low literacy levels. In fact, the regional variation presented in the next section is likely to be an underevaluation of the true variation. Furthermore, trends inferred from retrospectively reported data have little, if any, validity.

A discussion and presentation of the various indices of nuptiality and polygyny, their definitions and usage, is also necessary. Among the most commonly used indices are:

1. The proportion single among women aged 15–19 and men 20–24. These proportions show the highest regional variance and they are therefore ideal for mapping and illuminating contrasts. But, as shown, they are far from being free of error.

2. Hajnal's singulate mean age at marriage ($SMAM$) for both sexes can be produced from the age schedule of the proportions never-married by 5-year age groups. These values are strongly related to the proportions single women 15–19 (PSW) and men 20–24 (PSM) respectively, as shown in figures 6.2 and 6.3. For those who prefer the more familiar metric of ages at marriage rather than proportions single, $SMAM$ values can be obtained as:

$$SMAM\text{-}f = 15.0 + 16.5 \ PSW \qquad \text{(eq. 6.1)}$$

$$SMAM\text{-}m = 16.0 + 13.33 \ PSM \qquad \text{(eq. 6.2)}$$

These conversions are obviously shortcuts, but they illustrate when compared with $SMAM$s that little is to be gained from the usage of the entire age schedule of proportions never-married in sub-Saharan populations. The only exception to this fit in the entire data file pertains to Saharan nomads or Berber groups (for example, Woodabe

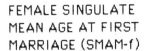

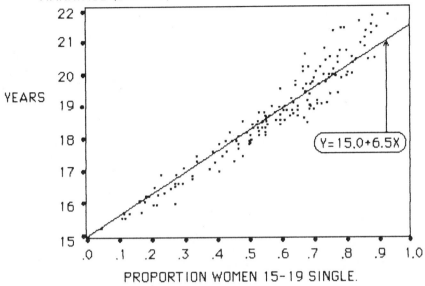

FEMALE SINGULATE MEAN AGE AT FIRST MARRIAGE (SMAM-f)

YEARS

$Y = 15.0 + 6.5X$

PROPORTION WOMEN 15-19 SINGLE.

FIGURE 6.2. Relationship between Proportions Single Women 15–19 and Female Singulate Mean Age at Marriage (*SMAM-f*). (Data for Benin, Burkina Faso, Burundi, Cameroon, Chad, Congo, Ghana, Kenya, Lesotho, Madagascar, Mauritania, Nigeria, Rwanda, Senegal, Somalia, North Sudan, Tanzania, Togo, West Zaire)

Fulani, Twareg, Hassania) with non-universal marriage among their caste of ex-slaves or servants.

3. The polygyny ratio (M), the classic index of polygyny, is the ratio of the number of currently married women (CMF) to the number of currently married men (CMM). As for all indices, only the population aged 15+ is used here in the computations.

4. Several indices mentioned above can be usefully combined: differences in ages at first union between the sexes can be measured through a ratio of proportions single women 15–19 to the proportion single men 20–24 (that is, the proportions single ratio or *RPS*). Alternatively, equations 6.1 and 6.2 can be used to estimate differences between *SMAM* values for both sexes. Of course, the directly calculated values of *SMAM* can be used in establishing such differences. The range in *SMAM* differences is of the order of 3 to 11 years and the age differences between the spouses at first marriage also displays a high degree of regional and ethnic variation.

MALE SINGULATE
MEAN AGE AT FIRST
MARRIAGE (SMAM-m)

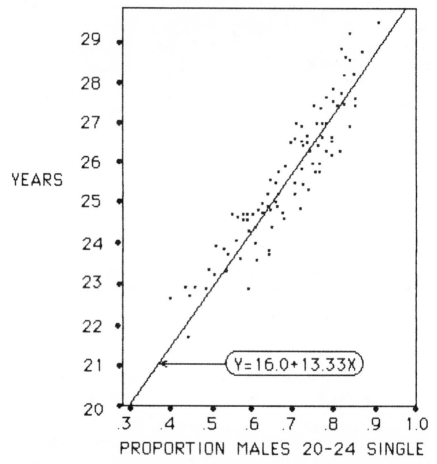

FIGURE 6.3. Relationship between Proportions Single Males 20–24 and Male Singulate Mean Age at Marriage (*SMAM-m*). (Data for Benin, Burkina Faso, Cameroon, Chad, Congo, Lesotho, Liberia, Madagascar, Mauritania, Rwanda, Senegal, Somalia, Tanzania, West Zaire)

In addition to these classic indicators, several new ones were employed:

1. The ratio of *proportions* ever-married (*L*), that is the ratio of *proportions* ever-married women 15+ of all women 15+, to the *proportions* of ever-married men 15+ of all men 15+:

$$L = (EMF/F)/(EMM/M) \qquad \text{(eq. 6.3)}$$

This ratio is different from the ever-married ratio (EMR), defined as

$$EMR = EMF/EMM \qquad \text{(eq. 6.4)}$$

in the sense that L takes the adult sex-ratio (F/M) into account. Obviously $L = $ EMR in a population with an adult sex ratio of unity. As shall be shown later on, sex-ratio distortions in the adult population are frequently encountered in sub-Saharan regions, mainly as a result of male migration. It is therefore advisable to have two sets of measures which deal with ratios between numbers and proportions respectively. When differences in ages at first marriage between the sexes are small, both *EMR* and L approach unity, and when the husband-wife age gap increases, both show a marked surplus of ever-married women. The two measures, however, diverge when sex ratios of adults are no longer balanced.

2. The ratio of proportions currently married (K) is the ratio of the *proportion* of currently married women 15+ of ever-married women 15+, to the equivalent *proportion* for men:

$$K = (CMF/EMF)/(CMM/EMM) \qquad \text{(eq. 6.5)}$$

K measures the *relative* deficit of widowed and divorced men. If the relative surplus of widows or divorcées is preferred, the reciprocal of K is simply used. The values of K are commonly lower than unity since widowhood is more frequent for women (effect of male surmortality, polygyny, and the husband-wife age gap) and since remarriage is generally slower for women than for men. Hence, the lower the value of K, the higher the relative proportion of currently widowed and divorced women, and generally, the slower the relative pace of female remarriage. From the definitions of the classic polygyny ratio M, K and L, it follows that:

$$M = K \cdot L \cdot \text{Adult sex-ratio } (F/M) \qquad \text{(eq. 6.6)}$$

or

$$K \cdot L = M/\text{sex-ratio} = (CMF/F)/(CMM/M) \qquad \text{(eq. 6.7)}$$

In other words, the product KL is the common polygyny ratio's counterpart adjusted to the sex ratio, so that $KL = M$ when the adult sex ratio F/M equals unity. Equation 6.6 breaks down the polygyny ratio M into a component L, which reacts to the sex differential in ages at first marriage, a component K, which corresponds to the sex differential in proportions currently widowed and divorced, and the adult sex ratio itself. The product KL can be labeled as the "polygyny multiplier" since it converts the sex-ratio into the classic polygyny ratio. A few further comments with respect to K and L are, however, warranted. Theoretically, K and L should be independent of the adult sex ratio. This is in practice not so: the polygyny multipliers KL and the adult sex-ratios are *jointly* influenced by differences with respect to sex– and marital status–related variations in age patterns of mortality, and especially, of migration. Emigration of young single men, for instance, raises the value of the sex ratio by causing a surplus of women, and concomitantly lowers the value of L (that is, emigration of single males increases the *proportion* of ever-married men in the denominator of L). Hence, significant inverse correlations between L and the sex-ratio are to be expected. This issue will be returned to during empirical analysis in the next section.

Finally, a number of indices of polygyny, introduced by van de Walle in 1968 and referred to by Goldman and Pebley in the previous chapter, are also used. They are the proportion of polygynists among married men (p), the average number of wives per polygynist (w), and the proportion of married females living in a polygynous union (f). They are related via eq. 6.8:

$$f = pw/(1 + p(w - 1)) \qquad \text{(eq. 6.8)}$$

Censuses and surveys inspired by the French and Belgian traditions of data collection generally provide the data needed for the calculation of p and w, but most data from anglophone countries do not. Parenthetically, the British colonial tradition of demographic data collection paid generally little attention to marital status information despite a rich anthropological legacy in studying marriage, nor has this been rectified during the postcolonial period. Given that only a subset of regions have information on p, w, and f, some complementary information of an equivalent nature was sought. The WFS recorded the number of polygynously married women, but in most instances only for women age 15–49. It was, however, found in the sources for which f is available for the aged group 15+ and 15–49 that the two values were sufficiently similar to be interchangeable. The plot presented in figure 6.4 testifies to this effect. The WFS figures were subsequently added to the series of f without alteration.

ADDITIONAL NOTES ON THE FORMAL DEMOGRAPHY OF POLYGYNY

In the preceding chapter Goldman and Pebley described the formal demographic conditions that enhance the potential for polygyny and document their findings with data for three countries (Senegal, Cameroon, and Sudan). With access to a much larger data file, it is possible to make some additional remarks, drawing especially on the data from East Africa and the components derived from the breakdown of the polygyny ratio (that is, $M = K \cdot L \cdot$ sex ratio). In setting up a framework for comparison, more attention will be paid to the roles of divorce, widowhood, and remarriage.

PROPORTION OF CURR
MARRIED WOMEN 15+
IN POLYGYGOUS UNION

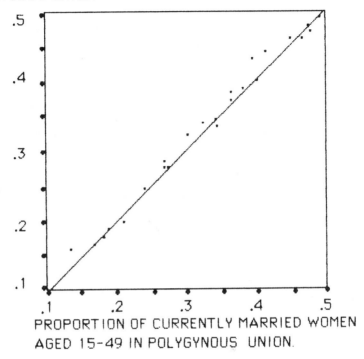

FIGURE 6.4. Relationship between Proportions Currently Married Women in Polygynous Unions in Two Age Categories (15–49 versus 15+). (Data for Cameroon, Central African Republic, Mali, Tanzania, West Zaire)

The age structure is again taken from a stable population. It corresponds with a gross reproduction rate of 3.0 daughters, a Princeton mortality level of 14 West with a life expectancy of 52.5 and 49.6 years for females and males respectively, a growth rate of 2.92 percent, and an adult sex ratio showing a 5 percent surplus of women. This stable age distribution was then combined with various age and sex-specific schedules of entry into first unions and proportions currently widowed and divorced. This parallels the strategy of Goldman and Pebley who used stable age distributions with similar mortality levels, but varying fertility levels and growth rates. The various combinations of age and sex-specific patterns of first marriage are given in table 6.3. The Coale-McNeil (1972) first marriage model, which allows for the reproduction of age-specific proportions ever-married based on three parameters, was used:

TABLE 6.3   Parameters Defining Age- and Sex-Specific Patterns of Age at
First Marriage Used in Polygyny Models

Combination	Females	Males	Sex Contrast
A	a_o = 12.0	16.5	RPS = .308
	k = 0.33	0.85	$SMAM$ difference = 10.3
	$SMAM$ = 15.8	26.1	
B	Idem	15.8	RPS = .362
		0.78	$SMAM$ difference = 8.9
		24.7	
C	Idem	15.0	RPS = .476
		0.70	$SMAM$ difference = 7.2
		23.0	
D	a_o = 13.0	16.5	RPS = .669
	k = 0.41	0.85	$SMAM$ difference = 8.4
	$SMAM$ = 17.7	26.1	
E	Idem	15.8	RPS = .758
		0.78	$SMAM$ difference = 7.0
		24.7	
F	Idem	15.0	RPS = 1.032
		0.70	$SMAM$ difference = 5.3
		23.0	
G	a_o = 14.0	16.5	RPS = .989
	k = 0.50	0.85	$SMAM$ difference = 6.4
	$SMAM$ = 19.7	26.1	
H	Idem	15.8	RPS = 1.163
		0.78	$SMAM$ difference = 5.0
		24.7	
I	Idem	15.0	RPS = 1.526
		0.70	$SMAM$ difference = 3.3
		23.0	

NOTE: Definitive celibacy at age 50 has been taken as 2 percent in all instances ($C = 0.98$).

- a_0: the minimum age at which first unions begin to occur
- k : the pace at which first marriage occurs relative to the Coale-McNeil standard
- C: the proportion ultimately marrying.

The value of k gives the tempo of entry into a union by relating the observed time scale to that of the standard. Since the latter approximates to the time scale of marriage in Sweden 1965–1969, African populations need a fraction of a year to achieve the same increment in proportions ever-married as the increment achieved in 1 year by the standard. Values of k are therefore substantially lower than unity for women. If $k = 0.50$, the pace of entry into a first union is twice as fast, and if $k = 0.33$ it is three times as fast as in the standard. As reported in table 6.3, values of a_0 are allowed to vary from 12.0 to 14.0 years for women and from 15.0 to 16.5 for men. The corresponding range for k is 0.33 to 0.50 for women and 0.70 to 0.85 for men. In all instances C was fixed at 0.98, implying nonmarriage for 2 percent only. These parameter values were chosen after having compared the proportions ever-married for the more extreme populations in the data file. Their range can be taken as an adequate representation of the observed spectrum. The corresponding *SMAM* values are also reported in table 6.3. The three schedules for males and females define the nine possible combinations, A through I, used in further analyses. For each combination, two indices of the sex differential are given: (1) the ratio of proportions single women 15–19 to single men 20–24 (*RPS*), and (2) the *SMAM difference*.

The joint impact of *RPS* and the differential age and sex patterns of proportions currently widowed and divorced on the polygyny multiplier *KL* is studied in figure 6.5. Restricting attention to just one pattern of widow-hood, divorce, and remarriage, that is, to one of the four planes in figure 6.5, it is clear how strongly the polygyny multiplier is determined by the sex differences in proportions single at young ages. The relationship can be clar-ified if *KL* is reviewed in *SMAM*-difference rather than with *RPS*. An incre-ment in the *SMAM* difference by 1 year results, on average, in an increment of approximately 0.06 in the polygyny multiplier *KL*. This increment is slightly larger than 0.06 if the increments in *SMAM differences are small* (3 to 4 years) and slightly smaller than 0.06 if the increment in *SMAM differences are large* (that is, 6 years or more). But, as a rule of thumb, one is not far off if the incremental value of 0.06 in *KL* per year for husband-wife difference in *SMAM* is maintained throughout. For instance, if two populations with (1) similar proportions currently widowed and divorced men and women, (2) similar stable age distributions with the typically African characteristics specified above, and (3) identical adult sex ratios have a difference in the husband-wife age gap at first marriage of 3 years (that is, populations corre-sponding with points A and C, D and F, and G and H in figure 6.5), they would show a difference in the polygyny multiplier of $3 \cdot 0.06 = 0.18$ and a difference in the polygyny ratio M of $0.18 \cdot$ sex ratio (F/M). Two such popula-tions with husband-wife age gaps at first marriage of 3 and 11 years respec-tively are 8 years apart, and the difference in their *KL* values would amount to 8×0.06 approximately. If their adult sex ratio equals 1.050, their polygy-ny ratios would differ by about 0.50. This contrast defines the real range encountered in sub-Saharan Africa, with polygyny ratios being comprised between 1.10 and 1.60, given balanced sex ratios. The populations A and I in

Polygyny ratio adjusted for
sex imbalance (1 * k) or
CMf/F15+ / CMm/M15+

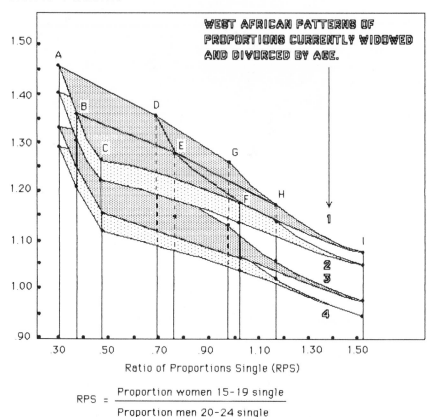

$$RPS = \frac{\text{Proportion women 15-19 single}}{\text{Proportion men 20-24 single}}$$

FIGURE 6.5. Relationship between the Ratio of Proportions Single and the Polygyny Multiplier (*L K*) in Different Situations with Respect to the Incidence of Union Dissolution and Remarriage

figure 6.5 sharing the same conditions with respect to proportions currently widowed and divorced are 7 years apart with respect to their *SMAM* difference, and one expects a difference in *KL* of 0.42. The actual difference is 0.38, illustrating that the rule of thumb is not far off the mark even for extreme cases. Furthermore, the four planes of figure 6.5 are virtually parallel, so that this simple rule is applicable to any two populations with identical proportions currently widowed and divorced, irrespective of the level of these proportions.

The matter is different when populations have varying patterns by age and sex of proportions currently widowed and divorced. Restricting the com-

PER CENT CURRENTLY
WIDOWED & DIVORCED   WEST AFRICAN SCHEDULES BY AGE

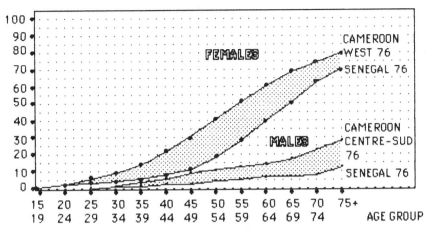

FIGURE 6.6. Age Schedules of Percentages Currently Widowed and Divorced Women and Men in Contrasting West African Populations

parisons to West African populations with similar age patterns but different levels of proportions widowed and divorced, four contrasting combinations were set up. For example, the lowest levels for both sexes in 1976 were found in Senegal and the highest in two regions of Cameroon (see figure 6.6). The four combinations in figure 6.5 are:

• *Pattern 1:* Low proportions currently widowed and divorced for females (Senegal) and high proportions for men (Cameroon, South-Central). For these conditions to materialize, widows and divorcées would have to remarry fast and predominantly marry men who are already polygynists. For specified values of *RPS*, the high polygyny multipliers for pattern 1 result mainly from a high average number of wives per polygynist (*w*). The death of a polygynist produces many widows who would all be absorbed quickly by other polygynous households. This reflects social conditions governed by gerontocrats and potentates with large harems. As indicated by many observers, "grande polygamie" is not the rule in sub-Saharan Africa and pattern 1 is rather extreme.

• *Pattern 2:* The Senegalese conditions prevail throughout and remarriage is fast for both sexes. More widowers and divorced men now compete for spouses than in pattern 1 and the incidence of "grande polygamie" diminishes in favor of more monogamously remarried men or more "petite polygamie."

- *Pattern 3:* The Cameroon West and South-Central conditions prevail with higher proportions widowed and divorced for both sexes; remarriage is slow by West African standards, which lowers the polygyny multiplier.
- *Pattern 4:* Males have low proportions currently widowed and divorced (Senegal), whereas women have high proportions (Cameroon West). Remarriage for men is obviously fast, but they do not draw as much from the pool of widows and divorcées as in the previous cases. This feature is less typical for West Africa, and pattern 4 constitutes the other extreme.

The effect of these four combinations appears in the form of parallel planes in figure 6.5. The difference in KL is about 0.14 for patterns 1 and 4, whereas that between Senegal and southwestern Cameroon amounts to about 0.08. With balanced sex ratios, it can be taken that West African patterns of divorce, widowhood, and remarriage rarely result in differences in KL multipliers in excess of 0.10. The effects of differing patterns of marriage dissolution and remarriage holds irrespective of the values of the ratio of proportions single at young ages (RPS). The effects of RPS and levels of proportions currently widowed or divorced on KL are additive. Furthermore, since only patterns 2 and 3 correspond with actual experience in West Africa, it is clear that the variation in KL multipliers is produced more by variation in sex differences of first marriage schedules, than by sex-differences in union dissolution and remarriage. This is further supported by the fact that the observed standard deviation of L is twice that of K so that the product KL reflects essentially variation in L.

A further consideration regarding the proportions currently widowed and divorced needs to be taken into account. It was found that the differences between West and East Africa could not be explained by differences in levels only, nor accommodated by parallel planes as in figure 6.5. Differing age patterns rather than levels are responsible. This can be shown in the following way. First, several schedules of proportions currently widowed and divorced women were standardized using the Senegalese schedule. Two families of curves emerged: West African populations (and Lesotho) were showing a bulge around age 40, whereas East African ones displayed a monotonically declining curve (see figures 6.7 and 6.8). Since divorce commonly occurs at younger ages than widowhood and most of the difference is produced prior to age 40, these two age patterns must be related essentially to differences in divorce patterns. Additional information is presented in figures 6.9 and 6.10 which relate the proportions of currently widowed and divorced women by age to the proportions for men in the two major regions. Senegal and the other West African countries have a large excess of divorced women over men at ages 20–24 (three to eight times as many), largely because young divorced males remarry extremely quickly. In East Africa, divorce is more

RATIO OF PROPORTIONS CURRENTLY
WIDOWED AND DIVORCED WOMEN TO
PROPORTIONS IN SENEGAL 76

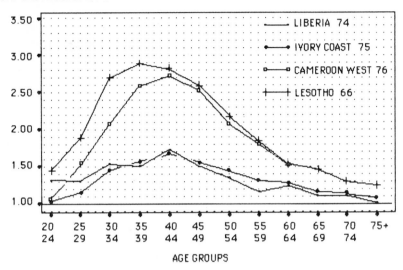

FIGURE 6.7. Age Schedules of Proportions Currently Widowed and Divorced Women (Selected Populations versus Senegal), West African Pattern

RATIO OF PROPORTIONS CURRENTLY
WIDOWED AND DIVORCED WOMEN TO
PROPORTIONS IN SENEGAL 76

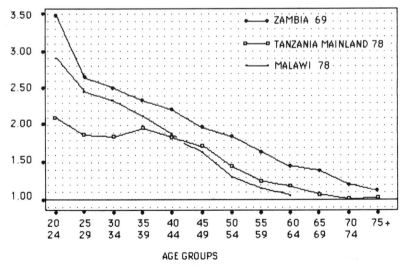

FIGURE 6.8. Age Schedule of Ratios of Proportions Currently Widowed and Divorced Women (Selected Populations versus Senegal), East African Pattern

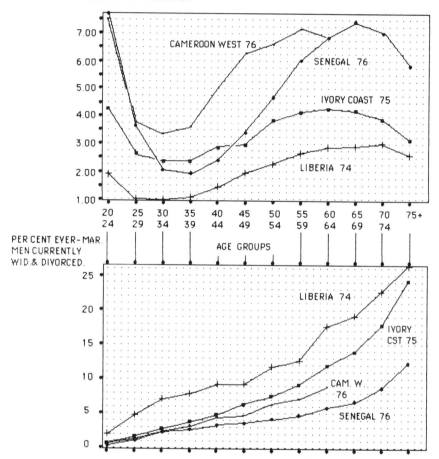

RATIO OF PROPORTIONS CURRENTLY
WIDOWED AND DIVORCED WOMEN
TO PROPORTIONS CURRENTLY
WIDOWED AND DIVORCED MEN

FIGURE 6.9. Comparison of Female and Male Schedules of Persons Currently
Widowed and Divorced, West African Pattern

common than in West Africa, and young males do not remarry at fast. The ratio
of divorced women 20–24 over divorced men 20–24 is therefore also much
lower in East than in West Africa. However, the fact that divorce is more
common among the young in East Africa implies that the standardization
of eastern proportions of women currently widowed and divorced using
the Senegalese proportions results in monotonically declining curves with age
(see figure 6.8).

The effect of the difference in age patterns of proportions currently

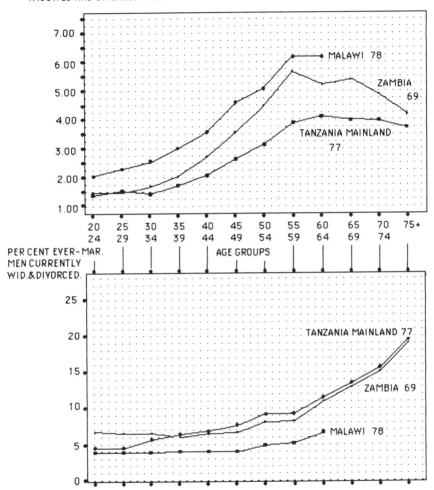

RATIO OF PROPORTIONS CURRENTLY
WIDOWED AND DIVORCED WOMEN
TO PROPORTIONS CURRENTLY
WIDOWED AND DIVORCED MEN.

PER CENT EVER-MAR.
MEN CURRENTLY
WID.&DIVORCED.

FIGURE 6.10. Comparison of Female and Male Age Schedules of Persons Currently Widowed and Divorced, East African Pattern

widowed and divorced between East and West Africa is shown in figure 6.11 using data for Senegal and Tanzania. The plane of the Tanzanian pattern no longer parallels the plane of the Senegalese pattern, and the additivity of the effects of *RPS* and of proportions currently widowed and divorced on *KL* holds no longer. If the age at marriage for women is very low (low *RPS* values) and Tanzanian conditions of marriage dissolution and remarriage

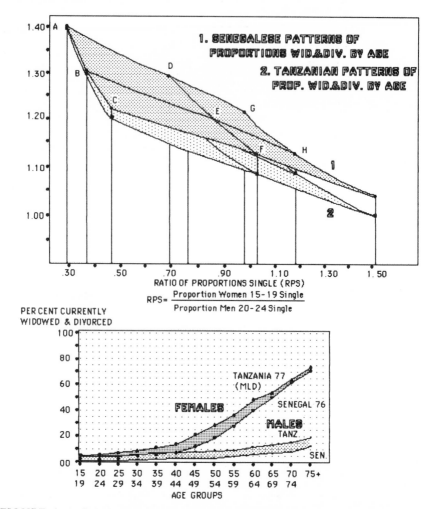

FIGURE 6.11. Relationship between Ratio of Proportions Single and Polygyny Multiplier (top) Given Senegalese and Tanzanian Patterns of Proportions Currently Widowed and Divorced (bottom)

prevail, a large supply of divorcées will be produced at young ages. However, as this stock of young divorced women is absorbed faster in Tanzania than in Senegal and since many second unions are presumably polygynous, the polygyny multiplier is increased in Tanzania. If female marriage is late (that is, *RPS* larger than 1.0), a similar supply of young divorcées is not formed, and the gap in *KL* remains, thereby reflecting the overall lower value of *K* for Tanzania. This leads to the conclusion that some East African populations have an extra contributor to polygyny in the form of the combination of early marriage for girls and high divorce followed by remarriage at young ages. The existence of this contributor is well worth pointing out as it can offset the effect of sex differences in proportions widowed. Nevertheless, its effect on the polygyny multiplier remains inferior to that of the sex difference in ages at first marriage.

Finally, the polygyny increasing effect of higher fertility is discussed. Goldman and Pebley documented this for growth rates up to 3 percent, and their figure can be extended for growth rates up to 4 percent: the growth rate in Kenya is already at this level and other populations in sub-Saharan Africa may have crossed the boundary of 3 percent as well. Two stable populations with a life expectancy of about 50 years, the age schedule of low proportions currently widowed and divorced (Senegalese schedule), and with gross reproduction rates of three and four daughters respectively (implying growth rates of almost 3 and 4 percent) differ with respect to the polygyny multiplier by about 0.10 (see figure 6.12). This difference is significant and larger than the effect of contrasting Senegalese and Cameroonian schedules of proportions currently widowed and divorced. But, as indicated by Goldman and Pebley, such an effect only comes into existence when very rapid population growth prevails. Several African populations meet these conditions and use their youthful populations to maintain high polygyny.

The ranking of the polygyny enhancing factors according to the magnitude of effects now appears as follows. The age difference at first marriage is by far the single most important contributor in all circumstances. If rapidly growing populations are considered (growth rates of 3 percent or more), then the youthfulness of these populations ranks second, followed by patterns of union dissolution and remarriage. In populations with slower growth, the ranking between these contributors is reversed. All of this presupposes the existence of balanced sex ratios. If these are distorted, an additional but more complicated effect is being produced. A surplus of women tends to enhance polygyny in West Africa, but not in Southern Africa. In the latter region female-headed households are being formed instead.

With these findings and caveats in mind, the geographical and ethnic patterns of the various parameters of the nuptiality regimes shall now be examined.

REGIONAL PATTERNS OF NUPTIALITY AND POLYGYNY

The measurement and collection of the nuptiality and polygyny indicators outlined above was attempted for as many regions (or, ethnic groups) as possible. The data were gathered from censuses and surveys. It should,

POLYGYNY RATIO ADJUSTED
FOR SEX IMBALANCE (1*k), OR:
CMf/F15+ / CMm/M15+

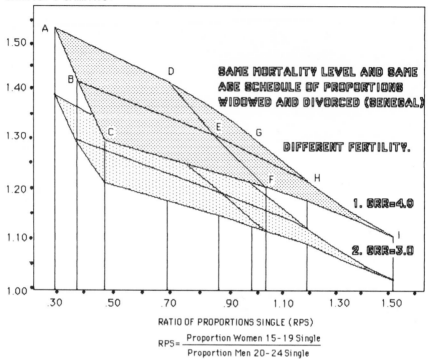

RATIO OF PROPORTIONS SINGLE (RPS)

$$RPS = \frac{\text{Proportion Women 15-19 Single}}{\text{Proportion Men 20-24 Single}}$$

FIGURE 6.12. Relationship between Ratio of Proportions Single and Polygyny Multiplier (*L K*) Given Different Fertility

however, be noted that dates of observation span a period of roughly 20 years, that is, from 1960 to 1980, and that this heterogeneity affects the cross-sectional regional comparisons. For all countries possessing multiple data sources the most recent information is presented. Where there are census and survey data covering the same period, the census data have been preferred. The reason for this is the difference in coverage. The information is summarized in a series of maps, each of which is subdivided into a West and East African part. Map 6.1 and its accompanying identification chart list the areas.

The first issues to be discussed are the ages at entry into a first union and the corresponding sex differential. The parameters used in map 6.2 are the proportions of single women 15–19 and the singulate mean age at marriage for women (*SMAM-f*), which corresponds to this proportion according to the link established in eq. 6.1. The following geographical pattern emerges:

1. A broad zone characterized by early marriage for women (*SMAM* values commonly below 18) lies in the western and central savannah and sahel regions, which contrast strikingly with a belt of later ages at marriage (commonly above 18 and often above 19.5) along the Atlantic. This Atlantic belt stretches all the way from Liberia to Namibia and is interrupted only in Gabon and Angola (provided that the data quality in these two countries was adequate in the 1960s). The inland boundary reaches from Monrovia in Liberia to Ilorin in Nigeria (Kwara state) and bends south to the Cameroon highlands, Congo, Bandundu province of Zaire, and Northwest Angola. The area of late female marriage continues with Southwest Angola until it reaches the Cape.

2. Several populations north of the sahelian strip of low female ages at marriage have higher values. This pertains particularly to Saharan nomadic groups who are often related to North African Berbers (for example, Hassania of Mauritania, Twareg).

3. There is a second strip of ages at marriage above age 18 for women covering much of East and South Africa. It contains pockets with *SMAM* values above 19 in Central Kenya, Rwanda, Burundi, and Northeast Tanzania. These pockets are welded together further south where ages at marriage above 19.5 become the rule in South African ethnic groups. Very recent survey data for the whole of Zimbabwe (1984) yield a *SMAM* value of just over 18, so that most of the blank area on map 6.2 for this country has presumably kept the Zambian pattern and has not yet adopted the South African system of very late marriage. Pockets of early marriage, that is, below 18, are also present in East Africa, for instance in Central Uganda, South Malawi, and North Mozambique.

4. It is not entirely clear whether the region of early female marriage in the western and central sahel still spreads along a north-south axis into Central Africa, as it did in the past. The data for Central, South, and East Zaire are old (that is, from 1955) and if a general trend toward later marriage has occurred, the contrast with West Zaire (data of 1975), Tanzania (1979), and Zambia (1969) may be artificial. Ages at marriage, however, in the Central African Republic, East Angola, and Northwest Zambia recorded in the 1960s further support the probable historical existence of such a central African area with *SMAM* values commonly lower than 18 years. If, on the other hand, mean ages at marriage have risen in central Africa, a general evolution towards a more simple dichotomy is probably underway, contrasting continued early marriage for women in the largely Islamized western and central savannah and sahel with mean ages at marriage over 18 for the rest of Africa.

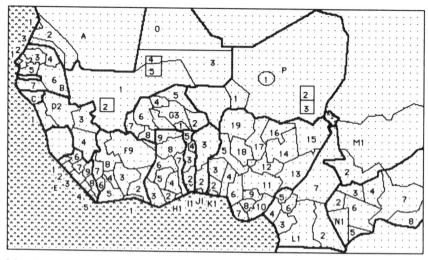

Map 6.1a. Statistical Areas, West Africa (see Key 6.1)

Key 6.1

Identification of Areas—West Africa

A. *Mauritania*: 1. Nouakchott; 2. Nomads/Other Rural; 3. Fleuve Rural/Settled Rural.

B. *Senegal*: 1. Dakar; 2 Thiès; 3. Louga & Diourbel; 4. Fleuve; 5. Sine Saloum; 6. Senegal Oriental; 7. Casamance.

C. *Guinea Bissau* (Total).

D. *Guinea Conacry*: 1. Maritime; 2. Fouta Djallon; 3. Upper; 4. Forest.

E. *Liberia*: 1. Grand Cape Mountain; 2. Montserrado; 3. Grand Bassa; 4. Sinoe; 5. Maryland; 6. Loffa; 7. Bong; 8. Grand Gedeh; 9. Nimba.

F. *Ivory Coast* (Ethnic Groups): 1. Lagunaires; 2. Agni and Related Akan; 3. Baoulé; 4. Guro; 5. Kru; 6. Guéré (Ngere); 7. Yacuba; 8. Malinke; 9. Senufo & Kulango.

G. *Burkina Fasso* (Ethnic Groups): 1. Bissa; 2. Gourmantche; 3. Central Mossi; 4. Yatenga Mossi; 5. Peul; 6. Bobo; 7. Senufo; 8. Lobi-Dagara.

H. *Ghana*: 1. Greater Accra; 2. Central; 3. Western; 4. Eastern; 5. Ashanti; 6. Brong-Ahafo; 7. Volta; 8. Northern; 9. Upper.

I. *Togo*: 1. Maritime; 2. Plateau; 3. Central; 4. Kara; 5. Savannes.

J. *Benin*: 1. Cotonou; 2. South & Central (Zou, Oueme, Atlantique, Mono); 3. Atacora & Borgou.

K. *Nigeria*: 1. Lagos; 2. Ogun; 3. Oyo; 4. Ondo; 5. Kwara; 6. Bendel; 7. Rivers; 8. Imo; 9. Anambra; 10. Cross-River; 11. Benue; 12. Plateau; 13. Gongola; 14. Bauchi; 15. Borno; 16. Kano; 17. Kaduna; 18. Niger; 19. Sokoto.

L. *Cameroon*: 1. Central-South; 2. East; 3. Littoral; 4. Southwest; 5. Northwest; 6. West; 7. North.

M. *Southern Chad*: 1. Central; 2. South.

N. *Central African Republic*: 1. Haute Sangha; 2. Nana Membere; 3. Ouham-Pende; 4. Ouham; 5. Lobaye; 6. Rest Western; 7. Central; 8. Fleuve.

O. *Mali*: 1. Rural; 2. Urban; 3. Nomads; 4. Delta Tamasheq Twareg & Bella; 5. Delta Bambara.

P. *Niger*: 1. Agadez & Tahoua; 2. Niger Peul (Wodaabe); 3. Niger Twareg

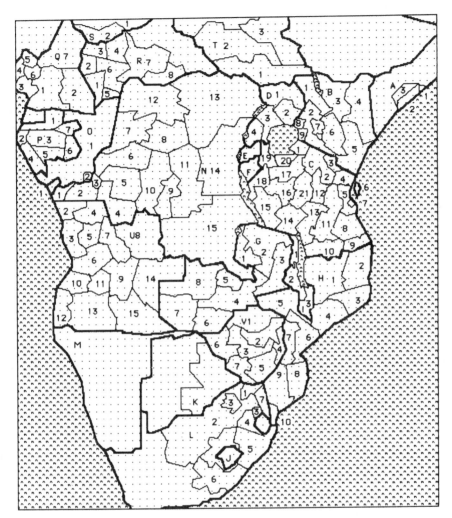

Map 6.1*b*. Statistical Areas, East Africa (see Key 6.1)

Identification of Areas—Central, Eastern, and Southern Africa

A. *Somalia*: Mogadishu & Urban Bay/Shebelle; 2. Benadir & Lower Shebelle Settled; 3. B. & LS-nomads.

B. *Kenya*: Rift Valley-Turkana; 2. Rift Valley Rest; 3. Eastern-Marsabit; 4. Northeastern; 5. Coast; 6. Eastern-Rest; 7. Central; 8. Western; 9. Nyanza; 10. Nairobi.

C. *Tanzania*: 1. Mara; 2. Arusha; 3. Kilimanjaro; 4. Tanga; 5. Coast; 6. Zanzibar; 7. Dar Es Salaam; 8. Lindi; 9. Mtwara; 10. Ruvuma; 11. Morogoro; 12. Dodoma; 13. Iringa; 14. Mbeya; 15. Rukwa; 16. Tabora; 17. Shinyanga; 18. Kigoma; 19. West Lake; 20. Mwanza; 21. Singida.

D. *Uganda*: 1. Northern; 2. Eastern; 3. Buganda; 4. Western.

E. *Rwanda* (Total).

F. *Burundi* (Total).

G. *Zambia*: 1. Luapula; 2. Northern; 3. Eastern; 4. Central; 5. Copperbelt; 6. Southern; 7. Western; 8. Northwestern.

H. *Mozambique*: 1. Niassa; 2. Cabo Delgado; 3. Moçambique; 4. Zambesia; 5. Tete; 6. Sofala; 7. Manica; 8. Inhambane; 9. Gaza; 10. Maputo (Laurenço-Marques).

I. *Malawi*: 1. Northern; 2. Central; 3. Southern.

J. *Lesotho* (Total).

K. *Botswana* (Total).

L. *South Africa* (Ethnic Groups): 1. Venda; 2. Tswana; 3. Ndebele; 4. Swazi; 5. Zulu; 6. Xhosa; 7. Thonga-Shangaan.

M. *Namibia* (Total).

N. *Zaire*: 1. Bas-Fleuve; 2. Cataractes (1 + 2 = Bas Zaire); 3. Kinshasa; 4. Kwango; 5. Kwilu; 6. Mai Ndombe (4 + 5 + 6 = Bandundu); 7. Equateur; 8. Tshuapa (7 + 8 = Equateur Prov.); 9. Lulua; 10. Kasai (9 + 10 = Kasai Occidental); 11. Sankura & Kabinda (Rest Kasai Prov.); 12. Ubangi & Mongala (Rest Equateur Prov.); 13. Orientale; 14. Shaba.

O. *Congo*: 1. Congo Overall or Villages + Centres Extracoutumiers; 2. Brazzaville.

P. *Gabon* (Ethnic Groups): 1. Fang; 2. Omyene; 3. Bakele; 4. Eshira; 5. Okande; 6. Mbede; 7. Bakota.

Q. *Cameroon*: See West Africa.

R. *Central African Republic*: See West Africa.

S. *Southern Chad*: See West Africa.

T. *Southern Sudan*: 1. Equatoria; 2. Bahr-el-Ghazal; 3. Upper Nile.

U. *Angola*: 1. Cabinda; 2. Zaire; 3. Luanda; 4. Uige; 5. Cuanza Norte; 6. Cuanza Sul; 7. Malange; 8. Lunda Norte & Sul; 9. Bie; 10. Benguela; 11. Huambo; 12. Mocamedes; 13. Huila & Cunene; 14. Moxico; 15. Cuando Cubango.

V. *Zimbabwe*: 1. North Mashonaland; 2. South Mashonaland; 3. Midlands; 4. Manicaland; 5. Victoria; 6. North Matabeleland; 7. South Matabeleland.

5. Sudan, Ethiopia, and Somalia have been omitted from the discussion until now. Fragmentary evidence suggests than *SMAM* values for women were lower than 18 years in the 1960s, but recent surveys in Somalia and North Sudan (WFS) suggest a substantial rise. For North Sudan it is highly likely that this rise can, at least partially, be attributed to marital status–related age misstatement (cf. figure 6.1). Hence it is too early to come up with a definitive judgment regarding a recent trend.

The map with the male proportion single 20–24 or male *SMAM* values based on these proportions differs greatly from the map with the comparable female values (see maps 6.2 and 6.3). There is no western sahelian pattern of early marriage for men and the "Atlantic crescent" no longer provides a continuous string of late age at marriage (that is, above 25). The Central African north-south strip of early marriage for males (that is, below 25) extends well into East Africa, even if data from the late 1970s are used. The only major similarity with the distribution of female marital behavior is an overall pattern of late marriage for both sexes in South Africa, Botswana, and Namibia. The proportions single for the two sexes can be contrasted by means of the *SMAM* difference computed via equations 6.1 and 6.2. As indicated above, the lowest difference in husband-wife ages at first marriage is 3 years and the highest 11. Taking 7 years as a cutoff point, one can readily see on map 6.4 that the largest husband-wife differences are especially concentrated in West Africa. Differences in excess of 9 years (omitting Sudan, Ethiopia, and Somalia) only exist in the western Islamized areas, such as in Senegal, Guinea, and Central Burkina Faso. In East and South Africa, husband-wife age differences at first marriages between 7 and 9 years are only found in North Kenya and the Kenyan Rift Valley, and among the Tswana, Ndebele, and Venda ethnic groups of South Africa. Age differences in excess of 7 years are hence the rule in West Africa and the exception elsewhere. *SMAM* values computed on the basis of the full age schedule of proportions never-married or ratios of proportions single (*RPS*) convey a similar picture.

The geographic distribution of *SMAM* differences is obviously related to the pattern of polygyny. The comparison of map 6.4 showing the *SMAM* differences between the sexes with either map 6.5, showing the proportion of women currently married to a polygynist (*f*), or map 6.6, with polygyny ratios (*M*), testifies to this effect. The Atlantic polygyny zone stretches far inland and incorporates all climatic and cultural zones of West Africa. The high polygyny zone extends further south to Angola. The only Atlantic areas with less than 40 percent of married women in polygynous unions and polygyny ratios below 1.3 are found in Southeast Ivory Coast and Southwest Ghana (that is, in matrilineal Akan ethnic groups) and in the border regions of Southeast Nigeria and Southwest Cameroon. Finally, sahelian nomads

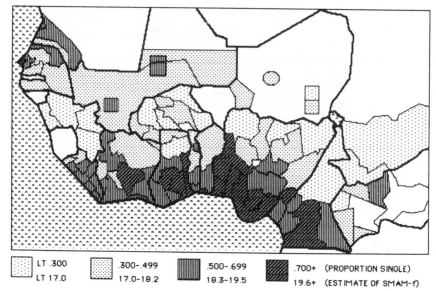

:::: LT .300	:::: .300-.499	▦ .500-.699	▨ .700+ (PROPORTION SINGLE)
LT 17.0	17.0-18.2	18.3-19.5	19.6+ (ESTIMATE OF SMAM-f)

Map 6.2a. Proportion Single Women Aged 15–19 and Approximate Values of the Female Singulate Mean Age at First Marriage (SMAM-f); Latest Available Data

and Berber groups have a very low incidence of polygyny and do not fit the sub-Saharan pattern at all (see, for instance, Randall on the Tamasheq Twareg, 1984, and the WFS-results for the Hassania of Mauritania).

In general, the incidence of polygyny in Central, Eastern, and Southern Africa is much lower than in the Atlantic zone and the western sahel. There are, however, a few exceptions. Polygyny ratios above 1.20 or percentages of women married to polygynists in excess of 30 (still modest by West African standards) are found in West Kenya, Central Tanzania, East Zambia, North Malawi, and North Mozambique, forming an East African polygyny ridge that stretches south from Kisumu on Lake Victoria to the Tete province of Mozambique. In places along the coast of the Indian ocean values of M larger than 1.20 or f larger than 30 percent are also found: for example, in the Kenyan Coast province; the Tanzanian districts of Tanga, Lindi, Mtwara, and Ruvuma; the Mozambique province of Manica-Sofala; and among the coastal Nguni (Zulu) of South Africa.

The polygyny multiplier KL (that is, the ratio of *proportions* currently married of both sexes) and its major component L (that is, the ratio of *proportions* ever-married women and men) change the information given by the polygyny ratio M and the proportion of women in polygynous unions f to a considerable extent. One may recall from the previous section that KL is not positively affected by the adult sex ratio F/M. Consequently, areas with high values of M and f, but also with a substantial surplus of adult women, no

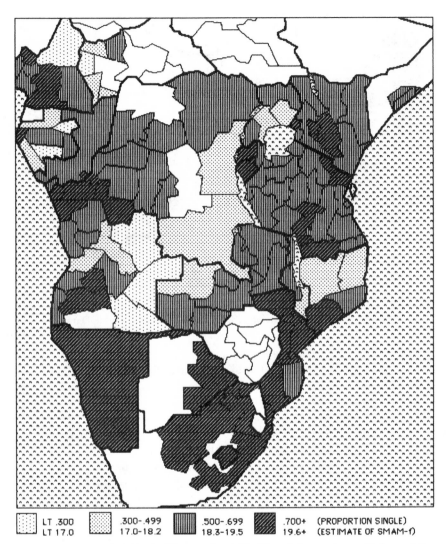

| LT .300 | .300-.499 | .500-.699 | .700+ | (PROPORTION SINGLE) |
| LT 17.0 | 17.0-18.2 | 18.3-19.5 | 19.6+ | (ESTIMATE OF SMAM-f) |

Map 6.2*b*. Proportion Single Women Aged 15–19 and Approximate Values of the Female Singulate Mean Age at First Marriage (SMAM-f); Latest Available Data

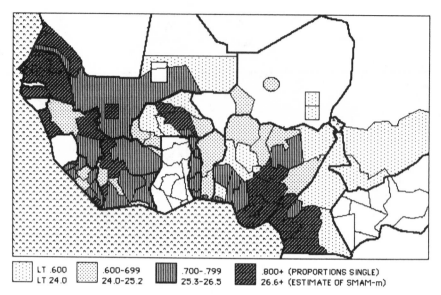

| LT .600 | .600-699 | ▓ .700-.799 | ▓ .800+ (PROPORTIONS SINGLE) |
| LT 24.0 | 24.0-25.2 | 25.3-26.5 | 26.6+ (ESTIMATE OF SMAM-m) |

Map 6.3*a*. Proportion Single Men Aged 20–24 and Approximate Values of the Male Singulate Mean Age at First Marriage (SMAM-m); Latest Available Data

longer show up with dark shadings in map 6.7 presenting the polygyny multipliers. This results in the total disappearance of the East African polygyny ridge. With very few exceptions, polygyny multipliers do not exceed 1.20 in Central, East, and South Africa.

The picture for West African polygyny, measured by M or f, undergoes similar modifications if the polygyny multiplier KL is used. It should be noted, in passing, that KL values larger than 1.20 are the rule in West Africa, which makes the East-West contrast even sharper in map 6.7 than in the preceding polygyny maps. The map with polygyny multipliers closely resembles the map with $SMAM$ differences (map 6.4). This is reflected in correlation coefficients: M and the sex difference in $SMAM$ have a coefficient of 0.42, whereas KL and the $SMAM$-difference have a coefficient of 0.60.

Several of the West African areas that had been singled out for their relatively low incidence of polygyny (that is, Akan groups, Nigerian-Cameroon border area), no longer stand out once the polygyny multiplier is used. The KL values act to smooth out the data and present a more even picture.

Map 6.7 contains, however, one major exception: several regions in southern Nigeria with high values of M and f, have low values of KL. It is suspected that this exception is artificial: Nigerian sex ratios were obtained in the WFS household survey, whereas sex ratios for other countries are derived from censuses or much larger surveys. Given the small samples by state in the Nigerian WFS and the focus of attention on the fertility-oriented indi-

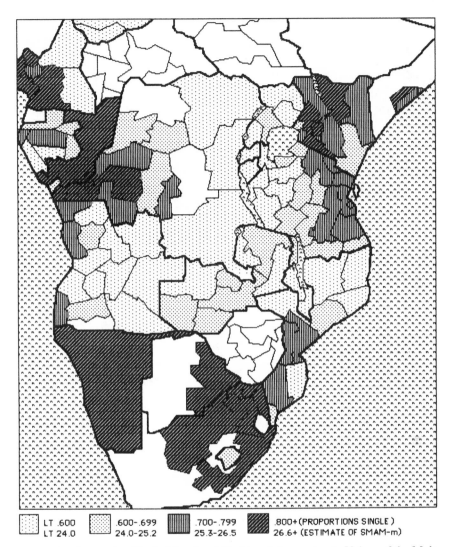

LT .600	.600–.699	.700–.799	.800+ (PROPORTIONS SINGLE)
LT 24.0	24.0–25.2	25.3–26.5	26.6+ (ESTIMATE OF SMAM-m)

Map 6.3*b*. Proportion Single Men Aged 20–24 and Approximate Values of the Male Singulate Mean Age at First Marriage (SMAM-m); Latest Available Data

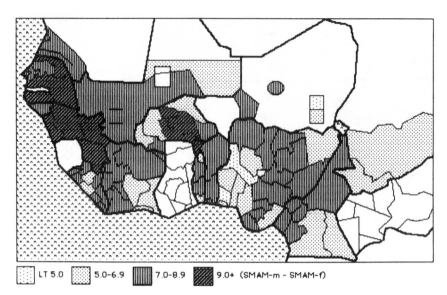

| :::: | LT 5.0 | :::: | 5.0-6.9 | ‖‖‖ | 7.0-8.9 | ▨ | 9.0+ (SMAM-m - SMAM-f) |

Map 6.4a. Husband–Wife Age Difference at First Marriage; Latest Available Data

vidual questionnaire, an accurate recording of men in the household or elsewhere was less likely. An idea of the size of the error can be obtained from comparing the adult sex ratios in Cameroon as measured through the Cameroon WFS of 1978 and the census of 1979. This comparison is illustrated in table 6.4. The areas are ranked by surplus of women, from high to low, and the ratio between the two series indicates the relative magnitude of the deviation. These Cameroon data indicate that the ranking is similar for both sources, but that deviations by area can be as high as 16 percent. The largest

TABLE 6.4   Comparison of Adult Sex Ratios (F/M) in Cameroon as Measured by the Census of 1976 and the WFS Household Questionnaire of 1978

Areas (Ranked)	Adult Sex Ratios		Ratio (1)/(2)
	WFS (1)	Census (2)	
West	1.597	1.447	1.104
Northwest	1.290	1.189	1.085
East	1.119	1.074	1.042
North	1.117	1.127	0.991
Central-South	1.080	1.092	0.989
Littoral	1.063	0.913	1.164
Southwest	1.046	0.908	1.152
Total Cameroon	1.139	1.110	1.026

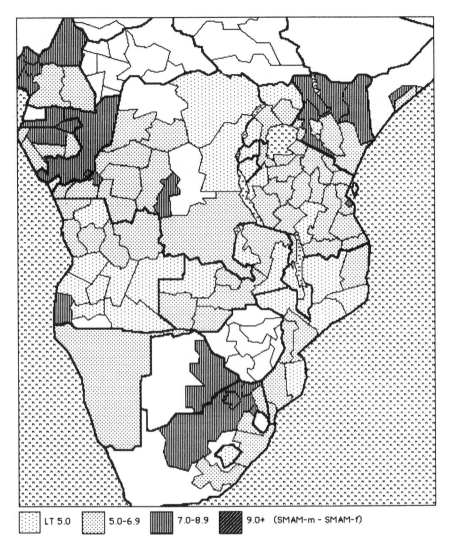

| | LT 5.0 | | 5.0-6.9 | | 7.0-8.9 | | 9.0+ (SMAM-m - SMAM-f) |

Map 6.4*b*. Husband–Wife Age Difference at First Marriage: Latest Available Data

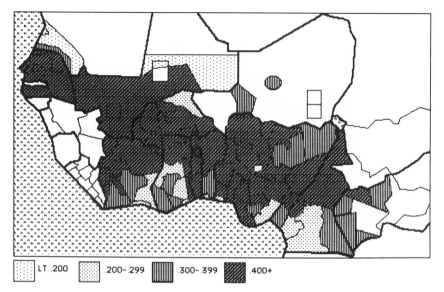

LT .200   .200-.299   .300-.399   .400+

Map 6.5*a*. Proportion of Currently Married Women Aged 15+ in Polygynous Unions

discrepancies are found in areas experiencing either considerable emigration (Western Highlands) or immigration (Southwest, Littoral). The WFS systematically produces a higher surplus of women, which is not surprising given that the main purpose of the household questionnaire was the identification of women of childbearing age. In Cameroon, greater care was taken to collect more detailed household-level information than in the other countries participating in the WFS, and it can be assumed that the WFS adult sex ratios for Cameroon are better than elsewhere. Morah (1985) compared the age specific sex ratios in the Nigerian WFS household data with those of the 1963 census and found a much larger excess of females in the age range from 15 to 60 in the national WFS-data set. In the age group 20–24, there were for instance 155 women per 100 men and in the age group 25–29 152 women. This anomalous pattern was less marked in the 1963 census with 119 and 114 women respectively. In view of this, it is entirely plausible to assume that the low *KL* values for southern Nigeria are the result of highly inflated sex ratios. Ogun state, for instance, has an adult sex-ratio for the entire population over 15 of 160 women per 100 men. The general conclusion is therefore that WFS data can be used to estimate values of *f*, but not for measuring *M*, *KL*, and sex ratios.

The issue of sex-ratio imbalances warrants further attention. There are two major sources of such imbalances: (1) measurement error as suspected, for instance, in the WFS household data, and (2) sex and marital status

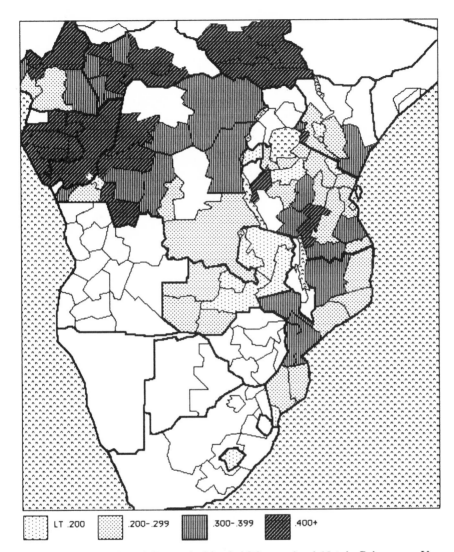

| | LT .200 | | .200-.299 | | .300-.399 | | .400+ |

Map 6.5b. Proportion of Currently Married Women Aged 15+ in Polygynous Unions

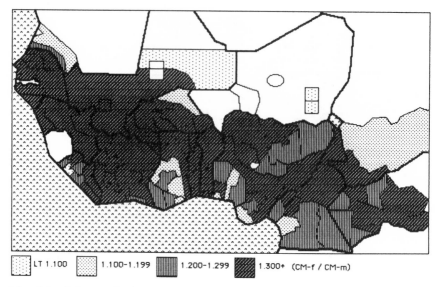

LT 1.100   1.100-1.199   1.200-1.299   1.300+ (CM-f / CM-m)

Map 6.6a. Polygyny Ratio; Latest Available Data

selective migration. Interaction between these two sources of variation may
also occur. For instance, husbands who have migrated may accurately report
the number of their wives but not specify their location. These women are
then assumed to have migrated with them. If the wives are, however, in the
area of origin, they risk being counted twice.

Most African migration streams are largely composed of men. The composition by marital status of the male migrants is more variable. The Vol-
taique migration to the Ivory Coast involves mainly single men, whereas the
labor migration in South Africa involves all men. To what extent can the
adult sex ratios of map 6.8 be explained in terms of migration? Table 6.5
contrasts the sex ratios of areas that are economically attractive with those of
either neighboring zones of labor recruitment or economically disadvantaged
areas. It is encouraging to find that the largest contrasts in adult sex ratios
within countries are strongly associated with known migration streams and
contrasts in regional population growth. Hence, the information in map 6.8
is not predominantly the product of measurement error.

The positive association between the polygyny ratio M and the adult sex
ratio F/M ($r = +0.50$) has been given a specific interpretation in West African populations with a high incidence of polygyny. Capron and Kohler
(1975) suggest that polygyny and male emigration are mutually reinforcing.
This thesis is supported by data from the Mossi of Burkina Faso. The absence of young Mossi men gave the older, wealthier men, who remained at
home, more opportunities for "monopolizing" the pool of available women.

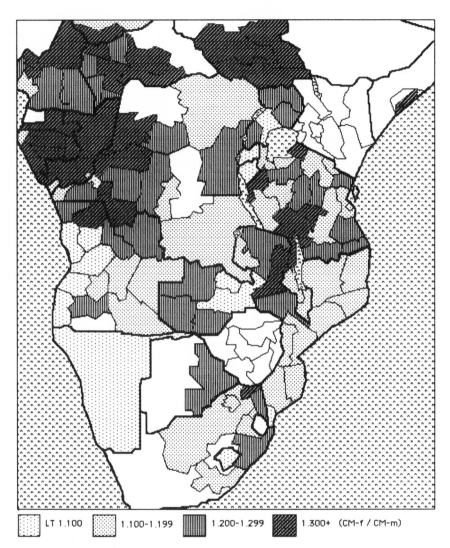

Map 6.6*b*. Polygyny Ratio; Latest Available Data

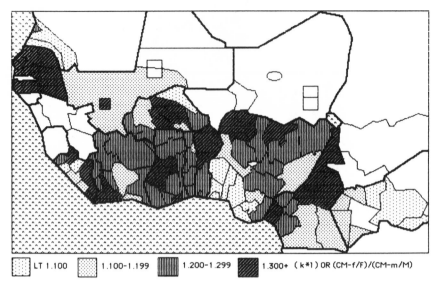

LT 1.100   1.100-1.199   1.200-1.299   1.300+ (k*1) OR (CM-f/F)/(CM-m/M)

Map 6.7a. Ratio of Proportions Currently Married 15+ or Polygyny Multipliers; Latest Available Data

This resulted in bridewealth inflation and enhanced polygyny, consequently pushing more young Mossi to emigrate to the Ivory Coast in pursuit of means for financing the acquisition of a first wife. Strong gerontocratic control, polygyny with early marriage for girls, emigration of single men, and subsequent male marriage postponement formed the basic ingredients of this particular nuptiality regime. It is possible to imagine the alternative, the young migrants earning enough independently to compete with the older men in the marriage market. However, independent earnings are so strongly connected with a period of exile that even if the earnings are large enough, time abroad is still being lost, thereby resulting in a longer period of marriage postponement.

It would be dangerous to interpret the positive association between the polygyny ratio (M) and the adult sex ratio exclusively in these terms. Alternatively, a surplus of married women is likely to be found wherever there is a surplus of women resulting from emigration of married males. Then, M is simply statistically contaminated by the adult sex ratio even in areas with much less polygyny.

The information presented in the various maps was compared and systematized through classic statistical procedures. First of all, it was considered fruitful to reduce the nine original indicators into a smaller number. This was done with a minimal loss of information by means of factor analysis. The underlying factors of the original set of indicators were defined in such a way

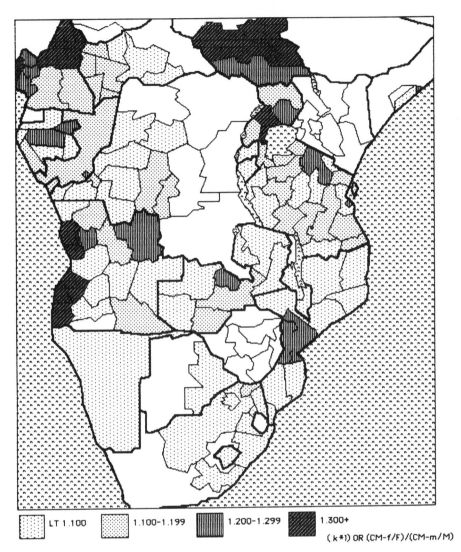

| | LT 1.100 | | 1.100-1.199 | | 1.200-1.299 | | 1.300+ |

(k*1) OR (CM-f/F)/(CM-m/M)

Map 6.7*b*. Ratio of Proportions Currently Married 15+ or Polygyny Multipliers;
Latest Available Data

TABLE 6.5   Adult Sex Ratios (F/M) of Economically Attractive Areas versus Those of Adjacent Areas or Economically Disadvantaged Areas

Country and Source	Receiving Areas		Sending Areas	
Angola, 1960 census	Cabinda	.966	Zaïre	1.321
	Luanda	.694	Uige	1.269
	Benguela	.734		
Botswana, 1971 census			Total Botswana	1.351
Burkina Faso, 1960 survey	Quagadougou	.998	Total Burkina Faso	1.221
Cameroon, 1976 census	Southwest	.908	West	1.447
	Littoral	.913		
	Yaounde & Douala (WFS)	.893		
Chad, 1962 census	N'Djamena	.956		
Congo, 1974 census	Brazzaville	.966	Rest Congo	1.170
Ghana, 1960 census	Accra	.840	Northern	1.159
	Eastern	.996	All rural	1.036
	All urban	.903		
Ivory Coast, 1975 census	All urban	.888	All rural	1.179
Ivory Coast, 1981 WFS	Abidjan	.805	Rural, forest region	1.068
	Urban, forest region	.869	Rural, savannah region	1.264
	Urban, savannah region	.982		
	Non-Ivoirien immigrants	.690		
Kenya, 1979 census	Nairobi	.543	Eastern	1.148
	Coast & Mombasa	.980	Western	1.189
	Rift Valley	.960	Nyanza	1.174
Kenya, 1962 census	Nairobi	.492	Nyanza & Western	1.060
	Coast & Mombasa	.951		
	Rift Valley	.930		
Lesotho, 1966 census	Absentee population	.202	De facto population	1.634

Source				
Malawi, 1977 census	Blantyre	.847	Northern	1.215
Mali, 1976 census	All urban	1.046	Rural settled	1.115
Mauritania, 1977 census	Nouakchott	.668	Rural settled	1.253
	Other urban	.730	Nomads	1.247
Mozambique, 1970 census	Maputo	1.030	Niassa	1.241
	Manica & Sofala	.959		
Rwanda, 1970 survey	Kigali	.989		
Senegal, 1976 census	Cap Vert & Dakar	.986	Fleuve	1.222
	Sine Saloum	1.034		
Somalia, 1980 survey	Urban & Mogadishu	1.079	Rural lower Shebelle settled	1.190
			Rural Bay settled	1.239
Sudan, 1973 census	All urban	.827	All rural	1.105
Sudan, 1979 WFS	Khartoum	.860	Kordofan	1.089
	Central (Gezira)	.944	Darfur	1.045
	Eastern	.875		
Tanzania, 1977 census	Dar Es Salaam	.772	Iringa	1.264
	Arusha	.955	Kigoma	1.222
	Tabora	1.038	Singida	1.182
Togo, 1970 census	Lomé	1.034	Kara	1.393
			Maritime (excl. Lomé)	1.287
			Centrale	1.252
Uganda, 1969 census	Buganda	.801	Northern	1.103
Zaïre (west), 1975 survey	Kinshasa	.877	Bas Zaire	1.206
			Bandundu	1.222
			Equateur	1.114
Zambia, 1969 census	Copperbelt	.830	Eastern	1.376
	Central & Lusaka	.902	Western	1.280
			Northern	1.274
			Northwestern	1.225

NOTE: Data for Nigeria are not reported as WFS is sole source of information.

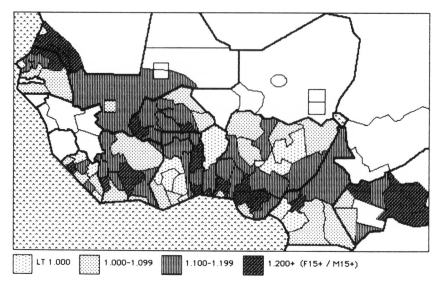

| ::::::| LT 1.000 | ::::::| 1.000-1.099 | ‖‖‖| 1.100-1.199 | ▓▓| 1.200+ (F15+ / M15+) |

Map 6.8*a*. Sex Ratios of Population Aged 15+ (Females/Males); Latest Available Data

that they bore no relation to each other (orthogonal factor extraction). In this instance, seven of the nine original indicators were used: the remaining two measure the differences in ages at marriage for men and women (*SMAM* difference and *RPS*) and they are derived algebraically from the indicators of age at first marriage belonging to the first set. It was therefore statistically impossible to introduce them simultaneously with their components. Correlation coefficients of the *SMAM* difference and *RPS* with the factors defined by the first seven indicators were obtained subsequent to the factor extraction, and these values are reported in the bottom section of table 6.6.

The factor analysis results point to the existence of three major factors that jointly explain almost 80 percent of the original variance. Factor identification can be achieved through the single best indicators:

1. Factor 1 correlates strongly with the two measures of polygyny *M* and *f*. As expected, the correlations with the measures of the age gap at first marriage (*SMAM* difference and *RPS*) are substantial. Those with the proportions single and with the adult sex ratio are equally logical in view of our previous discussion.
2. Factor 2 is identified by the adult sex ratio *F/M*. But, also a substantial negative association is found between *L*, that is, the main component of the polygyny multiplier, and factor 2. Moreover, this correlation is stronger than the one between *L* and the polygyny factor, which may seem surprising. At this point, it is necessary to recall that migration of

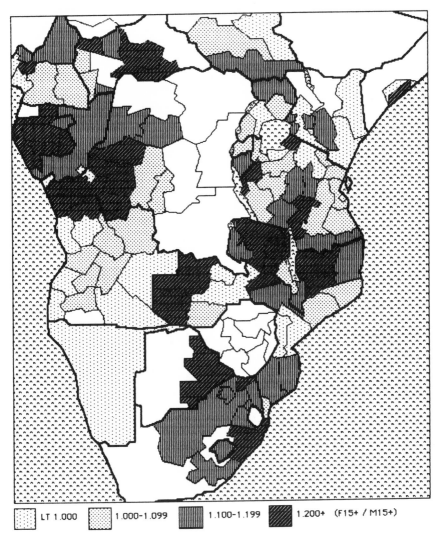

| | LT 1.000 | | 1.000-1.099 | | 1.100-1.199 | | 1.200+ (F15+ / M15+) |

Map 6.8*b*. Sex Ratios of Population Aged 15+ (Female/Males); Latest Available Data

TABLE 6.6   Major Underlying Dimensions of Sub-Saharan Nuptiality Indicators; Results from Factor Analysis

Indicators	Factor Coefficients (= Correlation Coefficients between Indicators and Factors)		
	Factor I	Factor II	Factor III
Proportion married women in polygynous unions (f)	.84	−.03	.10
Polygyny ratio (M)	.94	.15	.01
Ratio of proportions currently married (K)	.30	−.08	−.14
Ratio of proportions ever-married (L)	.31	−.66	.12
Adult sex ratio (F/M)	.34	.94	.06
Proportion women 15–19 single	−.42	.21	.74
Proportion men 20–24 single	.22	−.27	.82
Percentage of variance explained	33.7	24.4	20.8
Cumulative percentage of variance explained	33.7	58.1	78.9
	Correlation Cofficients Between Remaining Indicators and Factors		
$SMAM$ difference between sexes	.62	−.52	.35
Ratio of proportions single (RPS)	−.62	.42	.20

NOTE: Principle factoring (PA2) is used with VARIMAX and orthogonal rotation of factor axes.

single men distorts both the sex ratio and L in opposite directions: emigration of single men obviously raises the overall surplus of women and it increases the *proportion* of ever-married men, which is the denominator of L. Factor 2 can then be interpreted as carrying the effect of sex and marital status–differentiated migration. Equally noteworthy is the negative association between factor 2 and the $SMAM$ difference ($r = -0.52$). If the effect of polygyny is factored out, a typical migration and marriage market feature emerges: for the overrepresented sex in an area, the proportion single below age 20 for women or 25 for men tends to increase and for the underrepresented sex it tends to decrease. In the instance of a female surplus, the corresponding $SMAM$ values for women rise, whereas they fall for men. The correlation coefficients between factor 2 and the $SMAM$ difference or RPS are entirely in line with this. It should, however, be stressed that proportions single and $SMAM$ values are no longer valid indicators of ages at marriage in populations that are subject to substantial sex and marital status selective migration. Factor 2 correctly documents the concentration of young single men in immigration areas, but one should be cautious in interpreting this as indicative of late marriage for men.

3. Factor 3 is identified by the two indicators of ages at first marriage. Both factor coefficients are positive: if polygyny and sex ratios are factored out, a geographical pattern remains that describes the overall timing of marriage for both sexes *jointly*.

4. The only indicator with low factor coefficients throughout is K. Evidently, the geography of the sex differences in proportions currently widowed and divorced constitutes a dimension on its own and accounts for a portion of the variance not explained by the three previous factors.

The ratio of proportions currently married K needs further discussion. It may be recalled that high values of K indicate a small surplus of the proportion widowed and divorced women in relation to the proportion widowed and divorced men. This is typically produced by a rapid relative pace of remarriage for women. K is furthermore less affected by sex-ratio distortions ($r = -0.14$), in contrast to L, the other component of the polygyny multiplier. Areas with a small relative surplus of proportions widows and divorcées are commonly found north of the line running from Douala in Cameroon to Cabo Delgado in Mozambique (K larger than 0.90), and areas with the smallest surplus (that is, K larger than 0.95) are almost exclusively found in West Africa. Such fast remarriage is consistent with high levels of polygyny in West Africa. On the other hand, large relative surpluses of widows and divorcées, that is, low values of K, are common in Zambia, Namibia, Lesotho, South Mozambique, and Botswana. This is equally consistent with low levels of polygyny and the presence of female-headed households instead. Mauritania has also low levels of K, fitting the low level of polygyny among its Arab population.

But there has been an enigmatic finding in the dominance of low levels of K in the area made up by South Cameroon, Gabon, Congo, and West Zaire, which is neither characterized by the existence of female-headed households, nor by low polygyny. In fact, it is the existence of this zone which prevents K from falling into a closer relationship with the other indicators of nuptiality and polygyny; further, this zone is responsible for the low factor coefficients of K reported in table 6.6.

Factor analysis has enabled the basic dimensions underlying the various nuptiality and polygyny indicators to be teased out. A few determinants were also collected for the regions and their effects were examined by multiple regression. The most important covariate is female literacy. Where actual measurement of illiteracy was missing it was measured as the proportion of women without formal schooling, in both cases for women 15–19. The information was limited to the youngest age group, primarily because most first marriages for women occur before age 20. The proportion of illiterate women 15–19 also reflects the general level of illiteracy in the population and serves to distinguish those populations that have undergone a boost in female schooling and those which have not. The other covariates are the logarithm of population density and year of observation. Population density indicates the presence of urban concentrations, normally associated with higher ages at marriage for women and less polygyny. It also captures the presence of population concentration in rural areas which, often for geographic and climatic reasons, have had high population densities in the past (for example, Rwanda, Burundi, Central Kenyan Highlands, areas around Lake Victoria, and so forth). Population pressure in these rural areas is often considerable, and it is conjectured that this could result in the postponement of marriage. The year of observation is added to examine the effect of variation in the periods of observation.

The first set of dependent variables is made up of the indices of age at first marriage and the sex differences in these ages. The regression results are shown in table 6.7 in the form of beta-coefficients (that is, standardized regression coefficients). The zero-order correlations are provided for comparison. The results for the proportion of women single 15–19 and the ratio of proportions single (*RPS*) are of necessity similar, given that RPS is influenced more by the proportion of women single 15–19 than the *SMAM* difference. The strongest determinant was female illiteracy, which exhibited the classic inverse relationship with proportions single women 15–19 and *RPS*: areas with high female illiteracy have earlier marriage for girls than areas with better schooling. This not only supports but justifies the extension of the findings made in chapters 2 and 3 to the rest of sub-Saharan Africa.

The results for the variable "year of observation" were also significant: areas contributing recent observations tend to have later female marriage and higher *RPS*-values. But this should not be used as evidence of a rising trend in female age at marriage. Areas that are more developed socioeconomically also tend to have more recent data sources, while other, less developed areas are often described by a single, older source (such as Central African Republic, Chad, Bukina Faso, Mali, Guinea, South Sudan, East and North Zaire).

Male age at marriage and the *SMAM* difference were less affected by female literacy, but more so by polygyny. This reflects the fact that high male ages at marriage and the concomitant large age gap between spouses are almost exclusive to the West African polygyny belt. The extension of the study area beyond West Africa alters a finding of chapter 2, where a closer relationship between polygyny and female age at marriage was found. Hence, there is a plurality of factors associated with low ages at marriage for women and a more dominant single factor, that is, polygyny, associated with late marriage for men.

TABLE 6.7 Effects of Selected Variables on Measures of Age at First Marriage and Age Difference at First Marriage

Dependent Variable	Zero-Order Correlations and Beta-Coefficients						
	Proportion Women 15–19 Illiterate	Sex Ratio F/M	Proportion Married Women in Polygynous Union	Log of Population Density	Year of Observation	R^2	R
Proportion women 15–19 single							
zero-order	−.62	+.05	−.31	+.20	+.41		
x̄ = .57 σ = .20 beta	−.63*	+.03	+.06	−.07	+.39*	.52	.72
Proportion men 20–24 single							
zero-order	−.08	−.12	+.28	+.32	+.27		
x̄ = .69 σ = .13 beta	−.42*	−.28*	+.60*	+.21	+.01	.30	.54
Age difference at first marriage							
zero-order	+.40	−.21	+.53	+.19	−.01		
x̄ = 6.5 σ = 1.6 beta	+.04	−.36*	+.59*	+.04	−.06	.42	.65
Ratio proportion single women 15–19 to proportion single men 20–24 (RPS)							
zero-order	−.62	+.17	−.49	−.01	+.27		
x̄ = .83 σ = .27 beta	−.44*	+.23*	−.27*	−.11	+.30*	.53	.73

*Denotes significance at .05 level; N varies from 104 to 201.

Imbalances in adult sex ratios also have an impact on the proportion of single men 20–24 and the *SMAM* difference. A large surplus of women tends to lower male ages at marriage and the age difference between the spouses (cf. factor analysis results above). Population density, however, fails to produce significant results: the small positive zero-order correlations with both proportions single were as expected, but they vanish once literacy and polygyny are introduced.

The second set of dependent variables includes polygyny measures and the components of the polygyny multiplier. The regression results are shown in table 6.8. Attention is again directed to the effect of female schooling in view of the Westernization thesis of Goode and Caldwell. Despite the introduction of the proportion of women single 15–19, which is itself influenced by literacy, a strong positive and direct effect of female illiteracy on the polygyny indicators M and f is found. Areas with more literacy tend to have less polygyny, not only because women marry later in such areas, but also because of the direct polygyny-reducing effect of higher literacy. This is in line with Goode's hypothesis, but also consistent with Boserup's thesis that polygyny is a form of appropriation of female productive capacity in societies with traditional, low-technology agriculture. Given a negative relationship between subsistence agriculture and female education, one can indeed expect a negative association between female literacy and polygyny. The relationship between female illiteracy and the polygyny multiplier is smaller, but still in the direction suggested by Goode.

It is interesting to note the finding that higher female illiteracy is associated with higher K values, or with a smaller relative excess of widows and divorcées and faster remarriage of women. In other words, low literacy is associated with the minimization of the loss of reproductive capacity through celibacy, divorce, and widowhood.

The coefficients of proportions single are all in the expected direction and do not warrant further attention. Neither do the coefficients of the sex ratio since they show once more that the two types of polygyny measures (M and f versus KL and L) are distorted in opposite directions. The coefficients of "year of observation" are nonsignificant throughout, and the effects of density on f and K essentially measure the East-West contrast.

The regional information for the components of the sub-Saharan nuptiality regimes can be summarized by the following:

1. With the exception of Arabs and Berbers, West African populations have considerably higher levels of polygyny, larger age gaps between spouses and faster remarriage then Central, East, and especially South African ones.

2. Islamized populations in West Africa have particularly early ages at marriage for women. This is partially due to high levels of female illiteracy. Non-Islamized populations of the region often reach similar

TABLE 6.8 Effects of Selected Variables on Measures of Polygyny and Components of the Polygyny Multiplier

Dependent Variable	Zero-Order Correlations and Beta-Coefficients							
	Proportion Women Single, 15–19	Proportion Men Single, 20–24	Proportion Women Illiterate, 15–19	Sex Ratio F/M	Log of Population Density	Year of Observation	R^2	R
Proportion of married women in polygynous unions (f)								
$\bar{x} = .40$ $\sigma = .14$ zero-order	−.31	+.28	+.57	+.27	+.18	−.02		
beta	−.20	+.42*	+.54*	+.40*	+.28*	−.09	.65	.80
Polygyny ratio (M)								
$\bar{x} = 1.28$ $\sigma = .17$ zero-order	−.33	+.14	+.49	+.50	−.05	−.10		
beta	−.31*	+.36*	+.59*	+.37*	+.07	−.01	.63	.79
Polygyny multiplier (KL)								
$\bar{x} = 1.16$ $\sigma = .16$ zero-order	−.34	+.32	+.52	−.54	+.13	+.05		
beta	−.30*	+.30*	+.36*	−.44*	+.05	+.01	.60	.77
Ratio of proportion ever-married (L)								
$\bar{x} = 1.29$ $\sigma = .15$ zero-order	−.23	+.36	+.38	−.52	+.04	+.05		
beta	−.35*	+.50*	+.16	−.45*	−.15	+.09	.56	.75
Ratio of proportion currently married (K)								
$\bar{x} = 1.90$ $\sigma = .07$ zero-order	−.25	+.01	+.39	−.14	+.24	+.01		
beta	+.02	−.06	+.44*	−.07	+.36*	−.10	.26	.51

* Denotes significance at .05 level; N varies from 104 to 201.

polygyny levels, but these are based on higher ages at marriage for women.

3. First marriage for men tends to be early in East Africa, which is in line with the more modest levels of polygyny. But male ages at marriage are particularly high in southern Africa, despite low polygyny levels. This undoubtedly reflects the disruption of traditional nuptiality patterns by vast male labor migration and the concomitant social and economic constraints on household formation typical for this region (see also chapter 8).

4. Male emigration is associated with enhanced polygyny in West Africa, but not in Southern Africa, where the response to it has been the emergence of female-headed households.

5. Apart from polygyny, the regional distribution of proportions single is also affected by migration and sex ratio distortions, largely because of the sex and marital status specificity of migration streams. Male emigration and the resultant surplus of women usually lead to enhanced proportions single among women 15–19 in the sending area. Conversely, in the receiving areas, males form the overrepresented sex with large accumulations of single males aged 20–34. *SMAM* values for regions experiencing heavy migration, in or out, do not reflect the real ages at first marriage of their individuals because of the violation of the stationarity hypothesis underlying the calculation of *SMAM*.

6. The cross-sectional associations of female literacy with female ages at marriage and polygyny are impressive and in the direction expected by Goode's thesis. They are, however, not directly interpretable as supporting Goode's proposition, which postulates, first, a causal link, and second, a general trend towards later marriage and less polygyny. There are "common causes" at work in the cross-section used so far, and these simultaneously affect female literacy, female age at marriage, and polygyny. For instance, simple technology in agriculture (that it, hoe agriculture) with heavy involvement of women is also correlated with low female literacy, early marriage, and high levels of polygyny (cf. Boserup's thesis). Islamization too depresses female literacy and enhances early female marriage as a result of the tighter control over women and partner selection (cf. Goody's thesis). The causal interpretation of the cross-sectional correlations between female literacy and the components of the nuptiality regime is, therefore, partially spurious since other social organizational variables are involved. Without statistical controls for these variables, the cross-sectional results are of limited use in inferring trends towards later marriage and less polygyny. What happens if such statistical controls are provided and if the traditional patterns of social organization are allowed to play their role? Before answering this question, a reformatting of the data according to ethnicity is required. This is taken up in the next section.

THE CONSTRUCTION OF AN ETHNIC NUPTIALITY AND
SOCIAL STRUCTURE FILE

As illustrated in chapter 2, patterns of social organization can be documented on the basis of ethnographic descriptions, and here further use is made of Murdock's Ethnographic Atlas. It was necessary to merge the demographic file, which was mostly region specific, and the ethnographic file, which was ethnic specific. The following principles were used to achieve such a merger:

1. Murdock classified each ethnic group in an ethnic cluster, thereby re-grouping populations with similar linguistic, cultural, and organizational patterns. These clusters form the basic unit for establishing the correspondence between the two files.

2. Correspondence was first sought between individual ethnic groups and the regions for which demographic information was available. The matching was performed on the basis of ethnographic maps and the geographical coordinates given in the Ethnographic Atlas. This procedure works well in regions with a single dominant ethnic group. The matter is more complex, however, when a region holds a plurality of ethnic groups, or when an ethnic group is spread over several regions. To alleviate this problem, a nested design with differential weights was introduced.

3. The principles of this design were as follows. If an ethnic cluster was made up of, for example, four ethnic groups residing in areas with demographic information, each ethnic group was given a weight of 0.250. Within a cluster, weights always sum up to unity. If an ethnic group was spread over two regions with demographic information, its social structural characteristics were entered twice along with the two sets of demographic data for these two regions. The total weight for this ethnic group in the cluster was obviously maintained, but the two entries for the same ethnic group were given half this weight (for example, twice 0.125 instead of 0.250).

4. Two ethnic groups may reside in the same area. If they belonged to the same cultural cluster, as defined by Murdock, both received the same regional demographic information, either as their sole demographic input or as a partial input. In the latter instance, weights were further fragmented as outlined by principle 3. Regions with heterogeneity in terms of *cluster* membership were avoided as much as possible. This principle assured that the correspondence between regions and ethnic clusters was maximized in instances where correspondence between regions and ethnic groups was imperfect.

5. A few deviations were tolerated. The Fulani, Twareg and northern (or "nuclear") Mande groups are spread over much of the West African sahel and savannah, and the ethnic entries in the Murdock file for these

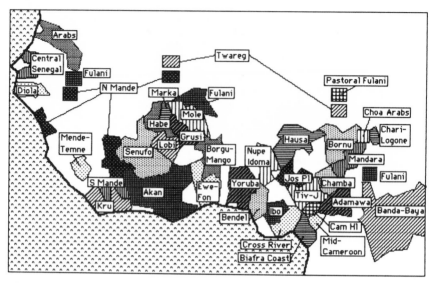

Map 6.9*a*. Correspondence Between Areas with Demographic Information and Location of Ethnic Clusters

groups pertain to three particular populations that fall outside the regions with demographic information. In these instances, the ethnographic information was maintained and coupled with demographic information from the Fulani, Twareg, and northern Mande groups elsewhere. A second alteration was performed on Murdock's "Coastal Nigeria" cluster, which was broken up into a new cluster (Bendel) and a set of ethnic groups which were attached to the existing "Cross River" cluster. This new configuration is ethnically more homogeneous and covered fully by demographic information.

6. In instances where demographic information was already ethnic specific (such as Burkina Faso, Gabon, South Africa, most WFS-participating countries) the above problems were absent and a direct match was made.

The outcome of the matching process is shown in map 6.9 for the clusters. The data file contains entries for 170 ethnic groups nested in 69 clusters. The ratio is 2.46 groups per cluster. In further statistical work, all weights were inflated by this ratio in order to respect the real sample size ($N = 170$) without distorting the nested design.

The following demographic variables were entered:

1. The proportions single women 15–19 and men 20–24. The approximate *SMAM* values were computed through the conversion formulae given earlier and an estimate of the sex difference in *SMAM* was added.

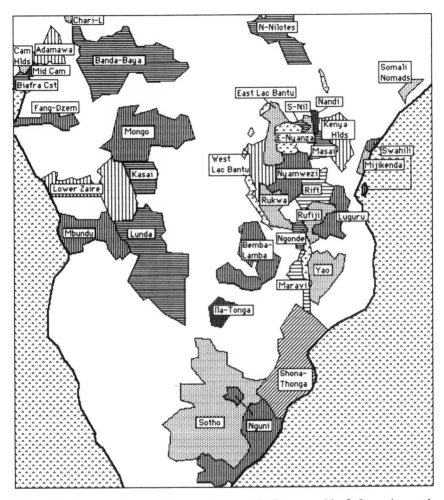

Map 6.9*b*. Correspondence Between Areas with Demographic Information and Location of Ethnic Clusters

2. Polygyny is measured through the same indices as before, but for the cases without entries for the proportion of married women in polygynous unions (f), values were estimated on the basis of the polygyny ratio (M) in accordance with the regression of f on M ($r = 0.75$; $N = 119$ entries). Obviously, this estimation was performed to reduce the number of missing values, which would otherwise lead to a serious selection bias. Hence, the selection bias associated with missing values was considered to be more hazardous than the approximation of f through M.

3. Additional demographic variables are the adult sex ratio (F/M) and population density. Also the period of observation was added.

The file contains the following ethnographic data:

1. The Murdock scales of the degree of subsistence dependence on respectively hunting/gathering, fishing, animal husbandry, and farming. These scales can be interpreted as the degree (expressed in percentages) of subsistence reliance on any of these sectors.

2. The pattern of exchange of goods and services on the occasion of marriage (EXCH MAR) was measured through the entries in column 12 of the Murdock file and recoded as follows:

   0: no exchange or token exchange only (O,T)
   1: prestations from the groom's lineage to the bride's lineage (i.e., bridewealth, bride-service, and sister exchange; B,S,X)
   2: reciprocal exchange of substantial gifts (G)
   3: transfers from the bride's lineage to the new household or the groom's lineage (i.e., dowry; D)

3. The pattern of residence of wives (MARRES) is based on Murdock's column 16 and recorded as:

   0: no common residence (O)
   1: uxorilocal or matrilocal (U,C,M,A)
   2: neolocal (N)
   3: virilocal or patrilocal (P,V,D)

4. Lineage organization (LIN) stems from columns 20, 22, and 25 (second digit):

   1: strong patrilineal (o in 22, not in 20, a in 25)
   2: patrilineal (o in 22, not in 20, not a in 25)
   3: matrilineal (o in 20, not in 22, not m in 25)
   4: strong matrilineal (o in 20, not in 22, m in 25)
   5: duo + bilateral (o in 20 and 22 or not o in 20 and 22)

In further statistical work codes 1 and 2 are merged to identify patrilinearity and 3 and 4 are regrouped to indicate matrilinearity.

5. The tolerance of or preference for cousin marriages (COUSMAR) are taken from column 25 and coded as follows:
   1: no cousin marriage of any kind (N,O,R,S)
   2: patrilateral cousin marriage (P,D)
   3: evidence of matrilateral cousin marriage (M,G)
   4: duolateral, trilateral, and quadrilateral cousin marriage (C,T,Q).
   Endogamous marriage is identified by combining the variables "Lineage organization" and "cousin marriage." All societies without cousin marriage of any sort are obviously exogamous. Those with patrilineal organization and patrilateral cousin marriage, matrilineal organization and matrilateral cousin marriage, and those with multilateral cousin marriage are considered as tolerating endogamy (it must be noted, however, that trilateral cousin marriage is an exception and is exogamous).

6. The degree of political complexity (POLCOMP) is obtained from column 32 (second digit):
   0: stateless societies
   1: existence of petty chiefs
   2: existence of large paramount chiefs
   3: states
   4: large states
   Note that Murdock has excluded patterns of political organization introduced by colonial authorities.

7. The variable describing "community size" was directly taken from the Murdock files (column 31), with codes ranging from 1 to 8. The distinctions between the lower codes (1 to 6) do not appear to be very meaningful and the scale can be dichotomized on the basis of the existence of indigenous cities (code 1–6 versus 7,8).

8. Murdock provides a code for the female involvement in agricultural work (FWAGRIC) (column 62). These were recoded as:
   0: agriculture of no importance
   1: males do more agricultural work than women (M,N)
   2: both sexes are equally involved (E,D)
   3: females do more agricultural work (F,G)
   This variable is important in testing Boserup's proposition (see later discussion), but, as argued by Goody (1976), the validity of this variable is reduced when the analysis is confined to sub-Saharan populations only. In many such societies with entries specifying less female agricultural involvement or equal division of labor, women are involved in trading as well, which enhances their "productive value."

9. The existence of caste and/or class stratification (CCS) is taken from Murdock's columns 67 and 69:

1: unstratified by caste or class (o in 67 and 69)
2: stratification by wealth only (W in 67, o in 69)
3: some despised social groups (o in 67, D in 69 or D in 67, o in 69)
4: moderately stratified (E in 67 or D,E in 69)
5: heavily stratified (C in 67 or 69)
For sub-Saharan populations, a dichotomy can be formed by adding the societies with despised groups, of which there are normally only one or two, to the category of unstratified societies. The numerical share of such groups is very small and the label "despised" is not always accurate since some groups (for example, blacksmiths) are often endowed with magic powers. Obviously, stratification by age grades or other forms of gerontocratic rule are not considered as forms of class or caste stratification.

10. The possibility of women inheriting property is given in Murdock's columns 74 for real property (REAL) and column 76 for movable property other than kitchen utensils and the like (MOVE). The codes are:
    1: women inherit (C,D)
    2: women do not inherit (M,N,O,P,Q)

MAJOR ANTHROPOLOGICAL THEORIES AND THEIR EMPIRICAL TESTING

At this juncture, it is necessary to review the anthropological theories that form the basis for the interpretation of the collected data. In figure 6.13, use is made of six explanatory variables measuring respectively the degree of subsistence dependence on agriculture and female labor inputs, the format of lineage organization, the presence of forms of diverging devolution of property through women, the degree of political complexity, the extent of social stratification, and female literacy. These factors are considered to influence male and female ages at marriage, either directly (paths A and C) or indirectly through the incidence of polygyny and its corollary, the age gap between spouses (paths B, D, G, and H).

Although anthropologists documented the existence and practice of polygyny in early research (see, for example, Radcliffe-Brown and Forde, 1950), little attempt was made to explain its occurrence. Inasmuch as structural functionalist anthropology drew elegant, holistic pictures of discrete societies, it tended not to engage in extensive comparative approaches. Only with the advent of the Murdock Ethnographic Atlas and demographic measurements did this become a real possibility.

It was an economist, Ester Boserup (1970), who first attempted a comparative overview of the relationship of social features such as nuptiality to organizational and economic variables. Boserup's thesis is straightforward:

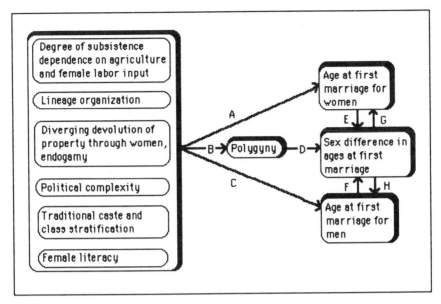

FIGURE 6.13. Variables Involved in Statistical Analyses of Ethnic Marriage Regimes

farming systems can be divided into male and female systems. In areas of low population density, such as sub-Saharan Africa, Boserup postulated that shifting cultivation using the hoe and female labor, would be practiced. Any other female economic contribution, such as trading in West Africa, would be added to the productive value of women. Women's high economic value would therefore be reflected in high levels of polygyny, fast remarriage for widows (appropriation of female labor in gerontocratically structured societies), and bridewealth. The alternative is a system where men do the agricultural work with more advanced technology (irrigation, plough) and the women's reduced contribution would be reflected in monogamy, less re-marriage, and dowry. In sum, Boserup viewed marital practice as being a function of the relative contribution of the sexes in agricultural production, and the operationalization of her thesis would essentially occur via paths B and D in figure 6.13.

As shown in chapter 1, Goody (1976) put Boserup's thesis to the test and found that, in general, it held well when run against Murdock's ethnographic information. In fact, Goody's own thesis is similar and goes one step further. For Goody, the transmission of property becomes the deciding factor in the social and economic system. In low-technology hoe agriculture, land is cor-porately owned and widely available, and its transmission is not a grave issue since all lineage members have access to it. Marriage payments in such a system, that is, bridewealth, are not so much concerned with the transmission of property, but with the transmission of the productive and reproductive value of women. In systems with more advanced plough agriculture, property, states, castes, and other forms of social stratification based on wealth are predicted. The system evolves away from the principle of circulation of resources towards concentration of wealth. In order to protect these interests, marriage tends to become endogamous. This is also an answer to the practice of bilateral inheritance. A father who wishes to protect his daughter's status with a dowry, but keep the family property intact, may solve the problem with caste or lineage endogamy. In-marriage implies strong parental control with respect to partner choice and avoidance of premarital conceptions or births. In many instances that are not characterized by neolocal residence, this leads to the marrying off of women at young ages. Goody's mechanism operates essentially via path A in figure 6.13.

Similarly, Goody's thesis divides the world essentially into two: those societies with diverging devolution of property through bilateral inheritance, dowry, monogamy, plough agriculture, complex polity, and social stratification, versus those with unilineal descent groups, bridewealth, polygyny, shifting cultivation with hoe technology, and high female labor inputs in agriculture. In this fashion, he also incorporates Boserup's dichotomy.

The testing of Goody's and Boserup's thesis with a sub-Saharan rather than a worldwide sample faces the problem of increased homogeneity with respect to the social organization variables. Bridewealth, for instance, constitutes by far the most common form of marriage prestation (86 percent of entries in our data file), irrespective of the form of lineage organization. The practice of dowry is virtually absent, and the remaining 14 percent of societies without bridewealth are distributed over the categories of no exchange, token exchange only, gift exchange, bride-service, or sister exchange. Inheritance for women is rare and occurs in 20 percent of the entries. Tolerance of or preference for endogamous forms of cousin marriage is more common (mostly of the bilateral, trilateral, or quadrilateral types) with 46 percent of entries, but the combination with inheritance for women results in few societies that manifestly counteract diverging devolution of property through endogamy. In fact, this combination is found in twenty-nine societies only, or seventeen percent of the entries. Hence, the few that have inheritance for women generally tolerate endogamous marriage, but those who tolerate cousin marriage do not necessarily practice inheritance for women. Of the twenty-nine societies with both diverging devolution of property and endogamy, twenty-one are thoroughly Islamized, which presumably explains the origin of this non-African combination. None of the remaining eight societies are patrilineal and hence they are exceptional in more than one respect.

As Comaroff (1980) pointed out, what is the use of the Boserup-Goody generalized distinction, when so much of Africa falls in a single category? Hence, additional explanatory variables have to be found with more discriminating power for this continent. Goody (1973) himself, in an earlier critique of Boserup, stressed that female involvement in agricultural production itself would not suffice to explain marriage patterns. As Comaroff underlines, the problem with assigning "value" to women according to their productive potential begs the question of what kinds of female and male activities are regarded as valuable. There may be a crucial distinction between the actual economic contribution of the sexes with respect to the production of means of subsistence and the socially perceived contribution. For example, in many African societies, which rely predominantly on agriculture, animal husbandry is also practiced, and in these the socially perceived value of female agricultural work is often lower relative to the inflated value ascribed to the male involvement in cattle raising and trading. This relationship is typical to East Africa, where cattle raising is common and women seldom engage in trading activities.

The relevant distribution characteristics in the data file are as follows: the modal category for reliance on agriculture is comprised of between 50 and 69 percent dependence on this sector and contains 61 percent of the entries. Of these, half the number of entries have scores indicative of greater female than male labor involvement in agriculture. The modal category for animal husbandry is 6–25 percent reliance with 55 percent of entries. Hence, the combination of a dominant farming sector with an additional cattle raising one is not rare and the same probably holds true for the social devaluation of women's economic contribution.

To sum up, the Murdock variables relating to the degree of subsistence reliance by sector and to the female work input in agriculture do not constitute an optimal measurement of the dimension of the *perceived* value of women. This is most clearly visible in the fact that the variable of female versus male farming does not discriminate between East and West Africa, whereas the social value of women's work and the social position of women are known to be weaker in East Africa. The reliance on animal husbandry versus agriculture may be a better proxy than the direct female work input in agriculture used by Boserup, because of the prestige associated with cattle owning accruing to men only. The hypothesis to be tested is then that increased reliance on farming and decreased importance of animal husbandry leads to greater perceived productive value of women and to more polygyny and larger age gaps between the spouses (paths B, D in figure 6.13).

Another essential element that should be included in the explanatory framework is the relationship between lineage organization and polygyny. One might predict that matrilineal societies would be less polygynous because of problems with household formation. Matrilineal societies that have matrilocal or uxorilocal residence of spouses impede polygyny since the husband would have to marry sisters. In the present data file, 18 percent of societies are matrilineal, of which two thirds have matri- or uxorilocal residence. As a consequence, one can indeed expect that societies with matrilineal descent systems would be less polygynous, have smaller age gaps between the spouses, and have either later marriage for women and/or earlier marriage for men (effect through paths B, D, G, and H in figure 6.13).

The effects shown in figure 6.13 were statistically tested and measured as follows. Two sets of tables were prepared, respectively excluding and including polygyny as a predictor. In the first set the direct effects A, B, and C in figure 6.13 proved of interest, whereas the results of the second set also take the existence of D, G, and H into account. Each set is composed of three tables. The first table in each set (that is, tables 6.9 and 6.12) gives the results of an analysis of variance and permits a comparison of the proportions of variance of each of the four dependent variables (proportions single women 15–19, proportions single men 20–24, SMAM difference inferred from these proportions, proportion married women 15+ in polygynous unions) accounted for by the independent variables listed in figure 6.13. The year of observation has been added to the set of predictors merely as a control for differential data quality over time. The five social organization variables are discrete (factors), whereas female literacy and the year of observation are continuous (covariates). In the second set of tables, the incidence of polygyny is added as a covariate. The second table in each set (that is, tables 6.10 and 6.13) contains the results of a Multiple Classification Analysis (MCA) corresponding with the analyses of variance. In all these analyses missing values have been deleted in a listwise fashion, which means that a missing value for any of the variables results in the deletion of the case from the file. Listwise deletion produces a substantial loss of cases and sample sizes are reduced from 170 to 107–121 depending on the dependent variable. The third table in each set (that is, tables 6.11 and 6.14) shows the unstandardized regression coefficients from a dummy regression analysis. As no interaction terms are considered, the column with "adjusted deviations" in the MCA tables and the regression coefficients should reveal, each in its own way, a similar picture. However, the dummy regression procedure used here is based on pairwise deletion of missing values, meaning that a case is only omitted from a bivariate relationship as a result of a missing value. The procedure minimizes the loss of cases, but bivariate relations are rarely computed on the basis of identical samples. These two different treatments of missing values serve to check whether results display sufficient robustness against the selection bias produced by missing data. Finally, one should be reminded of the fact that the nested design and its weighting procedure are used throughout these analyses (see earlier discussion).

The first set of tables which exclude polygyny as a predictor are now considered (tables 6.9 through 6.11). The independent variables provide the

TABLE 6.9 Proportions of Variance of Four Nuptiality Variables Accounted for by Social Organization Indicators and Female Literacy; Sub-Saharan Ethnic Clusters

	Proportion Women 15–19 Single	Proportion Men 20–24 Single	SMAM difference	Proportion Married Women in Polygynous Unions
A. Social Organization (Factors)				
Pastoralism/Agriculture (4 categories)	.01	.02	.05	.10*
Lineage (3 cat.)	.00	.01	.02	.13*
Diverging devolution (2 cat.)	.06*	.00	.05*	.00
Political complexity (2 cat.)	.06*	.00	.02	.03*
Social Stratification (2 cat.)	.01	.01	.05*	.00
All Variables	.13*	.05	.17*	.21*
B. Other (Covariates)				
Literacy	.28*	.01	.12*	.04*
Year of observation	.01	.04*	.02	.01
All Covariates	.33*	.07*	.13*	.04*
N	118	108	108	121
Total Variance Explained (R^2)	.46	.12	.30	.25
Multiple Correlation Coefficient (R)	.68	.34	.55	.50

NOTE: Results from classic analysis of variance, with factors introduced prior to covariates; sums of proportions of the variance explained by each factor (resp. covariate) do not equal the total proportions because of correlations and interactions between the factors (covariates) themselves. Values of N are based on *listwise* deletion of missing values. Asterisks denote significance at .05 level.

TABLE 6.10 Effects of Social Organization Indicators on Four Nuptiality Variables: Results of Multiple Classification Analyses Excluding Polygyny as a Covariate for Age-at-First-Marriage Variables; Sub-Saharan Ethnic Clusters

	Proportion Women single, 15–19 $\bar{X}=.57$, $N=118$			Proportion Men Single, 20–24 $\bar{X}=.70$, $N=108$			SMAM Difference $\bar{X}=6.61$, $N=108$			Proportion Married Women in Polygynous Unions $\bar{X}=.37$, $N=121$		
	Unadjusted deviation	Adjusted deviation	N	Unadjusted deviation	Adjusted deviation	N	Unadjusted deviation	Adjusted deviation	N	Unadjusted deviation	Adjusted deviation	N
Factors												
Pastoralism/Agriculture												
Pastoral	−.07	.06	(8)	−.07	−.03	(6)	−.67	−1.50	(6)	−.10	−.14	(9)
Mixed (pastoral, hunter-gatherer, agriculture	−.01	−.04	(28)	.02	.01	(25)	.43	.54	(25)	−.03	−.03	(28)
Medium agriculture	.01	.01	(74)	−.00	.00	(70)	−.08	−.06	(70)	.01	.02	(76)
High agriculture	.04	−.03	(7)	.01	.02	(7)	−.16	−.04	(7)	.07	.04	(8)
eta/beta	.10	.14		.13	.08		.17	.27		.25	.33	
Lineage Organization												
Patrilineal	−.01	−.00	(79)	.00	.01	(71)	.10	.09	(71)	.02	.03	(81)
Matrilineal	.02	.02	(23)	−.03	−.02	(23)	−.48	−.31	(23)	−.09	−.10	(23)
Bilateral and duolateral	−.00	−.02	(16)	.02	.00	(14)	.29	.07	(14)	.02	.01	(16)
eta/beta	.05	.06		.11	.08		.16	.10		.30	.35	

Diverging Devolution of Property											
No inheritance by women	.02	.01	(102)	.00	.00	(91)	−.13	−.08	(91)	.00	.00	(105)
Diverging devolution through women + endogamy	−.12	−.07	(16)	−.00	−.01	(16)	.76	.43	(16)	−.02	−.02	(15)
eta/beta	.23	.14		.01	.03		.20	.11		.04	.05	
Political Complexity											
No chiefs or minor local chiefs	−.03	−.04	(68)	−.01	−.01	(61)	.05	.11	(61)	.01	.02	(70)
Paramount chiefs and states	.05	.05	(50)	.01	.01	(47)	−.06	−.14	(47)	−.02	−.02	(50)
eta/beta	.19	.20		.09	.06		.03	.08		.12	.15	
Class and Caste Stratification											
Unstratified or despised group only	.02	−.00	(69)	−.02	−.02	(63)	−.36	−.20	(63)	.00	.00	(72)
Stratified (wealth or castes)	−.03	.01	(49)	.02	.03	(45)	.50	.28	(45)	.01	−.00	(49)
eta/beta	.13	.03		.15	.20		.27	.15		.01	.02	

NOTE: "Adjusted deviations" measure deviations from the overall mean adjusted for all other factors and 2 covariates (literacy women 15–19 and year of observation). See also note for table 6.9.

TABLE 6.11 Effect of Social Organization Variables and Female Literacy on Nuptiality and Polygyny in Sub-Saharan Ethnic Clusters; Unstandardized Regression Coefficients

	Proportion Women Single, 15–19	Proportion Men Single, 20–24	SMAM Difference in Years	Proportion Married Women in Polygynous Union
	X̄ = .55 σ = .22	X̄ = .69 σ = .14	X̄ = 6.57 σ = 1.52	X̄ = .36 σ = .14
Social Organization Variables				
Pastoralism/Agriculture				
Pastoral	Reference Group			
Mixed (pastoral, hunter-gatherer, agriculture)	−.08	+.00	+.82	+.14*
Medium dependency agriculture	−.06	−.00	+.56	+.20*
High dependency agriculture	−.07	−.01	+.45	+.21*
Lineage Organization				
Patrilineal		Reference Group		
Matrilineal	+.01	−.02	−.37	−.11*
Bilateral and duolateral	+.00	−.06	−.11	−.03
Diverging Devolution of Property				
No diverging devolution & exogamy			Reference Group	
Women inheritance, edogamy	−.07	−.02	+.13	−.04*
Political Complexity				
No chiefs or local chiefs only				Reference Group
Paramount chiefs or states	+.06*	+.09	−.23	−.05*

Class and Caste stratification
None or despised group only

		Reference Group		
Class or caste stratified	+.02	+.07*	+.13	−.00
Other Variables (Continuous)				
Female literacy (proportion)	+.441*	+.078	−2.019*	−.132*
Year of observation (55–82)	+.003	+.005*	+.042*	+.002
Regression Constant	.577	.352	1.625	.021
R	.68	.43	.51	.56
R²	.47	.18	.26	.31

NOTE: In contrast to MCA-results, regression outcomes are based on pairwise rather than listwise deletion of missing variables so that Ns are comprised between 142 and 170 (maximum). Asterisks denote significance at .05 level.

TABLE 6.12 Proportion of Variance of Three Nuptiality Variables Accounted for by Social Organization Variables, Female Literacy and Polygyny; Sub-Saharan Ethnic Clusters

	Proportion Women Single, 15–19	Proportion Men Single, 20–24	SMAM Difference
Social Organization (Factors)			
Pastoralism/Agriculture (4 cat.)	.01	.02	.06*
Lineage (3 cat.)	.00	.01	.02
Diverging devolution (2 cat.)	.05*	.00	.06*
Political complexity (2 cat.)	.06*	.00	.02
Social stratification (2 cat.)	.01	.02	.05*
All Variables	.11*	.06	.18*
Other (Covariates)			
Literacy	.25*	.03	.07*
Year of observation	.01	.03	.01
Polygyny	.01	.03	.05*
All Covariates	.35*	.10*	.17*
N	117	107	107
Total Variance Explained (R²)	.47	.16	.35
Multiple Correlation Coefficient (R)	.68	.40	.59

NOTE: Results from classic analysis of variance, with factors introduced prior to covariates; sums of proportions of the variance explained by each factor (resp. covariate) do not equal the total proportions because of correlations and interactions between the factors (covariates) themselves. Values of N are based on *listwise* deletion of missing values. Asterisks denote significance at .05 level.

best prediction in the instance of ethnic variation in proportions single women 15–19 ($R^2 = 0.46$). Much of this is attributable to the positive effect of female literacy, which accounts for 28 percent of the variance in proportions single. Ethnic variation in female ages at first marriage is consequently essentially related to the modernizing effect of higher female literacy in this cross-section. This is entirely in line with all the earlier findings (see chapters 2 and 3). The other significant, but much smaller, proportions of the explained variance stem from diverging devolution coupled with endogamy (6 percent) and political complexity (6 percent). Table 6.10 with the corresponding MCA results shows the magnitude and the direction of the effects. As expected, the few societies with both inheritance for women and tolerance and/or preference for endogamy have substantially lower proportions of single women 15–19. Not adjusting for the other variables, their mean proportion is $0.57 - 0.12 = 0.45$ as opposed to $0.57 + 0.02 = 0.59$ in societies without diverging devolution of property through bilateral inheritance. The original discrepancy of 14 percentage points is reduced to 8 percentage points if the other variables (including literacy) are controlled for, but the difference nevertheless remains significant. Since very much the same result is obtained in table 6.11, this finding does not stem from the specific treatment of missing values. Hence, Goody's variables of property transmission and control over young women identify the pattern of particularly early marriage for girls in societies that are mostly profoundly Islamized and perform exactly according to the theory. The effect of political complexity stems from later marriage in societies that have paramount chiefs or states. This is also in line with a similar (although nonsignificant) effect of enhanced stratification.

A quarter of the variance of polygyny is accounted for by the set of predictors used here. The effect of female literacy is much smaller (0.04) than in the instance of female age at first marriage (0.28), but the effects of subsistence dependence on cattle or agriculture and of lineage organization emerge more clearly (0.10), as would be expected from the theoretical propositions. The reduced effect of female literacy contrasts with the finding in chapter 2 where female schooling levels played a far more prominent role. Admittedly, literacy and schooling level are not identical variables, but the main source of the reduction in the explanatory power of literacy is the extension of the present sample to most of sub-Saharan Africa in contrast to the predominantly West-African sample used in chapters 2 and 3. However, as can be seen from the dummy regression results reported in table 6.11, polygyny and literacy are still negatively related. The magnitude of the coefficient (-0.132) indicates that a 10-percentage-point shift in female literacy produces on average a diminution of the percentage of married women in polygynous unions of 1.3 points. Considering that the respective means for polygyny and literacy are 36 and 45 percent, and the respective standard deviations are 14 and 30 percent, this cross-sectional slope indicates that polygyny would on average

TABLE 6.13 Effects of Social Organization Indicators on Three Nuptiality Variables: Results of Multiple Classification Analyses (Including Effect of Polygyny); Sub-Saharan Ethnic Clusters

	Proportion Women Single, 15–19 $\bar{X}=.57$, N3 = 117			Proportion Men Single, 20–24 $\bar{X}=.70$, N3 = 107			SMAM Difference $\bar{X}=6.60$, N = 107		
	Unadjusted deviation	Adjusted deviation	N	Unadjusted deviation	Adjusted deviation	N	Unadjusted deviation	Adjusted deviation	N
Factors									
Pastoralism/Agriculture									
Pastoral	−.07	.03	(8)	−.07	.01	(6)	−.66	−.78	(6)
Mixed (pastoral, hunter-gatherer, agriculture)	.00	−.04	(27)	.02	.03	(23)	.42	.66	(23)
Medium agriculture	.00	.01	(74)	−.00	−.01	(70)	−.07	−.14	(70)
High agriculture	.04	−.02	(7)	.01	−.03	(7)	−.15	−.16	(7)
eta/beta	.10	.11		.14	.11		.16	.24	
Lineage Organization									
Patrilineal	−.00	.00	(78)	.01	.00	(70)	.09	.00	(70)
Matrilineal	.02	.00	(23)	−.03	.00	(23)	−.47	−.03	(23)
Bilateral and duolateral	−.01	−.02	(16)	.02	−.01	(14)	.30	.02	(14)
eta/beta	.04	.05		.11	.03		.16	.01	
Diverging Devolution of Property									
No inheritance by women	.02	.01	(102)	−.00	−.00	(91)	−.13	−.09	(91)
Diverging devolution + endogamy	−.11	−.06	(15)	.00	.01	(15)	.78	.56	(15)
eta/beta	.20	.11		.01	.02		.20	.14	

Political Complexity

No chiefs or minor local chiefs	−.03	−.03	(66)	−.01	−.01	(60)	.04	.10	(60)
Paramount chiefs and states	.04	.04	(50)	.01	.01	(47)	−.05	−.12	(47)
eta/beta	.18	.17		.08	.05		.03	.07	

Class and Caste Stratification

Unstratified or despised group only	.02	−.01	(69)	−.02	−.03	(63)	−.35	−.25	(63)
Class or caste stratified	−.03	.01	(48)	.03	.04	(43)	.51	.36	(43)
eta/beta	.12	.04		.16	.24		.26	.19	

NOTE: "Adjusted deviations" measure deviations from the overall mean adjusted for all other factors and covariates (literacy women 15–19, year of observation, and proportion of married women in polygynous unions). See also notes for table 6.9.

TABLE 6.14 Effect of Social Organization Variables, Female Literacy, and Polygyny on Age-at-First-Marriage Variables in Sub-Saharan Ethnic Clusters; Unstandardized Regression Coefficients

	Proportion Women Single, 15–19		Proportion Men Single, 20–24		SMAM Difference	
	X̄ = .55 σ = .22		X̄ = .69 σ = .14		X̄ = 6.57 σ = 1.52	
Social Organization Variables						
Pastoralism/Agriculture						
Pastoral	Reference Group		Reference Group		Reference Group	
Mixed (pastoral, hunter-gatherer, agriculture)	−.04		−.02		+.34	
Medium dependency agriculture	−.01		−.03		−.13	
High dependency agriculture	−.01		−.05		−.29	
Lineage Organization						
Patrilineal			Reference Group			
Matrilineal	−.02		−.01		−.00	
Bilateral and duolateral	−.01		−.00		−.01	
Diverging Devolution of Property						
No diverging devolution & exogamy			Reference Group			
Women inherit, endogamy	−.08		−.02		+.26	
Political Complexity						
No chiefs or local chiefs only			Reference Group			
Paramount chiefs or states	+.05		+.02		−.04	
Class and Caste Stratification						
None or despised group only			Reference Group			
Class or caste stratified	+.02		+.07*		+.71*	

Other Variables (Continuous)

Female Literacy (proportion)	+.406*	+.100*	−1.557*
Year of Observation (55–82)	+.004	+.004*	+.035*
Married Women in Polygynous Unions (proportions)	−.262*	+.167	+3.494*
Regression Constant	.582	.349	1.552
R	.70	.45	.57
R^2	.48	.20	.32

NOTE: In contrast to MCA-results, regression outcomes are based on pairwise rather than listwise deletion of missing variables so that Ns are comprised between 142 and 170 (maximum). Asterisks denote significance at .05 level.

still occur at the 31 percent level in societies with 80 percent female literacy and at the 29 percent level in instances of complete female literacy. Hence, the sign of the slope is in line with Goode's expectation, but its size points in the direction of the robustness of the institution, as hypothesized by van de Walle and Kekovole (1984). This discussion on the relationship between literacy and polygyny cannot be complete without the warning that cross-sectional results are no substitutes for trends over time, notwithstanding the controls for traditional social organization variables.

The effect of the variable measuring the importance of cattle raising versus agriculture produces, as indicated, a major effect: it accounts for 10 percent of the variance in polygyny, and the differences between the extreme catego-ries (pastoral versus sole dependence on agriculture) amounts to an average of 18 percentage points more polygyny for the agricultural societies in the MCA analysis (table 6.10) and to 21 percentage points in the dummy regression analysis (table 6.11). Polygyny increases also monotonically with the growth of agriculture. This is clearly "within-Africa" evidence supportive of Boser-up's thesis that increased activity in low-technology swidden agriculture en-hances the productive value of women and fosters polygyny. The contrast with cattle raising societies, where women are perceived as "uneconomic" and polygyny is lower, accounts partially for the contrast in the incidence of polygyny between West and East Africa (cf. maps 6.5, 6.6, and 6.7).

The two organizational features that tend to reduce polygyny and which statistically curb the polygyny enhancing effect of greater involvement in low-technology agriculture are matrilineal kinship organization and aspects associated with the emergence of social stratification. The lineage factor ex-plains 13 percent of the variance of polygyny (table 6.9), which is as much as agriculture (0.10) and much more than female literacy (0.04). The entire effect of lineage is due to the category of matrilinearity as shown by the MCA and dummy regression results (tables 6.10 and 6.11). The order of magni-tude of the effect is equally important: matrilinearity produces on average a 13-percentage-point diminution in polygyny when compared to patrilineal descent systems. This is confirmed by the dummy variable regression with a shift of 11 percentage points. This corresponds almost to a full standard de-viation shift toward the lower end of the polygyny distribution. The finding is in accordance with the theoretical proposition that matrilineal systems would have an additional problem with polygynous household formation as a result of their tendency toward matrilocal or uxorilocal residence. The result also suggests that matrilineal descent should be added to the Boserup-Goody list of explanatory variables, especially when dealing with low-technology farming societies.

The three variables that are connected with the emergence of social strati-fication in function of wealth or descent (that is, diverging devolution and endogamy, political complexity, and class or caste stratification) also have a negative effect on polygyny, but the magnitudes are smaller. The finding is again in line with Goody's view that monogamy becomes the rule in more complex societies with bilateral transmission of property and a concern for endogamy and homogamy. There are several reasons accounting for this negative relationship:

1. A simple gerontocratic structure is most propitious for polygyny as this practice involves the appropriation of female productive and reproductive functions by older men. Deviations from such gerontocratic organization generally imply complications for the maintenance of high levels of polygyny.
2. A stratification system based on wealth and descent leads to the fragmentation of the marriage market and imposes problems in the recruitment of suitable brides.
3. If hypergamy is desirable, plural marriages increase the chances of hypogamy. If the top stratum is highly polygynous, more single men of this stratum may be inclined to take a bride from the next lower stratum rather than remain single for a longer time. This in turn creates a deficiency of available brides in the second stratum and in the presence of polygyny, more men of the second stratum may again have to resort to hypogamy. Each man who succeeds in recruiting a bride from a higher class or caste is effectively imposing a match with a woman of a lower stratum on someone else. This externality arising from a deviation from perfect homogamy is contained by monogamy and exacerbated by polygyny.

There are, however, several societies in the sample which have a dual caste system combined with high levels of polygyny. One of these, the sedentary Fulani or Peul, has been thoroughly studied by G. Pison (1982, 1986). Typical of Goody's "Asian" pattern is that the Fulani (Pison studies the Bandé subgroup located in Senegal) have a theoretical preference for endogamous patrilateral parallel cousin marriage, and caste homogamy. Typical of the "African" system is the existence of bridewealth rather than dowry and the presence of all the demographic prerequisites for the maintenance of high polygyny. The Bandé Fulani are in other words replicating the African system within the boundaries of each caste by preventing younger men from marrying earlier with women of a lower caste. As a result, the mean age at first marriage for men is 26 years, or 11 years later than for women. Only if such excessive differential ages at first marriage are tolerated can the polygynous system be sustained in combination with homogamy. Also, if the need for exogamy arises, foreigners are preferred to hypogamy. The example of the Bandé shows that this "Asian" form of endogamy is grafted uncomfortably on the African system.

To sum up, the findings of tables 6.10 and 6.11 support the general tendency towards the dichotomy suggested by Goody, but the orders of magnitude of the effects of diverging devolution and class/caste stratification and the Bandé Fulani example clearly show that a synthesis of the two contrasting systems can be made. In other words, Goody's dichotomy stems essentially from a geographical contrast between the Eurasian and sub-Saharan types, but these should not be taken as being completely mutually exclusive. If the demographic prerequisites of polygyny are strongly enforced in conjunction with strict homogamy, and if tensions within the stratified marriage circles can be solved by recruitment from outside rather than by hypogamy, the maintenance of highly polygynous nuptiality regimes within the various strata is a possibility. The main feature of such a system is an exaggerated age difference between the spouses. Finally, several ethnic groups in Senegal, such as the Wolof and Tukulor, have a similar combination of caste stratification and high polygyny, and this may partially account for the particularly large *SMAM* differences found in this region when compared to those of the Ivory Coast, Togo, Benin, Nigeria, and Cameroon (see map 6.4).

The MCA and dummy regression results for the age difference at first marriage (*SMAM* difference) are consistent with those for polygyny. As expected, the *SMAM* difference is reduced in pastoral societies and matrilineal ones, given their lower incidence of polygyny, and enhanced in caste- or class-stratified societies. Diverging devolution through bilateral inheritance combined with endogamy further increases the *SMAM* difference. Controlling for literacy and year of observation, the average *SMAM* difference for patrilineal societies with a medium-level involvement in agriculture and with diverging devolution and caste stratification is of the order of $6.61 - 0.06 + 0.09 + 0.43 + 0.28 = 7.47$ years according to the MCA results. That for a pastoral society without stratification or diverging devolution is 4.83 years. This difference of more than 2.5 years is appreciable given that the standard deviation of the *SMAM* difference is only 1.5 years. The corresponding difference between these two types of societies produced by the dummy variable regression and pairwise rather than listwise deletion of missing values is considerably less, namely 0.82 years, or half a standard deviation. Equally noteworthy and consistent is the negative effect of female literacy on the *SMAM* difference.

The age at first marriage for men remains inadequately explained: the analysis of variance (table 6.9) indicates that none of the social organization variables, individually or taken together, are significant. The dummy variable regression results only suggest a positive effect of class and caste stratification. This, at least, is consistent with the mechanisms described above concerning the organization of polygyny in stratified societies on the basis of enhanced age gaps between the spouses.

The second set of tables reports findings of similar analyses but includes polygyny among the independent variables. On the whole, the results presented in the first set of regressions are not systematically altered. The increase in R^2 resulting from the introduction of polygyny on the independent variable side is modest (compare tables 6.9 and 6.12) and roughly the same variables prove to be significant. The MCA results in table 6.13 compared to those of table 6.10 show a slightly attenuated effect of pastoralism versus agriculture and of lineage organization, and a slightly enhanced effect of diverging devolution and social stratification on the three age-at-marriage variables. The same holds for the dummy regression results with pairwise deletion of missing data (tables 6.11 and 6.14). This outcome seems logical: the arguments advanced for explaining contrasts in the ages at first marriage and the *SMAM* difference between pastoral and agricultural societies and between matrilineal and patrilineal ones hinges on the relatively large difference in the functionality and incidence of polygyny. A control for the difference in the incidence of polygyny must therefore reduce the effects of these social organization variables. The situation with respect to diverging devolution and stratification is different: societies with these characteristics have on average *less* polygyny than those without them, but are nevertheless characterized by enhanced age gaps between the spouses. This illustrates once more the particular situation of those sub-Saharan societies who have maintained polygyny while adopting a caste stratification and bilateral inheritance.

The next question pertains to the patterning of the residuals of the dummy variable regressions presented in tables 6.14 and 6.11. More specifically, it is interesting to inspect forms of geographical autocorrelation in these residuals. To investigate this, the residuals of individual ethnic groups were averaged by ethnic cluster using the weighted design. The residuals by cluster were subsequently divided over two broad geographical regions (West + Central versus East + South) and four categories for their direction and size. The frequencies are reported in table 6.15. Geographical autocorrelation emerges most clearly for polygyny, proportions single males 20–24, and the *SMAM* difference. It is least marked for proportions single females 15–19. In all instances there is a tendency for residuals to be skewed in the positive direction for West and Central ethnic clusters and in the negative direction for East and South. Hence, despite controls for major social organization variables and female literacy, West and Central groups still tend to exhibit *more* polygyny than expected on the basis of the variables in the regression, *higher* proportions single for both sexes, and *larger* age gaps between the spouses. For East and South, there is still an unexplained tendency toward less polygyny, earlier marriage for males and females, and a smaller *SMAM* difference. For proportions single women 15–19, the underlying autocorrelation pattern can be specified further: of the eight ethnic clusters with considerably smaller proportions single than predicted, that is, with particu-

TABLE 6.15 Distribution of Ethnic Clusters According to Size of Residuals from Regressions of Polygyny, Proportions Single, and Age-at-Marriage Difference on Selected Background Variables

Proportion of Married Women in Polygynous Unions (Actual versus Predicted)

	Much Less Polygynous	Less Polygynous	More Polygynous	Much More Polygynous
West & central ethnic clusters				
N = 35	2	10	17	6
percent	6	29	49	17
East & south ethnic clusters				
N = 23	5	9	7	2
percent	22	39	30	9

Proportion of single women 15–19 (Actual versus Predicted)

	Considerably Fewer Single	Fewer Single	More Single	Many More Single
West & central ethnic clusters				
N = 35	6	7	20	2
percent	17	20	57	6
East & south ethnic clusters				
N = 22	2	10	7	3
percent	9	45	32	14

Proportion of Single Men 20–24 (Actual versus Predicted)

	Considerably Fewer Single	Fewer Single	More Single	Many More Single
West & central ethnic clusters				
N = 34	4	8	16	6
percent	12	24	48	18
East & south ethnic clusters				
N = 20	4	9	5	2
percent	20	45	25	10

Age Difference at First Marriage (Actual versus Predicted)

	Much Smaller Difference	Smaller Difference	Greater Difference	Much Greater Difference
West & central ethnic clusters				
N = 34	4	8	16	6
percent	12	24	47	18
East & south ethnic clusters				
N = 20	6	6	8	0
percent	30	30	40	0

NOTES: The standard deviation of each series of residuals (σ_e) is used to set up the four categories: Much less than expected: $-1\sigma_e$ or more extreme
Less than expected: $-.01\sigma_e$ to $-.99\sigma_e$
More than expected: $0\sigma_e$ to $+.99\sigma_e$
Much more than expected: $+1\sigma_e$ or more extreme.

larly early marriage for women, three are not Islamized (Maasai, Bemba-Lamba, Cameroon Highlands). The others are Islamized and clustered in the western Sahel (Hausa, Bornu, Chari-Logone groups, Mandara hill groups, sedentary Fulani). There is no detectable effect of Islam in the patterning of the residuals of the remaining variables. The overall outcome is that the geographical contrast in female ages at first marriage can be adequately accounted for by the variables in the regression and Islamization, but that the West and Central versus East and South contrast persists with respect to polygyny, *SMAM* difference, and male age at first marriage. Either existing variables with some East-West differentiation have not been adequately measured, or new variables that similarly follow an East-West division need to be incorporated. Likely candidates are more precise measures of female economic value and social status, such as the strength of women's organizations and the customary involvement of women in trading activities (see chapter 1).

TRENDS IN POLYGYNY AND AGE AT MARRIAGE

Before inspecting census and survey data taken at different points in time, it should be recalled that the extent of marital status-related age misreporting has probably changed. Hence, even if the geographic coverage of two successive data sets was identical, differences in data quality may still hamper comparisons over time. As noted above, the typical errors are age overstatement for married women and age underestimation for single persons. These produce transfers across the boundary of 15 years in societies with particularly early ages at marriage for women and across age 20 for others. It is important to determine the effect of a decline in such transfers as a result of better age information in more recent sources. In older sources, a large upward transfer of married women across age 20 and a considerable downward transfer of single women results in the inflation of proportions single in the age group 15–19 and deflation in the age group 20–24. The inflation in the former age group may, however, be reduced if similar transfers occur across the boundary of 15. If the transfers across age 20 dimish in later sources and if no real change in ages at first marriage take place, the second source should show a drop in the proportion single aged 15–19 and a rise for the 20–24 group. In other words, a decrease in transfers across age 20 would result in a steepening of the line linking the proportions single in the two age groups. If, however, the proportions single increase in age group 15–19 as well as in the age group 20–24, a genuine increase in ages at first marriage for women may be assumed. This check is not entirely adequate as an artificial increase in proportions single 15–19 may still result from a reduction in the transfer of very young married women across the boundary of age 15. Nevertheless, one can reasonably infer that marriages below age 15 have diminished in most Afri-

TABLE 6.16 Changes in the Proportions Single in Countries with Two or More Censuses

	Proportions Single Women		Change 15–19	Proportions Single Men			Change 20–24
	15–19	20–24		15–19	20–24	25–29	
Angola							
C 1960	.564	.113		.920	.538	.243	
C 1970	.643	.172	+.079	.924	.583	.286	+.045
Kenya							
C 1962	.553	.126		.892	.568	.264	
C 1969	.636	.184	+.083	.956	.718	.321	+.150
C 1979	.712	.245	+.076	—	.720	—	+.002
Liberia							
C 1962	.435	.120		.962	.685	.400	
C 1974	.577	.214	+.142	.968	.744	.411	+.059
Tanzania (mainland)							
C 1967	.480	.092		.929	.565	.245	
S 1973	.555	.139	+.075	—	—	—	
C 1977	.632	.161	+.077	.964	.654	.286	+.089
Ghana							
C 1960	.459	.086		.964	.712	.367	
C 1971	.682	.160	+.223	.986	.796	.395	+.084
W 1979	.691	.154	+.009	—	—	—	

NOTE: Data for Ghana are from the postenumeration surveys based on censuses; 1973 data for Tanzania (S) are from the National Demographic Survey and they are inserted here for comparison with two census results. The same holds for the 1979 WFS data for Ghana (W).

TABLE 6.17 Changes in the Proportions Single in Countries with Data That Are Only Approximately Comparable

Country	Survey	Proportions Single Women 15–19	Proportions Single Women 20–24	Change 15–19	Proportions Single Men 15–19	Proportions Single Men 20–24	Proportions Single Men 25–29	Change 20–24
North Cameroon	S 1963	.155	.070		.890	.451	.102	
	C 1976	.221	.043	(+.066) ⎫	.925	.598	.305	(+.147) ⎫
	W 1978	.209	.032	(+.054) ⎭	.923	.564	.273	(+.113) ⎭
Congo	S 1960	.416	.072		.950	.568	.197	
	C 1974	.668	.205	(+.252)	.989	.817	.379	(+.249)
Ivory Coast	C 1975	.572	.228		.966	.747	.422	
	S 1978	.479	.178	(−.093)	.967	.753	.451	(+.006)
	W 1981	.514	.180	(+.035)	.987	.775	.432	(+.022)
Mali	S 1960	.210	.031		.984	.782	.373	
	C 1976	.476	.117	(+.266)	.951	.816	.470	(+.034)
Mauritania	S 1965 (rural)	.528	.289		.989	.844	.554	
	C 1977 (all)	.570	.244	(+.042)	.982	.805	.472	(−.039)
	W 1981 (all)	.615	.249	(+.045)	.988	.849	.465	(+.044)
Rwanda	S 1970	.824	.180		.967	.455	.100	
	S 1983	.876	.319	(+.052)	—	—	—	
Senegal	S 1960	.372	—		—	.853	—	
	S 1970	.566	.146	(+.194) ⎫	.992	.901	.560	(+.048) ⎫
	C 1976	.548	.206	(−.018) ⎬	.989	.864	.542	(−.037) ⎬
	W 1978	.452	.161	(−.114) ⎭	.983	.852	.501	(−.049) ⎭

Zaire

Bas Fleuve	S 1956	.719	.197	.991	.673	.228
Cataractes	S 1956	.864	.306	.995	.788	.265
Bas-Zaire	S 1975	.711	.238	.996	.835	.289
Equateur	S 1956	.649	.167	.989	.630	.290
Tshuapa	S 1956	.572	.113	.986	.643	.265
Equateur + Tshuapa	S 1975	.596	.160	.981	.686	.262

NOTE: C = census, S = survey, W = WFS; bracketed values pertain to a similar time period and are both compared to the earlier value; the Bas-Zaire region corresponds approximately to the earlier Bas Fleuve and Cataractes regions.

can societies, implying that proportions single at 15 or 16 may have undergone a genuine increase. This obviously contributes to a rise in female *SMAM* values. Hence, an increase in proportions single in *both* age groups for women (15–19; 20–24) an in *all three* for men (15–19; 20–24; 25–29) constitutes a valid criterion for the detection of rises in ages at first marriage.

Regional data from censuses and surveys have been used to assess the possibility of such overall rises in proportions single. The countries are grouped in separate categories depending on the comparability of the sources. Table 6.16 contains the proportions single for the five countries covered by at least two censuses. Table 6.17 presents the same information but the data sources are either mixed (surveys and censuses) or only surveys. Comparability is not optimal. The increment in the proportion single women 15–19 and single men 20–24 are therefore placed between parentheses in table 6.17.

It may be recalled from the empirical relationships between these proportions single and the *SMAM* values for the two sexes (see earlier discussion) that a 10-percentage-point rise in the proportion single women 15–19 (or single men 20–24) corresponds roughly to an increase in the female *SMAM* of 0.65 years and in the male *SMAM* of 1.33 years. The male *SMAM* value increases by the same amount as the female *SMAM* value for a rise in the proportion single males 20–24 that is half that for the proportion single women 15–19. For instance, a rise in the female proportion single 15–19 of 0.100 and in the male proportion single 20–24 of 0.050 produces approximately the same increase in the respective *SMAM* values and leaves the age gap between the spouses at first marriage (*SMAM* difference) essentially unaltered. These approximate conversion rules are useful for interpreting the data of tables 6.16 and 6.17.

In countries with two or more censuses, *all* proportions single, irrespective of sex or age group, tend to show an increase over time. In Angola, Kenya, and Tanzania the proportions single women 15–19 rise by approximately 0.080 per decade, implying an increase in *SMAM* of almost half a year. In Liberia and Ghana, the increment is of the order of 0.110 and 0.200 respectively for the decade of the 1960s, implying a *SMAM* increase of 8 and 13 months. Judging from the Ghanaian WFS (which is not fully comparable to the two postenumeration surveys), this rise seems to have come to a halt in the 1970s. The changes for the males aged 20–24 are furthermore often larger than half those for females 15–19, implying that the age gaps between the spouses have not diminished. This holds true particularly for the decade prior to 1975 and has significance for the trends in polygyny.

As expected, the second set of data, presented in table 6.17, produces less convincing patterns owing to the reduction in comparability. The pattern of a uniform increase in all proportions single is found in the Congo (but seems exaggerated), in Mali (equally large among women), and Rwanda (major increment is for women 20–24, given that ages at marriage for women were already very high to start with). Compared to 1963, the 1970s data for North Cameroon show an increase for men at all ages, but for women only for the first age group. The proportions single women 20–24 are, however, very low at all dates, and large sampling errors combined with imperfect comparability can easily result in such an outcome. In the Ivory Coast, the surveys of 1978 and 1981 produce lower proportions single women than the census of 1975 and very similar proportions for the men. An upward trend in both male and female ages at first marriage seems to be absent in the period after 1975. Unfortunately, no earlier data are available for the Ivory Coast. The problem with Mauritanian surveys is that the ethnic differences in ages at marriage between the Maures and the Wolof or Tukulor settled populations along the Senegal River are of long standing. Shifts in sample coverage involving these two groups can easily result in both upward or downward biases. The Mauritanian data suggest at most a small increase in female ages at marriage. The Senegalese survey of 1970 shows a major increase in the proportion single women 15–19 and single men 20–24 when compared to the 1960 survey, but the figures for 1970 were not confirmed by the census of 1976 and the WFS of 1978. The 1970 survey figures are probably too high, and the 1978 WFS data yields proportions for women that are probably too low (given the WFSs targeting of married women for further interviewing). In the end, much depends on the validity of the 1960 figure if a genuine increase in female age at first marriage is accepted. Given, however, that West African Islamic populations are known to have had very early marriages for women, a rise in female $SMAM$ in Senegal is acceptable. The Zairois regions, finally, do not seem to have had a rise in female ages at marriage over a 20-year period. Only ages at marriage for men in Bas-Zaire appear to have increased.

On the whole, the data of these two tables support the thesis of rising female ages at first marriage in the majority of countries surveyed here. Most of the rises, however, seem to have taken place prior to 1975 and correspond to a $SMAM$ increase for women by half to a full year per decade. Changes in male ages at marriage have also taken place and, in the countries where they occur, the upward shifts in male $SMAM$ values are seldom smaller than those for women. The age gap at first marriage between the two sexes therefore seems to persist, at least until the mid-1970s. Clearly, census returns for the 1980s will shed much more light on the continuity of such trends in age at marriage, especially since the number of countries with two censuses will increase considerably. Finally, the time data presented here are congruent with the cross-sectional relationship between ages at marriage for women and literacy and with the rises in female education the 1960s and early 1970s.

The evaluation of trends in polygyny is much more hazardous given the lack of information to compute suitable indicators such as f, p, and w. The

TABLE 6.18   Changes in Polygyny Indicators in Countries with two or
more Censuses

		Polygyny Ratio (M)	Polygyny Multiplier (KL)	Proportion Married Women Polygynous (f)
Kenya	C 1962	1.28	—	—
	C 1969	1.29	1.18	—
	C 1979	1.21	—	—
	W 1977	—	—	.295
Liberia	C 1962	1.38	1.30	—
	C 1974	1.29	1.28	—
Tanzania	C 1967	1.25	1.13	—
(mainland)	S 1973	1.18	1.17	.271
	C 1977	1.21	1.14	—
Ghana	C 1961	1.27	1.26	.454
	C 1971	1.24	—	—
	W 1979	1.24	—	.344
Mozambique	C 1955	.83	.94	—
	C 1970	1.15	1.05	.246
	C 1980	1.17	1.04	—

polygyny ratio (M) is affected by sex ratio distortions and so is the polygyny multiplier (KL) (but then in the opposite direction if sex ratio distortions are connected with marital status–related migration). The proportion of married women 15+ in polygynous unions (f) is more reliable, but it is seldom available for the countries with a British tradition of census-taking. As the countries with at least two censuses, that is, those of table 6.18, are predominantly former British colonies (Kenya, Tanzania, Ghana), there are few entries for f in table 6.18. Fortunately, Kenya, Liberia, and Tanzania have not been subject to large-scale international migration, so that M and KL do offer a basis for comparison. The same holds for Ghana in the 1960s. The general impression from M and KL in these four countries is that of no decline in the incidence of polygyny or of a small reduction only. The f value produced by the Ghanaian WFS in 1979 is considerably below that from the 1961 post-enumeration survey, whereas the polygyny ratio is not. This allows for the possibility of a larger decline in polygyny in Ghana since M for 1979 is likely to be inflated as a result of male emigration. The data for Mozambique show M and KL values below unity for 1955, corresponding with large segments of the male population involved in labor migration to Zimbabwe and the Republic of South Africa (RSA). The data for the subsequent censuses show more normal results, but these cannot be taken as indicative of a downward trend.

TABLE 6.19 Changes in Polygyny Indicators in Countries with Data That Are Only Approximately Comparable

		Polygyny Ratio (M)	Polygyny Multiplier (KL)	Proportion Married Women Polygynous (f)
North Cameroon	S 1963	1.28	1.09	.463
	C 1976	1.69	1.50	.442
	W 1978	1.35	1.21	.429
Congo	S 1960	1.46	1.07	.538
	C 1974	1.56	1.12	.381
Benin	S 1961 (rural)	1.42	1.24	.513
	W 1982 (all)	—	—	.346
Ivory Coast	C 1975	1.35	1.24	.414
	S 1978	—	—	—
	W 1981	1.31	1.28	.414
Mali	S 1960	1.41	1.29	.441
	C 1976	1.34	1.22	.463
Mauritania	S 1965 (rural)	1.04	—	.084
	C 1977 (all)	1.14	1.01	—
	W 1981 (all)	—	—	.180
Rwanda	S 1970	1.09	—	.161
	C 1978	1.25	—	.152
	S 1983	—	—	.184
Senegal	S 1970	1.41	1.32	.469
	C 1976	1.47	1.39	.518
	W 1978	1.48	1.38	.485
Zaire				
Kinshasa	S 1975	1.03	1.18	.102
	S 1983	—	—	.104
Bas Fleuve	S 1956	1.08 ⎱	—	.150 ⎱
Cataractes	S 1956	1.15 ⎰	—	.112 ⎰
Bas Zaire	S 1975	1.20	1.11	.272
Equateur	S 1956	1.24 ⎱	—	.347 ⎱
Tshuapa	S 1956	1.25 ⎰	—	.370 ⎰
Equateur + Tshuapa	S 1975	1.02	.83	.161

The second set, show in table 6.19, pertains to countries with less adequate data bases for temporal comparisons. The general pattern is of relative stability for the incidence of polygyny in North Cameroon, the Ivory Coast, Mali, Mauritania (cf. earlier discussion for the effect of the ethnic duality), Rwanda, Senegal, Kinshasa, and Bas-Zaire. A decline in f is found in the Congo, but it is not substantiated by a corresponding drop in M or

KL despite the fact that international migration is not a disruptive factor for this country. The value of f is also lowered in Benin, but the basis for comparison is extremely weak. A significant and more convincing drop in f occurs in the Zairois province of Equateur (including Tshuapa). This decline in polygyny can be understood in the context of a dramatic reduction in sterility and subfecundity (see Tabutin et al., 1981) and a rupture of the self-enforcing spiral linking polygyny and sterility. The very low value of M and the value of KL below unity signal, however, that an aberrant sex ratio may be partially responsible for the result of the survey of 1975.

On the whole, it seems that van de Walle and Kekovole (1984) were right in pointing out that there was no swift decline in polygyny in sub-Saharan Africa and that a horizontal trend or at most a slight downward one was closer to the mark. The instances of declines in table 6.18 and 6.19 are limited to Liberia, Ghana, Benin, Congo, and the Equateur province of Zaire. For four of the five cases the evidence from respectively f and M (or KL) is either contradictory (Ghana, Congo), insufficient (Benin), or suspect (M and KL in Equateur). These essentially negative findings with respect to the presumed existence of a marked downward trend are in line with the earlier finding pointing in the direction of higher rather than lower ages at first marriage for men and of the persistence of the age gaps at marriage between the spouses. Since male ages at first marriage are also positively related to literacy in the cross-sections (see earlier discussion), a rise in male age at marriage is plausible. In other words, both trend and cross-sectional data on male ages at marriage support the thesis that changes in male nuptiality have neutralized those in female ages at marriage as far as the age gap and polygyny are concerned.

The discussion on the future of polygyny is evidently not closed. There may be considerable differences in the evolution of polygyny between the urban and rural areas which are not adequately taken into consideration by the statistical analysis presented so far. Clignet (1984), for instance, has posited that urban polygyny levels are declining, but that polygyny is being replaced by illicit visiting unions (that is, the "outside wives" or "deuxièmes bureaux"). The title of Clignet's paper, "La polygamie est morte, vive la polygamie" suggests that the institution of polygyny is merely transformed and that a higher statistical incidence of monogamy is by no means to be taken as an indication of an evolution toward more conjugality. There are to our knowledge no data permitting a measurement of trends in the incidence of such unions, but it cannot be denied that urban polygyny levels are often lower than the rural ones, even if sex ratio distortions are taken into account, and that the practice of "outside wives" is an urban feature. This poses the question of the possibility of a geographical spread of the new phenomenon: is it likely to remain a typically urban characteristic predicated on urban anonymity, or can it be exported to settings where such anonymity is absent, either as a fashion or as a desirable functional alternative to polygyny? The fact that the practice is often illicit makes measurement particularly difficult and the spread of the phenomenon would hamper the interpretation of census results even more. All that can be said at present is that the emergence of the "deuxièmes bureaux" shows that polygyny in urban areas undergoes considerable strain, but that the outcome is a new arrangement rather than more monogamous and conjugal marriage of the Western type as hypothesized by Goode.

The current economic crisis in sub-Saharan Africa is also of relevance for the future of ages at marriage and polygyny. The formal sectors of the economy are no longer growing at rates comparable to those in the decade following independence and the demand for better educated labor often trails far behind the supply. The returns from investing in children's education are falling and school systems are under considerable strain for both financial and demographic reasons. Hence, the current economic crisis is not propitious for the enhancement of female education and a continuation of the female nuptiality transition. Male ages at marriage may stay at their present high levels given the increase in the jobless and landless among the younger cohorts. The crisis features would, therefore, support the maintenance of a large age gap at marriage between the spouses. The main threat to polygyny, that is, a convergence of male and female ages at marriage, is not likely to emerge in the 1980s.

PREMARITAL FERTILITY

The rise in the age at first marriage for women does not necessarily imply a corresponding reduction of the reproductive age span. The issue of premarital fertility is therefore of importance.

However, premarital sex or pregnancies do not constitute a new issue. According to the Murdock files, which reflect the traditional situation, one set of African societies had a strong preference for premarital chastity, probably because this facilitated the bargaining procedures connected with the transfer of women against bridewealth, but another set tolerated premarital sex, presumably because of their interest in transfers of young women with proven fertility. The role of Islamic and Christian penetrations have definitely operated in the direction of less tolerance toward premarital relations, but it would be hazardous to assume that these influences led to a uniform level of low "illegitimacy." Many African scholars would argue the contrary and maintain that African societies do not distinguish between "legitimate" and "illegitimate" births. Personally, we would be inclined to adopt an intermediate position, as there is evidence that premarital births have higher infant and child mortality rates, even after controls for urban versus rural residence and mother's education. Professor Adegbola of the University of

Lagos is currently pursuing this matter, but a first analysis of the WFS data (Lesthaeghe, Meekers, Surkyn, and Adegbola—unpublished as yet) confirms this expectation for the Ivory Coast, Ghana, Benin, southern Nigeria, Cameroon, and Lesotho. The infant and child mortality differential is much smaller or nonexistent in Senegal and northern Nigeria (where early female marriage precludes premarital births to a significant extent) and in Kenya.

Judging from this information it is presumably more accurate to say that many African societies at present do not have a preference for pregnancies or births occurring prior to marriage, but have a certain degree of tolerance towards the phenomenon. However, given low levels of contraceptive protection and a rise in ages at first marriage, premarital pregnancies and births are likely to become more visible and to be defined as problematic, especially when girls are still in school.

The figures on present levels are therefore worthy of consideration. In the WFS surveys of southern Cameroon, Benin, the Ivory Coast, and especially Kenya, 15 to 25 percent of parous women aged 15–24 admit to having had a premarital live birth. The hypothetical "marital" fertility rates for the age group 15–19, computed from the division of the overall fertility rate for this age group (as given by the WFS first country reports) by the proportion ever-married, exceeds 0.500 in the latter two countries. This rate corresponds to the marital fertility rate that would prevail if *all* births occurred within marriage. Levels of 0.500 or more are as high or higher than the *peak* marital fertility rates registered for women 20–24 in historical populations with particularly high natural fertility (such as, Hutterites, Amish, French Canadians). In Africa, such levels of marital fertility are extremely rare and they can only be obtained if large numbers of premarital births are counted as occurring in marriage. Figure 6.14 illustrates that the regions covered by the WFS with 10 percent or more of parous women 15–24 admitting to having had a premarital birth tend to exhibit higher age-specific fertility rates for a given proportion ever-married than regions with less than 10 percent premarital births. Moreover, the line corresponding to combinations leading to a "marital" fertility rate (ASFR/proportion EM) of 0.350 separates the two clusters of points fairly well. Table 6.20 gives an illustration of the outcome of such calculations for sixteen countries. The differences are substantial: six countries have rates between 0.300 and 0.350, which is within the range expected if premarital fertility is low; five countries have rates around 0.400 to 0.500; and five have rates of 0.500 or more, which is indicative of the existence of a major problem.

Admittedly, the data of table 6.20 are only rough approximations and they contain inconsistencies (cf. "marital" fertility rates and proportions admitting premarital births in Ghana or Benin). But, they nevertheless illustrate the fact that a rise in ages at first marriage for women may not necessarily be converted into a shortening of the reproductive age span. In other

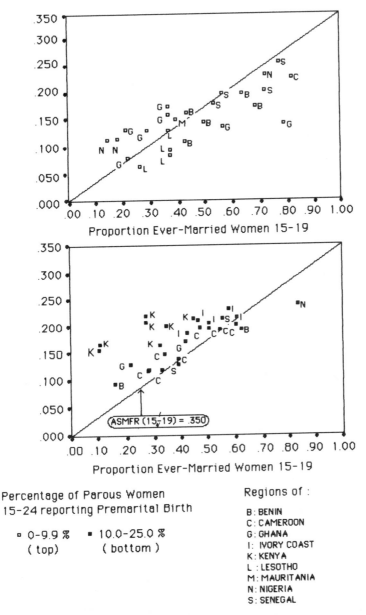

FIGURE 6.14. Effect of Premarital Fertility on the Ratio between the Age-Specific Fertility Rate and the Proportion Ever-Married among Women Aged 15–19 in Regions Covered by the World Fertility Survey, 1976–1982

TABLE 6.20   Indicators of Premarital Fertility in Selected Sub-Saharan Countries

	Fertility Rate 15–19 (1)	Proportion Ever-Married 15–19 (2)	Marital Fertility Rate Implied by (1)/(2) Assuming Zero Premarital Fertility	Proportion of Parous Women Admitting Premarital Birth (WFS)	Proportion of Parous Women Admitting Birth Within First 9 mos. of Marriage (WFS)
Botswana 1971	.096	.135	.711	—	—
Kenya 1977–1978 W	.168	.276	.609	20.2	18.6
West-Zaire 1975–1976 S	.190	.336	.565	—	—
Ivory Coast 1975 W	.216	.428	.505	16.7	14.1
Liberia 1970 C	.230	.460	.500	—	—
Ghana 1971–1980 W	.136	.309	.440	7.9	11.9
Burundi 1971 S	.051	.122	.418	—	—
Mauritania 1981 W	.155	.385	.403	3.6	—
Cameroon 1978 W	.194	.493	.394	17.9	11.5
Nigeria 1981–1982 W	.173	.440	.393	10.5	11.3
Tanzania Mld 1973 S	.154	.445	.346	—	—
Benin 1982 W	.151	.437	.346	15.2	18.7
Uganda 1969 S	.172	.499	.345	—	—
Senegal 1978 W	.197	.593	.332	3.7	4.9
Zambia 1974 S	.137	.423	.324	—	—
Lesotho 1977 W	.102	.315	.324	4.9	8.3

words, the fertility postponement effect of later marriage is partially counteracted by a high incidence of premarital teenage pregnancies in a number of
countries.

CONCLUSIONS

In historical Europe the modernization of marriage patterns proved to be a
prelude to or a correlate of the fertility transition, a pattern since followed by
many developing nations on other continents. The growth of a wage economy, the emergence or restructuring of a class stratification, and the spread
of education nearly always alter the patterns of household formation that
prevailed in earlier systems with kinship-based modes of production. As marriage precedes procreation in most instances, changes in nuptiality were, in
effect, a first indication of other changes to come.

In sub-Saharan Africa, however, the awaited nuptiality transition has
been slow. In several instances no change in age at first marriage has been
detected and in others it has been reduced to more plausible proportions.
The latter occurred primarily when such changes were inferred from data
collected in a single survey: the mixture of current status data, affected by age
misstatements and retrospectively reported ages at first marriage with overall low validity, was found to be particularly prone to producing illusions of
dramatic rises in ages at first marriage (see WFS data). In the majority of
countries with at least two comparable censuses and age schedules of proportions single, rises in ages at marriage were detected, but the orders of magnitude are mostly comprised between 6–12 months per decade.

Whenever there was a rise in the age at first marriage, it occurred for both
sexes. The age difference between the spouses at first marriage remains therefore essentially unaltered, which is consistent with the finding that the incidence of polygyny has not significantly declined. Admittedly, the institution
of polygyny is being replaced by other forms of union formation in urban
areas, but the outcome in the form of "outside wives" is just as far removed
from the Western conjugal and monogamous marriage as polygyny was.
Hence, van de Walle and Kekovole were correct to reject Goode's evolutionary prediction towards Western-style marriages.

The major feature that may have undergone change in the direction described by Goode is the form of partner selection. Although no new material
is presented on this issue in this chapter, fragmentary evidence from small-
scale studies suggests that partner selection has become a matter of greater
personal choice. Usually, such a tendency is associated with the disappearance of very early ages at marriage for girls (below 15), but in the absence of
contraception, diminished parental and lineage controls may also lead to
rising teenage premarital fertility. But no adequate data on trends in premarital fertility are available, and it is known that many sub-Saharan

populations did not have stringent restrictions on premarital sex. Hence, a great deal of caution is needed in interpreting current levels of premarital fertility as outcomes of rising trends.

The main correlate of higher ages at first marriage, both for individuals and regional or ethnic aggregates, is the level of female education. This is not surprising given that this is a recurrent pattern on other continents as well, and that female education is a proxy of major socioeconomic change. Higher levels of female schooling in sub-Saharan Africa are also strongly related to the penetration of Christianity, and low levels remain typical for Islamized populations. Hence, higher female education is the product of both socioeconomic structural change and a historical cultural component. It is, however, feared that the pace of educational expansion is currently slowing down and that relative school enrollment figures may even be declining as a result of the economic crisis, diminished returns of education, and rapid population growth. This would imply that the major motor of rising ages at first marriage is no longer operative. In this instance it would be unsurprising to find that the gradual evolution towards later marriage for girls witnessed during the 1960s and 1970s has not only been slowing down but has even come to a halt in several countries.

The effects of traditional social organization variables are still clearly detectable. They operate either directly or indirectly (via education) on various components of the nuptiality regime. Goody's hypothesis concerning the extension of kinship controls over women leading to earlier marriage and fast remarriage in societies with caste stratification and diverging devolution of property through bilateral inheritance is confirmed, but this feature is only relevant for a small minority of sub-Saharan societies. More important is Boserup's thesis that the productive value of women increases as African societies engage to a larger extent in swidden agriculture. More specifically, it seems that the presence of animal husbandry, chiefly a male activity, deflates the perceived economic utility and social status of women, whereas its absence increases them.

The difference in relative value would explain the high incidence of polygyny among unstratified farming populations who organize their economic exchange and social relations according to Goody's principle of circulation of property (bridewealth) and persons (exogamy) rather than on appropriation (endogamy, dowry). The cross-sectional ethnic data support this hypothesis, which therefore accounts at least *partially* for the difference in polygyny and husband-wife age gaps at first marriage between East and West Africa. In addition to animal husbandry, matrilineal kinship organization tends to reduce polygyny.

A third, major factor needs to be taken into account: labor migration and sex-ratio distortion. This factor is not only of direct relevance for the sending populations in the western Sahel or southern Africa, or for the receiving populations along the Atlantic, the Gulf of Guinea, and South Africa, but it is operative in many other parts as well, involving substantial migration streams within or between countries. These streams concern not only rural to urban, but also rural to rural migration. Whenever sex-ratio distortions result, demographic measures such as *SMAM* or the polygyny ratio become poor indicators of ages at first marriage and of the incidence of polygyny. Aside from substantial measurement error, also age-, sex-, and marital status–selective migration distort the functioning of traditional nuptiality systems. In the western Sahel, outmigration of single males may have enhanced polygyny in farming populations, whereas in southern Africa it has reduced polygyny among cattle keepers and led to the development of female-headed households instead. In short, the labor exporting economies of southern Africa and the black population of the RSA itself exhibit striking signs of a major disruption of the traditional marriage systems.

These three main clusters of influences, namely those associated with education, traditional social organization, and migration, only offer a partial explanation of regional and ethnic nuptiality patterns. Obviously a substantial portion of the residual variance is attributable to plain measurement inaccuracy in both dependent and independent variables, but, as geographic autocorrelation revealed, other factors must be at work as well. A possible avenue for further research is the more extensive and varied measurement of indicators of the economic and social position of women, the development of better regional indicators of the economic structure, and the explicit introduction of religious influences (such as various types of Christianity, Islam, survival of traditional religion). Data from the 1980s round of censuses are equally badly needed to update the information and recheck the empirical work presented here. In short, this exercise is merely a beginning that can and should be upgraded since too many crucial questions concerning patterns and trends have been left with partial answers.

ACKNOWLEDGMENTS

Financial support from USAID through the Population Council's International Awards Program (agreements CP84.12A and CP82.39A) is gratefully acknowledged. Additional support for the expansion of this analysis is being provided by the Rockefeller Foundation. The chapter benefited greatly from comments by Hilary Page and E. van de Walle.

BIBLIOGRAPHY

Boserup, E. 1970. *Women's role in economic development.* London: Allen and Unwin.
Caldwell, J. C. 1980. Mass education as a determinant of the timing of fertility decline. *Population and Development Review* 6(2): 225–255.

Casterline, J., and J. Trussell. 1980. Age at first birth. *World Fertility Survey Comparative Studies*, no. 15. Voorburg: International Statistical Institute.

Capron, J., and J. Kohler. 1975. *Migration de travail et pratique matrimoniale—Migrations à partir du Pays Mossi*. Ouagadougou, Burkina Faso: ORSTOM (mimeo).

Clignet, R. 1970. *Many wives, many powers—Authority and power in polygynous families*. Evanston: Northwestern University Press.

———. 1984. La polygamie est morte, vive la polygamie. Paper presented at the Conference on the Transformation of African Marriage—Customary Models in a New Setting. Nairobi: International African Institute.

Coale, A. J., and D. R. McNeil. 1972. The distribution by age of the frequency of first marriage in a female cohort. *Journal of the American Statistical Association* 67: 743–749.

Coale, A. J. 1973. The demographic transition reconsidered. In: *Proceedings of the World Population Conference*. Liège: Ordina for the International Union for the Scientific Study of Population.

Comaroff, J. L. 1960. Introduction. In: *The meaning of marriage payments*, ed. J. L. Comaroff. New York: Academic Press, 1–48.

Dries, H. 1985. De Afrikaanse familie: Structuro-functionalistische interpretatie in een context van modernisatie. *Afrika Focus*, 1(1): 89–121.

Eelens, F., and L. Donné. 1985. The proximate determinants of fertility in sub-Saharan Africa: A factbook based on the results of the World Fertility Survey. *Interuniversity Programme in Demography Working Papers*, no. 86–6. Brussels: Vrije Universiteit.

Goode, W. 1970. *World revolution and family patterns*. 2d ed. New York: Free Press.

Goody, J. 1973. Polygyny, economy and the role of women. In: *The character of kinship*, ed. J. Goody. Cambridge: Cambridge University Press.

———. 1976. *Production and reproduction—A comparative study of the domestic domain*. Cambridge: Cambridge University Press.

Gough, H. G. 1977. Further validation of a measure of individual modernity. *Journal of Personality Assessment* 41: 49–57.

Hajnal, H. J. 1965. European marriage patterns in perspective. In: *Population in history*, ed. D. V. Glass and D. Eversley. London: Edward Arnold, 101–143.

Henin, R. A., D. Ewbank, and H. Hogan n.d. *The demography of Tanzania—An analysis of the 1973 National Demographic Survey of Tanzania*. Dar Es Salaam, Tanzania: Bureau of Statistics and BRALUP.

Hunter, G. 1967. From the old culture to the new. In: *Modern Africa*, ed. J. M. McEwan and R. B. Sutcliffe. New York: Harper and Row, 315–325.

Kuper, A. 1985. *African marriage in an impinging world—The case of southern Africa*. Leyden: Afrika Studiecentrum.

Lesthaeghe, R. 1980. On the social control of human reproduction. *Population and Development Review* 6(4): 527–548.

Lorimer, F. 1969. *Culture and human fertility—A study of the relation of cultural conditions to fertility in non-industrial and transitional societies*. 2d ed. New York: Greenwood Press.

McCarthy, J. 1982. Differentials in age at first marriage. *World Fertility Survey Comparative Studies*, no. 19. Voorburg: International Statistical Institute.

McDonald, P. 1985. Social organization and nuptiality in developing countries. In:

Reproductive change in developing countries, ed. J. Cleland and J. Hobcraft. Oxford: Oxford University Press.

Meillassoux, C. 1981. *Maidens, meal and money—Capitalism and the domestic community.* Cambridge: Cambridge University Press.

Murdock, G. P. 1967. Ethnographic atlas: A summary. *Ethnology* 6(2): 109–234.

———. 1975. *Outline of world cultures*, 5th ed. New Haven, Conn.: Human Relations Area Files.

Morah, B. C. 1985. Evaluation of the Nigeria Fertility Survey 1981–82. *World Fertility Survey Scientific Reports*, no. 80. Voorburg: International Statistical Institute.

Notestein, F. W. 1945. Population—The long view. In: *Food for the world*, ed. T. W. Schultz. Chicago: University of Chicago Press.

Pison, G. 1982. *Dynamique d'une population traditionelle—Les Peuls Bandé du Sénégal Oriental.* Cahier de l'INED, no. 99. Paris: Presses Universitaires de France.

Radcliffe-Brown, A. R., and D. Forde. 1950. *African systems of kinship and marriage.* London: Oxford University Press.

Romaniuk, A. 1967. *La fécondité des populations congolaises.* Paris: Mouton.

———. 1968. The demography of the Democratic Republic of the Congo. In: *The demography of tropical Africa*, ed. W. Brass et al. Princeton: Princeton University Press.

Saucier, J. F. 1972. Correlates of the long postpartum taboo: A cross-cultural study. *Current Anthropology* 13(2): 238–249.

Schoenmaeckers, R., I. H. Shah, R. Lesthaeghe, and O. Tambashe. 1981. The child-spacing tradition and the postpartum taboo in tropical Africa: Anthropological evidence. In: *Child-spacing in tropical Africa—Traditions and change*, ed. H. J. Page and R. Lesthaeghe. London: Academic Press.

Schwimmer, B. 1979. Market structure and social organization in a Ghanaian marketing system. *American Ethnography* 6(4): 682.

Tabutin, D., M. Sala-Diakanda, Ngondo a Pitshandenge, and E. Vilquin. 1981. Fertility and child-spacing in western Zaire. In: *Child-spacing in tropical Africa—Traditions and change*, ed. H. J. Page and R. Lesthaeghe. London: Academic Press, 287–299.

van de Walle, E. 1968. Marriage in African censuses and inquiries. In: *The demography of tropical Africa*, ed. W. Brass et al. Princeton: Princeton University Press.

van de Walle, E., and J. Kekovole. 1984. The recent evolution of African marriage and polygyny. Paper presented at the annual meeting of the Population Association of America, Minneapolis, Minn.

Ware, H. 1981. *Women, education and modernization of the family in West Africa.* Changing African Family Project Series, no. 7. Canberra: Australian National University.

CHAPTER SEVEN

Polygyny and Fertility in Sub-Saharan Africa

Anne R. Pebley
Wariara Mbugua

INTRODUCTION

Polygyny is a common part of married life in many sub-Saharan populations, although its incidence varies considerably according to region and ethnic group. In non-African societies in which polygyny is, or was, socially permissible, only a relatively small fraction of the population is in polygynous marriages. Chamie's (1986) analysis of data for Arab Muslim countries between the 1950s and 1980s shows that only 5 to 12 percent of men in these countries have more than one wife. Similarly, as mentioned in an earlier chapter, Smith and Kunz (1976) report that less than 10 percent of nineteenth-century American Mormon husbands were polygynists. By contrast, throughout most of southern West Africa and western Central Africa, as many as 20 to 50 percent of married men have more than one wife (van de Walle, 1968; van de Walle and Kekovole, 1984; Kaufmann, Lesthaeghe, and Meekers, 1987). The frequency is somewhat lower in East and South Africa, although 15 to 30 percent of husbands are reported to be polygynists in Kenya and Tanzania (Kaufmann, Lesthaeghe, and Meekers, 1987). While there have been predictions that the frequency of polygyny would decline as African societies undergo social change, there is no evidence that such a decline has occurred in the decades since 1960 (Locoh, 1976; Clignet and Sween, 1974; van de Walle and Kekovole, 1984; Kaufmann, Lesthaeghe, and Meekers, 1987). In fact, rising incomes may increase the frequency of polygyny, at least in the short run, as more men are able to pay brideprice for and/or support two or more wives. Van de Walle and Kekovole (1984), for example, suggest that polygyny has increased in Senegal in the past two decades. Goldman and Pebley (1987) have shown that even if African populations experience substantial declines in the rate of growth over the

next several decades, they will have no difficulty in maintaining a large surplus of women required by a high frequency of polygyny, as long as large
differences in the ages at marriage of men and women continue.

Most carefully executed studies have found that the fertility of women
in polygynous marriages is lower than that of women in monogamous
marriages (van de Walle, 1968; Page, 1975; Ngongo a Pitshandenge, 1978;
Locoh, 1984; Garenne and van de Walle, 1985). The differential, however, is
generally small. Garenne and van de Walle (1985), for example, report age-
specific marital fertility rates for women in monogamous and polygynous
marriages of 7.5 and 7.0, respectively, for a population in the Fatik (formerly
Sine-Saloum) region of Senegal.

Polygyny may affect fertility both by changing fertility within marriage
and by altering the proportion of the fecund period women spend in marriage
or in a sexual union. These effects may operate at the societal or population
level, as well as at the individual level. In this chapter, our focus is limited to
the association between polygyny and the fertility of individual women *within
marriage*. Societal level effects are briefly discussed at the end of the chapter.

To examine this association, we use data from national fertility surveys
conducted in six sub-Saharan African countries in the late 1970s in connection with the World Fertility Survey program. Many previous analyses have
either employed detailed data for only one region or relied on very limited
information from a wide range of countries. A central objective of this analysis is to determine whether the associations between polygyny and fertility
are observed in all countries in our analysis, which would imply common
behavioral or biological differences between polygynous and monogamous
marriage across regional and cultural boundaries. The countries involved
in the analysis—Senegal, Ivory Coast, Ghana, Cameroon, Kenya, and
Lesotho—include a broad range of regions and cultures in sub-Saharan Africa. They also have widely varying frequencies of polygyny. The proportions
of married women at the time of the survey who were in polygynous
marriages ranged from a low of 9 percent in Lesotho to a high of 48 percent
in Senegal. This sample of countries, however, is not intended to be representative of the entire population of sub-Saharan Africa. It is also important
to note that an analysis of this kind, of necessity, ignores important cultural
differences both among and within countries in the types of marriage that
take place, and the meaning and function of marriage.

DATA AND METHODS

The data were collected from nationally representative samples of women
aged 15 to 49 in each country, using a modified version of the World Fertility
Survey core questionnaire. Details of the survey procedures used can be
found in the first country report for each country (Central Bureau of Statis-

tics, Kenya, 1980; Central Bureau of Statistics, Lesotho, 1981; Direction de la Statistique, Senegal, 1981; Direction de la Statistique et de la Comptabilité Nationale, Cameroon, 1983; Central Bureau of Statistics, Ghana, 1983; Direction de la Statistique, Côte d'Ivoire, 1984). The core questionnaire included a complete live birth history; questions on the respondent's age, characteristics, and contraceptive use; and a record of the dates of marriages and marriage dissolutions. For African countries, one or more questions were asked about polygyny. All six surveys used in this analysis included questions on whether a woman's husband had other wives, and all (except Ghana) asked wives in polygynous marriages about their rank (first wife, second wife, and so forth). Several countries also asked about the number of other wives in the marriage.

Each of the six survey questionnaires included versions of the "factors other than contraception affecting fertility" (FOTCAF) module designed by WFS to measure biological factors and traditional practices that affect fertility in countries with low levels of contraceptive use. The FOTCAF module includes questions on the lengths of: breastfeeding, unsupplemented breastfeeding, postpartum amenorrhea, and postpartum abstinence. Questions on postpartum abstinence and amenorrhea were omitted in Senegal.

Goldman, Rutstein, and Singh (1985) report wide variations in the quality of data collected in WFS surveys, with more serious deficiencies apparent in African and South Asian countries. Reports of age at interview are subject to considerable heaping and to distortions at oldest and youngest ages. Birth histories for several African countries appear to be incomplete: early births to the oldest cohorts seem to be especially likely to be omitted. However, Chidambaram and Sathar (1984) show that the completeness and accuracy of reporting of dates for the most recent birth is considerably better than for early births, in many WFS surveys.

The evidence concerning the quality of data on breastfeeding and postpartum abstinence and amenorrhea collected in these surveys is more limited. Distributions of these variables in all six countries are seriously heaped at multiples of 6 and 12 months. An analysis by Ferry (1981) of heaped breastfeeding data from other WFS surveys, however, suggests that the level of overall bias is low.[1] Ferry shows, for example, that median durations of breastfeeding estimated from reported lengths of breastfeeding in the last closed and open birth intervals are consistent with those estimated from current status reports. Data on postpartum abstinence and amenorrhea are likely to be more seriously flawed, however. Hobcraft and Guz (1985) report, for example, that significant proportions of women in African WFS surveys report durations of postpartum amenorrhea and abstinence which exceed the time between the previous birth and the next conception.

All studies of African marriage patterns using data from surveys and censuses are handicapped by the complexity of African marriage practices.

Marriage is often a process involving a series of steps taken over a period of months or years, rather than a single civil or religious ceremony (see, for example, Oppong, 1987). Thus, the point at which a woman is married is often difficult to define. Sexual relations begin at some point during the process, or in some situations, outside of the marriage process entirely. On the other hand, some married women are not in a sexual union. For example, a widow who is inherited by her brother-in-law and thus is technically married to him, may not have sexual relations with him, particularly if she is close to menopause or already has several children. For all these reasons, marital histories, and even current marital status and whether the current marriage is monogamous or polygynous, may be subject to considerable misreporting. We believe, however, that respondents' reports of their marital situation at the time of interview are likely to be more accurate than retrospective information about marriage events.

Even if there were no difficulties with the quality of data in these surveys, several aspects of the type of data collected limit the scope of the analysis. First, the only information available on polygyny concerns whether the marriages of women who were married at the time of the survey were monogamous or polygynous. Thus, for the small fraction of women not married at interview, we know nothing about whether they were ever in a polygynous marriage. Furthermore, for women in a particular type of marriage at interview, we do not know whether or not that particular marriage has always been of the same type, or whether previous marriages were monogamous or polygynous.

As a result, all of our comparisons between women by type of marriage are based on their marital status at interview. Of necessity, we assume that marriage type at the time of the survey also accurately characterized an arbitrarily chosen 3-year period before the survey, or the entire duration of the marriage, for women married for fewer than 3 years. The analysis is, therefore, limited to fertility that occurred in this time period. This restriction has the additional advantage that it avoids many of the more serious problems in birth histories, described above.

A second problem is that information on breastfeeding, contraceptive use, and postpartum amenorrhea and abstinence are only available for the intervals after the last two live births.[2] Thus, if we are to examine whether differentials in these proximate determinants account for the association between polygyny and fertility, the analysis must be limited to the open and last closed birth interval. Use of these data, however, poses a methodological problem, because the last closed interval is, on average, longer than the average birth interval. Hence, more fertile women will be underrepresented in an analysis based only on the last two intervals. To avoid this bias we have adopted a strategy used by Goldman et al. (1983) for calculating life tables and for our multivariate analysis, in which the observation is confined to a fixed period before the survey, in this case, 3 years. Since information on breastfeeding, contraceptive use, abstinence, and amenorrhea is available only for the last closed and the open interval, the analysis can include, at most, the conception leading to one live birth. However, by confining observation to a 3-year period, we are able to obtain the needed information for almost all pregnancies in the period. We assume that all reported pregnancies of at least 3 months duration at the time of interview will result in live births. Some women who do not report a current pregnancy in the survey may have become pregnant recently. For this reason, the observation period is terminated 3 months before interview; the 3-year observation periods, thus, encompasses months 3 through 39 before the interview.

In summary, because of the available data, we have confined our analyses to events occurring in the 3 years before the survey and to women who are married at the time of interview. We assume that the type of marriage in which a woman reported herself at the time of the survey was the type she was in during the 3 years before the survey, if she was continuously married to the same man, or during the entire duration of the marriage, if her current marriage began in the 3 years before the survey.

POLYGYNY AND FERTILITY

The population of women in polygynous marriages consists of two groups: women who originally married a monogomist and who later acquired a cowife or cowives, and women who married a husband who already had a wife or wives. For the most part, the first group will be first or senior wives at the time of the survey, while the second group will mainly be junior (second, third, or fourth) wives. Since the associations between polygyny and fertility may be quite different for the two groups, we examine the results for first wives in polygynous marriages separately from junior wives, in all countries except Ghana which did not collect information on wife's rank.

The top panel of table 7.1 shows total marital fertility rates calculated for all currently married women by type of marriage, for the 3 years prior to the survey.[3] In each country, marital fertility rates for all women in polygynous marriages combined are lower than for women in monogamous marriages, although the differences range from 0.16 in Lesotho to 1.8 in Kenya. When the polygynous group is divided by rank, there is no uniform pattern across countries in fertility rates. First wives have lower fertility than more junior wives in Kenya and Lesotho. However, the rate for senior wives in Lesotho is based on a very small number of cases. The differences between junior and senior wives are small and most likely not significant in Cameroon and the Ivory Coast. Senior wives have higher fertility than junior wives in Senegal. In fact, all of the fairly small fertility differential by marriage type in Senegal is due to the lower fertility of junior wives.

TABLE 7.1   Total Marital Fertility Rates for Women 15–49 during the
3 Years before the Survey, by Type of Marriage

All Married Women	Cameroon	Ghana	Ivory Coast	Kenya	Lesotho	Senegal
Monogamous	7.67	8.00	8.69	10.40	7.87	8.71
(N)	(3245)	(2562)	(2358)	(3675)	(2581)	(1476)
Polygynous	7.15	7.87	7.69	9.12	7.53	8.55
(N)	(2356)	(1430)	(1715)	(1518)	(246)	(1456)
Polygynous first wives	7.05	—	7.76	8.68	4.87	8.80
(N)	(850)		(751)	(544)	(26)	(662)
Polygynous Second+ wives	7.20	—	7.64	9.36	7.84	8.34
(N)	(1506)		(964)	(974)	(220)	(794)
Women With at Least 1 Live Birth						
Monogamous	8.05	7.38	8.77	10.07	7.63	8.71
(N)	(2491)	(2056)	(1880)	(3206)	(1980)	(1092)
Polygynous	7.73	7.37	7.76	9.01	7.17	8.79
(N)	(1785)	(1267)	(1479)	(1355)	(200)	(1263)
Polygynous first wives	7.21	—	8.03	8.73	4.95	8.92
(N)	(715)		(694)	(505)	(26)	(629)
Polygynous Second+ wives	8.07	—	7.52	9.18	7.50	8.67
(N)	(1070)		(785)	(850)	(174)	(634)

The differentials in marital fertility in table 7.1 must be the result of differences in one or more of the factors that have come to be known as the proximate determinants of fertility: fecundity, coital frequency, the length of the postpartum nonsusceptible period, fetal loss, and contraceptive use. One explanation for fertility differentials by type of marriage may be differences in female fecundity because of selection into polygynous marriages of sterile or subfecund women (Pison, 1986; Lesthaeghe, 1984; Clignet, 1969). This selection may occur in two ways. The sterility of a wife in a monogamous marriage is often an important factor precipitating the husband's marriage to a second wife. Husbands are also more likely to divorce subfecund or sterile wives. When these women remarry, they are more likely to become second or third wives in a polygynous household. Thus, we would anticipate that both senior and junior wives may be less fecund than wives in monogamous marriages, *ceteris paribus*.

TABLE 7.2 Differences between Monogamously and Polygynously Married Women*

	Mean Wife's Age	Mean Duration of Marriage	Mean Husband's Age*	Median Length of Breast-feeding**	Median Length of Full Breast-feeding**	Median Length of Amenorrhea**	Median Length of Post-partum Abstinence**	% Using Contraception in the Open Interval†	% Using Contraception in the Closed Interval†	% Coresiding with Husband
Cameroon										
Monogamous	30.2	11.3	38.8	18.7	4.9	12.1	14.8	6.8	6.4	—
Polygynous										
Senior wife	34.9	16.7	39.0	20.5	5.4	12.7	16.2	5.1	3.1	—
Junior wife	29.4	10.0	43.2	22.5	5.2	12.8	18.6	6.7	3.7	—
Ghana										
Monogamous	29.6	10.3	44.7	14.7	4.4	12.3	6.7	11.6	11.4	76.9
Polygynous	32.4	12.1	50.3	16.9	5.0	12.5	8.9	6.7	6.3	73.5
Ivory Coast										
Monogamous	27.9	9.3	38.9	18.2	6.2	10.7	12.4	2.7	2.0	90.8
Polygynous										
Senior wife	33.2	15.3	39.7	18.6	6.1	10.5	12.6	1.3	2.0	94.8
Junior wife	28.9	8.5	44.8	18.7	6.2	10.1	12.7	1.0	1.0	86.2
Kenya										
Monogamous	29.9	11.9	40.2	14.2	3.4	9.9	3.1	11.0	6.8	80.8
Polygynous										
Senior wife	36.3	19.3	41.1	15.8	3.5	12.0	3.2	9.5	3.6	73.0
Junior wife	30.4	11.9	49.9	14.5	3.6	10.0	3.0	8.2	4.4	82.7
Lesotho										
Monogamous	29.7	11.5	38.8	24.1	4.1	9.3	14.3	9.4	7.8	60.8
Polygynous	31.7	12.1	45.1	24.0	4.3	6.9	13.0	8.1	9.5	69.5

Senegal

Monogamous	30.8	10.0	47.7	20.5	5.5	—	—	7.3	5.4	—
Polygynous										
Senior wife	36.6	18.3	48.1	20.9	6.2	—	—	7.3	6.0	—
Junior wife	31.2	9.1	52.9	21.1	5.5	—	—	6.8	4.6	—

*Standardized for wife's age as follows: mean husband's age was calculated for each five year grouping of wife's age. Then these mean ages were averaged over all wife's age groups, assigning each wife's age group a weight of 1.

**These medians are calculated from lifetables based on exposure during the open and closed birth intervals in the 3 years before the survey. As explained in the text, women who had nonlive births during this period are excluded from the calculation because information on their last closed-birth interval was not available.

†This measure includes use of contraceptive methods other than abstinence. Use of the rhythm method *is* included.

In order to determine how much of the fertility differentials by marriage type are due to higher sterility of wives in polygynous marriages, we recalculated the total marital fertility rates for the 3-year period before the survey excluding women who had never had a live birth by the beginning of this observation period. The results are shown in the bottom panel of table 7.1. In the process of eliminating childless women, we also exclude a few, mainly younger, women who are newly married and thus have not had adequate time to have a child by the beginning of the 3-year period. However, during the period of observation itself, they generally experience relatively high fertility. Exclusion of these women accounts for the lower fertility rates, as in the case of Ghana, in the bottom panel of table 7.2 when compared with rates in the top panel.

Elimination of childless women from the calculation reduces the gap between the fertility of wives in monogamous and polygynous marriages in all countries except Lesotho. However, in some countries the change is only slight. In the Ivory Coast and Kenya, the difference by marriage type remains large: slightly more than one child, on average. A smaller difference also remains in Lesotho and Cameroon, but there is no longer any difference in Ghana and Senegal. In Cameroon and Kenya, senior cowives have the lowest fertility. In fact, in Cameroon the fertility of junior wives is about the same as that of wives in monogamous marriages. The situation is reversed in Ivory Coast and Senegal where senior cowives have higher fertility than junior cowives.

The classical hypothesis about fertility differences between wives in monogamous and polygynous marriages is that they are caused by differences in coital frequency (Muhsam, 1956). The usual argument is that if the husband's frequency of intercourse remains the same or increases only slightly if he marries another wife, then the coital frequency of each wife will decline as the number of wives increases. However, Garenne and van de Walle (1985) point out that models of coital frequency and fertility suggest that even substantial reductions in the frequency of intercourse may have a relatively minor impact on fertility. Furthermore, in societies in which women are frequently pregnant or abstinent, it may be relatively easy for each wife to be as sexually active as a wife in a monogamous marriage since cowives are likely to be abstinent at different times.

Data on coital frequency are difficult to collect and may be highly unreliable when available. In several of the surveys included in this analysis one or more questions were asked about whether a woman was sexually active at the time of the survey or about coital frequency. We will return to these data later on in the chapter.

The fertility differentials between women in monogamous and polygynous marriages may also be due to differences in postpartum variables and contraceptive use. Table 7.2 shows summary statistics for the distributions of several of these variables, by marriage type for each country. In Ghana, all women in polygynous marriages are again grouped together since no information is available on cowives' status or rank. We have also grouped all wives in polygynous marriages together for Lesotho, in this and all subsequent tables, since there are relatively few women in polygynous marriages and very few senior cowives.

The first three columns of table 7.2 show that the wife's age, her duration in her current marriage, and her husband's age, at the time of interview, all differ consistently by marriage type. Wives in monogamous marriages and junior cowives in polygynous marriages are, on average, very close in age in all countries in which rank can be determined. The results for Ghana and Lesotho are at least consistent with this pattern. Senior cowives are considerably older than the other two groups. Similarly, senior cowives have also been married for longer average durations than junior cowives and wives in monogamous marriages. The latter two groups have roughly equivalent durations of marriage.

The reason for these two related patterns is the operation of the marriage system itself. Since all marriages may potentially become polygynous, many wives in monogamous marriages are those whose marriages are not yet polygynous: that is, they tend to be younger and at shorter marriage durations. Junior cowives in polygynous marriages are also more recently married, by definition, than senior cowives and are, therefore, younger and at shorter marriage durations. In fact, junior cowives at any given age are more likely to have shorter marriage durations in the current marriage than wives in monogamous marriages, because they are more likely to have been divorced or widowed than wives in monogamous marriages.[4] Thus, one possible explanation for the lower fertility of senior cowives in Kenya and Cameroon may be the longer average marriage duration of these women. We have eliminated effects on the fertility differentials by marriage type of differences in primary sterility by excluding women who never had a live birth from the bottom of table 7.2. However, women at longer marriage durations may have lower coital frequency.

In the third column of table 7.2, we compare the mean ages of husbands to whom wives of each union type are married. However, substantial proportions of the sample did not report a husband's age in Cameroon and the Ivory Coast. In Senegal, a question on husband's age was not included in the individual questionnaire. To obtain husband's age information, we matched husbands and wives using information on the household schedules. Unfortunately, we were unable to match all currently married women with husbands. Even when matches were made, information on the husband's age was not always available. The proportion of wives for whom we have no husband's age information is shown in Appendix J. In Cameroon and the Ivory Coast, this information is more frequently missing for wives in polygynous marriages. Thus, the means shown in table 7.2 for husband's age are averaged only across wives for whom husband's age information is available. These means are standardized for the wife's age since wives in different types of marriage have different age distributions. The standardization procedure used is analogous to calculating a total fertility rate. A separate mean husband's age was calculated for each 5-year wife's age group. These means were then averaged again across all wife's age groups, which has the effect of giving each wife's age group equal weight. The resulting mean husbands' ages reflect primarily the age difference between husbands and wives at marriage since wife's age is held constant.

The results indicate that when wife's age is held constant, wives in monogamous marriages and senior cowives in polygynous marriages are married to men of roughly the same mean age. This is not surprising, since the women in both groups are generally the first wives that these men married. Junior cowives, on the other hand, are at any given age married to much older husbands. The means for Ghana and Lesotho show that when all wives in polygynous marriages are grouped together, they are, on average, married to older men. But we can see from the means for other countries that the entire effect is most likely due to the fact that junior co-wives have older husbands.

Recent research on a population in Senegal by Garenne and van de Walle (1985) and on nineteenth-century American Mormons by Bean and Mineau (1986) suggests that the fact that husbands of junior cowives are older may be part of the reason for lower fertility among these wives. Two possible explanations for these effects of husband's age may be reduced coital frequency and reduced fecundity among older husbands.

In the next four columns of table 7.2, we examine differences in breastfeeding, amenorrhea, and abstinence by marriage type. Each median is calculated using life table methods[5] and exposure in the open birth interval (the interval since last live birth) and the last closed birth interval, which occurred during a 3-year observation period. The sample of birth intervals is the same one used for multivariate analysis and was described in the preceding section. Because of the sample on which they are based, the medians pertain to a period of observation shortly before interview.

Many observers argue that polygyny may be associated with fertility in part because it allows wives to breastfeed and to observe the postpartum sexual taboo for a longer time after giving birth, since polygynists have other legitimate sexual partners while monogamists do not. Wives in polygynous marriages may also breastfeed and abstain from sex for longer periods because they come from more traditional backgrounds than wives in monogamous marriages. This longer median duration of breastfeeding for senior cowives is at least consistent with the fertility differentials by marriage type and rank observed for Kenya in table 7.2. Thus, one of the hypotheses we will test in the next section is that longer breastfeeding for senior cowives accounts for their lower fertility relative to other women.

The median duration of breastfeeding is generally shortest for women in monogamous marriages, longer for senior cowives in polygynous marriages, and longest for junior cowives, although the differences among these three groups are very small in the Ivory Coast and Senegal. The exception to this pattern is Kenya, where senior cowives have the longest median duration of breastfeeding. The median duration of full breastfeeding shows no strong association with marriage type, although in most countries the medians for wives of polygynists are slightly higher.

The median lengths of postpartum amenorrhea vary relatively little by marriage type within each country. It is encouraging to note that for the most part these variations follow the same patterns as those in the median length of breastfeeding. For example, in Kenya, the median length of postpartum amenorrhea is highest for senior cowives, as in the median length of breastfeeding. Questions on postpartum amenorrhea and postpartum abstinence were not included in the Senegal questionnaire.

The median durations of postpartum abstinence vary markedly from country to country, with high median durations reported in Cameroon and the Ivory Coast, and very low median durations reported in Kenya. The relatively long durations of postpartum abstinence in Lesotho are less the result of strict observance of a postpartum sexual taboo than of the frequent absence of substantial portions of the male population who leave home to work in South Africa. Postpartum abstinence does not appear to differ significantly by marriage type and rank in the Ivory Coast and Kenya, where fertility differentials are the greatest. In Cameroon and Ghana, women in polygynous marriages report abstaining 2 to 3 months longer than wives in monogamous marriages. In Lesotho, however, wives in monogamous marriages abstain for about a month longer, on average, than those in polygynous marriages.

The last three columns of table 7.2 indicate the frequency of contraceptive use and the proportion of wives coresiding with their husbands by type of marriage and rank. Since contraceptive use in the open and last closed birth intervals is generally higher among wives in *monogamous* marriages in most countries, differential contraceptive use can not be an explanation of the lower fertility among wives in polygynous marriages. In fact, differentials in contraceptive use in some countries such as Kenya may tend to reduce the size of fertility differentials by marriage type. However, even in Kenya, contraceptive use is not common and the differentials in use by marriage type are not large.

In many African societies, separate residence of spouses does not necessarily imply the lack of sexual relations. However, spouses who are not coresident may have a lower frequency of intercourse than spouses who coreside. As the figures in table 7.2 show, the vast majority of women coreside with their husbands, except in Lesotho where male labor migration to South Africa makes coresidence of spouses more difficult. The proportion of wives coresiding with husbands is also low in Ghana primarily because separate residence of spouses is traditional in several Ghanaian cultures. No information on coresidence of spouses is available for Cameroon or Senegal. In the Ivory Coast, junior cowives are the least likely to coreside with their husbands. The situation is reversed in Kenya, where senior cowives are least likely to live with their husbands.

Thus, differentials in several of the variables shown in table 7.2 may explain the fertility differentials by marriage type and rank shown in table 7.1. Marriage duration and husband's age all vary consistently with marriage type. Differences in the length of breastfeeding may be important in Cameroon, Ghana, and Kenya, as may be many differences in postpartum abstinence in Cameroon. The patterns of contraceptive use suggest that fertility differentials by marriage type might actually be larger if there were no contraceptive use. Finally, the lower proportions of senior cowives in Kenya and junior cowives in the Ivory Coast who coreside with their husbands may be associated with lower fertility for these two groups. We have not investigated differentials in one other proximate determinant of fertility—fetal loss— because of apparently severe problems of underreporting. However, there is no reason to believe that fetal loss rates would differ sufficiently by type of marriage to contribute to the fertility differentials between women in monogamous and polygynous marriages.

MULTIVARIATE RESULTS

In order to determine whether differences in fertility by marriage type can be accounted for by the intermediate variables discussed above, we use multivariate statistical methods. Our basic strategy is to determine whether the association between marriage type (monogamous, polygynous—senior wife, polygynous—junior wife) and fertility remains sizable and statistically significant once intermediate variables are held constant.

As described in the methods section, we focus on the probability of fertile conception (a conception that results in a live birth) in the portion of the open and last closed birth intervals which occur in a 3-year observation period prior to the interview.

The analytic technique we use is a hazard model, which is analogous to a regression model with life table rates as the dependent variable. More detailed descriptions of hazard models can be found in Trussell and Hammerslough (1983), Trussell et al. (1985), and Pebley and Stupp (1987). In our analysis, each woman can contribute, at most, two observations, that is, an open and a last closed birth interval to this life table. For each birth interval, a woman contributes exposure to the life table beginning at the duration since last live birth that she had attained by the beginning of the three year observation period. In other words, if, at the beginning of the observation period, a woman's last live birth had occurred 15 months before, she would begin contributing exposure to the life table at duration 15 months. She would continue to contribute exposure until she was either censored, by the interview, or until she conceived. In order to avoid problems associated with the period between marriage and first birth and the possibility of selection into polygynous marriages of sterile women, we exclude from the analysis the interval between marriage and first birth. This exclusion has the effect of limiting our analysis to women of proven fecundity.[6]

The hazard model allows us to estimate the direction and magnitude of the effects of independent variables on the probability of conception, in a multivariate framework. The functional form of the hazard model is:

$$ln\ [c_i(t)] = a(t) + X_i(t)\ b(t)$$

where $c_i(t)$ is the risk of conception during duration interval t for woman i, the exponentiated first term $(e^{a(t)})$ is the underlying vector of age-specific risks of conception, $X_i(t)$ is a set of characteristics, and $b(t)$ is a set of estimated coefficients. Note that in a hazard model the set of independent variables, $X_i(t)$, may be different in each duration interval, t. Similarly, separate coefficients, $b(t)$, can be estimated for the same variable at each duration (t). Coefficients are estimated using maximum likelihood methods and we use t-statistics (the coefficient divided by its standard error) to assess whether a coefficient is statistically significantly different from zero. For ease of presentation, we summarize the results by using the relative risks of conception for women with specific characteristics. The risks are calculated as e^b where b is the coefficient for a given independent variable. Actual coefficients and tests of significance are given in Appendices K and L.

The first question to be answered is whether the fertility differences by marriage type shown in table 7.1 are statistically significant once age and marriage duration are held constant. Table 7.3 presents the relative risks of conception for women with different characteristics for each country. The variable included for wife's age compares women younger than 35 with those 35 years and older, since the underlying physiological decline in female fecundity appears to begin in the mid-30s (Menken et al., 1986). Marriage duration is divided into four categories as shown in table 7.3. Both age and marriage duration are measured as of the beginning of the birth interval under consideration. The first marriage duration category includes women who were not married, or were in another marriage when the birth interval began, but subsequently married their current husband before the interview.

The risks of conception for wives in polygynous marriages at the top of table 7.3 are shown relative to wives in monogamous marriages and reflect

TABLE 7.3   Relative Risks of Fertile Conception during the 3 Years
before Interview by Marriage Type, Woman's Age, Marriage Duration,
and Duration since Last Live Birth

Variables	Cameroon	Ghana	Ivory Coast	Kenya	Lesotho	Senegal
Monogamous	1.00	1.00	1.00	1.00	1.00	1.00
Polygynous first wife	.91	.98	.90	.88**	.95	.99
Polygynous junior wife	1.05		.82*	.89*		1.00
Wife's Age						
Less than 35	1.00	1.00	1.00	1.00	1.00	1.00
35+	.63*	.66*	.56*	.69*	.68*	.49*
Marriage Duration						
Not married at Beginning†	1.00	1.00	1.00	1.00	1.00	1.00
0–5 Years	1.07	.84	1.04	.96	1.02	1.07
5–15 Years	.92	.71*	.95	.77*	.86*	1.01
15+ Years	.71*	.52*	.75*	.54*	.59*	.79
Duration in Months since Last Birth††						
0–2	.01††	.00	.01	.01	.01	.00
3–5	.01	.01	.01	.02	.01	.01
6–8	.01	.01	.01	.02	.01	.01
9–11	.02	.02	.02	.04	.01	.02
12–17	.04	.04	.04	.07	.03	.04
18–23	.06	.05	.06	.08	.05	.07
24–35	.06	.06	.08	.07	.07	.08
36–47	.03	.06	.05	.05	.05	.04
48–59	.02	.04	.03	.03	.03	.02
Number of Birth Intervals	5174	4651	4412	5648	2954	3070

*statistically significantly different from zero at .05 level, using two-tailed t-test.
**Statistically significantly different from zero at .10 level, using two-tailed t-test.
†These women married during the birth interval period. They begin contributing exposure at the data they report their marriage to have occurred, or the beginning of the observation period, whichever is more recent.
††All figures in this section are statistically signficantly different from zero at .05 level, using two-tailed t-test.

the effects of polygyny and rank, holding the woman's age and marriage duration constant. The results show that fertility differences by marriage type and rank are statistically significant only in the Ivory Coast and Kenya. In the case of the Ivory Coast, it is only junior cowives who have significantly different fertility, while both junior and senior cowives have significantly different fertility in Kenya. These results confirm the observation in table 7.1 that fertility differences by marriage type are small for Cameroon, Lesotho, and Senegal and nonexistant for Ghana.

The results also show that age and marital duration, as expected, generally have important effects on fertility. The relative risks at the bottom of the table show the shape of the probability of conception distribution by duration since last birth. As is usually observed, the probability increases up until roughly 24 months and then declines.

The figures in table 7.2 suggested that the pattern of contraceptive use in some countries might obscure the association between marriage type and fertility, since wives in monogamous marriages are generally more likely to use contraception. We, therefore, reestimated the coefficients after excluding all birth intervals in which contraceptives[7] were used. The results are virtually identical to those shown in table 7.3, except in the case of Kenya where the strength and significance of the negative association between polygyny and fertility increases when contraceptive use intervals are excluded. As shown in the first column of table 7.4, the relative risk of conception for senior cowives changes from 0.88 to 0.83 and there is a smaller change for junior cowives.

INTERMEDIATE VARIABLES: KENYA

Since fertility differences by marriage type are not statistically significant in Cameroon, Ghana, Lesotho, and Senegal, the remainder of the analysis focuses on Kenya and the Ivory Coast. Our objective is to determine the mechanisms through which marriage type affects fertility in these two populations.

In the case of Kenya, both junior and senior cowives in polygynous marriages have lower fertility than wives in monogamous marriages. Our earlier examination of table 7.2 suggests that: (1) the lower fertility of junior cowives in Kenya may be associated with the fact that they are married to much older men, and (2) the lower fertility of senior cowives may be associated with longer breastfeeding and less frequent coresidence with husbands. To test these hypotheses, we have estimated a series of models in which these variables are introduced as controls. In all of these models, the wife's age and marriage duration are also held constant. Intervals in which contraception is used are excluded from the analysis for Kenya.

The results are summarized in table 7.4. In the first column, we show the relative risks by type of marriage when only wife's age and marriage duration

TABLE 7.4   Relative Risks of Fertile Conception during the 3 Years
before Interview by Marriage Type, Controlling for
Other Independent Variables, Kenya WFS Data*

| Marriage Type | Holding Constant: | | | |
	Wife's Age & Marriage Duration	Breast-feeding**	Husband's Age	Proximate Determinants†
Monogamous	1.00	1.00	1.00	1.00
Polygynous				
Senior wife	.83††	.83††	.83††	.83††
Junior wife	.86††	.87††	.95††	.94

*Contraceptive users are eliminated from the analysis, as are women who never had a live birth.
**Wife's age, marriage duration, and this variable are held constant.
†Including wife's age, marriage duration, breastfeeding, husband's age, and coresidence.
††Statistically significant at .05 level.

are held constant. The second column shows the results when breastfeeding is also held constant. We used a set of breastfeeding variables that differ for each duration category. Each variable indicates whether or not a woman was still breastfeeding at the beginning of the duration interval.[8] As would be expected, the coefficients for breastfeeding are strongly and significantly related to the probability of conception in all but the longest durations since last birth. Despite the fact that senior cowives have a median duration of breastfeeding which is 1.5 months longer than other women, the results in table 7.4 indicate that this difference does not account for their lower fertility. In fact, the association may be the reverse: the lower fertility of senior cowives may allow them to continue breastfeeding, at least partially, for a longer time.

In the third column of table 7.4, we show relative risks of conception by marriage type holding constant wife's age, marriage duration, and husband's age. The husband's age categories are: less than 40 years, 40–54 years, and 55 or more years.[9] The estimated coefficients show that husband's age is strongly and significantly associated with the probability of conception. The relative risk in the third column of table 7.4 indicates that having an older husband accounts for most of the difference in fertility between junior cowives and wives in monogamous marriages. When husband's age is held constant the difference in conception probabilities between these two groups is no longer statistically significant.

The fourth column summarizes the results of holding constant simultaneously all of the variables that we hypothesized might explain differences in fertility by type of marriage: wife's age, marriage duration, breastfeeding, husband's age, and coresidence of spouses. Our results indicate that these

TABLE 7.5   Proportion of Currently Married Women Who Report
Not Being Sexually Active by Type of Marriage and Marriage Duration,
Kenya WFS Data*

Marriage Duration (Years)	Monogamous	Polygynous	
		Senior Wife	Junior Wife
Less than 5	17.6	—**	15.8
5–9	18.9	18.5	17.8
10–14	18.5	22.5	15.0
15+	18.9	22.9	17.2
Total	18.5	22.8	16.6

*Women who reported themselves to be practicing postpartum abstinence are excluded from these calculations.
**Fewer than 50 cases.

variables do not jointly account for the lower fertility of senior cowives in polygynous marriages. In fact, the coefficient on coresidence of spouses is not statistically significantly related to the probability of conception. This is, perhaps, not surprising since the information we have concerns coresidence *at the time of the survey* and may not accurately reflect coresidence during the preceding 3 years.

As a final attempt to explain lower fertility among senior cowives relative to wives in monogamous marriages, we examine information on sexual activity at the time of the survey in table 7.5.[10] Like the information on coresidence, these data may pertain only to the time period close to interview and not the entire prior 3-year period. Furthermore, answers to this question may be suspect because of the ambiguity of time period to which the question referred. Nevertheless, the differentials shown in table 7.5 by type of marriage and marriage duration are consistent with those in table 7.2 for coresidence: senior cowives are both less likely to coreside with their spouses and less likely to be sexually active, at least at marriage durations of greater than 10 years. The differences between senior cowives and wives in monogamous marriages are fairly small. However, they suggest the possibility that part of the explanation for the lower fertility of senior cowives may be reduced sexual activity, possibly due to terminal abstinence, among senior cowives at later marriage durations. Unfortunately, the limitations of the data do not permit more detailed investigation of this hypothesis.

The proportions in table 7.5 also suggest that reduced sexual activity on the part of older husbands may not be the reason that junior cowives have lower fertility than wives in monogamous marriages. In fact, junior cowives are more likely to be sexually active at any given marriage duration than other wives. When husband's age or wife's age is held constant instead of marriage duration, junior cowives are also more likely to be sexually active.

While these data concern whether or not a woman is sexually active rather than her coital frequency, they are consistent with Garenne and van de Walle's (1985) argument that the lower fertility of junior cowives is due more to declining fecundity of older husbands than reduced sexual activity.

INTERMEDIATE VARIABLES: IVORY COAST

In the case of the Ivory Coast, only junior cowives have significantly lower fertility than wives in monogamous marriages. Our earlier examination of table 7.2 and the results of the analysis for Kenya suggest that the fact that junior cowives have substantially older husbands may account for their lower fertility. We also investigated the possibility that longer breastfeeding or postpartum abstinence might account for some of the difference. Although the variation in median lengths of these two behaviors among marriage types is small, they play an important role in determining the timing of fertility in this population. Since junior cowives are also less likely to live with their husbands than other wives in the Ivory Coast sample, our analysis also examines the potential role of coresidence. The results of analyses in which these hypotheses are tested are shown in table 7.6.

The first column again shows the association between fertility and marriage type, holding constant wife's age and marriage duration, for purposes of comparison. In the second and fourth columns, breastfeeding and postpartum abstinence, respectively, are held constant, as well. As in the analyses for Kenya, the breastfeeding variable used is different for each duration and indicates whether a woman was still breastfeeding at the beginning of the

TABLE 7.6   Relative Risks of Fertile Conception during the 3 Years
before Interview by Marriage Type, Controlling for Other Independent
Variables, Ivory Coast WFS Data*

	Holding Constant:				
Marriage Type	Wife's Age & Marriage Duration	Breast-feeding**	Husband's Age[†]	Abstinence	Proximate Determinants[††]
Monogamous	1.00	1.00	1.00	1.00	1.00
Polygynous					
Senior wife	.90	.91	.91	.91	.92
Junior wife***	.82	.83	.83	.84	.84

*Women who never had a live birth are excluded.
**Wife's age, marriage duration, and this variable are held constant.
[††]Proximate determinants include wife's age, husband's age, marriage duration, breastfeeding, and abstinence.
[†]This variable was divided into the following categories: <40, 40–54, 55+, and husband's age unknown.
***Statistically significant at .05 level.

duration category. A similar strategy is followed for postpartum abstinence: the variable for each duration category indicates whether a woman was still abstaining at the beginning of that duration category. Coefficients for both variables indicate that they have a significant impact on the probability of conception, at most durations. However, as the relative risks in table 7.6 show, the association between fertility and marriage type does not change when either of these variables is held constant.

The results for husband's age are shown in the third column. As we have seen, more than half of currently married respondents in the Ivory Coast survey did not report their husband's age, and the degree of nonresponse is higher among women in polygynous marriages. In order to include all currently married women in the analysis, we used a four-category variable to indicate husband's age: less than 40, 40 to 54, 55 or more, and age unknown. The results in table 7.6 show that when this variable is held constant, along with wife's age and marriage duration, the association between junior cowife status and lower fertility remains unchanged.

In a separate analysis not shown in table 7.6, we examined the associations among the probability of conception, polygyny, and husband's age for the subsample of women in the Ivory Coast survey who had reported their husband's age. When marriage duration and wife's age alone are held constant, the association between polygyny and the probability of conception is small and not statistically significant. The fact that the association between polygyny and fertility in the full sample is not also seen in the subsample means that additional analysis of the subsample cannot shed any more light on the reasons for lower junior cowife fertility in the full sample.

Thus, there is no direct evidence—either from the results in table 7.6 or from our subsample analysis—that the fact of having older husbands accounts for the lower fertility of junior cowives in the Ivory Coast, as it appears to in Kenya. The available data are inadequate to test this hypothesis, since information on husband's age is unavailable for a high proportion of wives. An examination of the husband's age distribution among wives who do report an age suggests that a disproportionate number of husbands whose ages are unknown were older men. It is also clear from Appendix J that junior cowives are the least likely to report their husband's age. Furthermore, there is no significant association between polygyny and fertility once cases without husband's age information are removed from the sample. These observations are, at least, consistent with the possibility that an older average husband's age is, in fact, the reason behind lower junior cowife fertility in the Ivory Coast and that if adequate data were available, we would find such an association in the Ivory Coast as well as Kenya.

In the final column of table 7.6 we introduce, simultaneously, wife's age, marriage duration, breastfeeding, husband's age, postpartum abstinence, and whether the wife lives with her husband. As in the Kenya data, coresi-

TABLE 7.7   Currently Married Women who Report *Not* Being
Sexually Active by Type of Marriage and Marriage Duration,
Ivory Coast WFS Data*

Marriage Duration (Years)	Monogamous	Polygynous	
		Senior Wife	Junior Wife
Less than 5	11.7	—**	12.6
5–9	15.6	16.7	12.8
10–14	15.5	10.3	12.7
15+	16.4	12.6	17.6
Total	14.3	13.7	13.9

*Women who reported themselves to be practicing postpartum abstinence are excluded from these calculations.
**Fewer than 50 cases.

dence is not statistically significantly related to the probability of conception. Furthermore, although junior cowives are less likely to coreside with their husbands, this factor does not appear to account for their lower fertility, at least given the data available.

The questionnaire for the Ivory Coast also included a question on current sexual activity. Table 7.7 presents the proportions who were not sexually active by marriage duration and marriage type. Although junior cowives report themselves more likely to live separately from their husbands, they are no less likely to be sexually active than other wives, overall. However, at 15 or more years of marriage, they are less likely to be sexually active than senior cowives and slightly less likely than wives in monogamous marriages.

DISCUSSION

Our results indicate that the association between polygyny and fertility is small in four out of the six countries included in the analysis and that in these countries the association is not statistically significant once childless women are excluded and the wife's age and marital duration are held constant. Thus, polygyny cannot be said to result in universally lower marital fertility in African populations, at least on the individual level.

However, in Kenya and the Ivory Coast, wives in polygynous marriages do have significantly lower fertility than wives in monogamous marriages. Total marital fertility rates for wives in polygynous marriages are roughly one child lower in both populations. In Kenya, both senior cowives and junior cowives have significantly lower fertility in comparison with wives in monogamous marriages. In the Ivory Coast, only junior cowives have significantly lower fertility.

Earlier research has suggested that lower fertility among junior cowives in polygynous marriages may be due to their marriage to older husbands (Garenne and van de Walle, 1985; Bean and Mineau, 1986). In both the Kenyan and Ivory Coast samples, junior cowives have substantially older husbands, on average, than other wives. Multivariate results for Kenya indicate that the fact of having an older husband does appear to account for lower fertility among junior cowives. In the case of the Ivory Coast, on the other hand, there is no evidence that older husbands' ages are the reason for lower fertility among junior cowives. We have suggested, however, that this outcome may be due at least in part to the inadequacy of data on husbands' ages for the Ivory Coast sample. In both the Kenyan and Ivory Coast populations, data on sexual activity indicate that junior cowives are generally as likely as, or more likely than, other wives to be sexually active. Thus, if the explanation for lower junior cowife fertility is that they are married to older men, this very limited evidence suggests that the mechanism may be a decline in male fecundity with age rather than reduced sexual activity. It is impossible, however, given the data available, to draw firm conclusions on this issue.

Our results do not provide a satisfactory explanation for the lower fertility of senior cowives in Kenya. Evidence on coresidence and sexual activity, however, suggests that senior cowives at later marriage durations may be somewhat less likely to be living with their husbands or to be sexually active.

Among the factors that we have not taken into account in the analysis is secondary sterility. The reason is that determining whether a woman is subfecund or has become sterile after having one or more children is clearly difficult. However, part of the explanation for fertility differentials by marriage type may be a selection process by which *subfecund* women are more likely to be divorced and remarried as junior cowives, or are more likely to precipitate a subsequent marriage and become a senior cowife. Another possible explanation may be higher rates of disease-induced secondary sterility among women in polygynous marriage because of the greater number of sexual partners their husband has. However, it seems likely that this effect would operate on a societal level rather than at the individual level.

SOCIETAL EFFECTS

In this chapter, we have limited our focus to the association between polygyny and fertility within marriage, at the individual level. The practice of polygyny may also have societal-level effects on fertility that may in fact be equally or more important than those on the individual level. We conclude by briefly considering these potential associations.

Two effects that we have considered on the individual level may work on the societal level to reduce fertility. First, a high frequency of polygyny, especially if it is associated with frequent marriage dissolution and remarriage

and multiple sexual partners, may increase the incidence of sexually transmitted disease, which is an important cause of sterility in many African
populations (Adadevoh, 1974; Retel-Laurentin, 1974). We have little information, however, about whether the average number of sexual partners
is higher in a traditional African population practicing polygyny than in
societies in which polygyny is not socially sanctioned but multiple informal
sexual unions are common, as in many non-African societies. Unless the
number of sexual partners is greater, there is no reason to believe that the
transmission rates will be higher in a polygynous marriage system.

A second factor that may operate in populations where polygyny is frequent is a stricter observance of postpartum sexual taboos by members of
the population, regardless of the type of marriage they themselves are in.
Societies in which polygyny is common may tend to have a greater control
over the relations between husbands and wives, and may, therefore, practice
postpartum abstinence to a greater degree.

There are also two aspects of polygynous marriage systems that are likely
to increase the fertility of populations that practice polygyny. First, in order to
maintain a high frequency of polygyny in a population, women must marry
at relatively young ages. An alternative interpretation is that polygynous
marriage systems are well designed for high fertility, since at least on an
aggregate basis, all women have the chance of marrying as soon as they
become fecund. In practice, the average age at which women marry in most
African societies is delayed well beyond puberty. However, in populations
with very high levels of polygyny, such as Senegal, the average age at
marriage for women is relatively young, both for social and cultural reasons
(Lesthaeghe, 1984), and because it would otherwise be difficult to maintain
such a high frequency of polygyny, as the chapter by Goldman and Pebley in
this volume shows.

A second and closely related aspect of polygynous marriage systems is
that they permit divorced and widowed women to remarry quickly since,
at least theoretically, all men are potential mates whether or not they are
married. Thus, despite a high incidence of divorce and widowhood in many
polygynous societies, relatively little of the fecund period is lost to marital
dissolution.

Lesthaeghe (1984) carried out an aggregate-level analysis in which he
investigated the association between these four societal-level effects and the
frequency of polygyny. His analysis shows, in general, that all four of these
effects seem to be operating. The frequency of polygyny appears to be positively associated, on an aggregate basis, with early female ages at marriage,
rapid remarriage after marriage dissolution, longer observance of the postpartum sexual taboo, and higher rates of both sterility and subfecundity.

What is the net effect of these four factors, on a societal level, of a polygynous marriage system on fertility? Comparisons between monogamous

societies and those practicing frequent polygyny is difficult because of the large number of related and unrelated differences in social organization between these two populations with very different marriage systems. Pison (1986) provides one example: the marriage and fertility experience of Sahelian populations who have high and low frequencies of polygyny, based on data from Randall (1984). In Sahelian Africa, nomad populations are usually monogamous or practice polygyny only infrequently, whereas settled populations often have high frequencies of polygynous marriages. Pison argues that at least part of the reason for lower fertility among the nomads may be that they practice monogamy. For example, the total fertility rate of nomadic Touareg women in Mali is 6.6 children, whereas their settled Bambara neighbors, who practice polygyny, have a TFR of 8.1 children. However, the difference in fertility is due in large part to substantially lower exposure among Touareg women: had Touareg and Bambara women both been continuously married throughout their fecund years, the situation would have been reversed. The TFR would have been 10.1 for Touareg and 8.9 for Bambara women, respectively. While the differences in fertility between the two groups are unlikely to be related entirely to their marriage systems, this example suggests that, at least in the Sahel, the longer marital exposure associated with the greater chances for marriage in a polygynous marriage system may outweigh the potentially counterbalancing effects of increased subfecundity and longer birth spacing, which may also be associated with polygyny. Thus, to the extent that polygyny is associated with fertility, its effects on the individual level and the societal level may be quite different. On the individual level, polygyny appears to reduce fertility, though in most populations included in this analysis the difference is not statistically significant. However, at the societal level, a polygynous marriage system may contribute to the achievement of high fertility.

ACKNOWLEDGMENTS

This research was conducted under a grant from The Population Council's Program on Determinants of Fertility in Developing Countries, funded by USAID. The authors are grateful to Noreen Goldman and James Trussell for suggestions that substantially improved the analysis, and to Barbara Vaughan and Stan Stein for assistance in preparing the data files.

NOTES

1. Ferry's analysis, however, is flawed by sample selection bias. See John et al. (1987).

2. In fact, the FOTCAF module includes questions on breastfeeding, postpartum amenorrhea, and abstinence only for the open and last closed *pregnancy* (not *birth*)

intervals, while contraceptive use questions continue to be asked for the open and last closed birth intervals. Collecting information in this way complicates the analysis considerably. For example, no information on the breastfeeding of the last two live born children would be available for a woman who had had two miscarriages right before the survey. To avoid these problems in our analysis of the association between polygyny and fertility, we exclude from the analysis all women who report that either their last closed or their open pregnancy interval did not result in a live birth. The numbers of intervals excluded from the multivariate analysis for this reason are: 405 in Cameroon, 162 in Ghana, 363 in the Ivory Coast, 287 in Kenya, 127 in Lesotho, and 258 in Senegal.

3. Neither these rates nor subsequent results have been weighted in surveys that used weighted sampling schemes, since the objective is to make comparisons among individual women rather than to describe the national population.

4. In a separate analysis, we looked at the probability of entering a monogamous marriage (as a junior cowife, since it is rare to enter as a senior cowife), for all women married in the 3 years before the survey. Holding constant age at marriage, childhood residence, residence at interview, whether the respondent was Muslim, school attendance, ethnicity, and whether she had any children before this marriage, we found that previous marriage significantly increased a woman's chances of entering a polygynous marriage in all six countries.

5. We use life tables in which exposure for a given birth interval begins at the duration since last birth which a woman reached by the beginning of the 3-year observation period. Two types of decrements are possible: censoring at the time of interview, and termination of the particular behavior under investigation.

6. In other words, these women do not suffer from primary sterility. Some of these women may, of course, have subsequently become sterile after their first live birth.

7. Our definition of contraceptive use does not include postpartum abstinence or breastfeeding.

8. This type of variable is generally known as a time varying covariate. For the duration interval 0–2 months the breastfeeding variable indicates whether a woman ever breastfed; for the interval 3–5 months it indicates whether she was still breast-feeding at 3.0 months. No distinction is made between full and partial breastfeeding, since the length of full breastfeeding does not appear to vary greatly by marriage type.

9. The small fraction of wives not reporting their husband's age are excluded from all multivariate analyses for Kenya.

10. Women who reported themselves to be practicing postpartum abstinence, when asked how long they abstained from sex after their last birth, were excluded from the calculations in table 7.5.

BIBLIOGRAPHY

Adadevoh, B. K., ed. 1974. *Sub-fertility and infertility in Africa*. Ibadan, Nigeria: Claxton Press.

Bean, L. L., and G. P. Mineau. 1986. The polygyny-fertility hypothesis: A re-evaluation. *Population Studies* 40(1): 67–82.

Chamie, J. 1986. Polygyny among Arabs. *Population Studies* 40(1): 55–56.

Chidambaram, V. C., and Z. Sathar. 1984. Reporting ages and dates. *World Fertility Survey Comparative Studies*, no. 5. Voorburg: International Statistical Institute.

Clignet, R. 1970. *Many wives, many powers—Autonomy and power in polygynous families.* Evanston: Northwestern University Press.

Clignet, R., and J. Sween. 1974. Urbanization, plural marriage and family size in two African cities. *American Ethnologist* 1: 221–241.

Ferry, B. 1981. Breastfeeding. *World Fertility Survey Comparative Analyses*, no. 13. Voorburg: International Statistical Institute.

Garenne, M., and E. van de Walle. 1985. Polygyny and fertility among the Serrer of Senegal. ORSTOM and University of Pennsylvania manuscript.

Goldman, N., A. R. Pebley, C. F. Westoff, and L. Paul. 1983. Contraceptive failure in Latin America. *International Family Planning Perspectives* 9(2): 50–57.

Goldman, N., and A. R. Pebley. 1981. The demography of polygyny in sub-Saharan Africa. In *Reproduction and social organization in sub-Saharan Africa*, ed. R. Lesthaeghe. Berkeley, Los Angeles, London: University of California Press.

Goldman, N., O. Rutstein, and S. Singh. 1985. Assessment of the quality of data in 41 WFS surveys: A comparative approach. *World Fertility Comparative Studies*, no. 5. Voorburg: International Statistical Institute.

Hobcraft, J., and D. Guz. 1985. Lactation and fertility: A comparative analysis. Paper presented at the annual meeting of the Population Association of America, Boston, Mass.

John, A. M., J. Menken, and J. Trussell. 1987. The use of current status data to estimate mean duration of status. Stanford, Calif.: Stanford University, Food Research Institute, manuscript.

Kaufmann, G., R. Lesthaeghe, and D. Meekers. 1987. Marriage patterns and change in sub-Saharan Africa. Paper presented at the IUSSP seminar on Changing Family Structures and Life Courses in LDCs, Honolulu, Hawaii.

Lesthaeghe, R. 1984. Fertility and its proximate determinants in sub-Saharan Africa: The record of the 1960s and 70s. Paper presented at the WFS seminar on Integrating Proximate Determinants into the Analysis of Fertility Levels and Trends, London. Liège, Belgium: Ordina for the International Union for the Scientific Study of Population.

Locoh, T. 1976. La nuptialité au Togo, évolution entre 1961 et 1970. *Population* 2: 379–398.

————. 1984. *Fécondité et famille en Afrique de l'Ouest: Le Togo méridional contemporain.* Cahier de l'INED, no. 107. Paris: Presses Universitaires de France.

Menken, J., J. Trussell, and U. Larsen. 1986. Age and infertility. *Science* 233: 1389–1349.

Ngondo a Pitshandenge. 1978. Polygamie et fécondité dans la société Zairoise—L'example des Yaka de la zone de Popokabaka. *Département de démographie working paper*, no. 58. Louvain-la-Neuve, Belgium: Université Catholique de Louvain.

Oppong, C. 1987. Traditional family systems in rural settings in Africa. Paper presented at the IUSSP seminar on Changing Family Structures and Life Courses in LDCs, Honolulu, Hawaii.

Page, H. J. 1975. Fertility levels: patterns and trends. In: *Population growth and socioeco-*

nomic change in West Africa, ed. J. C. Caldwell. New York: Columbia University Press.

Pebley, A. R., and P. W. Stupp. 1987. Reproduction patterns and child mortality in Guatemala. *Demography* 24(1).

Pison, G. 1986. Démographie de la polygamie. *Population* 41(1): 93–122.

Randall, S. 1984. A comparative demographic study of three Sahelian populations: Marriage and child-care as intermediate determinants of fertility and mortality. Ph.D. dissertation. London: London School of Hygiene and Tropical Medicine.

Republic of Ghana. 1983. *Ghana fertility survey: 1979–1980*. Accra: Central Bureau of Statistics.

Republic of Kenya. 1980. *Kenya fertility survey: 1977–78*. Nairobi: Central Bureau of Statistics, Ministry of Economic Planning and Development.

Republic of Lesotho. 1981. *Lesotho fertility survey, 1977*. Maseru: Central Bureau of Statistics, Ministry of Planning and Statistics.

République de la Côte d'Ivoire. 1984. *Enquête Ivoirienne sur la fécondité, 1980–81*. Abidjan: Direction de la Statistique, Ministère de l'Economie et des Finances.

République du Sénégal. 1981. *Enquête Sénégalaise sur la fécondité, 1978*. Dakar: Direction de la Statistique, Ministère de l'Economie et des Finances.

République Unie du Cameroun. 1983. *Enquête nationale sur la fécondité du Cameroun, 1978*. Yaoundé: Direction de la Statistique et de la Comptabilité nationale. Ministère de l'Economie et du Plan.

Retel-Laurentin, A. 1974. *Infécondité en Afrique noire*. Paris: Masson et Cie.

Trussell, J., and C. Hammerslough. 1983. A hazard-model analysis of the covariate of infant and child mortality in Sri Lanka. *Demography* 20(1): 1–26.

Trussell, J., L. Martin, R. Feldman, J. Palmore, M. Conception, and D. N. L. B. Abu Baka. 1984. Determinants of birth interval length in the Philippines, Malaysia and Indonesia: A hazard-model analysis. *Demography* 22(2): 145–168.

van de Walle, E. 1968. Marriage in African censuses and inquiries. In: *The demography of tropical Africa*, ed. W. Brass et al. Princeton: Princeton University Press.

van de Walle, E., and J. Kekovole. 1984. The recent evolution of African marriage and polygyny. Paper presented at the annual meeting of the Population Association of America, Minneapolis, Minn.

CHAPTER EIGHT

Labor Circulation, Marriage, and Fertility in Southern Africa

Ian Timaeus
Wendy Graham

INTRODUCTION

Throughout Southern Africa, circulation of members of the labor force between rural areas and the major centers of wage employment is an important and long-established feature of people's lives. In some areas, such as the "homelands" of South Africa, Lesotho, and parts of Botswana, labor migration involves a large proportion of the adult male population and affects nearly every household. Although such movement is usually temporary, it frequently entails the prolonged separation of migrants, especially young men, from their immediate families and other relatives. The effects on relationships between close kin, on marriage systems, and on household structure have been wide ranging and to some extent are only now becoming apparent. Equally the pattern of labor migration has been influenced by, and integrated with, the domestic institutions and economies of the indigenous populations of the region as well as by wider economic and political relationships and inequalities. Thus, in order to fully understand the reproductive regimes of this part of Africa, it is essential to consider them in the context of the migrant labor system and the political economy of the region as well as in their local and familiar institutional framework.

One aspect of labor circulation with which we are concerned is its direct effects on the proximate determinants of fertility. By direct effects we mean those aspects of labor circulation that influence only the fertility of migrants and their sexual partners. Such effects may have an immediate impact on fertility, for example, through the separation of spouses at times when the woman would otherwise be exposed to the risk of conception, or a longer-term impact, for example, through women whose husbands work as miners having an increased chance of being widowed at a young age. We also consider the indirect impact of labor circulation on the fertility of entire populations. Contextual effects on the domestic economy and attitudes to reproduction are important. In addition, in the longer term, the impact of labor circulation on the development of social institutions has to be considered. In particular, we argue that the economic opportunities and roles for both men and women associated with widespread migratory wage employment have contributed to the constitution of distinctive marriage systems. The main features of these systems are documented in chapter 6 of this book. Throughout the region, ages at marriage for both sexes are late and the prevalence of polygyny is low compared with other sub-Saharan African countries. Moreover in Botswana a growing proportion of women never marry. Marital breakdown has become increasingly common and divorce, separation, and widowhood are seldom followed by remarriage for women. These trends help explain changes in and the increasing diversity of the structure of domestic groups and, in particular, the emergence of households headed permanently by women.

The discussion that follows commences with a brief description of the development of the migrant labor system within and between the countries of Southern Africa. Against this background we discuss the marriage systems of these countries and the effect of labor circulation on each of the determinants of the proportion of women of childbearing age who are living in conjugal unions. It is the household that is the locus of the labor circulation and marriage systems. The developmental cycle of domestic groups forms a framework that shapes, and is shaped by, its members' migrant careers, marital histories, and fertility. Following our analysis of these interrelationships, we examine the direct impact of labor circulation on levels of fertility. Finally we discuss the extent to which the migrant labor system is related to the adoption of modern methods of contraception in the region, and we assess the prospects for fertility decline. Throughout, the discussion concentrates on Botswana and Lesotho and on the large majority of their inhabitants whose permanent homes are in the rural areas. In part this reflects the authors' familiarity with these countries and in part the availability of data. Where appropriate we draw on surveys conducted in South Africa and Zimbabwe but, while aspects of the discussion may be relevant to these countries, their massive internal migration flows undoubtedly have different demographic implications from the international movements on which we concentrate. We would also be very cautious about extending our arguments to the matrilineal kinship systems and different domestic economies characteristic of much of Zambia and Malawi.

THE MIGRANT LABOR SYSTEM

The populations of Southern Africa are frequently described as "migratory societies," and an extensive literature exists on all aspects of this mobility—

from its historical roots to its pervasive impact on the politics, economics, and social structure of these countries (for example, Bell, 1986; Kowet, 1978; Magubane, 1975; Mitchell, 1985; van Binsbergen and Meilink, 1978). The presentation of a profile of migration for this region of Africa is complicated by the commutation of determinants and consequences, by the interplay of historical and contemporary forces, and by the variety of types of movement grouped under the term migration. We therefore limit ourselves to introducing important dimensions of the patterns and processes of migration in Southern Africa that are relevant to fertility.

It is important to begin by clarifying a couple of terms. Much of the literature on mobility makes a basic distinction between migration and circulation (Prothero and Chapman, 1985). The former implies some form of permanency—or intention to stay permanently—at a destination, while the latter describes short-term, repetitive movements. While this distinction is difficult to adhere to strictly, since migration is also the term used colloquially to describe mobility in Southern Africa, it is important to emphasize that the majority of movement with which we are concerned is circulation. It is the historical development of this circulation and the political, economic, and social setting in which it takes place that helps to explain its character.

There are several major works on the origins of the migrant labor system (see, for example, Bundy, 1979; Cliffe, 1977; Parsons, 1977; Schapera, 1947). The early evidence suggests that although migrations took place in the traditional societies of Southern Africa, often related to season or to tribal conflicts or environmental pressures, an increase in the volume and diversity of movements can be linked to contact with Europeans. Several authors have indicated that the initial migrants were age regiments of young men sent by the local chief to work on nearby settler farms in exchange for guns and other European commodities. By the midnineteenth century, however, much of Southern Africa was being absorbed into a monetary economy in which cash was required to meet new needs and to pay the taxes imposed by European administrations. Many of the migrants were young single men who oscillated between their parents' homesteads and nearby farms. Indeed a period of earning cash became a form of rite de passage into manhood. Although young women were reported to have worked as agricultural laborers or domestic servants on European farms, this was comparatively rare. Indeed there is evidence that chiefs and elders often prohibited the outmigration of women (Molenaar, 1980). It is hard to generalize about these early movements as they took a great variety of forms. Nevertheless, in the areas covered today by Botswana, Lesotho, South Africa, and Swaziland, it was primarily individuals who migrated while, in the regions of white settler agriculture in Zimbabwe and Zambia, whole families tended to move to take up employment.

Although farm work played an important role in the initial development of the migrant labor system and remains numerically significant in areas

TABLE 8.1   Migrant Labor from Botswana, Lesotho, and Swaziland to South Africa, 1911–1975 (in thousands)

Date	Botswana	Lesotho	Swaziland
1911	2.6	25.0	8.5
1921	3.3	47.0	6.0
1936	10.4	101.0	9.6
1946	NA	127.0	8.1
1956	NA	155.0	11.7
1966	45.0	117.0	19.2
1975	60.0	200.0	18.0

SOURCE: Kowet, 1978.

such as the Transvaal and southern Botswana (Wylie, 1981), it was the establishment of mining and manufacturing industries that provided the major stimulus to the system's growth. Exploitation of the unskilled labor of temporary migrants from neighboring territories and distant tribal areas has been the basis of South Africa's industrial and commercial growth for a very long time. The practice can be traced back to the opening of diamond mines in Kimberley in the 1870s and of gold mines on the Witwatersrand from the mid-1880s, but it was the early part of this century that saw a massive upsurge in numbers migrating as can be seen from table 8.1. The interplay of environmental and economic factors contributing to this trend is well documented in the literature (for instance, Colclough and McCarthy, 1980; Leggasick and Le Clerq, 1978; Palmer and Parsons, 1977; Skinner, 1985). Although the precise combination of factors varied over time and between populations, among the most influential were: the lack of local wage-labor opportunities; recurring droughts and cattle disease; serious land shortages following appropriations for white settler farming; the introduction of the hut tax, tribal levies and fines; and the destructive effect on the domestic economy of the loss of manpower and skills that arose from outmigration itself. Although an extensive catchment area developed, with workers being drawn to the Republic of South Africa (RSA) from as far north as Malawi and Northern Mozambique, it was the territories abutting the RSA that came to be regarded as labor reserves. Even within this area, however, there have always been regional and ethnic variations in the extent of labor migration. Some recent figures are presented in table 8.2. In Lesotho as a whole in 1975, 60 percent of the male labor force was employed in the RSA and 81 percent of them were working in the mining sector; 90 percent of men had worked in the RSA at some point in their lives (van der Wiel, 1977). In Botswana it has been estimated that, until the mid-1970s, 50 percent of those employed in the RSA worked in the mines, 10 percent in agriculture, and the rest in manufacturing and the service sectors (Cooper, 1979; Kerven, 1979a).

TABLE 8.2   Percentage of Men Aged 15–54 Absent at the Time of Census or
Survey, According to District, Botswana and Lesotho

Botswana, 1971		Lesotho, 1977	
District*	% Absent	Region	% Absent
Barolong	29.9	Lowlands	45.1
Central	26.9		
Chobe	12.9	Foothills	39.3
Ghanzi	12.3		
Kgalagadi	20.8	Mountains	33.0
Kgatleng	38.0		
Kweneng	38.6	Orange R. Valley	48.2
Ngamiland	19.4		
Ngwaketse	40.0		
Northeast	32.3		
Southeast	35.4		

*Excluding town population.
SOURCE: Botswana, Central Statistics Office, 1972; Lesotho Fertility Survey, household data.

The complex process by which migrant labor in Southern Africa was institutionalized by the labor-recruiting agencies and developed into a self-perpetuating system has been extensively studied (for instance, Clarke, 1977; Mitchell, 1985; Parsons, 1977). The social and economic interdependence of migrant workers and their rurally based kin is crucial to the maintenance of the system. Low mine wages and South African policies of apartheid and separate development have restricted movement to adult laborers and excluded their families (Colclough, 1980; Taylor, 1982; Wilson, 1972). Conversely loss of manpower in the rural areas reduced the productivity and viability of farming and helped to create rural dependency on migrants' remittances. Kin in the areas of outmigration, in turn, provide for the long-term security of the migrants, maintaining rights to land and raising the next generation of the labor force.

One aspect of the migrant labor system that is relevant to the discussion that follows is the arrangements operated through the Chamber of Mines for the recruitment of foreign labor. Mine workers are employed on fixed-term contracts, usually of 9 months duration, and must return to their home country on completion of their contract even though they usually take up another one a few months later. Circulation between the laborers' homes and the mine dominates the working lives of these men and their families. In these circumstances, household structure is in a constant state of flux, with marked differences existing between de jure and de facto household composition and headship. For example, in Botswana over 10 percent of households are headed by women whose husbands are temporarily absent (Izzard, 1981).

Schapera (1947) provides some of the earliest insights into the social implications of labor circulation and many of his observations remain relevant today. Writing primarily about the Tswana, he noted that 90 percent of male absentees were between 15 and 44 years old and that they spent about 12 years of their working lives in the mines. A mine contract often marked entry into manhood, and migrants continued to take up contracts until their sons were old enough to migrate themselves. At this point they could expect some support from their sons and tended to retire from wage employment to their rural homes.

The characteristics of the dominant migrant streams are reflected in the demographic structure of the areas of outmigration, which have high dependency ratios and a marked predominance of women—often referred to as the "women left behind." There is an extensive literature on the role these women play in the maintenance of the migrant labor system and on how the overall status of women has developed in response (Bozzoli, 1983; Brown, 1979; Gay, 1980; Gordon, n.d.: Izzard, 1982; Kooijman, 1978; Meillassoux, 1975; Murray, 1981; Wolpe, 1972). As mentioned previously, rurally based kin offer an incentive and opportunity for migrants to return, and their value is implicitly recognized in the system of Voluntary Deferred Pay that operates to ensure that miners remit part of their wages to these kin. In Botswana, such remittances may contribute nearly half of the total income of a family as well as injecting cash into the rural economy (Kerven, 1982; Lucas, 1982). On the other hand, constraints on entry, residence, and movements in the RSA, and insecurity of employment arising from withdrawal of contracts, redundancy, or ill-health, require migrants to maintain strong contacts with their place of origin. However, the links between a migrant and his kin are not solely economic. Social obligations are also important, particularly with regard to the interdependence of generations and expected patterns of support in old age.

Although the pattern of labor migration in Southern Africa at the end of the 1970s was in many ways similar to that observed for the previous 50 years, more recently there have been a number of significant changes. Two of them require brief discussion; first, the change in the pattern of mine labor recruitment, and second, the growth in opportunities for wage employment within some of the labor-exporting countries. Table 8.3 reveals the expansion in the recruitment of black South Africans for mine work between 1973 and 1985 and the concomitant decline in the employment of foreign workers. A number of authors have identified similar falls in the demand for foreign labor in other sectors of the RSA's economy (Clarke, 1977; Davies, 1978; Wylie, 1981). To some extent the fall in the employment of foreigners in the RSA has been offset by the growth of employment opportunities in the black African states, in particular Botswana and Zimbabwe. This upsurge in formal sector employment is a postindependence phenomenon and is concen-

TABLE 8.3   Origins of Black Workers Employed in Gold Mines in South
Africa (in thousands)

Country	1973	1985
South Africa	81	240
Botswana	20	18
Lesotho	76	97
Malawi	109	16
Mozambique	83	50
Swaziland	4	12
Others	2	—
Total	375	433

SOURCE: Chamber of Mines, 1985.

trated in urban areas. In Botswana the development of the mining sector, in particular, led to a 53 percent increase in the number of people in formal employment between 1972 and 1976. Although it is estimated that between a quarter and a half of all rural Batswana households still have at least one member working in the RSA, the emergence of internal townward migratory flows is an important development. Two of its features that are relevant here are the continuing importance of circulatory movement and the comparatively high proportion of female migrants involved.

So far the discussion has concentrated on male migration. While female labor circulation is numerically less significant, as indicated in table 8.4, it is an important indicator of the changing social and economic roles of women in Southern African societies (Bryant, 1977; Chaney, 1980; Izzard, 1981 and 1985; Marks and Unterhalter, 1978; Murray, 1981). In the earlier part of this century outmigration was a means of 'escape' for women and was often a response to extramarital pregnancy, infertility, or marital breakdown. In-

TABLE 8.4   Origins of Foreign-Born Women Working in South Africa, 1970

Country of Origin	Number of Women
Botswana	12,060
Lesotho	53,740
Malawi	1,140
Mozambique	3,780
Namibia	300
Swaziland	12,320
Zimbabwe	940
Others	240
Total	84,520

SOURCE: Marks and Unterhalter, 1978.

creasingly, it has become part of the diversification of women's roles to encompass the positions of breadwinner and household head. The predominant occupation of women in the major centers of employment is as unskilled workers in the service sector and, in particular, as domestic servants (Cock, 1980). Three-quarters of the Basotho women interviewed by Gay (1980) who had worked in South Africa had been employed as servants. The equivalent figure from a study in Botswana was 57 percent (Izzard, 1982). While the unregulated nature of employment in domestic service has enabled many women to avoid some of the tight controls on entry and movement experienced by mine workers, they have suffered from the absence of standards concerning hours of work, wages, job security, and accommodation. Many female migrants have to supplement their income with informal activities such as beer brewing and must delay or delegate to others their role as mother. Insecurity of employment and multiple roles and activities lead women, like men, to maintain strong links with their rural kin and to circulate, throughout their working lives, between the centers of employment and their rural home. While their pattern of movement may resemble that of men, the distinctive feature of rural–urban interdependence for women is its association with the development of family forms in which the role of the father is marginal in both social and economic terms and of households headed permanently by women (Gay, 1980; Izzard, 1982). In Botswana the growth of local employment opportunities has affected women as well as men. Townwards migration has been dominated by women since the mid-1970s, although rising domestic formal-sector employment of Batswana women has been roughly paralleled by a fall in numbers working abroad (Izzard, 1982).

THE MARRIAGE SYSTEMS OF BOTSWANA AND LESOTHO

In this section we discuss the marriage systems of the Basotho and Tswana in their wider social context. We speak of marriage systems to emphasize that each aspect of marriage patterns, for instance, ages at marriage or proportions widowed, is related to all the others. This is exemplified by the discussion of polygyny in earlier chapters of this book. Similar considerations apply to the interrelationships between nuptiality and fertility. For example, while polygyny probably lowers the fertility of young wives, it may also be linked to the remarriage of a higher proportion of older widowed and divorced women (van de Walle, 1985). Moreover, when discussing the historical development of marital institutions, it is probably misleading to consider modification of any single aspect of the marriage system as the cause of changes in its others. Rather explanations should be sought in wider circumstances that lead people to alter their patterns of behavior in ways that gradually affect all aspects of marriage. Having said this, we discuss each facet of marriage patterns separately in order to impose some structure on the argument.

An apparent contradiction in the development over the last 100 years of the marriage systems of Botswana and Lesotho has been the continuity of the basic structure of marital institutions despite massive changes in marriage patterns and disruption of family life (see, for example, Kuper, 1985; Molenaar, 1980; Murray, 1981). A brief outline of some of these structural aspects of marriage is essential to the discussion that follows. While lineages are not corporate property-owning groups, residential groups have always been and remain constituted according to patrilineal premises. In line with these, residence on marriage is virilocal, that is to say that the woman moves into her husband's household or that of his parents (Preston-Whyte, 1974). The jural component of marriage is still the transfer of bridewealth reckoned in cattle in exchange for rights in the woman's children. Marriage without cattle remains very rare, at least in rural areas, but the payment of bridewealth may only be completed years after the initiation of the sexual and domestic components of the marital relationship. Therefore getting married is a protracted process rather than a single event (Comaroff and Roberts, 1977). As a result, in the event of marital dispute or disruption, people's marital status may become hard to define. A man is expected to provide a dwelling, agricultural land, and cattle for his wife to support her and her children (Poulter, 1976). In a polygynous union each wife has to be provided for separately. Inheritance and the circulation of bridewealth transfers are concentrated within a woman's "house" (Preston-Whyte, 1974). She forms the nucleus of a set of patrimonial property and the pattern of marital relationships defines rights over productive wealth (Gluckman, 1971).

Polygynous marriages are now rare among the Basotho and Batswana. According to the 1977 Lesotho Fertility Survey (LFS) only 8.5 percent of married women were living in polygynous unions and only 1 percent of them had more than one cowife (Bureau of Statistics, 1981). The resilience of polygyny in the face of social and economic change in most of sub-Saharan Africa has been documented in this book (see chapter 6). In Southern Africa the practice was a far less durable feature of the marriage system. In Botswana, nobles initiated between 1830 and 1860 married an average of 3.3 women and commoners 1.9 women. Subsequently such marriages became less and less common and men initiated after 1920 married an average of only 1.1 women. (Kuper, 1985). There are no nineteenth-century data for Lesotho, but census statistics for the early part of this century reveal that the proportion of married men with more than one wife fell from 18.7 percent in 1911 to 8.9 percent in 1946 (Murray, 1981). These developments occurred so early that it is probably futile to attempt to assess the relative importance of the factors underlying them. The list of those that were probably relevant, however, seems fairly clear. The influence of the Christian missions was one such factor. It affected not only individual converts but also underlay attempts at the legal abolition of polygyny in Botswana in the early part of this century. Second, polygyny was integrated with traditional relationships of clientage whereby chiefs and other political figures, who controlled rights to land and citizenship, amassed wealth in the form of cattle and the productive and reproductive capacities of women. Polygynous marriages enabled better-off men to enlarge the size of the kin group over which they had influence. The diffusion of political power, initially to colonial officers and later to elected politicians and official bodies, led to the breakdown of these relationships of clientage. As a result traditional political leaders lost the opportunity to express and reinforce their position by accumulating wives and offspring (Kuper, 1985; Murray, 1981). Third, the importance of women's contribution to agricultural labor is one factor closely associated with the prevalence of polygynous marriage in sub-Saharan Africa (see chapter 6 and Boserup, 1970). The period of colonial expansion led to the confinement of the Basotho in a mountainous and increasingly overpopulated area and of the Tswana in one much more suited to pastoralism, a male activity, than to farming. Agriculture became less viable at the same time as new opportunities for wage employment developed. In addition, the adoption of the plough in the late nineteenth century increased men's contribution to agricultural work. As a result, polygynous families became less economically advantageous for men in comparison with the cost of bridewealth and the difficulty of acquiring an independent provision of land for each wife (Kuper, 1985; Murray, 1981).

Ages at marriage are high for both sexes throughout almost all of Southern Africa. For Lesotho, the LFS household data shown in table 8.5 yield a singulate mean age at marriage of 20.1 years for women and 24.8 years for men (Bureau of Statistics, 1981). Nearly 70 percent of women marry by age

TABLE 8.5   Percent Distribution of Women According to
Marital Status by Age

Marital Status	*Age*						
	15–19	20–24	25–29	30–34	35–39	40–44	45–49
Botswana, 1971							
Single	87	56	37	27	20	17	13
Married	8	38	56	63	67	66	65
Widowed	0	1	2	3	5	9	13
Divorced	4	5	6	7	8	9	9
Lesotho, 1977							
Single	69	19	9	6	4	3	3
Married	29	76	83	81	81	76	68
Widowed	0	1	2	5	8	16	24
Divorced/Separated	1	4	6	8	6	6	5

SOURCE: Botswana, Central Statistics Office, 1972; Lesotho Fertility Survey, household data.

25 and 95 percent by age 30 (Timaeus and Balasubramanian, 1984). Late marriage is not a recent development. A detailed assessment of the LFS marriage histories and census data suggests that for women it dates back to at least the 1940s. In fact ages at marriage declined slightly between the mid 1960s and mid 1970s (Timaeus and Balasubramanian, 1984). Moreover anthropologists conducting fieldwork in the 1930s reported that men married at between 23 and 26 years and women at ages 18 to 24 (Ashton, 1967). In Botswana the pattern of first marriage is different. Village studies conducted by Schapera in the 1930s and 1940s suggest that ages at marriage were already very high, in their early twenties for women and their late twenties for men (Kuper, 1985), and appreciable numbers of women never married (Molenaar, 1980). The picture revealed by the 1971 Census data shown in table 8.5 is even more striking. The singulate mean age at marriage is 24.3 for women and 29.3 for men (Central Statistics Office, 1972). Moreover some 17 percent of men and women aged between 35 and 50 have never married.

In view of the link between female education and marriage patterns throughout sub-Saharan Africa (see chapter 6), one factor that may be related to late marriage is the high level of schooling of the populations of Botswana and Lesotho. The Christian missions were responsible for the early development of the school system and the LFS data on older women suggest that by the 1920s and 1930s a majority of girls in Lesotho were receiving some formal education. Today about 95 percent of girls attend school. In Botswana around 30 percent of girls attended school in the prewar period, rising to about two-thirds more recently (Central Statistics Office, 1972). Notably, fewer men than women receive elementary education. In Lesotho, about 30 percent and in Botswana a majority of boys never go to school. The importance of labor migration is one explanation of this pattern. On the one hand mothers and, in particular, female household heads favor the education of their daughters as they are more likely to remain attached to their natal households than sons and as knowledge of English is often required of domestic servants (Allison, 1979; Gay, 1980). On the other hand, education is not essential for mine work and the shortage of male labor means that boys are often removed from school to herd cattle.

Considering that the pattern of late marriage had already been established in Botswana and Lesotho by the 1930s and 1940s, it is also plausible to link its development to the decline in polygynous marriage. Other things being equal, a decline in polygyny will bring about delayed entry into marriage for women. Moreover the economic disincentives to polygynous marriage for men would also have discouraged them from marrying at young ages. Today men who lack other sources of income can only afford to marry after they have spent one or more periods as migrants earning a cash income. In Lesotho bridewealth transfers are high and are no longer drawn from a wide variety of a man's kin and distributed among his wife's relatives (Murray, 1981). They now represent a transfer between two households and are largely funded by the cash earnings of the man concerned. Furthermore, Basotho men aim to establish an independent household as soon as possible after they marry (Gay, 1980). One major expense that this involves is the acquisition of a dwelling, but it also implies access to agricultural land and cattle as the household's subsistence basis. Arable land in both countries is vested in the nation; it cannot be bought or sold. Rights to cultivate land are a prerogative of citizenship and are allocated to household heads by chiefs advised by land committees in Lesotho (Murray, 1981) and by landboards in Botswana (Molenaar, 1980). In theory they are allocated on the basis of need and ability to use the land and there is some expectation that men will gain access to their fathers' fields. In practice, particularly in Lesotho, the shortage of land makes obtaining rights to it difficult. Influencing the land committee in one's favor involves time, effort, and money (Murray, 1981). Moreover successful agricultural activities now require investment that most households can only fund by migrant earnings (Molenaar, 1980; Murray, 1981). Thus late male marriage, leading to late female marriage in the absence of polygyny, is at least in part a function of the interrelationship of labor migration and the domestic economy. To quote one of Murray's informants (1981, Sesotho translations omitted):

> On your first trip to the place of the whites you support those who brought you up. On your second trip you take out money that counts as cattle for marrying a wife. On your third trip, you look after everything in your own homestead.

In line with this analysis, the slight decline in ages at marriage between the mid-1960s and mid-1970s coincided with a period of rapid growth in mine earnings that would have made it easier for men in their twenties to marry.

Despite the economic obstacles to marrying early, most Basotho do establish a conjugal relationship at a fairly young age, whereas in Botswana marriage often occurs at much later ages. Kuper (1985) has suggested that this is linked to the different rural economies of the two countries rather than to variation in their cultures. As we have already outlined, the insecurity of wage employment and restrictions on permanent migration encourages migrants to maintain close links with their place of origin. Their long-term security depends on investment in the rural economy and the next generation. In Lesotho marriage is essential to this (Gay, 1980). Only married men can gain access to land and land has to be cultivated to be retained. In general, a man has to have a wife to acquire and maintain a farm for his old age. In contrast, in Botswana pastoralism is the central component of the rural economy. Agriculture is far less important than in Lesotho, and labor migration has never become as common. In order to provide for their old age men are likely to invest in cattle. The rural economy is stronger than in Lesotho and some men continue to exploit the opportunities offered by marriage for investment in internal political and economic enterprises. They tend to marry at young ages and often contract polygynous unions (Comaroff and Roberts, 1977). Migrant workers, however, often remit funds to their fathers or brothers who will buy cattle for them and tend them with their own herds. In this situation there is little incentive to marry before retiring from wage employment (Gulbrandsen, 1986; Kooijman, 1978; Kuper, 1985).

Another aspect of marriage patterns of significance for fertility and women's life courses is the high level of female widowhood in both countries. As can be seen from tables 8.5 and 8.6, appreciable numbers of young women are widows and the majority of women who marry are widowed before they reach old age. This pattern results from the abnormally high level of male compared with female mortality in both countries, from differences in ages at marriage, and from the infrequency of remarriage for widowed women. At the mortality rates prevailing in Lesotho in the mid-1970s, 35 percent of 25-year old men would die before age 55 while, in contrast, only 14 percent of women aged 20 would die before their fiftieth birthday (Timaeus, 1984). In Botswana adult male mortality is lower but still unusually high compared with the level of adult female mortality (Central Statistics Office, 1972). Unfortunately it is impossible to unravel with the data available either the exact contribution of labor migration to excess adult male mortality or the history of mortality differentials. However, a wealth of evidence attests to the appalling impact of minework on the health of the labor force earlier this century, and to the continuing dangers of accidents at work and occupationally related disease (Doyal, 1979; van Onselen, 1976).

Traditionally divorce was very rare in Botswana and Lesotho. A prolonged debate within social anthropology about the determinants of divorce rates in African societies concluded that this was linked to the inheritance system. The property allocated to a married woman's "house" passes to her sons and divorce has a very disruptive effect on rights over property (Gluckman, 1971). Both the families of an estranged couple and the traditional courts exert considerable pressure on them to maintain their relationship (Ashton, 1967; Schapera, 1940). However, as can be seen from table 8.5, marital breakdown is now quite common, although much less prevalent than in the West African countries surveyed by the World Fertility Survey (McDonald, 1985). Moreover it is likely that statistics gathered in large-scale demographic enquiries underestimate the extent of marital disruption. The hostile attitude of the courts means that marriages often end in separation rather than formal divorce, and some women who are still living in their marital home have been effectively deserted by their husbands (Gay, 1980). For example, the LFS household data show that 6 percent of women who said that they were married did not have a partner associated with their household. In addition, as we have outlined, the process of marrying someone is only completed after the entire bridewealth transfer has been made. If

TABLE 8.6   Percent Distribution of Women According to Household Circumstances by Age, Lesotho, 1977

Household Circumstances	Age											
	15–19	20–24	25–29	30–34	35–39	40–44	45–49	50–54	55–59	60–64	65+	15+
Single, related to head	67	18	8	8	3	2	2	1	1	1	1	16
Married, husband not head	21	32	16	8	4	2	1	1	0	1	0	11
Married, absent husband head	3	19	31	31	30	25	16	12	8	4	2	28
Married, husband head & present	3	19	31	39	44	46	48	43	36	28	13	17
Widowed household head	0	0	1	3	6	12	19	27	36	47	55	14
Divorced/separated, related to head	1	3	6	6	5	4	2	2	2	1	1	3
All other women	5	8	7	8	8	10	12	15	16	18	28	11

SOURCE: Lesotho Fertility Survey, household data.

marital disruption occurs before this point, respondents may redefine themselves as not having been married, even if the domestic and sexual components of the relationship had been well established, and fail to report the union. On the one hand, the economic opportunities and roles associated with wage employment and labor migration have weakened the social sanctions that used to inhibit marital breakdown. On the other hand, prima facie one would expect the prolonged separation of spouses stemming from labor migration to increase the likelihood of marital breakdown. Ethnographic studies support this conclusion. As Murray (1981) argues:

> A man's absence as a migrant labourer is a condition of his family's survival. But his absence also undermines the conjugal stability from which his family derives its identity.

Women have a heavy responsibility for household management in the absence of their husbands but are dependent on reliable cash remittances. Not suprisingly disputes about how money is spent are common. Moreover women regard it as inevitable that their husbands will have affairs, especially when they are working away from home, and women often have affairs themselves (Gay, 1980).

The other factor contributing to the large number of widowed, divorced, and separated women is the exceptionally low level of female remarriage. The LFS marriage histories indicate that 15 percent of ever-married women of childbearing age had experienced the dissolution of their first marriage but only 29 percent of divorced and separated women and 5 percent of widows remarried within 5 years (McDonald, 1985). In part this reflects demographic factors. As fewer men now contract polygynous marriages, excess male mortality and the more or less permanent emigration of a minority of men make it difficult for an older woman to find a new husband. Social structural factors are also important and help to explain why almost no widows remarry. In jural terms widows remain under the authority of their husband's (and sons') agnatic kin. Traditionally they would have become the wife of one of his close relatives, ideally his younger brother (Ashton, 1967; Schapera, 1940). Like divorce, remarriage of widows raises problems about the group membership and inheritance rights of the next generation. Poulter (1976) reports that most widows in Lesotho believe that remarriage is illegal, although the actual legal position is less clear-cut. In addition, a widowed woman has rights to, and effective control over, the building, fields, and property that, together with her offspring, constitute her "house" (Gay, 1980; Kerven, 1979*b*; Poulter, 1976). She can also expect support from her affines in farming her land. In Botswana, they will tend her cattle for her, although this often leads to disputes about ownership with widows claiming that their husband's brothers have "eaten" their cattle (Molenaar, 1980). Many widows experience great hardship. Nevertheless, if they remarry, they lose both their independence and control of the productive wealth that they manage on behalf of their dead husband's heirs.

The marriage systems that we have described are intimately interlinked with the developmental cycle of domestic groups and shape the household circumstances of women of childbearing age. Moreover, as we have outlined and as a number of workers have elucidated in detail, migrants' careers and the developmental cycle are also closely interrelated (Izzard, 1982; Mitchell, 1969). In Lesotho, Gay (1980) has outlined six common domestic situations that women are likely to experience in the course of their lives. The first is that of the single woman who remains subordinate to her parents even if she resides elsewhere. The second is a usually brief period spent as a married woman in her parents-in-law's household. The third is married life in her husband's household acting as the de facto household head while he works in RSA. The fourth occurs when her husband retires and returns to live with her permanently, and the fifth when he dies and she becomes a household head in her own right. Finally there are divorced and separated women who usually become reattached to their natal home. Clearly this model ignores the complexity of some women's lives. However, although one must be careful about inferring longitudinal experience from cross-sectional data, table 8.6 reveals the importance of the categories distinguished by Gay and the way in which women's domestic circumstances are likely to change during the course of their lives. Thus the structure of the households that women live in are liable to change as the wider domestic group responds to changing opportunities and constraints. Migration is one such response. The domestic situations described by Gay are also characteristic of women's experience in Botswana (Izzard, 1982). What is distinctive about the current situation there is that household fission now occurs at a far later stage in the developmental cycle than in Lesotho. In the ward studied by Molenaar (1980), average household size increased from 5.6 people in the 1930s to 10.4 in the 1970s. National data reveal that the mean de jure size of households is 9.5 (Izzard, 1979), compared with an equivalent figure of 4.9 in Lesotho. This reflects two facts. First, delayed marriage in Botswana means that large numbers of adult men and women now remain members of their natal household till quite advanced ages. While many of them will be absentees, children of a migrant woman will usually be fostered with her kin. Second, the relative importance in Botswana of cooperation among men in cattle herding, as opposed to setting up an independent household, means that brothers often continue to live together after they marry and even after the death of their parents. Male migrants in particular frequently delay setting up their own household until they retire from wage employment (Molenaar, 1980). As a result women are less likely to spend a lot of their adult lives as de facto household heads in Botswana than in Lesotho. On the other hand, while the majority of de jure female household heads in Lesotho are widows, in Botswana older single women with regular employment or economically active children also tend to establish their own households (Izzard, 1985). In both countries most women spend at least some part of their lives as household heads.

MARITAL STATUS AND FERTILITY

The relationships between marital status and lifetime and current fertility are examined in tables 8.7 and 8.8. The impact of late marriage, frequent marital dissolution, and low rates of female remarriage on fertility is less than one might expect. Although many women of reproductive age are not formally married, childbearing outside marriage is common. The Botswana Family Health Survey conducted in 1984 enquired about informal unions (Manyeneng et al., 1985).[1] As can be seen from table 8.9, the responses reveal that many women have informal relationships. It would be misleading to consider these relationships as socially equivalent to marriages. The ethnographic literature emphasizes the transitory and exploitative nature of many of them (Molenaar, 1980) and often they do not imply membership of the same household. According to the LFS household survey, 16 percent of widowed women of childbearing age do have a partner who is a member of their household. However, recalculation of the current fertility rates reveals that whether or not women are living with a partner has even less of an effect on their fertility than their marital status. Ever-married women who were not living with a man had 94 percent of the number of births in the preceding year of an equivalent group of women with partners in the household.

The level of premarital fertility is markedly different in the two countries.

TABLE 8.7   Mean Number of Children Ever-born According to Age and Marital Status of Mothers

Marital Status	Age						
	15–19	20–24	25–29	30–34	35–39	40–44	45–49
Botswana, 1971							
Single	0.1	1.0	2.2	3.4	3.9	4.2	3.9
Married	0.6	1.7	3.1	4.4	5.2	5.9	6.0
Widowed/divorced	0.2	1.6	3.0	4.3	5.0	5.3	5.3
Lesotho, 1977							
Single	0.0	0.3	1.1	1.7	2.6	2.9	2.8
Married	0.5	1.4	2.6	3.9	4.8	5.5	5.8
Widowed	0.7	1.6	2.7	3.8	5.1	5.4	5.4
Divorced/separated	0.6	1.4	2.2	3.1	3.9	3.3	4.2

SOURCE: Botswana, Central Statistics Office, 1972; Lesotho Fertility Survey, household data.

TABLE 8.8 Age-Specific Fertility Rates According to Marital Status, Lesotho, 1976–1977

Marital Status	15–19	20–24	25–29	30–34	35–39	40–44	45–49	Standardized Incidence Ratio
Single	0.01	0.06	0.11	0.05	0.06	0.03	0.11	0.13
Married	0.20	0.31	0.29	0.22	0.17	0.08	0.04	1
Widowed	0.12	0.27	0.24	0.20	0.16	0.07	0.03	0.86
Divorced/separated	0.25	0.22	0.21	0.16	0.11	0.06	0.02	0.73

SOURCE: Lesotho Fertility Survey, household data.

TABLE 8.9   Percent Distribution of Women According to Union Status by Age, Botswana, 1984

Union Status	Age						
	15–19	20–24	25–29	30–34	35–39	40–44	45–49
Never in union	47	4	1	0	0	0	0
Legally married	3	22	43	53	60	63	54
In consensual union	43	62	45	36	29	28	30
Previously in union	6	12	11	10	11	9	17

SOURCE: Manyeneng et al., 1985.

Single women in Lesotho have fewer children than those of comparable ages in Botswana and had only 13 percent of the births in the year before the survey that one would have expected if they had been married. Moreover, according to the birth histories collected in the LFS, only 5 percent of women had a birth before they married and only another 5 percent were pregnant when they married (Bureau of Statistics, 1981). In Botswana, according to the preliminary results of the 1981 census, 7 percent of single women aged 15–19 and 14 percent of those aged 20–24 have a birth each year (Lesetedi, 1984 quoted in Fako, 1985). This pattern is related both directly to labor migration and to late marriage. Traditionally prohibitions against premarital sex and pregnancy were very strong (Schapera, 1933). By the 1930s they were already collapsing as Christianity, schooling, and labor migration disrupted the mechanisms whereby parents and the community maintained their authority over the young. Today young people are almost completely free of such control—often they provide the income that supports the older generation—and almost all of them have sexual relationships (Comaroff and Roberts, 1977). For many young women, especially those without jobs or who already have chidren, the presents and assistance they get from their boyfriends are an economic necessity (Molenaar, 1980).

The current fertility data for Lesotho reveal that divorced, separated, and widowed women also have high levels of fertility. Widowed women had 86 percent of the births in the year before the survey that they would have done if they were married. For divorced and separated women the equivalent figure is 73 percent. Given the small number of unmarried men in Lesotho, it is clear that many of these women have married lovers. Some of these relationships are a recognized form of concubinage known as *bonyatsi* (Murray, 1981). This is a long-term and open relationship in which the man provides a measure of support for his mistress. Such relationships are also common in Botswana. The 1930s village studies link the spread of concubinage to the decline of polygyny and emphasize that the woman had nearly always been married previously or was regarded as too old to marry (Schapera, 1940). In

Lesotho it is fairly acceptable for widowed women to conduct discreet affairs although any overt relationships may threaten their rights to the house-property complex established by their dead husband. Any children that they bear are considered the legal heirs of their dead husband (Gay, 1980). The somewhat lower fertility of divorced and separated women is probably related to their more insecure social and economic position. In jural terms they become reattached to their natal household and they usually lose all rights to the dwelling, land, and productive wealth of the "house" established by their marriage (Gay, 1980). Some deserted women may be able to remain in their marital home and the fathers or brothers of divorced and separated women may be in a position to allocate them some land. Even women with access to fields, however, are unlikely to have the cash resources needed to farm successfully. Moreover, there is still considerable stigma attached to returning to live in the natal home (Gay, 1980). As a result divorced and separated women are particularly likely to become migrants. To interpret their fertility patterns we need to consider the interrelationships between migration and childbearing for women.

FEMALE MIGRATION AND FERTILITY

The extent to which the migration of women from Lesotho is related to their marital status and household circumstances can be seen from table 8.10. The absolute number of married female migrants is large, but married women are much less likely to migrate than single, divorced and separated women. Bearing in mind that not everyone who slept elsewhere the previous night is a migrant—or every migrant currently an absentee—it is clear that, for

TABLE 8.10   Percentage of Women Absent by Marital Status and Relationship to Household Head by Age, Lesotho, 1977

Marital Status	Age						
	15–19	20–24	25–29	30–34	35–39	40–44	45–49
Single	10	23	27	27	31	29	26
Married	11	8	7	7	6	7	7
Widowed	0	19	9	12	9	6	8
Divorced/separated	14	18	20	29	29	20	19
Relationship to Head							
Daughter/sister/ mother	10	20	24	29	31	25	29
Daughter-in-law	13	14	20	24	25	22	19
Wife	8	4	4	5	6	7	7
Self head	5	4	5	3	6	5	7

SOURCE: Lesotho Fertility Survey, household data.

women, migration is incompatible with maintaining their own household at their place of origin. Those married women who do migrate are almost all living with their parents-in-law and those unmarried women, mainly widows, who head households in the rural areas are highly unlikely to be migrants themselves. Female labor migration is concentrated among the minority of women whose marital status tends to exclude them from access to both agricultural land and remittances from male migrants (Gay, 1980). Writing about Botswana over 40 years ago, Schapera (1940) noted the tendency for unmarried mothers, divorcees and separated women to be pushed into migration in order to obtain support for their children. The migration of such women reflects their lack of alternative sources of income. In this respect the economic situation of divorced and separated women is similar to that of the small minority of single women with children in Lesotho and the much larger number of such women in Botswana. In the Basotho village studied by Gay (1980), 49 percent of single women and 54 percent of divorced and separated women had some form of wage employment compared with 8 percent of married women and 14 percent of widows. Such work as is available both in the formal and in the informal sectors, for example beer brewing, is largely insecure and poorly paid. For some women, moving to an urban area may be an attractive opportunity, but female migrants with children usually have to foster them with their mother or other relatives. They migrate because they are forced to as the only way of fulfilling their maternal responsibilities.

The links between female migration and fertility are neither simple nor unidirectional. Not only are unmarried women with children pushed into migration but women living in the townships of the Republic of South Africa are both less subject to the social pressure militating against premarital pregnancy and less likely to meet potential husbands than those who remain at home (Murray, 1981). In the short term, however, the links between female migration and fertility operate in the opposite direction. Migrants who become pregnant may lose their jobs and women breastfeeding young children are unable to take up work away from home (Izzard, 1985). In this light the fertility differentials shown in table 8.11 are hard to interpret. Clearly much of the reduction in the fertility of widowed and divorced women in Lesotho is associated with their involvement in labor migration. What is less clear is to what extent migrant women are restricting their fertility through contraception and abstinence and to what extent caring for an infant prevents migration.[2] To us it seems highly likely that both factors are important.

MALE MIGRATION AND MARITAL FERTILITY

The direct impact of spousal separation on the level of fertility within unions depends to a considerable extent on its timing relative to birth intervals (Hill, 1985; Millman and Potter, 1984). The LFS household data in table 8.12

TABLE 8.11   Standardized Ratio of Births in the Last Year According to Marital Status and De Facto Residence Compared with Present, Married Women, Lesotho, 1977

Marital Status	Residential Status	
	Present	Absent
Single	0.15	0.10
Married	1	0.99
Widowed	0.49	0.28
Divorced/separated	0.85	0.32

SOUCE: Lesotho Fertility Survey, household data.

TABLE 8.12   Age-Specific and Total Fertility Rates (TFR) According to De Facto Residence of Partner, All Women with Partners in the Household, Lesotho, 1977

Residence of Partner	Age							
	15–19	20–24	25–29	30–34	35–39	40–44	45–49	TFR
Present	0.17	0.28	0.27	0.21	0.17	0.07	0.04	6.1
Absent	0.18	0.32	0.31	0.23	0.17	0.09	0.07	6.9

SOURCE: Lesotho Fertility Survey, household data.

show that in Lesotho women whose husbands were absent the previous night had higher fertility over the previous year than women whose husbands were present. To some extent this may be because migrants are drawn preponderantly from high fertility groups of the population. Probably more importantly, spells of labor migration often follow the birth of a child. In part this correlation arises simply because most births are conceived during periods of leave. It also seems likely that the birth of a child provides an extra economic incentive to migration. In addition Basotho and Tswana culture prescribe a period of separation of husband and wife after birth (the woman normally returns to her natal home for several months) and prolonged postpartum abstinence (Gay, 1980; Manyeneng et al., 1985). Thus migration in the period following birth is in accordance with local values.

Information on the frequency of spousal separation at times when the woman would otherwise be exposed to the risk of conception is available from the LFS. It enquired about absences of three or more months during the open birth interval whenever the respondent was married and not pregnant, sterilized, or abstaining after a birth. Analysts who have considered the retrospective data have judged them incomplete and difficult to interpret (Casterline et al., 1984; Mpiti and Kalule–Sabiti, 1985). However, if women reported any absences, they were asked if their husband was still away. These current status data are probably more accurate and are easier to interpret. From them one can identify the number of exposed women whose husbands are absent. Using this figure one can calculate a prevalence-incidence mean duration of absence during the period of exposure in each birth interval.[3] In all, 16.5 percent of otherwise exposed married women said that their husband was absent. This suggests that women's husbands are away on average for about 3.4 months between the end of the postpartum nonsusceptible period and when they become pregnant, lengthening birth intervals by an equivalent amount. This is very much a minimal estimate of the direct impact of labor circulation on martial fertility. The questions posed in the survey asked about absences of 3 or more months, but even short periods of separation will affect fertility if they occur on a wide enough scale. The 1978/1979 Labour Force and Migration Survey of Lesotho showed that 20 percent of currently absent miners had visited home two or more times in the last 6 months (UN Economic Commission for Africa, 1982). Almost none of them would be detected by the LFS questions although on average they had spent only 1 month at home in this period. Moreover, even if the average interval between periods of leave for the 80 percent of migrants who return home less often was as long as 9 months, a third of them would have been omitted from the LFS statistics. According to the LFS household survey, only 54 percent of married men aged less than 55 slept at home the previous night. Therefore, even though migration is concentrated in women's postpartum nonsusceptible period, it seems likely that the LFS questions picked up less than half the demographically significant episodes of spousal separation and that male migration adds at least 6 to 7 months to the length of birth intervals.

There is a second way in which spousal separation affects the length of birth intervals. Not only prolonged breastfeeding but also a prolonged period of postpartum abstinence is still normal in Botswana and Lesotho (Manyeneng et al., 1985; Mpiti and Kalule–Sabiti, 1985). Data from the Botswana Family Health Survey shown in table 8.13 demonstrate that women with absent husbands whose last birth occurred more than 6 months ago were much more likely to report that they were abstaining than women whose husbands were present. In Lesotho, women who were abstaining were not asked about spousal separation and part of the reduction in fertility attributed to abstinence could more reasonably be attributed to labor migration. The published data on Botswana do not permit one to make exact calculations but the mean duration of postpartum abstinence estimated from data on women whose husbands were present at the time of the survey is about 9 months, compared with an estimate of 12 months based on all women.[4] In Lesotho the mean duration of postpartum abstinence reported was about 15 months (Mpiti and Kalule–Sabiti, 1985). As prolonged periods of spousal separation are much more common in Lesotho than in Botswana, it seems

TABLE 8.13   Percentage of Women in Unions Not Having Resumed Sexual Relations by Duration since Last Birth and De Facto Residence of Partner, Botswana, 1984

Months since Birth	Total	Partner Present	Partner Absent
0–3	94	91	96
4–6	70	68	72
7–9	52	36	68
10–12	50	41	61
13–18	40	36	44
19–24	22	16	29
25–36	18	11	27

SOURCE: Manyeneng et al., 1985.

likely that anything between 3 and 6 months of the lengthening of birth intervals ascribed to postpartum abstinence in Lesotho occurs only because of the separation of married couples resulting from labor circulation.

MODERN METHODS OF FERTILITY CONTROL

Several southern African countries are experiencing the initial phases of fertility transition. In the RSA the total fertility rate of the black population probably declined from around seven to just above five children during the 1960s and 1970s (Science Committee of the President's Council, 1983). A fertility survey conducted in 1982 showed that 45 percent of married women were currently using contraception (van Tonder, 1985).[5] Surveys conducted in Botswana and Zimbabwe in 1984 showed that 28 percent and 38 percent respectively of women currently in a union were using contraception (Manyeneng et al., 1985; National Family Planning Council, 1985). Although the LFS revealed fewer users of contraception, the position could have changed greatly during the last decade and even in 1977 there was evidence of fertility decline among educated women (Timaeus and Balasubramanian, 1984). A preliminary examination of the provisional results of the recent censuses of Botswana and Zimbabwe suggests that, so far, the adoption of modern methods of contraception has had little impact on the overall level of fertility. The total fertility rate in both countries is still in the range 6.5–7.0 children (Central Statistics Office, 1972; Manyeneng et al., 1985; National Family Planning Council, 1985). Moreover the mean completed family size expected by women, although lower than in many sub-Saharan African countries, remains as high as six children (Manyeneng et al., 1985; National Family Planning Council, 1985). A similar figure was reported in the LFS (Lightbourne, 1985). As in the RSA, where black women still want 4.4 children on average (van Tonder, 1985), fertility decline may proceed more slowly than it has in other parts of the world.

It is impossible to quantify the extent to which the migrant labor system has encouraged the adoption of modern methods of contraception. None of the published reports on the fertility surveys conducted in Southern Africa investigates differentials in contraceptive use according to whether women or their partners are involved in labor migration. Furthermore none of them examine the influence of marital status on recent fertility or contraceptive use. Most of the tables are restricted to currently married women. Yet, despite the lack of statistical evidence, there are reasons for supposing that the pervasive influence of labor migration on southern African society extends to this development. We would not disagree with those, such as Cleland (1985), who see the onset of control of marital fertility as a cultural innovation. But, as Cleland implies, there are at least two reasons why this represents an incomplete explanation. First, other social changes may be important preconditions for the diffusion of the idea of family planning. The populations of Southern African countries have been involved in wage employment and migration to urban areas for several generations. Although female migration is not very prevalent, a substantial proportion of women spend some period of their life working in a town. Moreover, whether or not they work outside the home, the wives of migrants are accustomed to making decisions, managing their households, and controlling their own lives. Partly in response to the emergence of large numbers of female-headed households, the rights of women to own productive wealth and be independent of men are being recognized gradually (Gay, 1980; Molenaar, 1980; Poulter, 1976). In addition, levels of female education are high in Southern Africa. Thus the wide-ranging series of changes in the status of women associated with labor migration and the long and profound exposure of the indigenous population of Southern Africa to Western ideas and values have probably removed any institutional barriers to the adoption of new attitudes to family building. Second, we would argue that, as Cleland (1985) admits, there are strong cultural supports for high fertility in Africa which may be based on social structural factors. Cleland suggests that the importance of the numerical strength of kin groups may be relevant. In Botswana and Lesotho, the growth of wage earnings in combination with their distinctive land tenure systems mean that such considerations no longer apply. While political and economic incentives to maximizing fertility appear to have existed in the nineteenth century, they probably ceased to operate as long as 50 years ago. It may be, as we have already speculated, that despite this women in Southern Africa will continue to want large families. If most women are using contraception to control the timing and spacing of their births, rather than to reduce the size of their families, the overall impact on the level of fertility will be slight. On the other hand, the strong and immediate economic disincentives to childbearing for single, divorced, and separated women in Botswana and Lesotho suggest that even this pattern of contraceptive use could lead to a substantial decline in fertility outside marriage.

THE OVERALL LEVEL OF FERTILITY

In order to assess the overall significance of labor circulation for fertility it is helpful to examine the impact of the more important proximate determinants of fertility on its level using the model developed by Bongaarts (Bongaarts, 1978; Bongaarts and Potter, 1983). The data required are only available for Lesotho. We would emphasize that such an analysis does not permit one to make counterfactual predictions. While the development of widespread migration and late marriage were associated, it does not follow that a reduction in the extent of migration would lead to earlier marriage. More generally, the impact of the total and permanent cessation of labor migration on Lesotho's population would be disastrous and the implications for fertility impossible to determine.

Estimates of the fertility-inhibiting effects of the proximate determinants of fertility are shown in table 8.14. Our model is a revised and extended version of the one presented by Mpiti and Kalule-Sabiti (1985). We prefer to base our estimates of overall fertility and marital fertility on the WFS household survey (Timaeus and Balasubramanian, 1984) and have included spousal separation in the model. The total fertility rate of 5.4 is extremely low for a sub-Saharan African country. Even our minimal estimate of the extent of spousal separation at times when women would otherwise be exposed to the risk of conception suggests that it reduces the level of marital fertility by 9 percent. If we assume that the LFS questions underestimated such separation by a factor of two and that abstinence arising from spousal separation lengthens the postpartum nonsusceptible period by 3 months, a 24 percent reduction in fertility results. In other words, a hypothetical country with

TABLE 8.14   Indices of the Impact of the Proximate Determinants on Fertility, Lesotho 1977

Progressive Fertility Reduction due to:	Percent Reduction	Fertility Level	
Factors such as sterility and frequency of intercourse		Total Fecundity Rate	= 12.8
Lactational amenorrhea	37.3		9.2
Postpartum abstinence	24.4	Total Natural Fertility Rate	= 7.5
Spousal separation	10.7		6.8
Contraception	4.9	Total Marital Fertility Rate	= 6.5
Widowhood and divorce	2.4		6.4
Age at first marriage	20.2	Total Fertility Rate	= 5.4

NOTE: The corresponding Bongaarts' indices are: $C_{amen.} = .723$; $C_{abst.} = .809$; $C_{separ.} = .911$; $C_{contr.} = .958$; $C_{cm} = .979$; $C_{em} = .839$

SOURCE: Mpiti and Kalule-Sabiti (1985); Lesotho Fertility Household data.

similar marriage and fertility patterns to Lesotho but no labor migration would have a total fertility rate of at least six children and more probably one of around seven children.

The low level of premarital fertility in Lesotho means that the high mean age at marriage of women exerts an appreciable downwards influence on the level of fertility. In contrast marital dissolution has a trivial impact on the total fertility rate. It is worth emphasizing that this is not because there are few widowed, divorced, and separated women or because they are concentrated at the upper end of the reproductive age range. It is because of the high level of extramarital fertility. If no births occurred outside marriage, the current pattern of marital dissolution would result in an 11 percent reduction in the level of fertility in Lesotho (Casterline et al., 1984). Given that female migration is concentrated among divorced and separated women, it follows from the unimportance of marital dissolution for fertility that labor migration of women has little effect on the national level of fertility.

DISCUSSION

It is sometimes argued that because childbearing often occurs outside marriage in sub-Saharan African nuptiality is irrelevant to the analysis of fertility.[6] We believe that this is a misconception for the following reasons. First, even when there are few sanctions against extramarital childbearing, the fertility of unmarried women is lower than that of those who are married. In Lesotho premarital pregnancy remains fairly uncommon despite high ages at marriage of women. Second, in Southern Africa at least, the increase in childbearing outside marriage is a fairly recent development. In Botswana and Lesotho extramarital fertility and the transformation of marriage patterns are two aspects of the same process of change. If we wish to explain why births occur outside marriage, we have to understand the marriage system (Comaroff and Roberts, 1977). Third, marital status has important implications for women's social and economic circumstances. It determines the recruitment of children to social groups, the allocation of responsibility for their upbringing, and rights to their labor as they grow older. In Botswana it seems likely that a group of elderly men who have never married and have no legitimate children will emerge, raising new issues concerning support of the old. The social significance of childbearing inside and outside marriage is different as are the implications for the welfare of children and even their mortality. As a result, adoption of modern methods of fertility control may have different implications for the fertility of married and unmarried women.

As well as having a direct impact on fertility, the growth of widespread labor migration in Botswana and Lesotho played a major part in the development of the contemporary marriage systems of these countries. At the individual level we have shown how, for both men and women, involvement in and the timing of labor migration shape and are shaped by their marriage and fertility histories. Late marriage, the decline of polygyny, increased marital disruption, and frequent extramarital sexual relationships are a series of interrelated changes that have reinforced one another and are all linked to labor migration. Other factors, in particular the spread of education, especially of women, the influence of the Christian church, and wider aspects of the development of a money economy and of the emancipation of women, are also relevant to the process of change. However the influence of labor migration is pivotal. It lies at the heart of a transformation of the role marriage plays in the social system and, more generally, of relationships between men and women and successive generations.

In traditional society, which we would loosely locate in the nineteenth century, women's lives were dominated by their key contribution to subsistence agriculture and their subordination to men (Izzard, 1981). Their participation in the political and ritual life of the community was restricted and they could neither own nor control productive wealth. For men marriage was an avenue to the control of the economic and political resources represented by women's productive and reproductive capacities. The payment of bridewealth transferred these irrevocably to the husband's family. Polygynous marriage, the accumulation of cattle, and the establishment of relationships of clientage were related practices that could be used to amass wealth and power. The monopoly over economic resources held by senior men lay at the root of their control over both women and the younger generation. We would argue from the anthropological record that maximizing fertility, and therefore for men their number of wives, was economically advantageous. This stemmed at least as much from the speculative dynamics of the political, land-tenurial, and technological context as from the net wealth flow obtained directly from the labor of children (Caldwell, 1982).

Labor migration disrupted traditional relationships of authority both directly, by removing elders and young men from their households, and by providing new avenues for gaining a livelihood and accumulating wealth (Murray, 1977). As the importance of wage earnings grew, other political and cultural changes initiated by contact with Europeans undermined the viability of traditional means of amassing resources. As a result marriage lost much of its economic and political rationale for men while at the same time sanctions against sexual relationships outside marriage weakened and conjugal relationships came under increasing stress as many men began to spend most of their young adult life away from their permanent home. The defining characteristic of marriage remains the exchange of bridewealth for social paternity. A decline in the significance of rights in the younger generation underlies both the transformation of marriage patterns and the increase in other forms of sexual relationship. The apparent continuity in the structure of marital institutions, which remain shaped by Basotho and Tswana cultural premises, is belied by a change in their purpose. To quote Murray (1981) again:

> it is often more realistic in contemporary practice to represent marital transactions as the result of bargaining conducted by senior women over the earning capacity of men, than as the result of bargaining conducted by senior men over the productive and reproductive capacities of women.

In both countries most men's long-term security still depends on investment in the rural economy. They desire heirs and marry eventually. The earnings and contribution to domestic work of the younger generation are an important source of support in old age (Murray, 1977). But, in Botswana, ages at marriage are dispersed, reflecting the diversity of economic options available to different groups of men and women. For migrants there is little incentive to marry early. In contrast, in Lesotho, involvement in migration is more widespread and marriage patterns are more uniform. Marriage occurs at younger ages as only married men can begin to establish viable farming enterprises to provide for their retirement. There is nothing inevitable about these developments in the marriage system. As well as being shaped by the systematic exclusion of women from work in the RSA, they are contingent on the cultural and legal premises of Basotho and Tswana society. In particular, they are underpinned by differentiation between male and female labor, men's privileged access to land and cattle, and the identification of marriage with the transfer of bridewealth (Kuper, 1985).

The development of the migrant labor system created new roles and responsibilities for the wives of migrants and for migrant women. To a considerable extent these have become accepted and institutionalized both culturally and legally. This and related developments, such as the spread of female education, have greatly enhanced women's status. Nevertheless, their responsibility for child rearing, restricted access to land, exclusion from inheritance, and lack of opportunities for paid employment mean that most women, whether married or not, remain dependent on relationships with men to obtain the means of survival. Kraeger (1982) has suggested that:

> demographic facts may in important respects constitute groups in some of their most distinctive features. In characterizing different demographic regimes we should ask: To what social purposes are demographic relations organized?

What we would emphasize is that the social purposes underlying demographic patterns may vary between groups of the population that differ in their economic situation and social status. A reproductive regime represents a negotiated or imposed resolution of such conflicts. In both countries a central concern of men in marriage and reproduction is to establish their rights in a farm and the next generation in order to provide for their retirement. For women in Lesotho and also many women in Botswana, it is crucial to gain and maintain access to economic resources controlled by men. For the parental generation, the marriage of their daughters is an opportunity to obtain bridewealth cattle from younger men. Prolonged spousal separation adds to the stresses imposed on the conjugal relationship by these conflicting interests. Whether it survives or collapses, it is often women with young children who lose the most.

The differences between the marriage systems of Botswana and Lesotho are a telling caution against assuming that our analysis can be extended in every detail to other Southern African countries. On the other hand, many migrants in such countries also retain links with their village of origin despite long periods of absence. Moreover patrilineal kinship systems and marriage with bridewealth are found throughout most of the region to the south of Zambia and Malawi, although the focusing of property rights on a woman's "house" is confined to the area south of the Limpopo River. Tentatively we would suggest that Lesotho may typify areas where it remains important for male migrants to retain a link to a rural farming enterprise whereas elsewhere, including urban areas, the disruption of family life will be even greater. The data that are available about marriage and fertility patterns in other Southern African countries are consistent with our expectations. In the RSA the mean age at marriage of black women is above 20 years and polygynous unions are rare and had already become uncommon by the 1940s (see chapter 6 and Clignet, 1970). According to the fertility survey conducted in 1982, 44 percent of both Sotho and Nguni women had borne a child before they were married (van Tonder, 1985). Anthropological evidence also attests to the disruption of marital institutions and high level of fertility outside marriage in the Republic of South Africa (Dubb, 1974; Pauw, 1973). Similarly in Zimbabwe only 27 percent of 15 to 19-year-old women are married but 11 percent of all women of reproductive age are living in informal unions (National Family Planning Council, 1985). Thus there is some wider evidence that the complement of the distinctive Southern African marriage pattern identified by Lesthaeghe and his colleagues (see chapter 6) consists of other forms of sexual relationship and extramarital fertility.

Our attempts to measure the direct impact of labor migration on fertility have been bedeviled by lack of data, inadequacies in the questions used to investigate the subject, and difficulties in establishing the direction of causality. In Lesotho, the only country for which we could make estimates, almost every household is involved in migration. It is therefore impossible to measure any but the most short-term differentials between the fertility of migrants and their spouses and that of nonmigrants. Nevertheless we have firm evidence that male migration reduces the level of marital fertility by at least 9 percent and some grounds for suggesting that the actual reduction in fertility is very large, perhaps in the region of 25 percent. In Botswana patterns of breastfeeding, postpartum amenorrhea, and abstinence, on the one hand,

and of migration, on the other, are broadly comparable with those in Lesotho. The proportion of the male population involved in labor migration is about half of that in Lesotho. While we would not attempt to estimate a figure, it seems likely that spousal separation has an appreciable impact on fertility. In contrast, although migrant women have a low level of fertility, such migration is not common enough in Lesotho for it to have any significance for the overall level of fertility. Effects operating in the opposite direction are very important. Women's marital and reproductive histories are major determinants of their direct involvement in the migrant labor system.

Use of modern methods of contraception is now common in at least Botswana, the RSA, and Zimbabwe. This contrasts with the slow adoption of contraception in other sub-Saharan African countries including those such as Ghana and Kenya with active family planning campaigns. One can only speculate as to whether labor migration is the crucial feature distinguishing Southern Africa from the rest of the continent in this respect. Certainly the political and economic history that has transformed the indigenous population of South Africa and its periphery into an impoverished rural proletariat has destroyed many potential obstacles to the spread of the idea of controlling fertility. It remains to be seen whether a rapid decline in fertility is resulting, as it has elsewhere in the world, or whether women will continue to have large families. One theme of our argument has been that changing economic opportunities and social disruption resulting from labor migration led to the replacement of a reproductive regime in which marriage for women was early and universal by one in which a variety of forms of sexual relationship without payment of bridewealth are common. The result was a high level of fertility outside marriage. Use of modern methods of contraception makes it possible for unmarried women to be sexually active without having children. If for no other reason, the desperate economic plight of many such women may be leading them to adopt this course.

ACKNOWLEDGMENTS

We would like to thank Allan Hill and Colin Murray for their comments on an earlier version of this paper.

NOTES

1. The exact meaning of these data is unclear. While the text describes those in an informal union as living with a partner, the English translation of the relevant question merely asks whether they have a partner. This makes interpretation of the subsequent questions about whether the partner spent the previous night in the household and how long he had been absent very difficult.

2. We are also concerned about sampling errors and whether all the recent births

of absent women have been reported. However, we feel that the differentials are sufficiently large and consistent to accept that they have some basis in reality.

3. The monthly incidence of women entering the period of exposure can be estimated from the mean number of births per month. The calculations and assumptions involved in making such estimates from current status data are discussed in Mosley et al. (1982).

4. These very approximate estimates have been made by calculating a trimean from a plot of the unsmoothed current status data.

5. It should be noted that this survey did not cover the populations of the ten "homelands."

6. This explains why no question on marital status was included in the 1976 census of Swaziland (Central Statistical Office, n.d.).

BIBLIOGRAPHY

Allison, C. 1979. The determinants of primary schooling in the Kweneng with special reference to cattle and mine labour migration. *Working Paper of the National Migration Study*. Gaborone, Botswana: Central Statistics Office.

Ashton, C. H. 1967. *The Basotho*, 2d ed. Oxford: Oxford University Press.

Bell, M. 1986. *Contemporary Africa*. London: Longman.

Bongaarts, J. 1978. A framework for analyzing the proximate determinants of fertility. *Population and Development Review* 4(1): 105–132.

Bongaarts, J., and R. Potter. 1983. *Fertility, biology and behavior: An analysis of the proximate determinants*. New York: Academic Press.

Boserup, E. 1970. *Women's role in economic development*. London: Allen and Unwin.

Bozzoli, B. 1983. Marxism, feminism and South Africa studies. *Journal of Southern African Studies* 9(2): 139–171.

Brown, B. 1979. Women's role in development in Kgatleng District. *Working Paper of the African Studies Center*. Boston: Boston University.

Bryant, C. 1977. Women migrants, urbanization and social change: An African case. Paper presented at the meeting of the American Political Science Association, Washington, D. C.

Bundy, C. 1979. *The rise and fall of the South African peasantry*. London: Heinemann.

Caldwell, J. C. 1982. *Theory of fertility decline*. London: Academic Press.

Casterline, J. B., S. Singh, J. Cleland, and H. Ashurst. 1984. The proximate determinants of fertility. *World Fertility Survey Comparative Studies*, no. 39. Voorburg: International Statistical Institute.

Chaney, E. 1980. *Women in international migration: Issues in development planning*. Washington, D. C.: U.S. Agency for International Development.

Clarke, D. C. 1977. *Foreign migrant labour in southern Africa*. Geneva: International Labour Organization.

Cleland, J. 1985. Marital fertility decline in developing countries: Theories and evidence. In: *Reproductive change in developing countries*, ed. J. Cleland and J. Hobcraft. Oxford: Oxford University Press.

Cliffe, L. 1977. Labour migration and peasant differentiation: Zambian experiences. *Journal of Peasant Studies* 5: 326–346.

Clignet, R. 1970. *Many wives, many powers—Autonomy and power in polygynous families.* Evanston: Northwestern University Press.

Cock, J. 1980. *Maids and madams.* Johannesburg, South Africa: Raven Press.

Colclough, C. 1980. Some aspects of labour use in southern Africa—Problems and policies. *IDS Bulletin* 11(4): 29–39.

Colclough, C., and S. McCarthy. 1980. *The political economy of Botswana: A study of growth and distribution.* Oxford: Oxford University Press.

Comaroff, J. L., and S. Roberts. 1977. Marriage and extra-marital sexuality: The dialectics of legal change among the Kgatla. *Journal of African Law* 21(1): 97–123.

Cooper, D. C. 1979. Economy and society in Botswana: Some basic national socio-economic coordinates relevant to an interpretation of the National Migration Study statistics. *Working Paper of the National Migration Study.* Gaborone, Botswana: Central Statistics Office.

Davies, R. 1978. Demand trends for foreign workers and employment strategy in South Africa. Paper presented at the Economic Commission for Africa, Conference on Migratory Labour in Southern Africa, Lusaka, Zambia.

Doyal, L. 1979. *The political economy of health.* London: Pluto Press.

Dubb, A. A. 1974. The impact of the city. In: *The Bantu-speaking peoples of southern Africa,* ed. W. D. Hammond-Tooke. London: Routledge and Kegan Paul.

Fako, T. T. 1985. *Youth education and services for health and family life.* London: International Planned Parenthood Federation.

Gay, J. 1980. Basotho women's options: A study of marital careers in rural Lesotho. Ph.D. dissertation. Cambridge University.

Gluckman, M. 1971. Marriage payments and social structure among the Lozi and Zulu. In *Kinship,* ed. J. Goody. London: Penguin.

Gordon, E. n.d. Towards a final report: The women left behind—The wives of migrant workers of Lesotho. Geneva: International Labour Organization.

Gulbrandsen, O. 1986. To marry—or not to marry. *Ethnos* 51(1–2): 7–28.

Hill, A. G. 1985. A practical guide to estimating the Bongaarts indices of the proximate determinants of fertility. In *Population factors in development planning in the Middle East,* ed. F. C. Shorter and H. Zurayk. New York: The Population Council.

Izzard, W. J. 1981. The impact of migration on the roles of women. Paper presented at the National Migration Study Conference, Gaborone, Botswana.

———. 1982. Rural-urban migration in a developing country: The case of women migrants in Botswana. Ph.D. dissertation. Oxford University.

———. 1985. Migrants and mothers: Case studies from Botswana. *Journal of African Studies* 11(2): 258–280.

Kerven, C. 1979a. Botswana mine labour migration to South Africa. *Working Paper of the National Migration Study.* Gaborone: Central Statistics Office.

———. 1979b. Urban and rural female-headed households, dependence on agriculture. *Working Paper of the National Migration Study.* Gaborone: Central Statistics Office.

———. 1982. The effects of migration on agricultural production. In *Migration in Botswana: Patterns, causes and consequences,* ed. C. Kerven. Gaborone: The Government Printer.

Kingdom of Swaziland. n.d. *Report on the 1976 Swaziland population census.* Mbabane, Swaziland: Central Statistical Office.

Kooijman, K. 1978. A report on the village of Bokaa. Gaborone, Botswana: Botswana Extension College.

Kowet, D. K. 1978. *Land, labour migration and politics in southern Africa: Botswana, Lesotho and Swaziland*. Uppsala: Scandinavian Institute of African Studies.

Kraeger, P. 1982. Demography in situ. *Population and Development Review* 8(2): 237–266.

Kuper, A. 1985. *African marriage in an impinging world—The case of southern Africa*, Leyden: Afrika Studiecentrum.

Leggasick, M., and F. Le Clerq. 1978. The origins and nature of the migrant labour system in southern Africa. Paper presented at the Economic Commission for Africa, Conference on Migratory Labour in Southern Africa, Lusaka, Zambia.

Lesetedi, D. 1984. *Education—1981 population and housing census*. Gaborone: Central Statistics Office.

Lightbourne, R. E. 1985. Individual preferences and fertility behaviour. In *Reproductive change in developing countries*, ed. J. Cleland and J. Hobcraft. Oxford: Oxford University Press.

Lucas, B. 1982. Outmigration, remittances and investment in rural areas. In *Migration in Botswana: Patterns, causes and consequences*, ed. C. Kerven. Gaborone: The Government Printer.

McDonald, P. 1985: Social organization and nuptiality in developing societies. In *Reproductive change in developing countries*, ed. J. Cleland and J. Hobcraft. Oxford: Oxford University Press.

Magubane, B. 1975. The "native reserves" (Bantustans) and the role of the migrant labour system in the political economy of South Africa. In *Migration and development: Implications for ethnic identity and political conflict*, ed. H. I. Safa and B. M. Dutoit. The Hague: Mouton.

Manyeneng, W. G., P. Khulumani, M. K. Larson, and A. A. Way. 1985. *Botswana family health survey, 1984*. Columbia, Md.: Westinghouse Public Applied Systems.

Marks, S., and E. Unterhalter. 1978. Women and the migrant labour system in southern Africa. Paper presented at the Economic Commission for Africa, Conference on Migratory Labour in Southern Africa, Lusaka, Zambia.

Meillassoux, C. 1975. *Maidens, meal and money*. Cambridge: Cambridge University Press.

Millman, S. R., and R. G. Potter. 1984. The fertility impact of spousal separation. *Studies in Family Planning* 15(3): 121–126.

Mitchell, J. C. 1969. Structural plurality, urbanization and labour circulation in southern Rhodesia. In *Migration: Sociological studies*, ed. J. A. Jackson. Cambridge: Cambridge University Press.

———. 1985. Towards a situational sociology of wage-labour circulation. In *Circulation in third world countries*, ed. R. M. Prothero and M. Chapman. London: Routledge and Kegan Paul.

Molenaar, M. 1980. Social change within a traditional pattern: A case study of a Tswana ward. Leyden, Netherlands: Institute of Cultural and Social Studies.

Mosley, W. H., L. Werner, and S. Becker. 1982. The dynamics of birth-spacing and marital fertility in Kenya. *World Fertility Survey Scientific Reports*, no. 30. Voorburg: International Statistical Institute.

Mpiti, A. M., and I. Kalule-Sabiti. 1985. The proximate determinants of fertility in Lesotho. *World Fertility Survey Scientific Reports*, no. 53. Voorburg: International Statistical Institute.

Murray, C. 1977. High bridewealth, migrant labour, and the position of women in Lesotho. *Journal of African Law* 21(1): 79–96.

———. 1981. *Families divided.* Cambridge: Cambridge University Press.

National Family Planning Council, Zimbabwe. 1985. *Zimbabwe reproductive health survey 1984.* Columbia, Md.: Westinghouse Public Applied Systems.

Palmer, R., and N. Parsons. 1977. *The roots of rural poverty in central and southern Africa.* London: Heinemann.

Parsons, N. 1977. The economic history of Khama's country in Botswana, 1844–1930. In *The roots of rural poverty in central and southern Africa*, ed. R. Palmer and N. Parsons. London: Heinemann.

Pauw, B. A. 1973. *The second generation*, 2d. ed. Oxford: Oxford University Press.

Poulter, S. 1976. *Family law and litigation in Basotho society.* Oxford: Clarendon Press.

Preston-Whyte, E. 1974. Kinship and marriage. In: *The Bantu-speaking peoples of southern Africa*, ed. W. D. Hammond-Tooke. London: Routledge and Kegan Paul.

Prothero, R. M., and M. Chapman, eds. 1985. *Circulation in third world countries.* London: Routledge and Kegan Paul.

Republic of Lesotho. 1981. *Lesotho fertility survey 1977, first report.* 2 vols. Maseru, Lesotho: Bureau of Statistics.

Schapera, I. 1933. Premarital pregnancy and native opinion: A note on social change. *Africa* 45: 258–279.

———. 1940. *Married life in an African tribe.* London: Pelican.

———. 1947. *Migrant labour and tribal life: A study of conditions in the Bechuanaland Protectorate.* Oxford: Oxford University Press.

Science Committee of the President's Council, Republic of South Africa. 1983. *Report on demographic trends in South Africa.* Cape Town: The Government Printer.

Skinner, E. P. 1985. Labour migration and national development in southern Africa. In *African migration and national development*, ed. R. Lindsay. University Park: Pennsylvania State University Press.

Taylor, J. 1982. Changing patterns of labour supply to the South African gold mines, *Tijdschrift voor Economische and Sociale Geografie* 73(4): 213–220.

Timaeus, I. 1984. Mortality in Lesotho: A study of levels, trends and differentials based on retrospective survey data. *World Fertility Survey Scientific Reports*, no. 59. Voorburg: International Statistical Institute.

Timaeus, I., and K. Balasubramanian. 1984. Evaluation of the Lesotho fertility survey 1977. *World Fertility Survey Scientific Reports*, no. 58. Voorburg: International Statistical Institute.

United Nations Economic Commission for Africa. 1982. Lesotho—A demographic, socio-economic profile. Paper presented at the seminar on Population Planning for Development, Maseru, Lesotho.

van Binsbergen, W. M. J., and H. Meilink, eds. 1978. *Migration and the transformation of modern African society.* Leyden: Afrika Studiecentrum.

van der Wiel, A. C. A. 1977. *Migratory wage labour: Its role in the economy of Lesotho.* Lesotho: Mazenod Book Centre.

van de Walle, E. 1985. Community-level variables and institutional factors in the Study of African nuptiality. In *The collection and analysis of community data*, ed. J. B. Casterline. Voorburg: International Statistical Institute.

van Onselen, C. 1976. *Chibaro: African mine labour in southern Rhodesia—1900–1933*. London: Pluto Press.

van Tonder, J. L. 1985. *Fertility survey 1982: Data concerning the black population of South Africa*. Pretoria: Human Sciences Research Council.

Wilson, F. 1972. *Migrant labour in South Africa*. Johannesburg: South African Council of Churches.

Wolpe, H. 1972. Capitalism and cheap labour power in South Africa: From segregation to apartheid. *Economy and Society* 1: 425–456.

Wylie, D. 1981. Migration to freehold farms and to farms in South Africa. Paper presented at the National Migration Study Conference, Gaborone, Botswana.

CHAPTER NINE

Childrearing versus Childbearing: Coresidence of Mother and Child in Sub-Saharan Africa

Hilary J. Page

INTRODUCTION

Producing Successive Generations of Adults: Biological versus Social Reproduction
Most demographic studies restrict their analysis of reproduction to *biological* reproduction; either there is no mention of *social* reproduction, or it is assumed to be fully congruent with biological reproduction in the sense that the actors are assumed to be the same. Thus, for example, we find analyses of fertility in terms of the "costs and benefits" of children, or in terms of the demand for children, all cast in a model in which the childbearer (or begetter) is assumed to be the person responsible for bringing the child to full adult status. Not only academic and policy discussions but also programmatic activities are dominated by the simplest of possible decision-making models: fertility decisions are made by individual bearers and begetters, who are assumed to be those who will have the direct rights and responsibilities associated with socializing as well as producing the next generation.

Such a model is quite inappropriate for most of sub-Saharan Africa. Indeed, one of the most striking features of the region is a seemingly paradoxical combination. On the one hand, there is the tremendous importance attached to parenthood. There is, for example, an exceptionally high desire for biological parenthood. This finds its expression in large desired family size, in reluctance to cease childbearing, and in a horror of subfertility in general and of barrenness in particular. There is also a particularly strong bond between children and their parents: in addition to the affective links and/or strong sense of moral obligation toward parents that are common to many cultures, there is also the respect due to parents in their capacity as the link with the ancestors, especially the fear of invoking the ancestors' wrath and of bringing down an ancestral curse.[1] On the other hand, there is a very high incidence of children being reared by persons other than their biological parents. And these "foster" parents may assume not only the responsibilities of childrearing but also the rights associated with it.

This seeming paradox is, however, quite simple to explain. A first part of the explanation lies essentially in the nature of the family systems prevailing in Africa. Most important here is the absence of a long-established nuclear-family tradition (or of clearly defined nuclear-family units within an extended family) and of a strong husband-wife bond. Lineage links are traditionally more important than the husband-wife unit. One can question the extent to which one can even speak of a husband-wife-child unit since neither economic nor kinship links are traditionally thus defined. Along the economic dimension, the subsistence unit is commonly the woman and the children living with her, whereas along the kinship dimension the children belong to the husband's lineage, to which the wife does not belong (or, in matrilineal groups, to her lineage, to which he does not belong). In such cases where the broader lineage rather than the direct line is important, it is only normal that a wide range of other kin may exercise not only *joint responsibilities* in children but also *joint rights* in them.

Some recognition of the role of others in social reproduction is apparent in the demographic literature. One finds references, for example, to the fact that the grandparental generation may exert a not insignificant influence on fertility decisions and childrearing, or to the fact that various kin may help parents financially (for example with school fees) or may themselves press claims for economic assistance. By and large, however, this recognition has remained limited, with these features being perceived as affecting the parent-child relationship only marginally rather than fundamentally. The role of others in social reproduction has been seen largely as comparable to grace notes, or ornaments in a piece of baroque music—as forming a characteristic aspect of the whole but not impinging on the basic structure. Much more than this is involved, however. Rights and responsibilities may not merely be *shared*, they may also be *transferred*; not only may they be *delegated* to others, they may also be *preempted* by others. As a Mende saying puts it, "A child is not for one person" (Bledsoe, 1985).

The second part of the explanation lies in the commonly overlooked implications of the potential *segmentation* of parental roles. Not all aspects of social reproduction need be vested in the same adult or be transferred together: it is possible to transfer just some of them, or just one, along with the associated rights and responsibilities. Segmentation greatly facilitates the spreading of social reproduction beyond the primary parents to "proparents." Moreover, although transfers often occur within the kin group, segmentation of parental roles facilitates transfers beyond the bounds of the kin group. The result is that social reproduction constitutes a very flexible system in which the distribution of children and of parent-child relationships brought about by fertility can be extensively manipulated socially.

The concept of a unitary parental role, however, dies hard in population studies. This is partly because it lends itself to relatively simple analytical models. But it is also because most practitioners come from other culture-regions where a unitary role is almost everywhere the norm and strongly segmented parental roles are culturally almost unimaginable. Before proceeding further, it is, therefore, useful to give a brief review of the various components of social reproduction *sensu lato* and to see how they are often segmented in sub-Saharan Africa. Our overview is based on the classic work of Esther Goody (1982), to which the reader is referred for a detailed discussion.

PATTERNS OF PARENTING

The Components of Social Reproduction

Next to the biological aspect of reproduction, that is, the bearing and begetting of children, Goody distinguishes four universal components of social reproduction.

1. Provision of civil and kinship identity and status (including residence rights and inheritance/succession rights)
2. Nurturance
3. Training for an adult role
4. Sponsorship into the adult community as a full member of it.

These four components are quite distinct from each other and do not have to be located in the same adult.

Provision of Identity

Civil and kinship identity is derived from one's social parents, almost invariably defined as the biological mother and/or a clearly defined male. In most societies that male is defined as the woman's husband; in some (e.g., the Gonja [E. Goody, 1982, p.9] and the Mossi [Gruenais, 1981]) it is the child's biological father. The identity provided by these parents can be transmuted to an identity derived from others only through adoption, that is, through a change of jural identity.

Although adoption is found in other regions, it is virtually unknown in tropical Africa. Most references to "adoption" in the literature seem to refer in fact to transfer of childrearing or of sponsoring rather than to transfer of identity. In general the identity a child acquires by birth cannot be manipulated subsequently in sub-Saharan societies.[2] The nonmanipulability of this aspect of parent-child relationships is explained in large part by its cultural importance within the region. Religious beliefs concerning the importance of the ancestors, and the importance of descendants for performing ancestor rites, are probably highly significant here. These alone are insufficient, however. In other cultures that stress the importance of the ancestors and/or continuation of the line, adoption may be used to ensure descendants. Sub-Saharan Africa, however, is rich in other mechanisms for ensuring descendants (J. Goody, 1976) that mesh with the other cultural features and institutions typical of the region—especially the absence of strong nuclear-family forms in general and of a strong husband-wife bond in particular, on the one hand, and the importance of the kin *group* rather than just the direct line, on the other. Most striking here is the widespread institution of polygyny. Divorce and remarriage form a second common mechanism. Finally there are a large number of other, somewhat less common, mechanisms. Here we may mention the transfer of sexual and reproductive rights to another member of the descent group in the event of apparent infertility or widowhood, or the raising of seed for the individual by another member of the descent group (e.g., levirate and sororate); retention of a daughter to bear children for a father who has no sons (e.g., among the Krobo [Huber, 1963, cited in E. Goody, 1982, p. 11]); and "woman-marriage" to provide children when a father or a husband has had no sons (e.g., among the Lovedu [Krige, 1974]). Expressed another way, there is no need for adoption to ensure descendants; instead, reproductive rights need not be restricted to marriage with just one partner. Significant too is the widespread practice of bridewealth, by which the reproductive capacity of the woman is transferred from her natal kin to her husband's lineage. Adoption is sometimes seen as being incompatible with bridewealth, especially where the latter is high and nonreturnable and its payment diffuse; too many parties then have an interest in a woman's child either to necessitate or to permit his/her ready transfer to another group. This is, however, merely a reflection of a more general principle, namely that children traditionally belong to the lineage rather than just to their parents. And this applies not only to societies where, traditionally, rights *in genetricem* are transferred out of the woman's natal kin group (through acceptance of bridewealth), but also to those where they are retained by her natal kin group.

Adoption would be inconsistent with this constellation of institutions. Not surprisingly, therefore, it often appears quite alien and is even viewed with horror. At the same time, the absence of adoption may be linked to the redistribution of the other components of social reproduction. It may indeed be the case, as Esther Goody suggests, that the very immutability of identity in tropical Africa contributes to the ease with which the other three components of reproduction can be manipulated. If the child's identity and the rights and responsibilities between parent and child established by it cannot be called into question, then redistribution of other rights and responsibilities concerning children is facilitated.

Childrearing and Sponsorship

Nurturance. The task of nurturance is almost everywhere normatively allocated to the biological mother, especially in the case of very young children. The physiological constraints of breastfeeding are obviously dominant here—though the classic case of nurturance by others is precisely that of wet nurses in nineteenth-century Europe. Wet nurses are rarely used in sub-Saharan Africa: the biological mother is responsible for suckling her child, and also, in most cases, for care of the child in other respects too.

Once the child is weaned, these physiological constraints fall away and fostering becomes a possibility. However, up to the age of about 6 or 7, nurturance continues to be allocated typically to the mother. According to Goody, children under 6 or 7 are unlikely to be cared for by anyone other than their biological mother, even in those areas of West Africa where proparenthood for older children is widespread. The major exception she notes in Africa itself is widespread fostering of young children under family "crisis" conditions—widowhood, divorce, or remarriage. Where the children belong to her husband's lineage, they will be claimed by that lineage if he dies or the parents divorce. Where they belong to the mother's lineage, they may stay with her for a while. If she remarries, however, it may be considered preferable for her to delegate responsibility to one of her female kin than to take the children with her into the new marriage. The only other exceptions Goody notes involve the fostering of young children of West Africans studying overseas, who find it difficult to combine their study/work schedule with child care. Several more recent studies suggest, however, that even quite young children may leave their mother (see below, Differentials by Age and Sex).

Training. Children above the age of about 6 or 7 are ready to start either formal or informal preparation for an adult occupation and role. They are also able to supply useful labor. Their parents, however, are not necessarily the best-placed persons to provide the type of training desired. Nor are they necessarily those who can make the best use of the child's labor.

Looking first at the training aspect, we see that proparenthood is often used to enable children to acquire training of a kind the parents are not able to furnish themselves. Obvious examples are sending children away to attend school (educational fostering, Creole wardship) or to become apprentices in a particular craft or trade (apprentice fostering). They may also be sent away in order to acquire contacts or to establish or reinforce social ties that will be useful to them (or their family) later (alliance fostering). In the first case, such children provide little by way of labor to their proparents; in the second, however, they may provide considerable labor inputs. This is particularly true for some apprentices and for housemaids, where the child's labor input may be considerable relative to the practical training given.

But proparenthood in sub-Saharan Africa is not limited to situations where the proparents provide a type of training that is different from what the parents can provide. Kin may claim, or may be given, children to rear even when the type of rearing they provide is not fundamentally different. The stated reasons for this among the Gonja are that the proparents are better placed to insist on the discipline necessary for good upbringing (and for good labor productivity). Children may also be sent to proparents in need of a child's services: provision of assistance and companionship to grandparents by a foster child is common. So too is the giving of a child to a childless woman. Finally, as with younger children, widowhood, divorce, or remarriage may lead to children being reared by a proparent.

Sponsorship. Like training, sponsorship into adult society can take many forms. In Europe it traditionally involved marriage and the establishment of an independent economic unit; today it still involves achievement of economic independence, although the link with marriage has at least partially disappeared. In sub-Saharan Africa sponsorship for girls has traditionally involved celebration of puberty rights marking the threshold of womanhood and reproduction (more particulatly in matrilineal societies), or the actual transition to wife or mother (especially in patrilineal societies). For boys it most typically meant initiation. In all cases a range of kin could be involved as sponsors. Increasingly, and particularly in the more modernized areas, it is taking a more explicitly economic form—the provision of the training and, where necessary, the startup capital or the equipment needed to establish oneself in a particular profession. Here training and sponsorship tend to be intimately linked, with those who provide the training either indirectly or directly acting as full or partial sponsors. Thus the relative who acts as proparent or who has helped finance schooling is an indirect sponsor, whereas the master who provides skills to his apprentice is a more direct sponsor. Where the child's labor has been a relatively important element (as is the case with many apprentices and with most housemaids), the proparent/employer may be responsible for providing tools (e.g., a sewing machine) or startup capital, which effectively marks economic sponsorship into adult society.

Thus effective sponsorship can be seen to come from a wide range of proparents as well as from parents themselves.

Conclusions

Whatever the form it takes, proparenthood involves both rights and responsibilities for all the parties involved—parent, proparent, and child. In particular, it either establishes new sets of rights and responsibilities between child and proparent and between parent and proparent, or it reinforces existing ones. In the latter case especially, the resulting reciprocities may be diffuse and long term in nature. The child, in particular, is likely to carry long-term responsibilities towards his or her proparent, especially where the proparent played a significant role in training or in sponsorship.

There is a resonance evident between the absence of adoption in sub-Saharan Africa and the widespread segmentation of other parent-child reciprocities. Adoption was seen as redundant because descendants and the associated jural/religious reciprocities are assured in tropical Africa by the possibility of extending rights in reproduction beyond the single husband-wife unit. Similarly, both rearing and sponsorship into adult life can be assured for the child (even an orphan)—and also access to the rights accruing from rearing and sponsoring children can be assured for all adults—by extending rearing and sponsoring beyond the initial parent-child unit. In both cases, both the extent to which the potential is taken up and the way in which it is taken up may vary depending on other aspects of the social structure. Given the internal heterogeneity of the region one would expect considerable variation. Both features are, however, common throughout the region, and constitute one of the constellations of characteristics that may be peculiarly African.

DATA

The concept of proparenthood—particularly for children beyond the age of about 5 or 6—permeates daily life over large parts of the region. This is especially true in Western Africa where it appears to reach its highest levels and to manifest the greatest variety of forms. Even the most superficial outside observer can hardly fail to notice two of its more modern forms—both children living with foster parents while they attend school, and the preoccupation of well-to-do urban women with acquiring the services of reliable young girls as live-in housemaids/nannies, are readily apparent. In addition, references to proparenthood abound in African literature, both fiction and nonfiction. In the best-known childhood autobiographical works, for example, fostering as an institution is presented as both a common and a quite unremarkable part of everyday life. In an autobiographical work by Wole Soyinka (1981), a stream of children come and go from the Yoruba schoolmaster's household, sent to further their education and/or work as housemaids. In Laye's retelling of his early childhood experience in the Fouta Djallon (Laye, 1954), there are repeated references to the boys who lived in the compound as apprentices to his father, the village blacksmith; moreover, Laye's going to live with distant kin in order to pursue his schooling outside the village is among the key events of his story. In all cases, however, although the move to proparents may be a source of considerable personal upheaval, the institution itself is nowhere brought into question. It is probably precisely because of its normality that it has not yet formed the study object of many African social scientists (Fiawoo [1978] and Isiugo-Abanihe [1985] are exceptions), and most of the systematic studies on it have come from outsiders.

Previous Studies

Until recently, most of the studies that focused on child circulation were anthropological (e.g., Esther Goody primarily though not exclusively on the Gonja; Oppong on Dagbon [1971]; Skinner on the Mossi [1960,1961]; Schildkrout in southern Ghana [1973] and on the Hausa in Nigeria; Lallemand on the Mossi [1976] and Kotokoli [1980]; Etienne on the Baoulé [1979]; Brydon for Avatime [1979,1985]; Bledsoe and Isiugo-Abanihe on the Mende [1985, and this volume]; and Sanjek also on southern Ghana [1986]). In addition, there are numerous references to it in more general anthropological works (e.g., Fraenkel [1968] on Liberia). Despite the growing body of material provided by these studies, they largely failed to attract demographers' attention until very recently. As a result, the implications of extensive child circulation have been remarkably slow to penetrate the demographic literature.

The problem has not simply been a question of one discipline being unaware of work in another, although this factor doubtless played a role. That this was not the sole factor is shown by the fact that even Kreager's overview of the literature on fostering and adoption worldwide, prepared for IPPF (Kreager, 1980), largely failed to stir chords among people working in population studies. A second contributing factor is that these studies were largely unable to communicate effectively the *quantitative* importance of the phenomenon. Although they are often extremely rich in insights, they are also necessarily limited in scale, and many are limited in generalizability. The material ranges from the anecdotal (e.g., Smith's biography of Baba of Karo [1954]) to surveys of at most several hundred children (Isaac and Conrad [1982] on the Mende of Upper Bambara Chiefdom in Sierra Leone), with the majority of the individual studies focusing on a couple of dozen or fewer households. Moreover, with the exception of Goody, few of the authors have analyzed comparative material from more than one area and formulated theoretical generalizations from this. Thus it is perhaps not surprising that even Frank (1984) addressing specifically an audience of demographers, although able to alert them to the issues involved, was not fully able to convince many of those with little or no experience in Africa that the distinction between childbearing and childrearing is not only sufficiently *deep-rooted* but also sufficiently *widespread* to constitute a crucial element in discussions of reproduction in sub-Saharan Africa.

Large-scale data sets that might demonstrate the quantitative significance of the phenomenon more effectively have indeed been rare. Furthermore, the few available analyses based on them have tended to use summary indicators based on indirect data. Most demographic surveys in Africa have collected information on the number of children each woman has borne. To reduce the omission of children living elsewhere or of children who have died, three separate questions (the number of her children living with her, the number living elsewhere, and the number dead) have routinely been asked instead of just one direct question on the total number of children. Although not always coded and published separately, the answers to the second question, where available, yield information on the numbers or proportions of children living elsewhere. These are the data that have most often been proposed for analysis of mother-child coresidence patterns. Only Isiugo-Abanihe (1985) has attempted to go beyond this, using data contained in the Ghana census on individuals' relationship to the household head for a part of his work.[3]

This type of summary data is extremely frustrating, however. First, these data indicate which mothers' children have moved away but give no information about where they have moved to. Second and more importantly, they are not specific by age of the child; often they are not sex-specific either. Yet coresidence of mother and child may vary markedly by age or sex of the child. Thirdly, and equally importantly, they refer on average to very young children. In order to exclude grownup, married children, the analysis must be limited to women married less than, say 15 years (or to women under, say, 30 years of age). Young children are inevitably overrepresented in such data because although the oldest women in this group can have children of any age up to about 15, younger women can only have young children. The result is that although children born to women married less than 15 years can be any age between 0 and about 15, their average age is well under 5. Since the residence patterns of very young children are not likely to be the same as those of older children—very young children are more likely to be with their biological mother in nearly all societies—the results obtained may be quite seriously misleading.

In other words, for study of child-residence and childrearing patterns there is an urgent need for comparative data that are both large-scale and representative on the one hand, and also age- and sex-specific on the other hand, in order to complement the anthropological work.

New Data and Their Potential

The surveys conducted in Africa in the context of the World Fertility Survey (WFS) provide, for most of the countries concerned, not only the above type of summary measures but also a unique set of unexploited data. Not only are these data both age- and sex-specific, they also refer to large and representative samples of children in each age-sex group.

The surveys included not only an Individual Questionnaire administered to women of reproductive age, but also a Household Questionnaire in which all household members were recorded. Unfortunately in the Individual Questionnaire, although information was sought about each child the woman had given birth to, no information at all was collected about the child's residence. The Household Questionnaire, however, provides a unique source of information. For each child enumerated in a household, it was standard practice in the WFS to identify the child's mother, if present in the same household, and then to provide a code linking the child with that mother. The information was originally included in the design of the WFS to provide data for estimating recent levels of fertility: for example, allowing for mortality, the proportion of women aged 34 with a child aged 4 estimates the fertility rate 4 years before the survey of women then aged 30. Strangely enough, the procedure was retained in nearly all the surveys carried out in Africa in the context of the WFS (except Senegal), despite the fact that the method is largely inapplicable in these countries precisely because so many children are not living with their mothers (and also because of the limited knowledge of ages). Its inclusion turns out to be a windfall, however, because it provides a unique source of information on whether mother and child coreside. For children whose mother was not in the household a special code indicating that the mother was not enumerated in household was used.

The possibilities offered by these data are enormous. Firstly, sample sizes are unusually large. A total of nearly 300,000 young persons under age 20 are included in the WFS Household Files for the seven countries for which we have permission to use these data (Cameroon, Ghana, Ivory Coast, Kenya, Lesotho, Nigeria, and Sudan). Even if we restrict attention to children under 15 in order to facilitate exclusion of those who are already married or otherwise independent of their parents (and if we also exclude the few persons under 15 who were already married or recorded as a household head), there are still 225,000. The Cameroon survey in particular is a tremendous resource, with nearly 80,000 children under 15. These sample sizes are large enough to permit reliable age- and sex-specific estimates for major subgroups and regions representing a wide variety of populations.

Second, we can link the information on mother and child coresidence with a large range of other information. Through record linkage *within* each Household File, it is possible to link both the children and the information on their mother's residence with household composition variables and with characteristics of the household head. Some of the WFS Household Questionnaires included rather detailed information on the household and/or the socioeconomic characteristics of all household members: again Cameroon stands out here for its wealth of information, although the Ivory Coast, Nigeria, and Sudan should also be mentioned for their range of data. In these countries extensive analyses by socioeconomic subgroup should be possible. Furthermore, in all countries—even those with only limited information in their Household Questionnaires—it is possible through file linkage to link the data for children contained in the Household Files with the data collected in the Individual Questionnaire for women of reproductive age, available in standard form for all participating countries in the Standard Recode Files. In other words, it is possible not only to estimate the *prevalence* of nonmaternal residence and differentials by region or socioeconomic group, but also to analyse the *patterns* of child circulation. These data should, for example, permit us to assess two aspects of child redistribution that are of considerable demographic importance. We can examine not only the redistribution of children between socioeconomic groups but also the extent to which irregularities in the "natural" distribution of children—either between individuals or over the individual's life course—are smoothed out by redistributing the children from households with an abundance of children to those experiencing a shortage either as a result of subfecundity or because of advanced age. Put another way, we can examine the extent to which the distribution of children provided by fertility is socially manipulated.

In this chapter we present the first results from the first stage in analysis of these data, that is, estimation of the prevalence of nonmaternal residence and examination of its determinants. Our purpose is simply to document the extent of nonmaternal residence and to set the stage for subsequent work on the details of child-circulation patterns and on their implications.

Some Qualifications

Before presenting the results, we should mention a couple of cautionary notes:

Conceptual Issues.   Our data refer to nonmaternal residence; this is not synonymous with child-fostering, although it is often referred to as though it were. *Fostering* refers to the assumption by someone other than a social parent of the rights and responsibilities associated with domestic provision of one or more of the functions of childrearing. It does not refer to residence as such, although by definition the child is unlikely to live in the same household as his or her social parent.

1. Fostering typically involves the child residing away from both social parents. *Nonmaternal residence* refers only to the mother; in some cases children may be living with their father. Fostering arrangements can thus be seen as a subset of nonmaternal coresidence patterns.
2. Lack of common residence does not necessarily mean lack of contact or full transfer of the maternal role. It can happen that a child who is not living with his or her mother is living close by. If this occurs in a case where the maternal role was already relatively limited (for example, an older boy in a society where the father is the adult primarily responsible for the upbringing and training of boys), residence nearby rather

than actual coresidence may have only a small impact on the mother-child relationship. Thus whereas transfer of the parental role is the essential element in fostering, it is not necessarily present in non-maternal child residence. Where mother and child do not live together, however, it commonly means that the mother is no longer the primary childrearing agent: someone else has primary authority over and responsibility for the child.

These two considerations imply that nonmaternal residence is a phenomenon of interest in its own right; one which incorporates fostering but which is broader in scope.

Data Issues. As is the case with marriage and, indeed, with all the most interesting phenomena in African demography, the data should certainly not be treated as perfect.

1. *Reporting on a social rather than a biological mother* may occur in surveys, either as a result of genuine ignorance as to the identity of the biological mother or as a result of misunderstanding of the intent of the question. However, we suspect that the former is infrequent even if not entirely absent and that in the context of the WFS, with its strong emphasis on biological motherhood, errors of the second type were probably kept relatively low. To the extent that such errors are present they will lead to conservative estimates of the proportions of children not living with their mother.

2. The data refer to *residence in the same household* and thus are sensitive to the definition of household used. Again, in the context of the WFS—this time because of its strong emphasis on comparability—although differences in the definition of household may have occurred, they are likely to be less serious here than with most other data sets. Some differences may remain, however, particularly in the treatment of polygynous unions.

3. Given the difficulty sometimes experienced in defining who constitutes a "usual" resident, preference is often given to a de facto population definition in demographic analysis. Here, however, that could lead to overestimates of the phenomenon of interest: children of women who had gone away for just a short time on business or to visit their families would be counted as not residing with their mother. We have, therefore, not adoped a de facto definition here. We have considered the mother to be residing in the same household of the child if she was listed as either a de jure or a de facto member of it. As a result, our estimates of the levels of nonmaternal residence are likely to be slightly conservative the more so since respondents are more likely to have used overgenerous than overrestrictive definitions of "usual" residents of their households.

4. Finally we should note that the original WFS Household Files were not standardized or edited as intensively as the Standard Recode Files. We have, however, made systematic checks of the main variables used for this analysis, correcting any obvious errors.

Overall, we believe the data to be perfectly usable. The fact that we find quite good correspondence when we compare estimates for adjacent, related populations that were enumerated in the separate national surveys of two different countries is most reassuring.

FIRST RESULTS: THE PREVALENCE OF NONMATERNAL RESIDENCE

Overall Prevalence by Region

Proportions of children not living with their mother by age and sex are given in table 9.1 for each of the major regions used in the WFS reports. The corresponding sample sizes can be found in table 9.2. Figure 9.1 gives an overall impression: it maps the percentages of all children under 15 who are not living with their mother for some fifty-five regions (Lesotho is excluded only for reasons of space).

A distinct regional pattern is observed. The percentages are less than 10 percent throughout Sudan, in Eastern Kenya, and parts of Northern Nigeria. Ten to 20 percent is typical for most of Kenya and much of Cameroon, as it is for all the rest of Nigeria and the north of the Ivory Coast.[4] More than 20 percent of children are not living with their mothers, though, in parts of Southern Cameroon and throughout Southern Ivory Coast. The general pattern that emerges from these data is quite plausible, being in broad agreement with other, more fragmentary information indicating that child circulation is more limited in Eastern than in Western Africa, and agreeing with the fact that, within West Africa, particularly high levels of child circulation in Ghana and Southern Ivory Coast have drawn comments from several anthropologists (in addition to those already cited, see Clignet [1970]).

The percentages not *currently* residing with their mother among all children under 15 are of course well below the percentages who *ever* live away from their mother: in general, children are relatively unlikely to leave their mother in the very first years of life, and even older children who leave their mother do not necessarily spend all the rest of their childhood years away from her. The percentages *ever* living elsewhere are probably more closely approached by the percentages away from their mother in our oldest category, children aged 10–14. There are mapped in figure 9.2. A similar general pattern emerges here as in figure 9.1, though at markedly higher levels and with more marked differentials. Whereas the figures for Sudan and Kenya here are nearly all in the range of 10 to 19 percent (as are those for Northern Nigeria too), the whole of Cameroon, Ghana, and Ivory Coast, together with

TABLE 9.1 Percentage of Children Not Residing with Their Mother, by Sex and Age, Major Regions

Age	0–14			0–4			5–9			10–14		
Sex	T	M	F	T	M	F	T	M	F	T	M	F
CAMEROON												
South-Central & Yaounde	24.4	24.4	24.4	16.7	16.0	17.4	27.2	27.3	27.0	32.2	32.8	31.6
Coast & Douala	19.0	18.5	19.5	7.5	7.3	7.7	21.8	21.4	22.2	34.8	34.2	35.3
East	18.6	18.8	18.3	8.7	9.0	8.4	21.9	21.5	22.3	30.5	32.0	29.0
Southwest	17.2	17.1	17.4	6.3	5.6	6.9	17.8	17.0	18.6	32.5	34.0	31.0
West	17.2	16.8	17.5	8.1	8.0	8.2	20.0	18.4	21.5	26.7	27.3	26.0
North	17.0	17.2	16.8	7.4	6.5	8.3	20.4	20.1	20.7	28.7	30.4	26.5
Northwest	13.0	12.4	13.7	6.3	5.6	7.0	15.1	14.4	15.8	20.2	19.6	20.8
GHANA												
Volta	27.0	27.9	26.0	14.3	15.4	13.3	27.5	27.7	27.3	40.3	40.7	39.8
Western	25.6	22.9	28.4	14.0	12.6	15.5	28.3	26.3	30.2	38.0	33.1	42.6
Eastern	24.5	23.9	25.0	17.1	17.1	17.1	25.8	25.4	26.3	31.7	30.9	32.4
Central	23.7	22.4	25.2	14.9	13.8	16.2	26.8	24.9	28.9	31.5	31.2	31.7
Brong-Ahafo	23.0	21.6	24.5	15.3	15.5	17.1	26.6	25.5	27.9	27.4	25.7	29.1
Greater Accra	22.6	18.5	24.4	9.7	8.3	11.0	21.6	20.8	22.6	38.8	30.7	45.8
Ashanti	22.0	20.9	23.3	10.8	9.6	12.1	26.0	23.4	28.7	34.2	33.7	34.6
Northern	14.6	14.4	14.7	4.1	3.2	5.1	17.7	18.3	17.3	26.5	26.7	26.2
Upper	13.6	11.6	13.3	6.1	6.2	6.0	11.9	11.2	12.6	21.7	19.2	24.4
IVORY COAST												
Forest	21.2	20.5	22.0	7.4	6.8	8.2	24.6	22.9	26.2	39.9	39.6	40.3
Savannah	21.3	22.2	20.5	7.3	7.7	6.8	26.7	28.0	25.5	35.3	35.3	35.2

KENYA												
Western	16.1	15.4	16.8	10.2	12.4	8.1	17.8	16.0	19.4	22.2	18.9	25.1
Nyanza	14.6	14.3	15.0	6.9	7.9	5.9	16.1	14.8	17.4	22.6	21.8	23.2
Rift Valley	11.8	10.6	12.8	5.6	4.9	6.3	12.5	12.2	12.8	19.6	17.6	21.1
Coast incl. Mombasa	11.7	11.4	11.9	6.2	6.7	5.7	14.0	12.3	15.5	17.3	18.3	16.7
Central & Nairobi	11.3	10.2	12.3	6.0	6.1	6.0	11.2	10.4	12.2	18.3	15.6	20.8
Eastern	9.8	10.3	9.2	7.0	7.4	6.7	9.9	11.2	8.7	13.0	13.0	13.0
LESOTHO	20.7	20.8	20.5	11.6	11.3	11.9	22.9	23.0	22.8	29.0	30.0	27.9
NIGERIA												
Southwest	12.9	12.0	13.8	5.4	4.9	5.9	14.3	14.2	14.4	21.6	19.5	23.7
Southeast	12.9	12.2	13.6	6.5	7.4	5.7	13.6	11.4	15.8	20.1	18.9	21.1
Northeast	10.5	11.0	10.1	5.9	6.6	5.2	12.1	12.5	11.6	15.9	15.9	15.9
Northwest	9.0	8.8	9.3	5.1	4.3	5.8	10.8	10.8	10.9	13.1	12.7	13.6
SUDAN												
Darfur	8.8	8.8	8.7	3.5	3.0	4.0	9.6	9.7	9.6	14.3	15.3	13.3
Kordofan	6.6	6.2	7.1	3.0	3.5	2.5	6.6	5.9	7.3	10.9	9.9	11.9
Eastern	6.2	6.6	5.8	2.4	1.9	3.1	6.4	7.2	6.1	11.0	11.3	8.6
Central	5.2	5.4	4.9	1.7	1.8	1.6	5.5	5.9	5.0	8.6	8.8	8.3
Khartoum	4.7	4.7	4.6	1.8	1.6	2.1	4.7	5.1	4.3	7.6	7.4	7.7
Northern	4.4	4.0	4.7	1.3	1.2	1.4	2.6	2.2	3.1	8.8	8.5	9.0

NOTES: —Exclusively urban areas have been linked to the surrounding/neighboring region.
—Children recorded as ever-married or as living with a spouse are excluded, as are those recorded as a household head.
Source: World Fertility Surveys, household files.

TABLE 9.2   Sample Size: Number of Children under Age 15 Recorded in the WFS Household Surveys by Major Regions

Region	N	Region	N
CAMEROON		*KENYA*	
South Central & Yaounde	11,691	Western	2,835
Coast & Douala	12,278	Nyanza	4,418
East	3,791	Rift Valley	4,793
Southwest	7,098	Coast (incl. Mombasa)	1,635
West	12,347	Central & Nairobi	5,428
North	20,881	Eastern	3,948
Northwest	11,624		
		total	23,057
total	79,710		
		LESOTHO total	36,960
GHANA			
Volta	1,555	*NIGERIA*	
Western	1,105	Southwest	4,879
Eastern	2,318	Southeast	7,612
Central	1,037	Northeast	6,278
Brong-Ahafo	1,213	Northwest	5,378
Greater Accra	1,284		
Ashanti	2,921	total	23,947
Upper	1,332		
Northern	947	*SUDAN*	
		Darfur	6,165
total	13,712	Kordofan	4,516
		Eastern	4,451
IVORY COAST		Central	9,450
Forest	10,846	Khartoum	3,718
Savannah	4,292	Northern	2,532
total	15,138	total	30,832
		TOTAL	223,356

NOTE: The few persons under 15 recorded as ever-married/living with a spouse or as a head of household are excluded.

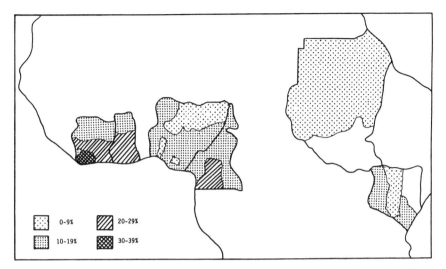

FIGURE 9.1. Percentage of Children under Age 15 Not Residing with Their Mother, by Administrative Region

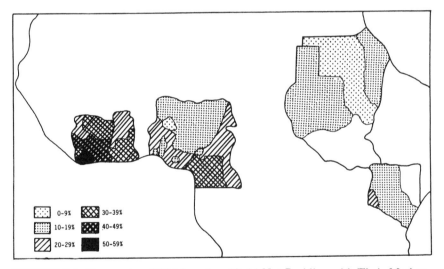

FIGURE 9.2. Percentage of Children Age 10–14 Not Residing with Their Mother, By Administrative Region

parts of Southern Nigeria, record figures in excess of 30 percent. In Southern Ivory Coast, more than 40 percent of children aged 10 to 14 (and in one area over 50 percent) were not living in the same household as their mother.

Clearly it is the case that over very wide areas, large numbers of children spend considerable portions of their childhood in another household than their mother's.

Differentials by Age and Sex

It is worth looking more closely at the pattern by age and sex, and at rural-urban differentials. Figure 9.3 plots selected quantiles from the frequency distribution of the regional percentages for each age-sex group. For the youngest children (ages 0–4), the percentage not living with their mother is typically in the range 5 to 12 percent, although even at this young age higher percentages are found. There are only limited indications of differences between sons and daughters. For age group 5–9, the percentage of children not living with their mother rises to typical values in the range 10 to 22 percent. Again there is little indication of a marked sex differential. By age group 10–15, however, not only have typical values risen to 20 to 30 percent, with some very high values, but there is also a slight but clear tendency for girls to be away more than boys.

More information on this differential is given in figure 9.4, which portrays rural-urban differentials.[5]

Figure 9.4 shows that for the youngest age group (0–4 years), the percent-

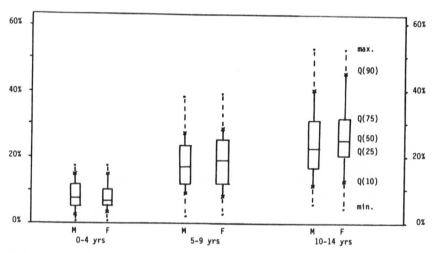

FIGURE 9.3. Distribution (Selected Quantiles) of Regional Percentages of Children Not Residing with Their Mother, by Age and Sex (56 Regions)

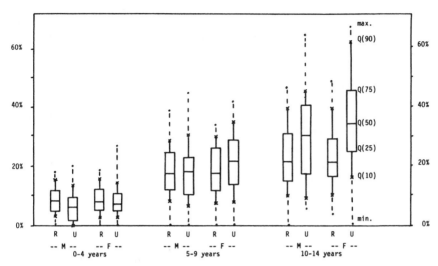

FIGURE 9.4. Rural-Urban Differentials in the Frequency Distribution for the Percentage of Children Not Living with Their Mother, by Age and Sex (55 Regions)

age of children not residing with their mother is systematically higher in rural than in urban areas. Either there is more circulation of young children in rural than in urban areas, or young children are being sent out of the urban areas. Although it is impossible with these data to disentangle these two possibilities, we suspect that the second may be increasingly important. Out-fostering of very young children from urban to rural areas has now been observed for several regions—for the Mende by Bledsoe (Bledsoe and Isiugo-Abanihe, in this volume), the Avatime by Brydon (1985), and in Zambia by Hansen (personal communication, 1986). There is a growing body of evidence that women find it hard to make child care arrangements for young children in urban areas, and that many find the presence of young children a financial, logistic, and even a social burden. Although the well-to-do may be able to employ housemaids, nannies, or *ayahs* to look after their young children, other women appear to prefer sending their children elsewhere, including to rural areas, at least until they reach school age. Some mothers say that rural conditions provide a better environment for their young children than do the towns. It may indeed be in the interests of the young child of a polygynously married woman or divorcée who cannot care for her child herself, to be left in the care of kin or with a neutral party rather than with a cowife or the husband's new wife (both persons commonly perceived as not having the child's welfare at heart, or even as being plainly hostile toward the child). Sending the child to a rural area may also be financially advantageous to the parents. Finally, sending the child to the home village may help reinforce links there and hence the position of both parent and child within the village.

Whatever the underlying reasons, it is certainly true that declines in breast-feeding in general and the increasing availability of bottle-feeding, of infant formula, and of various milk products and other weaning foods mean that physiological constraints necessitating coresidence of babies and very young children with their mothers are weakening.

For children aged 10–14 there are large rural-urban differentials for both sexes, particularly for girls. The proportions of both boys and girls not with their mothers are significantly higher in urban than in rural areas. This is probably largely the result of actual rural-urban movement related to the concentration of secondary schools in urban areas (see Gould [1985] for a discussion of education circulation in East Africa, Saint-Vil [1981] or Antoine sexes, particularly for girls. The proportions of both boys and girls not with their mothers are significantly higher in urban than in rural areas. This is probably largely the result of actual rural-urban movement related to the concentration of secondary schools in urban areas (see Gould [1985] for a discussion of education circulation in East Arica, Saint-Vil [1981] or Antoine [1983] on the Ivory Coast, and Sanjek [1986], for example), related to the better training and employment possibilities in the towns and, above all, for girls, to the demand for housemaids.

It is abundantly clear from these data that child circulation is a major phenomenon affecting sizable proportions of the population and that there are significant differentials to be explained. The extent of nonmaternal residence among very young children suggests in addition that child circulation may take forms other than the traditional ones of fostering originally studied. Before proceeding further, however, we need to consider the adequacy of the approach adopted so far. Analysis just by administrative region and by level of urbanization is in fact inadequate, for both methodological and substantive reasons.

Child circulation is a form of relocation or migration, and to analyze it most effectively using geographical units we need to have information on the place of origin of the children. Alternatively we need to use analysis units that form closed populations. Here we have neither. There is no indication of where the children originated, only of where they were residing at the time of the survey. Moreover, although administrative regions may be relatively closed in terms of their population (at least for many of the areas covered), not all are closed, and a breakdown of them into separate rural and urban areas is a clear contravention of the methodological requirements. We have already mentioned the impossibility of distinguishing differentials in circulation within two subregions from circulation from one to the other.

Moreover, categories based on "administrative regions" and the distinction "urban–rural" are both poor proxies for a host of social organization variables of key relevance for the study of child circulation in Africa.

SOCIAL ORGANIZATION AND THE PREVALENCE OF NONMATERNAL RESIDENCE

A Model

Esther Goody's classic work on fostering developed a model in which fostering is a function of kinship, marriage, and inheritance systems on the one hand, and of social and political complexity on the other. In essence, the first group of variables determines both the extent to which the members of the lineage(s) to which the child belongs, have an interest in exercising direct rights over the child and the extent to which a child has property or other rights elsewhere. (It can also, through the intermediary of residence patterns, affect the extent to which it is in the direct interest of the parents, particularly the mother, to send a child elsewhere to live with kin in order to maintain close contacts and/or support there later—for example, in those societies where marital residence is neither uxorilocal or matrilocal but where women return to live near their own kin in old age). The second set determines the extent to which circulation of children, not only to kin but also to nonkin, can be used to develop or strengthen patron-client or alliance relationships either for training or to enhance social mobility.

Goody summarized the general implications of these considerations with three broad propositions concerning traditional fostering patterns (E. Goody, 1982, p. 275):

1. In undifferentiated segmentary societies, parental roles are unitary and there is little delegation of childrearing; these societies are characterized by very little, if any, fostering other than as response to family "crises" such as divorce or widowhood. In undifferentiated societies with matrilineal or double-descent systems, parental roles are not unitary; generally, however, only jural status and reciprocities involve anyone other than the biological parents (e.g., the mother's brother), while childrearing is still vested primarily in the biological parents and there is little occasion for fostering outside crisis situations.

2. Differentiated states are characterized by fostering extending beyond response to family crises. Goody makes in addition a distinction between simple differentiated states and more complex hierarchical states:

3. *Simple differentiated states* are characterized by fostering primarily to kin.

4. *Complex hierarchical states* are characterized by a greater importance of fostering to nonkin as well as to kin and by fostering for social mobility and for forging alliance or patron-client relations.

As Goody also indicated, this model can readily be extended beyond traditional social structures to include the effects of increasing social and economic differentiation associated with contact with other populations (particularly trading and colonial contacts) and with modernization. Indeed, her model implies increasing levels of child circulation, especially circulation to nonkin for education, training, and sponsorship purposes, with the increasing social differentiation associated with modernization. The model could also be extended to include changes in kinship, marriage, and inheritance systems, although this seems less urgent given the slower pace at which these appear to be changing.

In Goody's model, modernization was not treated as a separate dimension but rather as an extension of the complexity variable. Figure 9.5 shows a simple extension that incorporates not only modernization as distinct dimension but also the fact that our data relate to nonmaternal residence rather than to fostering. Two sets of primary variables are distinguished. In the first are found the intensity and patterns of child circulation. In the second are found a series of variables reflecting other aspects of social organization. These are grouped under three headings:

Kinship and Marriage Variables

1. The form and strength of the lineage organization and inheritance systems provide an indicator of the potential interest of other lineage members in childrearing.

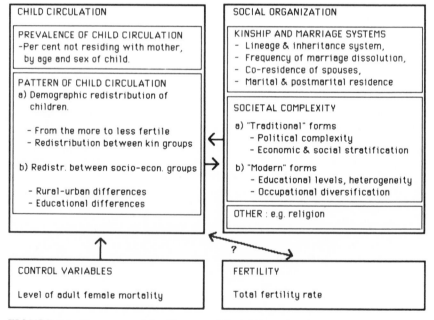

FIGURE 9.5. Nonmaternal Residence and Social Organization

2. Women's marriage and residence patterns affect both the possibility for her children to reside with her and the desirability of having at least one raised elsewhere. We distinguish three key variables here:

3. Coresidence of spouses may constrain the possibilities for coresidence of children and their mothers since, where spouses do not live in the same household, it is not uncommon for the older children, more particularly the boys, to live with their father rather than with their mother.

4. Frequency of marriage dissolution also constrains the possibilities for mother-child coresidence, since older children of both sexes are then unlikely to stay with their mother: in patrilineal societies they are most likely to follow the husband or to go to a member of his lineage; in matrilineal ones they are more likely to go to one of their mother's kin.

5. Marital residence rules *in combination* with the residence patterns of women in old age, after divorce, or following widowhood determine the desirability of sending at least one child to be raised in the place the mother will later live.

"Traditional" Forms and Levels of Societal Complexity

1. Complexity of the traditional political structure.
2. Socioeconomic stratification as reflected in the traditional occupational or class structure.

"Modern" Forms and Levels of Complexity

1. Educational levels and heterogeneity.
2. Occupational diversification related to modernization.

Finally, two additional sets of variables have been included in figure 9.5 to complete the overall model, namely a control variable (the level of female adult mortality) and fertility itself.

Obviously regional and rural–urban breakdowns are as inadequate to handle this type of model as they are methodologically limited. The use of *ethnic group* as a unit of analysis, however, provides a solution to both substantive and methodological problems. Our further analysis proceeds, therefore, on the basis of results for ethnic groups.

Ethnic Group as Units of Analysis

Using ethnic groups with the WFS Household Questionnaires is not straightforward. We need, therefore, to describe our procedures in some detail.

Direct information on ethnic groups is available for all children only in Cameroon, although we can assume that practically all the children in the Lesotho survey are Sotho. In the Ivory Coast, ethnic group was asked only for persons over age 15; we have linked the household head's data to each child and made the simplifying assumption that children were of the same ethnic group as their head of household.[6] In Sudan, too, ethnic group was not ascertained for individuals but at the level of the household; here, unfortunately, the meaning of the codes used for ethnic group is not available, so Sudan must be dropped from the analysis.[7]

In countries where ethnic group was not ascertained at all in the Household Questionnaire, we must use instead information from the Individual Questionnaire administered to women of reproductive age. In other words, we must link the data from two files. One possible procedure would be to identify for each child in the Household Files the data for his or her mother (if present) in the Standard Recode Files and then to assign to each child the ethnic group of the mother. Where the mother was not present one might assign the ethnic group of, say, the oldest woman interviewed in the household. Unfortunately, quite apart from any errors that might be introduced by interethnic marriages, this procedure would have the effect of excluding all children enumerated in households where there was no woman of eligible age interviewed. Since we suspect that a not insignificant portion of child circulation is movement of children to elderly persons, to help them in their household tasks and to provide companionship, this would be a potentially very serious loss. We have, therefore, opted for an alternative approach. We first split the Standard Recode Files into the smallest sampling areas used (there are between 150 and 250 areas per country in the countries concerned) and examined the ethnic distribution of women of reproductive age in each area. We then assigned to each child in the Household Files a probability of belonging to each ethnic group equal to the proportion of women in that ethnic group in his or her sample area. In other words, when making estimates for ethnic group A, each child has received a weight equal to the proportion of women in his or her sampling area who were from group A. Since the ultimate sampling units were usually small and rather homogeneous ethnically, this works rather well. In terms of the ethnic groupings used here, on average over 80 percent of the women in an area belonged to the same group; just over one-quarter of the areas were fully 100 percent homogeneous, and in over half, 90 percent or more of the women interviewed belonged to a single group.[8]

Finally, we should note that data on ethnic group can be quite hard to collect. The amount of assistance given the interviewers and coders (e.g., lists of the various names used for the different ethnic groups and subgroups, and detailed instructions concerning the way in which subgroups were to be recorded) varied considerably between countries. Moreover, ethnic group data can be extremely sensitive. Given the difficulties involved, it is perhaps not surprising that we cannot present results by ethnic groups for all the countries. Not only are ethnic group codes not available for Sudan, as we have already mentioned, but, in addition, permission to use the Nigerian data does not extend to publication of any data by ethnic group.

For this chapter we have used for each country the broadest ethnic groupings given in the Standard Recode Files (apart from a few exceptions related mainly to sample-size considerations). The disadvantages of using these particular groups stem from the fact that many are broad language groups rather than ethnic groups per se; some are, therefore, highly heterogeneous internally (e.g., the Northern Ghanaian groups). For these cases our data are rather bland averages over quite highly contrasting groups. The main advantage of using these groups is ready comparability with other analyses based on the WFS data, including analyses found elsewhere in this volume.

Our estimates of proportions of children not living with their mother, specific by the children's age and sex, are documented for the five countries where documentation is possible in table 9.3. Our subsequent analysis attempts to relate the age- and sex-specific levels of nonmaternal residence to selected social organization variables. More specifically we relate them here to the following:

1. Among the *kinship and marriage* variables we have used lineage organization, coresidence of spouses, and the frequency of marriage dissolution.

2. For *complexity of the "traditional" society* we have used an indicator of political complexity and a measure of caste and class stratification.

3. For *"modern" forms of societal complexity* we first examined four indicators of educational and occupational heterogeneity—the proportion literate among women aged 15–49, their average years of schooling, the proportion of their husbands working in high-level jobs or as employers themselves, and the proportion of husbands in the traditional self-employment sector. A factor analysis showed that the proportion literate loads much more heavily on the first factor than do any of the other three variables. For simplicity of interpretation, therefore, we have simply used the proportion literate. Proportion urban is also included as a separate variable in some analyses, since it is not strongly correlated with educational or occupational differentiation between ethnic groups.

Our covariates—*literacy, urbanization, marital residence,* and *coresidence of spouses*—were all derived from the WFS files. They are thus derived from the same sample of households as our child-residence variables. The first three can be derived immediately from the Standard Recode Files, which refer to women of reproductive age located in the households covered by the Household Questionnaire.[9] They were operationalized as follows:

1. *Literacy:* percentage reporting themselves as literate, women aged 15–49

TABLE 9.3 Percentage of Children Not Residing with Their Mother By Sex and Age; Major Ethnic Groups

Age	0–14			0–4			5–9			10–14			N
Sex	T	M	F	T	M	F	T	M	F	T	M	F	
CAMEROON													
Bakosi-Mbo, Bakundu-Balundu	17.0	17.1	16.8	6.8	6.3	7.2	17.2	17.2	17.2	31.4	32.5	30.4	3525
Douala	23.3	22.6	24.1	9.0	11.0	6.8	27.2	25.8	28.6	36.6	33.8	39.5	1028
Bafia	15.9	16.0	15.8	9.2	10.2	8.3	17.5	16.8	18.3	23.8	23.6	24.0	4237
Bassa	26.2	25.4	27.2	14.0	11.7	16.3	29.0	31.8	26.2	40.6	36.9	44.4	2168
Boulou, Fang	28.2	26.5	29.9	19.5	15.5	23.4	32.1	32.2	31.9	35.8	34.5	37.1	2675
Kaka	17.0	16.2	17.7	8.1	8.5	7.7	20.9	19.4	22.2	25.3	25.6	24.9	734
Maka	23.4	23.6	23.2	12.8	10.7	15.0	27.2	28.2	26.1	34.1	37.6	31.0	1616
Sanaga, Pygmy	22.1	23.1	20.9	15.3	16.4	13.8	20.9	21.6	20.2	33.3	33.3	33.3	471
Yaounde	24.8	24.9	24.6	16.8	16.6	17.0	27.2	27.6	26.8	33.2	33.3	33.0	6610
Bamenda	13.6	12.8	14.4	6.5	5.3	7.6	15.8	14.6	17.0	21.2	21.0	21.4	8636
Bamileke	16.5	16.0	16.9	6.2	5.9	6.6	19.0	17.2	20.8	29.3	30.6	27.9	15619
Bamoun	20.6	20.8	20.4	11.0	11.9	10.9	24.1	24.1	24.1	31.0	29.5	32.8	2871
Mbembe, Ekoi, Efik	15.1	14.3	15.9	6.8	6.6	7.0	18.0	16.1	19.9	24.1	25.1	23.3	3881
Widekun	16.5	17.9	14.9	5.5	6.1	5.0	17.0	18.7	15.3	31.6	31.0	32.4	1433
Adamawa, Benoue, Baya	20.7	21.4	19.9	9.9	8.3	10.0	23.7	23.1	24.4	34.4	37.2	30.3	4090
Fulani	22.9	22.5	23.4	10.0	9.6	10.4	28.5	27.4	29.6	36.8	37.1	36.5	4344
Logone, Chari	11.2	10.4	12.1	5.3	4.8	5.8	14.4	12.2	16.9	17.1	17.6	16.4	1590
Mandara, Wandala	15.5	16.4	14.5	17.0	17.3	16.6	19.5	20.6	18.3	25.9	26.9	24.6	4707
Shoa, Hausa	17.0	16.7	17.4	8.9	6.0	12.0	20.3	20.5	20.1	24.9	27.5	21.8	1661
Toubouri, Guiziga	12.1	12.1	12.2	4.6	3.4	5.8	13.9	13.6	14.2	22.9	24.1	21.3	4980
GHANA													
Fante	23.2	22.2	24.1	12.8	12.0	13.7	26.2	25.8	26.7	33.5	32.5	34.6	1232
Twi	23.2	21.7	24.8	13.4	12.2	14.6	25.4	23.3	27.7	33.1	31.6	34.6	5403
Other Akan	21.1	19.4	22.7	11.0	9.0	12.7	22.8	22.8	23.4	32.6	29.5	35.5	476
Ewe	25.4	25.6	25.2	14.1	14.0	14.2	27.4	27.4	27.5	36.5	37.2	35.7	1863
Ga-Adangbe	24.3	23.0	25.6	15.9	14.4	15.5	26.2	25.8	26.7	35.1	32.6	37.5	932

Guan	20.2	20.0	20.3	9.7	8.9	10.6	21.6	22.1	21.2	33.5	34.4	32.7	419
Mole, Dagbani	16.0	15.2	16.9	7.0	6.6	7.4	17.4	17.0	17.9	27.0	24.7	29.6	1917
Other	18.4	17.2	19.6	8.4	8.1	8.7	18.3	17.2	19.3	32.2	28.8	36.3	980
IVORY COAST													
Abe, Attie, Ebri	27.5	27.2	27.9	12.8	13.8	12.1	30.4	25.1	34.7	42.4	44.4	40.3	775
Agni	24.6	24.3	24.9	8.9	9.0	8.8	27.2	26.5	27.9	43.7	40.4	47.3	1360
Baoule	29.9	31.2	28.5	13.0	14.3	11.8	35.0	37.5	32.4	47.5	45.7	49.5	2644
Bete, Dida	33.1	32.8	33.4	10.5	7.5	13.8	38.0	38.0	38.1	52.8	54.7	50.7	1455
Gouro, Yacouba	22.6	20.4	25.1	6.0	5.6	6.4	25.2	23.6	26.8	49.4	45.0	53.8	823
Guere	19.3	19.3	19.4	9.0	10.0	8.3	20.6	20.7	20.4	32.7	28.8	37.8	729
Koulango, Senoufo	20.2	21.3	19.0	5.1	6.4	3.8	26.1	26.1	26.2	34.9	37.6	32.2	1678
Malinke	15.7	15.5	15.8	5.4	3.6	7.3	18.4	17.0	19.9	28.4	31.8	24.5	2542
Other (non-Ivoirien)	10.5	8.2	12.7	3.7	3.3	4.1	12.8	9.2	16.2	24.8	20.8	28.6	3059
KENYA													
Kikuyu	9.4	9.0	9.8	5.9	5.4	6.5	9.2	10.1	8.3	13.9	12.0	15.6	6194
Luo	15.8	14.6	16.9	6.2	6.4	6.1	17.9	15.8	20.2	25.4	24.2	26.6	3574
Luhya	16.4	15.9	17.0	10.0	12.2	8.0	18.3	16.4	20.0	23.0	20.4	25.4	3352
Kamba	10.8	10.6	11.0	7.7	7.0	8.4	11.5	12.5	10.6	13.8	12.9	14.7	2794
Kisii	11.0	11.5	10.5	7.1	9.5	4.8	12.5	11.9	13.1	14.3	13.8	14.7	1738
Meru, Embu	8.6	10.2	7.2	5.5	7.2	3.9	7.8	9.6	6.4	13.7	14.9	12.6	1724
Mijikenda	12.8	13.8	11.8	6.2	7.4	4.7	16.3	15.2	17.1	18.6	23.4	14.0	1151
Kalenjin	11.3	9.6	12.9	4.4	3.8	5.0	13.1	10.9	15.3	18.3	16.4	19.8	1746
Other	10.8	10.5	11.1	5.7	4.7	6.6	11.4	11.9	10.2	18.2	18.2	18.1	1110
LESOTHO													
Sotho	20.7	20.8	20.5	11.6	11.3	11.9	22.9	23.0	22.8	29.0	30.0	27.9	36960
NIGERIA	—	—	—	—	—	—	—	—	—	—	—	—	
SUDAN	—	—	—	—	—	—	—	—	—	—	—	—	

NOTES: —Children recorded as ever-married or as living with a spouse are excluded, as are those recorded as a household head.

—Sample sizes refer to weighted samples (see text).

SOURCE: World Fertility Survey household files, supplemented for Ghana and Kenya by ethnic group distributions from the WFS Standard Recode files.

2. *Urbanization:* percentage residing in urban areas, women aged 15–49
3. *Marriage dissolution:* percentage of all ever-married women aged 15–49 who have ever been divorced or widowed.

Our fourth covariate is defined analogously:

4. *Coresidence of Spouses:* percentage of all currently married women aged 15–49 recorded as living in the same household as their husband.

Unlike the first three, however, this fourth covariate was not derived directly from the Standard Recode Files. These files do include data from a question asked each currently married woman as to whether her husband usually lived in the same household as she did. However, the question used varied in content between countries. Moreover, the data obtained were not included in the Standard Recode Files for all the countries. We have, therefore, used an alternative source of information located in the Household Files. On each Household Questionnaire, a link was made between each husband and his wife or wives, and a code identifying him and his wife/wives (the "couple code") was included routinely in the Household Files. Women with no husband present received a special code. In some countries, an explicit distinction was made between those with no husband present because they did not have a husband at the time of the survey (single, widowed, and divorced women) and those whose husband was elsewhere; this distinction can also easily be made by drawing upon data for a separate variable on marital status. In these countries it is a simple matter to estimate the percentage of currently married women whose husbands were enumerated in the same household, using just the Household Files. Not all countries included information on marital status in their Household File, however. For Kenya and Ghana, for example, there is no separate variable for marital status, and for the couple code no distinction is made between women who have no husband and those whose husband is elsewhere. For these countries we have used the proportion of women not currently married obtained from the Standard Recode File to adjust the proportion of women with no husband present recorded in the Household File. The estimated proportion of currently married women whose husbands are elsewhere is given simply by:

$$\frac{[\% \text{ with no husband present (HH File)}] - [\% \text{ not currently married (SR File)}]}{[\% \text{ currently married (SR File)}]}$$

The data for our factors—*lineage organization,* traditional *political complexity,* and *stratification*—were extracted from Murdoch's Ethnographic Atlas (1962–1967, with updates through 1983), after identification of the ethnic group(s) in the Atlas corresponding most closely with the categories used in the WFS surveys. Since the number of observations incorporated in this analysis is rather small (sixty broad ethnic groups), we have reduced all the factors to simple dichotomies:

1. For our variable *lineage*, the small number of groups exhibiting bilateral or duolateral traits have been combined with the matrilineal groups:[10] our variable thus contrasts patrilineal societies (75 percent), with all the others (25 percent).

2. *Political complexity* contrasts societies with no chiefs or only petty chiefs on the one hand (65 percent), with states and with societies with paramount chiefs on the other hand (35 percent).[11]

3. *Stratification* contrasts societies with no stratification (or only despised, usually small, "caste" groups) (65 percent) with those exhibiting stratification by wealth or other more complex stratification (35 percent).[12]

Results

By way of exploration we pursued two lines. On the one hand, we conducted a factor analysis on the proportions of children not living with their mother in order to identify common patterns by age, sex, and rural-urban residence. On the other hand, we examined the effect of our social organization variables on nonmaternal residence levels using multiple classification analysis (MCA). First we did this on a very exploratory basis using the proportions by age; MCA is not the most appropriate technique in this regard, but it should suffice for the present exploratory purposes. Then we applied MCA to the factors extracted from the factor analysis. The results are presented in tables 9.4 through 9.6.

Turning first to the most exploratory MCA statistics on the proportions of children not residing with their mother, by age (table 9.4), we can note the following:

1. As expected, the explanatory power of our social-organization variables increases with the age of the child. The proportion of the variance in nonmaternal residence that they explain increases from 47 percent (39 percent, after adjustment for the large number of variables relative to the number of observations) for children under 5 years to 70 percent (66 percent after adjustment) for those aged 10–14. The effect of differences in social organization is clearly stronger for older than for younger children, who still tend to live with their mothers even in those ethnic groups that have social organization characteristics associated with high levels of nonmaternal residence in general.

2. Among the factors, lineage type is usually the most important factor in terms of zero-order associations, and it remains so when all variables are introduced simultaneously. Societies with matrilineal characteristics and those exhibiting any bilateral or duolateral traits tend to have slightly higher proportions of children not living with their mother. When the other variables are introduced, however, the effect generally becomes less marked (especially for the older children), although the beta values are statistically significant.

TABLE 9.4 Effect of Selected Social Organization Indicators on the Percentage of Children Not Living with Their Mother, by Age of Child

Age of child	0-4 ($\bar{X}$ = 8.96)		5-9 ($\bar{X}$ = 20.18)		10-14 ($\bar{X}$ = 27.64)		0-14 ($\bar{X}$ = 17.86)	
	Unadjusted deviation from $\bar{x}$	Adjusted deviation from $\bar{x}$	Unadjusted deviation from $\bar{x}$	Adjusted deviation from $\bar{x}$	Unadjusted deviation from $\bar{x}$	Adjusted deviation from $\bar{x}$	Unadjusted deviation from $\bar{x}$	Adjusted deviation from $\bar{x}$
1. *Factors*								
Lineage Organization								
Patrilineal	-.52	-.24	-1.52	-5.60	-1.90	-.04	-1.24	-.30
Matrilineal/bilateral	1.65	.76	4.82	1.78	6.06	.12	3.93	+.96
(eta/beta)	(.26)	(.12)*	(.39)	(.14)***	(.34)	(.01)***	(.37)	(.09)***
Political Complexity								
Minor or no chiefdoms	.08	-.10	.00	.05	.38	.68	.09	.14
Paramount chief- doms, states	-.15	.18	-.01	-.10	-.70	-1.28	-.17	-.26
(eta/beta)	(.03)	(.04)	(.00)	(.01)	(.05)	(.09)	(.02)	(.03)
Caste & Class Stratification								
None, or despised groups only	-.40	-.20	-.10	.05	.15	.36	-.13	.10
Stratified	.75	.38	.19	-.09	-.27	-.68	.25	-.18
(eta/beta)	(.16)	(.08)	(.02)	(.01)	(.02)	(.05)	(.03)	(.02)

2. *Covariates*

Percent urban	−.03	.10	.20***
Percent literate	.06**	.04	.02
Frequency of marital dissolution	.21**	.50***	.79***
Coresidence of partners	.05	.18*	.22

3. R^2

Unadjusted	.473	.646	.703
Adjusted	.392	.592	.657

***Significant at .001 level; **significant at .01 level; *significant at .05 level.

TABLE 9.5   Factor Analysis of Proportions of Children Not Living with
Their Mother, by Sex and Age (60 Ethnic Groups)

No Distinction between Rural and Urban Areas: Factor Loadings

	Factor 1
Boys 0–4	.718
Girls 0–4	.780
Boys 5–9	.965
Girls 5–9	.946
Boys 10–14	.917
Girls 10–14	.896
Eigenvalue	4.59
% of variance	76.6

Distinguishing Between Rural and Urban Areas: Factor Loadings

	Factor 1	Factor 2	Factor 3
Rural			
Boys 0–4	.867	.015	.226
Girls 0–4	.889	.002	.057
Boys 5–9	.862	.364	.179
Girls 5–9	.826	.401	.260
Boys 10–14	.617	.617	.273
Girls 10–14	.681	.554	.107
Urban			
Boys 0–4	.258	.103	.766
Girls 0–4	.138	.183	.885
Boys 5–9	.146	.714	.506
Girls 5–9	.128	.727	.530
Boys 10–14	.108	.864	.155
Girls 10–14	.225	.842	−.046
Eigenvalue	6.62	1.88	1.21
% of variance	55.1	15.6	10.1
Cumulated % of variance	55.1	70.8	80.9

NOTE: Factor analysis type PA1 in SPSS (varimax).

3. Somewhat surprisingly, political complexity and class/caste stratification—two variables one might expect to be of considerable importance in the light of Esther Goody's model of traditional child
fostering—do not exhibit significant systematic effects in the expected
direction. The deviations are often small (especially for the central age
group of children), and even where they are larger they do not reach
the 5 percent significance level. The irregular pattern may, of course,
be the result of relatively weak operationalization of these variables. It
is also possible, however, that "modern" forms of social differentiation
may be taking over from "traditional" ones.

TABLE 9.6 Effect of Selected Social Organization Indicators on the 3 Principal Components of Nonmaternal Residence Levels by Sex and Age of the Child

Component	"Rural" ($\bar{X} = 0.22$)		"Training" ($\bar{X} = 0.02$)		"Urban Nurturing" ($\bar{X} = -0.09$)	
	Unadjusted deviation from x̄	Adjusted deviation from x̄	Unadjusted deviation from x̄	Adjusted deviation from x̄	Unadjusted deviation from x̄	Adjusted deviation from x̄
Factors						
Lineage Organization						
Patrilineal	−.28	−.14	−.12	.15	−.29	−.30
Matrilineal/bilateral	.73	.36	.30	−.39	.74	.79
(eta/beta)	(.26)	(.13)*	(.17)	(.23)	(.52)	(.56)**
Political Complexity						
Minor or no chiefdoms	−.09	.18	.09	.16	−.08	−.10
Paramount chiefdoms, states	.17	−.36	−.18	−.31	.15	.20
(eta/beta)	(.07)	(.15)	(.12)	(.21)	(.12)	(.16)
Caste & Class Stratification						
None, or despised groups only	−.14	−.04	.13	.03	.17	.14
Stratified	.25	.07	−.23	−.05	−.29	−.24
(eta/beta)	(.11)	(.03)	(.16)	(.03)	(.25)	(.20)
Covariates						
Percent Literate		.03*		−.01		.00
Frequency of Marital Dissolution		.11***		.07***		.01
Coresidence of Partners		.05*		−.00		−.01
R^2						
Unadjusted	.609		.446		.392	
Adjusted	.544		.354		.291	

***Significant at .001 level; **significant at .01 level; *significant at .05 level.

4. Among the covariates measuring forms of heterogeneity associated largely with modernization, however, education does not appear to have a very strong effect. The beta coefficients for literacy are generally small and cannot be said to exhibit the pattern we had hypothesized, namely that higher levels of literacy would be associated, through greater educational heterogeneity, with more child circulation, especially for older children. The beta values for the two older age groups are negligible. The coefficient for the youngest age group, however, is not entirely negligible (and reaches the 1 percent significance level). Although higher levels of literacy do not appear to lead to more child circulation among older children, they do appear to lead to slightly higher proportions of very young children living away from their mothers. Presumably this is a reflection of the increasing difficulty in caring for very young children already discussed in the context of rural-urban differentials. It could also be related to the sending of children to their grandmothers when they are to be weaned—especially if they are to be weaned relatively young—as referred to by Isiugo-Abanihe (1985).

5. The estimated effects for degree of urbanization are however somewhat larger, particularly for older children, as was expected. For young children, higher levels of urbanization appear to have little impact on the proportion of children not living with their mother; perhaps any effect they have has already been taken up in the effect of literacy. For the oldest children the levels have a noticeable impact, as hypothesized: more urbanized ethnic groups have higher proportions not living with their mothers.

6. Our nuptiality variables play a more important role. As expected, coresidence of husband and wife has no effect for younger children, but it has a clear (and highly significant) effect for children above age 5. The magnitude of its effect is comparable to that of urbanization.

7. By far the largest effects of all are recorded for the variable measuring frequency of marriage dissolution. This variable is highly significant for all age groups and, as expected, increases markedly with age.

Overall, the marriage and kinship variables dominate over our social-complexity variables. Before jumping to conclusions, however, we should look at tables 9.5 and 9.6.

Table 9.5 shows the results of the factor analysis. When no distinction between rural and urban areas was made within each ethnic group (top panel), only one factor emerged: "all age and sex groups" loads relatively heavily on this factor (although the factor loadings are perceptibly lower for children under 5). When a distinction was made between rural and urban areas (bottom panel), three main factors emerged. The first is dominated by variation in rural values, the second by variations in values for older children (especially older urban children), whereas the third factor predominantly reflects variation among very young children in urban areas. Rural, presumably more traditional, variations in child circulation levels thus emerge as the most important component of interethnic variability. Next comes a dimension capturing differences in child-training and child-labor patterns, especially although not exclusively in urban areas. And this is followed by a dimension reflecting interethnic differences in child-nurturing patterns in urban areas.

Table 9.6 takes the three components derived from the factor analysis and submits them to an MCA. Since an explicit distinction was made between rural and urban areas in creating the components, the variable *urbanization* can be dropped. Before discussing the results we should note that statistical significance is slightly harder to reach here than in table 9.4, because of a slightly smaller sample size: ten ethnic groups with a very small number of observations for a particular age–sex–rural/urban residence group were excluded. Not surprisingly, the results for the first component—the general, predominantly rural, prevalence of nonmaternal residence—are quite similar to those shown in table 9.4. The proportion of the variance explained is about 60 percent (54 percent after adjustment). Frequency of marriage dissolution is the only variable to be significant at the 1 percent level, although both the other covariates—*coresidence of spouse*, and *literacy*—and the *lineage* factor are significant at the 5 percent level. For the second and third factors, which load heavily on particular age groups and on urban areas, the model performs less well overall here, with proportions explained around 30 to 40 percent. The beta values are, in general, smaller than in table 9.4, and the 5 percent significance level is rarely reached. As in table 9.4, however, systematic deviations in the expected direction are observed for *lineage organization* and for frequency of *marriage dissolution* (although, as expected, the latter has no impact on the "urban nurturing" factor). Comparing table 9.6 with table 9.4 shows that the main features of table 9.4 are confirmed at least in the rural patterns where the model performs best.

These results draw attention to two issues. First, they confirm the prime importance of kinship and marriage patterns in general, and of the prevalence of marriage dissolution in particular, for the prevalence of child circulation. Their importance should come as no surprise. Esther Goody has already identified the importance of lineage organization in general, and there are ample grounds for expecting marriage dissolution to play a major role: (1) To begin with, there is the *direct* effect of divorce (and widowhood) already referred to—what Esther Goody refers to as crisis fostering. The anthropological literature contains numerous references to children, especially older children, living with their father or with other relatives after a marriage is dissolved. (2) There may be *indirect* effects leading to nonmaternal residence even when the parents' marriage is still intact. For example there may be "insurance" against marital dissolution in societies marked by high instability of marriage (Frank, 1985). Where a married woman returns to her own kin at widowhood or divorce, there may be a greater tendency to ensure that at least one child is raised there in order to make certain that she always has a child to return to who will help support her; the child is also more likely to have rights there. Or, as Lallemand (1976) described for the Mossi, older women in the lineage may use a high risk of divorce as an argument for taking a child away from a woman who has not been married long in the compound, on the grounds that the child should be reared by women who have proven to be loyal and stable members of it. (3) Finally and more generally, as the Goodys suggested nearly 20 years ago in the context of child-fostering (J. Goody and E. Goody, 1967), circulation of children and circulation of women may be two intertwined elements of a single system. Where either marriage itself and/or the transfer of rights in a woman's reproductive capacity to her husband's lineage on marriage are essentially irreversable, neither children nor women circulate; where marriage and rights in a woman's reproduction are more flexible, both circulate.

The second finding is the rather surprising absence of systematic marked effects related to educational levels (at least as measured by literacy) and the only moderate effect of urbanization. These are found to play only a relatively minor role in determining differences *between* ethnic groups—although urbanization *is* significant for older children. However, this does not rule out the possibility that these variables exercise their influence *within* ethnic groups, affecting the pattern rather than the prevalence of child circulation. As figure 9.6 illustrates for literacy—which had almost no effect on between-group differences—within ethnic groups these variables indeed play a strong role. Within ethnic groups there are marked differentials in the proportion of children not living with their mother, depending on the literacy level of the area where the child lives. The prevalence of nonmaternal residence is nearly always higher for areas that have intermediate or high levels of literacy, indicating either more circulation within, or movement of children to, the more privileged areas. These variables can, therefore, be seen as constituting important determinants of internal redistribution *patterns*, even if they have only a small impact on the overall *level* of redistribution.

CONCLUSIONS

We certainly would not claim that these rather exploratory analyses are definitive. Much more remains to be done. Some points are, however, already clear.

First, these data demonstrate convincingly what several anthropologists have argued for some time, namely that nonmaternal residence is a widespread phenomenon and that it reaches such high levels over wide areas that

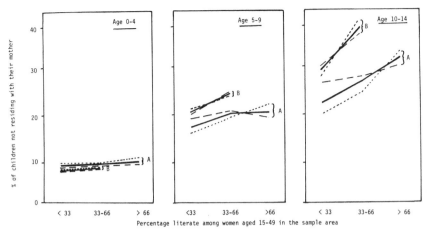

—— Boys
----- Girls
—— Total

A: Based on 20 ethnic groups with observations (N>30) in each of the age–sex subgroups for all three categories of literacy

B: Based on 22 ethnic groups with observations (N>30) in each of the age–sex subgroups for the lowest and middle categories of literacy only

FIGURE 9.6. *Within* Ethnic Group Differentials in Percentage of Children Not Residing with Their Mother, by Literacy Level of Women Aged 15–49 in the Sample Areas Where the Children Reside

to ignore its existence is to risk making nonsense of discussions of childrearing itself. By extension, ignoring it risks making nonsense of discussions of both fertility and child health as well.

Second, they confirm the fundamental importance of family systems, as opposed to education and, to a lesser extent, urbanization, in determining the prevalence of nonmaternal residence. The latter variables exert their impact on the pattern of child circulation rather than on its prevalence. The overwhelming importance of lineage and marriage patterns for the level of child circulation is of considerable importance because it suggests that child circulation and proparenthood are likely to remain common for quite a long time. In general, family systems and the underlying familial values they reflect change much more slowly than such socioeconomic characteristics as educational and occupational diversity or urbanization (Mead and McNicoll, 1986). Indeed, although there are some indications that lineage, for example, is slowly losing its influence through such changes as the privatization of land, the process has not yet advanced very far: privatization of birdewealth payments, for example, still appears to be found only in relatively restricted areas. Moreover, it is not clear that the changes involved are leading toward a nuclear family model with emphasis on a strong and long-term husband-wife link; they may be moving more toward more flexible union and family types with informal polygyny (*deuxièmes bureaux* or "outside wives") closer to those found in the Caribbean (Lacombe, 1983; Clignet, 1986; see also Wa Karanja, 1986). If change is in the direction of the nuclear family, then one would expect the prevalence of child circulation to decline considerably, but one would predict continuing high levels of child circulation (albeit with different patterns perhaps) in the latter case.

Finally, we should draw attention to what this particular analysis has not shown. It has restricted itself largely to the overall prevalence of child circulation and has not addressed the patterns of circulation in any detail. The extent to which proparenthood is used to redraw the pattern of access to children that is created by fertility has not yet been examined. Last but certainly not least, the social meaning of child circulation simply cannot be addressed with purely demographic data. Only anthropological studies can elucidate the extent to which child circulation changes the "costs and benefits" of bearing children, for example. Basically, therefore, the bottom line in terms of reproduction—"What effect, if any, does child circulation have on fertility?"—remains to be filled in.

ACKNOWLEDGMENTS

I am indebted to Yvan Wijnant for his programming work, especially the very extensive work on data cleaning, record linkage, and development of contextual variables involved in the preparation of the data files used in this paper. I would also like to thank the authorities in the countries concerned (Cameroon, Ghana, Ivory Coast, Kenya, Lesotho, Nigeria, Sudan) for permission to use their WFS data.

The work reported on here was supported by grant CP82.39A from the Population Council International Research Awards Program funded by USAID. The Vrije Universiteit in Brussels also provided both staff support through its Research Council and generous computer time.

An earlier version of this chapter was presented at the annual meeting of the Population Association of America in San Francisco, 1986. Esther Goody and Lynne Brydon provided comments on the earlier version, some (but not all) of which I have already been able to take into account here.

NOTES

1. See Caldwell and Caldwell (1985) for a discussion of the implications of this for fertility.

2. Esther Goody (1982), citing Fortes, refers to the possibility among the Tallensi of transferring paternity from the husband to the genitor where they are not the same person, but this seems to be merely a bringing into line of physiological and social paternity in exceptional cases.

3. Antoine and Guillaume (1984) and Locoh (1985) have collected direct information in demographic surveys in smaller areas (Abidjan and Southern Togo, respectively).

4. Since the Ivory Coast did not include detailed regional breakdowns, we have assigned data specific by ethnic group to the areas these groups largely occupy, as indicated in the survey report.

5. Ghana's Northern region is excluded here because it lacks data for urban areas.

6. The use of relatively broad ethnic groups should help reduce the number of errors introduced by this assumption.

7. This is less serious than it might at first appear, because the Sudan survey covered only the Northern Sudan, which differs in many respects from the countries further south.

8. The percentage distribution of the sample areas concerned is as follows:

Distribution by Sample Size		Distribution by Ethnic Heterogeneity	
No. of Women	Percent of Areas	Percent in modal ethnic group	Percent of Areas
01–09	6.4	1– 9	0
10–19	17.3	10–19	0
20–29	20.8	20–29	1.2
30–39	20.1	30–39	5.9
40–49	14.7	40–49	4.3
50–59	10.2	50–59	10.2
60–69	6.8	60–69	7.2
70–79	2.0	70–79	7.4
80–89	0.7	80–89	12.2
90–99	0.3	90–99	25.7
100+	0.8	100	25.9

9. In Lesotho and Cameroon, the sample of households to which the Household Questionnaire was administered was much larger than in the other countries. The sample of households used to identify women eligible for the Individual Questionnaire was in fact a subsample from it.

10. Based on columns 20 and 22 in Murdock.

11. Based on the second digit of column 32 in Murdock.

12. Based on columns 67 and 69 in Murdock. More specifically, the ethnic groups were first classified as follows:

1. Unstratified by caste or class (code O in both column 67 and column 69)

2. Stratified by wealth only (W in column 67, O in column 69)

3. Some despised groups (O in column 67, D in column 69, or vice versa)

4. Moderately stratified (E in column 67, D or E in column 69)

5. Heavily stratified (C in either column 67 or column 69)

BIBLIOGRAPHY

Antoine, P. 1983. Urbanisation et taille des ménages: Le cas d'Abidjan. *Cahiers d'OR-STOM*, Série Sciences Humaines, 19(3).

Antoine, P., and A. Guillaume. 1986. Une expression de la solidarité familiale en Abidjan: Enfants du couple et enfants confiés. In *Les familles d'aujourd'hui*. Paris: Association International des Démographies de Langue Française, 289–297.

Bledsoe, C. H. 1985. The politics of polygyny in Mende child fosterage transactions. Paper presented at the meeting of the American Anthropological Association, Washington D.C.

Bledsoe, C. H., and U. C. Isiugo-Abanihe. 1985. Strategies of child fosterage among Mende grannies in Sierra Leone. Paper presented at the meeting of the Population Association of America, Boston (also included in this volume).

Brydon, L. 1979. Women at work: Some changes in family structure in Amedzofe-Avatime, Ghana. *Africa* 49(2): 97–111.

————. 1985. The Avatime family and circulation, 1900–1977. In *Circulation in third world countries*, ed. R. M. Prothero and M. Chapman. London: Routledge and Kegan Paul, 206–225.

Bukh, J. 1979. *The village woman in Ghana*. Uppsala: Scandinavian Institute of African Studies.

Cain, M., and G. McNicoll. 1986. Population growth and agarian outcomes. *Working Paper of the Center for Policy Studies*, no. 128. New York: The Population Council.

Caldwell, J. C., and P. Caldwell. 1988. Is the Asian family planning program model suited to Africa? *Studies in Family Planning* 19(1): 19–28.

Clignet, R. 1970. *Many wives, many powers: Authority and power in polygynous families*. Evanston: Northwestern University Press.

————. 1986. On dit que la polygamie est morte: Vive la polygamie! In *Transformations in African marriage*, ed. D. Parkin and D. Nyamwaya. Manchester: Manchester University Press.

Etienne, M. 1979. Maternité sociale: Rapports d'adoption et pouvoir des femmes chez les Baoulé (Côte d'Ivoire). *L'Homme* 19(3–4): 63–107.

Fiawoo, D. K. 1978. Some patterns in foster care in Ghana. In *Marriage, fertility and parenthood in West Africa*, ed. C. Oppong et al. Canberra: Australian National University.

Fraenkel, M. 1964. *Tribe and class in Monrovia*. London: Oxford University Press.

Frank, O. 1984. Child-fostering in sub-Saharan Africa. Paper presented at the annual meeting of the Population Association of America, Minneapolis, Minn.

————. 1985. La mobilité des enfants et l'autosuffisance économique des femmes dans le milieu patriarcal africain. In *Femmes et politiques alimentaires*, ed. J. Bisilliat et al. Paris: ORSTOM-CIE. 641–652.

Goody, E. 1982. *Parenthood and social reproduction: Fostering and occupational roles in West Africa*. Cambridge: Cambridge University Press.

Goody, J. 1976. *Production and reproduction*. Cambridge: Cambridge University Press.

Goody, J., and E. Goody. 1967. The circulation of women and children in northern Ghana. *Man* (1967)(2): 226–248.

Gould, W. T. S. 1985. Circulation and schooling. In *Circulation in third world countries*, ed. R. M. Prothero and M. Chapman. London: Routledge and Kegan Paul, 262–278.

Gruenais, M.-E. 1981. Famille et demographie de la famille en Afrique. Collectif de Travail sur la Famille, Document de travail, no. 1. Paris: ORSTOM.

Isaac, B. R., and S. R. Conrad. 1982. Child-fostering among the Mende of Upper Bambara Chiefdom, Sierra Leone: Rural-urban and occupational comparisons. *Ethnology* 21: 243–257.

Isiugo-Abanihe, U. 1985. Child-fosterage in West Africa. *Population and Development Review* 11(1): 53–73.

Kreager, P. 1980. Traditional adoption practices in Africa, Asia, Europe and Latin America. Research for Action, no. 6. London: International Planned Parenthood Federation.

Krige, E. J. 1974. Woman-marriage with special reference to the Lovedu—Its significance for the definition of marriage. *Africa* 44(1): 11–37.

Lallemand, S. 1976. Génitrices et éducatrices Mossi. *L'Homme* 16(1): 104–124.

———. 1980. L'adoption des enfants chez les Kotokoli au Togo. *Anthropologie et Sociétés* 4(2): 19–37.

Laye, C. 1954. *L'enfant noir.* Paris: Plon.

Locoh, T. 1985. La migration des enfants rapportée par les mères: Application au Sud-Togo. In *Chaire Quételet: Migratione internes.* Louvain: Ordina Editions for Département de Démographie, Université Catholique de Louvain.

Murdock, G. 1962–1967. World ethnographic atlas. *Ethnology* vols. 1–6 (with addenda and corrigenda also through vol. 19).

Oppong, C. 1973. *Growing up in Degbon.* Legon: University of Ghana.

Saint-Vil, J. 1981. Migrations scolaires et urbanisation en Côte d'Ivoire. *Cahiers d'Outre Mer* 34(133): 25–41.

Sanjek, R. 1985. Maid servants and market women's apprentices in Adabraka. Paper presented at the American Anthropological Association Annual Meeting, Washington, D.C.

Schildkrout, E. 1973. The fostering of children in urban Ghana: Problems of ethnographic analysis in a multicultural context. *Urban Anthropology* 2: 48–73.

Skinner, E. P., 1960. The Mossi *Pogsioure. Man* 60: 20–23.

———. 1961. Intergenerational conflict among the Mossi: Father and son. *Journal of Conflict Resolution* 5: 55–60.

Smith, M. F. 1954. *Baba of Karo: A woman of the Muslim Hausa.* London: Faber.

Soyinka, W. 1981. *Aké: The years of childhood.* London: Collings.

Wa Karanja, W. 1986. "Outside wives" and "inside wives" in Nigeria: A study of changing perspectives in marriage. In *Transformations in African marriage,* ed. D. Parkin and D. Nyamwaya. Manchester: Manchester University Press.

CHAPTER TEN

Strategies of Child-Fosterage among Mende Grannies in Sierra Leone

Caroline Bledsoe
Uche Isiugo-Abanihe

INTRODUCTION

As shown in the previous chapter by Hilary Page, one of the most striking institutional features of West African families is that support for, and benefits from, raising children are rarely borne exclusively by parents, but are shared by many people. A prime case of this in West Africa is child-fosterage, in which children are sent to be raised by nonnatal caretakers: friends, relatives, neighbors, or patrons (see, e.g., Goody, 1982; Schildkrout, 1973). Yet despite the prevalence of fosterage in Africa, its demographic significance is largely unrecognized.

Fosterage (and other practices that redistribute the costs and benefits of children to people other than biological parents) bears important implications for fertility, whether one favors the supply or the demand side of the fertility debate.[1] In terms of the supply of children, fosterage may increase fertility through its proximate determinants. That is, fostering out small children may bring on earlier cessation of breastfeeding, earlier resumption of postnatal fertility, and so on. For girls sent to be raised in the household of their future husbands, a common practice among some African groups, their own fosterage may precipitate earlier nuptiality and earlier fecundity. On the other hand, for women who sometimes breastfeed young foster children they have received, this may decrease their own fertility.[2]

Second, fosterage questions the standard notion that the "demand for children" should be applied only to biological parents. Because of the magnitude of the topic, this paper is restricted to the latter: how fosterage affects—and is affected by—the demand side of fertility, in other words, the costs and values of children.

Demographic approaches to this issue usually make two assumptions that our data question: first, parents are taken as the unit of analysis, thereby focusing attention on why parents want children, how they pay costs, at what point they derive benefits, and so on. Conversely, the children whom parents bear biologically are seen as the only ones from whom parents will in turn draw support.

Alternative approaches (e.g., Caldwell, 1978; 1982; Fapohunda, 1978; Cain, 1981) have sought to expand the analysis of child costs and benefits to the individuals outside the nuclear household, especially elder family members who may support children and receive benefits from them, thereby influencing high childbearing by younger people.

This paper, concerning older women as caretakers of young children, draws on a theme in the germinative work of Caldwell. Whereas most analysts, including Caldwell himself (e.g., 1977, 1978), have focused on his notion of intergenerational wealth flows (as an explanation of why parents seek to limit or increase their offspring), we believe that even this analytical unit may prove too narrow. Ultimately his greatest contribution, at least for Africa, may be his elaboration of the theme this paper addresses: that support for children need not be restricted to parents (Caldwell, 1977, p. 16; for a discussion of developing areas in general, see Davis, 1955, pp. 34–35).

> As long as children are helped by their older siblings, by grandparents, uncles and cousins, and, indeed, by the other parent when that parent has a separate income and budget, the parent will not bear the full cost of the large family, and will not escape expenditure on other children by limiting his or her fertility.

This means that support for children can come from a wide network of kin, friends, and patrons—many of whom, we stress, may not even be related to the children by blood or marriage. Moreover, we believe that many people provide support for children because children are useful to invest in, rather than simply because they must be supported somehow. That is, fosterage is not always a measure of last resort: it can have strong positive incentives as well.

Second, most approaches examine prenatal means for regulating family size and composition such as birth control devices, family planning programs, local cultural methods, and so on. A notable exception to this is the work of scholars such as Scrimshaw (1978), who posit that infanticide provides a way for couples without access to prenatal forms of birth control to curtail the number of children they have. In our perspective, this is only one way—albeit an extreme one—of adjusting family size and composition postnatally.

It is clear that an individual's own fertility is limiting, given his or her needs for different kinds of social support, at different times in the life cycle. We suggest, therefore, that fertility is part of a much wider issue: the regulation and purposive management of family size and composition through a variety of means, only some of which are prenatal and primarily biological in nature. Perhaps the majority are socially managed and are postnatal: for example, transferring legal ownership of children through adoption, fostering out children on a nonpermanent basis, or accepting support for children in a variety of ways from other people. All provide ways for parents to mitigate the economic burdens of raising children. Conversely, these same means allow other individuals to foster in children from whom they can attempt to claim benefits in the present, such as labor, or future benefits such as cash assistance (see also Frank, 1984; Isiugo-Abanihe, 1985).

From the guardians' perspectives, fosterage has obvious advantages for subfertile people or those at the end of the life cycle, when labor and other support acquired through children are still needed but are unavailable through their own fertility. This chapter analyzes one such fosterage relationship: elderly Mende women in Sierra Leone who take in young children. We describe how this mitigates the cost of high fertility to childbearers at times in their lives when raising many young children would pose difficulties. Conversely, for older women who provide care for children, (or "mind" them, in the local British idiom), who may be past the age of childbearing—or, indeed, childless or neglected by their own children—we show that fostering small children gives them far more possibilities for support than their own fertility would dictate.

In focusing on this particular fosterage relationship, we also draw attention to the fact that even young children can be fostered: not simply older ones. Although the prevalence of this practice in other parts of the world is not well described, we believe its incidence and correlates deserve demographic attention.

On a more general level, we show that because biological reproduction is limited, relative to people's desires for assistance, family structure must be treated as a social outcome, as well as a biological one. The assumption that children are irrevocably assigned to a household (usually the one into which they were born) fails to take account of how individuals continually redefine their rights and obligations with respect to particular children, based on the children's changing potentialities as well as their own changing circumstances. Because the demands of childrearing are socially constructed and negotiable, costs as well as benefits of this task may be absorbed by a variety of people.

Besides exploring these micro-level patterns, we argue that the scope of the analysis of children's costs and benefits should be spread even further. We examine an important rural-urban (or subsistence-cash) tie through which costs of child rearing are absorbed, and we suggest that such regional modes of spreading costs and benefits of children merit further attention.

THE STUDY

The Mende people of Sierra Leone were chosen for the study because they have extraordinarily high rates of child-fosterage. They were also chosen because fosterage is known to begin very early: in some areas, children under the age of 2 are as likely to be found with women who are not their biological mothers as with their mothers. Data for this chapter come from an ethnographic study conducted by Bledsoe during 1981–1982 in a semiurban Mende town of about 4,500, in the Eastern Province.

The Mende, a Mande-speaking group, comprise one of the two largest ethnic groups in Sierra Leone. They number 799,905, or 30 percent of the country's population of 2,659,074, according to a recent analysis of the 1975 census (Thomas, 1983). The Mende traditionally grew upland rice, supplemented by occasional swamp rice farms (Richards, ms.). Polygyny is allowed, although gerontocracy and lack of wealth prevent most men from acquiring more than one wife until middle age. The Mende have a partilineal ideal, in which children legally belong to the husband's lineage. Actual practice, of course, often deviates. For example, although the husband is theoretically responsible for cash costs that his children incur, other people frequently contribute to these, in terms of food, school fees, and so on. Moreover, the husband may insist that the mother pay most of her children's expenses out of her separate income resources. On the other hand, she may want to pay these expenses when she can, because this gives her more leverage to retain custody of the children, should she divorce.

The area where the study was conducted had substantial diamond wealth, which local people have been exploiting since the early 1950s. The town studied was the headquarters for the chiefdom. It had a daily market, several primary schools, one secondary school, a hospital, and several stores. A number of men were employed in nearby diamond and lumbering industries. Other people gained a living from these industries indirectly by providing services to employees. Many others grew cash crops such as coffee, cacao, and groundnuts. Perhaps half still had subsistence rice farms, but rarely depended on them exclusively. The majority profess Islam, and most of the remainder Christianity.

Since the strength of the study is qualitative, this chapter relies primarily on open-ended interview data and observations of household subsistence activities. We also use quantitative data from a survey that sampled 154 households in the town. Concerning foster children, household heads were asked about unmarried children under 18 who were in the household with no mothers present—defined as "in-fosters" for the purpose of the survey— while women were asked about their unmarried children under 18 who were currently in the household as well as those who were away: "out-fosters."

Although the size of the sample was relatively small (155 in-fosters and 117 out-fosters), we use descriptive statistics to illustrate points.

MENDE FOSTERAGE

Fosterage is common among the Mende (see also Isaac and Conrad 1982). Of all the children under 18 currently in the households being surveyed in the present study, 39 percent were in-fosters—while 34 percent were out-fosters. Of the children under 5 who were born to women in the survey, 23 percent of these were currently fostered out, as were 28 percent from ages 6 to 10 and 46 percent from the 11 to 15 age group. A preliminary description of older children's fosterage will put that of small children in perspective.

Fosterage of Older Children

The reasons for fostering out older children are varied. Parents occasionally admit economic hardship as a reason for sending certain children out, but most have positive incentives. Parents usually hope to improve the quality of their children or the quality of their relationships with individuals such as distant or highly placed kinsmen by sending them children. They also give children to prestigious patrons, when possible, as a token of their dependence. But in many cases, parents hope that the education and contacts gained from fosterage will allow one or more of their children to rise in the national government or business bureaucracy or to contract advantageous marriages. Those children will then help the rest of the family to achieve economic progress in the modern world. They can help to forestall trouble with government authorities or tax collectors. They can also forestall lawsuits that village rivals may bring against their parents. Such lawsuits, a growing phenomenon, can wipe out the savings and property of rural people who have few urban patrons. Without such aid, rural people have little chance of hiring lawyers, if necessary, or of gaining access to higher government patrons for appeal purposes, and so on.

Families usually arrange for children about age 6 and over, particularly boys, to take up formal education, trade apprenticeship, or training in Arabic literacy. For this "learning" (kaa, which translates "training for life"), parents often send these older children to live with relatives, friends, and patrons who live in large towns with modern opportunities such as good schools. This is done, parents say, because children learn best with nonparental caretakers who are less likely to indulge them and more likely to discipline them. Girls, on the other hand, may be sent for education or (occasionally) Arabic literacy, but they are also sent for "household training" (maake) in which they learn to perform household chores such as cooking and housekeeping and learn childcare skills. Again, however, parents prefer that their daughters obtain this training in houses more modern than their own, to improve the girls' chances of marrying men with educations and jobs in the modern sector.

For a guardian, of course, there is much to gain, potentially, from fostering children. Foster children usually work hard, performing household and marketing chores, taking care of smaller children, and so on. Besides this, guardians can invest in promising children for future reciprocal assistance. The minder, or guardian, can make claims on a former minded child's monetary and political assistance much like a parent can. Typically, people who made any sort of contribution at all to a young wage earner's upbringing—school fees, food, even a bowl of rice one day when he was hungry—will claim assistance because of their own assistance (or claimed assistance) to him during his formative years. This is a critical fact for older women who mind children.

Young Children

The Mende send children out at very young ages. The youngest in-foster in the survey was 4 months old, although several people reported receiving children immediately after they were born. The first set of columns in Table 10.1 shows the distribution of in-fosters by the ages when they reportedly first came into the present house. The second two columns show the ages when children who were currently out-fosters first left their mothers.

Compared with some parts of Sierra Leone that the Mende occupy, these percentages are low. In some southern chiefdoms, over 50 percent of the children under 2 were away from their mothers, according to 1975 national census figures. (For purposes of clarity, children staying with fathers only—because of marital dissolution, mother's death, and so on—are excluded from the rest of the analysis of foster children. Also, numbers of out-fosters and in-fosters may vary slightly in different tables, because missing data are excluded.)

TABLE 10.1   Distribution of Fosters by Age of Fostering

	In-Fosters: Age When They Arrived		Out-Fosters: Age When They First Left Mothers	
	N	Percent	N	Percent
23 mos. or less	63	40.7	32	23.7
24–35 mos.	26	16.8	29	21.5
36–47 mos.	14	9.0	10	7.4
48–59 mos.	17	11.0	10	7.4
60–71 mos.	12	7.7	14	10.4
72+ mos.	23	14.8	40	29.6
Totals	155	100.0	135	100.0

While older children are usually fostered out to be trained for later life, younger children, as young as 4 months in the household survey, are simply sent out "to raise them up" (to learning age). The Mende maintain that a child cannot learn much before the "age of sense," around 6 or so. Therefore, they are willing to send younger children out to people who have little status or access to schools. Very commonly, such a minder is an older woman, a "granny" in the local English translation (in Mende, "mama"). People adamantly insist that a child sent to a granny is not there as a "learning child" (kaa-lopoi) or—in most cases—even as a "household training child" (maakɛ-lopoi). He is simply a "granny child," a *mama-loi*.

A granny is not necessarily the child's own biological grandmother. She may be a distant relative of the child's parents or may even be unrelated. Ages and generations can vary also. Older women in the same generation as one's parent can be called "granny." And since women may begin childbearing at 15 or 16, 34-year-old grannies are not rare. However, grannies can be very old: several grannies in the survey were in the fourth ascending generation from the small children they were minding. Because of the broad ways in which these kinship terms can be applied, therefore, this paper uses the terms "granny" and "grandchild" loosely, as the Mende do, to refer to the relationship between an older woman and the child she minds. We focus particularly on young children: those about 5 and younger.

There are, of course, many differences among the grannies who take in young children. Grannies may live in the same towns or villages with the parents of the children they mind, or in towns of similar size. A few live in areas more urban than the younger people. But because of increasing migration of young people to areas that can offer off-farm employment, many grannies remain in rural areas, where they engage in subsistence rice cultivation, sometimes in combination with a bit of vegetable gardening or small-scale cash cropping. This, together with the very young ages at which children are fostered out to these grannies, has far-reaching implications for patterns of migration and health of small children, in an area that may have the highest rates of child mortality in the world.[3]

Regional differences among grannies are mirrored by economic differences. A fair number of grannies seem well off. Some live with husbands and some are fairly young. Some divorced or widowed grannies come to live in large towns with their young relatives, where they help with child care and household duties in return for support. Some middle-aged grannies in more modern areas even head their own households as wealthy market women, owners of cash crop plantations, or diamond merchants. Many older women live as legal dependents of one of their deceased husbands' male kinsmen, whom they call "husbands." However, many old women who have passed their reproductive years can no longer rely on support from spouses, although they remain legally married to men (see Potash et al. 1986 for a general discussion of older African women). Although we focus on rural grannies with fewer means, many of the points we will raise pertain to grannies who have wealthy husbands or are themselves wealthy.

Grannies typically derive support from many sources. One women in the town had ties to the local paramount chief, whom she claimed, through remote ties, as her "husband" and occasionally pressed for cash. But she was living with the family of her sister's son, helped occasionally with this family's farm, and got her daily food from its members. She got money during the dry season, a time of relative plenty, from the parents and sponsors of girls who were initiated into the local Sande society chapter that she headed. She received gifts of "appreciation" from some of these sponsors at other times of the year. She also presided over several childbirths a year, for which she received fees, and minded a small child upon whose father she placed frequent demands. And after the project's investigator, Bledsoe, arrived in the town and made her acquaintance, the old woman put the anthropologist's house on her itinerary of places to visit and began to ask for cash, cloth, an umbrella, and so on.

Unlike this woman, however, many grannies experience considerable economic hardship, particularly those living in rural villages. And whereas subsistence rice farms and vegetable gardens provide most of these grannies' sources of food, rural villagers report increasing pressure to sell their subsistence foods to obtain cash.

Even grannies living in urban or semiurban areas worry about economic support. Many who go to other men after they become widows have quite tenuous support because men tend to regard older women they have inherited as burdensome. But even grannies living with long-time husbands can find subsistence difficult because spouses usually keep their incomes separate, aside from mutual participation on family farms. In many cases, a daily meal at most is all an old woman can expect from her husband. If she needs cash she must beg it from him or from her kinsmen or neighbors, or sell a bit of her garden produce.

Because of present economic insecurities as well as those anticipated with yet increasing age, grannies attempt to diversify their sources of potential support. One of the most important of these is minding children, an arrangement with mutual benefits to grannies as well as to parents.

WHICH PEOPLE SEND CHILDREN TO GRANNIES?

Just about anyone may send a child to a granny to be raised, though reasons vary. Older girls attending boarding school or a school in another town who become pregnant usually leave their children with their mothers or elder kinswomen if they want to return to school. In some cases, an unmarried girl gives birth, leaves the child, and returns to school almost immediately. Likely examples of this appeared in a survey of admission records at a mission hospital, which revealed three cases of babies under one month being raised by people other than their mothers (the exact relationships had not been recorded). Such arrangements may be kept secret, since pregnancy can result in the girl's dismissal from school, making it difficult to ascertain the real mother of a baby. The granny is young enough to appear to be the child's real mother and is not eager to endanger the real mother's school career by identifying the girl as the child's mother. Similar patterns occur when a woman is not married. In order to enhance her eligibility to a man, a woman may send her children born out of wedlock or to a previous husband to her mother to raise.

Young married women bring their young children to their mothers as well. A woman may bear her first child in the household of her mother, or whoever raised her, where she gains advice and assistance. Eventually she may leave the child to be weaned while she goes back to her husband to resume her sexual life. (She need not have borne the child in her mother's home, but may simply bring him to her mother for weaning.) Here, fosterage serves admirably an important cultural end. A woman anxious to have another child quickly fears social censure for resuming sexual relations with her husband while her young child is still nursing, since this is believed to contaminate her milk. Fosterage, combined with leaving her mother some money to buy the now ubiquitous infant formula, allows her to shorten the time of breastfeeding—and, therefore, sexual abstinence. This, in turn, allows her to speed up the arrival of her second child (Bledsoe, 1987).

After she bears another child or two, the one that was left with the granny may be ready to start school. So the parents take him back, perhaps keeping him themselves if they are in an area with a school, or even sending him on to yet another minder where schooling opportunities are better. At the same time, they leave the second child with the granny to raise until he, too, is ready for other training.

Other women who may send children to grannies include mothers of several young children who need child care, especially when their children are closely spaced. Although this can pose problems for grannies, particularly when they have young children of their own, grannies rarely refuse these grandchildren.

Women in polygynous unions, which are highly susceptible to competition and jealousy, are also likely to send children to grannies. A woman may fear that her cowife is trying to bewitch her child because their husband seems to favor him (Bledsoe, in process). Under these circumstances, her best option may be to send the child, especially if he is small, to her mother to mind.

Benefits to Parents in Sending Children to Grannies

For parents, sending a young child to a granny reduces many of the expenses they would have to bear. It is true that parents are expected to pay for at least some of the expenses that grannies incur on behalf of the children, as well as to send food and clothes for the children. But particularly when the mother is not married or her husband denies that the child is his, the granny herself must provide a great deal for the child out of her own resources.

The economic effect of these arrangements is to mitigate the expenses to parents that small children incur, at a time when supporting them fully would be difficult—such as when the parents are young, burdened with several small children, needing time to work, or lacking cash in a more urban environment. Other circumstances under which parents send children to grannies are seasonal hardships. Rainy season is the hardest time of year in rural as well as urban areas, because the rice is still growing and cash crops cannot be harvested until later. But many parents feel—whether rightly or not—that grannies living in rural areas have reserved rice and probably have access to green vegetables and to cassava, a crop that can be harvested at any time of the year. Hence, a number of small children seem to be sent to grannies during rainy season.

It is important to note, moreover, that sending children to grannies can be a very short-term parental strategy: one that is used when the day's household resources are in short supply, such as when checks fail to come to wage earners at the end of the month, an increasing phenomenon in the national economy. During an interview, one local teacher who had not received his check for a month reported that he had sent his children to his mother just that morning because he lacked enough to feed them that day. He had sent them to her with one leone (then about 85 cents U.S.), knowing that she would either feed them with her farm produce or beg additional money from someone else to buy their food.

Second, women often find it hard to care for their children while they work. Sending young children to grannies gives women time to work at farming, marketing, or, sometimes, at wage employment. They also gain time to care for the household and their other children. Although the advent of Western schooling is now welcomed almost universally by women as well as men, sending children to school has precipitated a severe loss of older children's labor for women, making it necessary for women to find other ways to care for their small children.

Transactions in Sending Children to Grannies

When someone receives a child from its parents, he or she does not receive legal custody, in the sense of "adoption" (see, however, Etienne, 1983, for a contrasting perspective). This has sometimes provoked misunderstanding when children of West African parents in England have been given to white foster parents (see, e.g., Goody and Groothues, 1977).

A mother or father may ask a granny to take a child. In many cases, however, grannies themselves ask their young relatives for children to mind.

In many cases, they attempt to evoke sympathy. Like infertile women, an old woman is seen as lonely and piteous: she has no children "by her," and needs a child as a "walking stick." Old women living under especially difficult circumstances may be given a child out of pity. Someone may give a blind old woman a girl who may be nearly blind or have some other physical problem herself. However, many grannies are quite demanding, insisting that it is their right to take these children, since they raised the women who are now bearing the children. This is a strong argument to a man, who ideally should demonstrate gratitude to his wife's kin for raising the woman who became his wife.

Grannies also stress the obligations of junior kinsmen to them as respected elders in the family and define their requests as legitimate in light of putative extended family obligations. They rally social support, accusing the parents of being stingy and lacking concern for their helpless—but revered—elder kinswomen. Guilt and shame are powerful levers, and grannies play on people's sympathies, as one man explained:

> The mother of my wife [the woman who raised her—not the actual biological mother] came and said, "I would like to take that child." They removed him by force. I couldn't object at all. The lady who brought up my wife is barren. The most sorrowful word the lady uttered is, "Yes, I know you will not allow the child to go because I am barren. I don't have a child. Therefore, you don't want your child to be with me." That made me feel very bad. If I didn't give her the child, it would mean I wasn't appreciative to her for bringing up my wife. And I got my wife through the help of that lady. So it's a matter of appreciation. If I give her my child, that would encourage her, and help her to forget that she is barren.

One long-time medical missionary related that when she asked nurses in her hospital as well as other professional women why they gave their children to grannies to raise, they usually replied:

> What can we do? If we don't send them, they [the grannies] say we don't like them; we don't love them anymore; we don't trust them with our children. And we will be in trouble if we don't. They'll say we're proud, we don't trust them, that we're backward because they didn't go to school.

If emotional levers do not work, however, a granny may hint of the consequences of refusing her a child. In her position as a powerful elder, she can invoke ancestral curses on ungrateful junior members (see also Oppong, 1973), or, if not given a child before her death, she can threaten to take it with her when she dies.

More concretely, she could influence male elders to withold farmland from young urban workers who increasingly find urban employment insecure. They sometimes find themselves unemployed, by losing favor with their employer/patrons, getting caught embezzling too many funds without sharing the rewards of the job with employers, and so on. More important, because of the government's growing economic problems with inflation, meeting debt payments, and obtaining foreign currency, wage earners frequently go months without pay. This compels many to supplement their urban employment with subsistence and cash crop farming in the home area, on land that is generally held by communal family groups, with access controlled by elders.

Not only must urban workers be assured of land, they must be assured that it is fertile and not rocky land on a steep slope or land that is far away from roads and streams. Even if they stay in the city during hard times, they must be able to persuade rural relatives to send them large bags of rice and other subsistence goods. For young urbanites on shaky economic grounds, maintaining good will with rural people—among whom grannies are quite influential—is essential.

Parents with children they cannot support, however, may exploit the norms, sending grannies with wealth and prestige many children to mind. In one instance, a granny, herself barren, was minding five small children, as well as several older ones who were going to school and working for her, doing housework, hawking, and diamond digging. She charged that all her poorer friends and relatives seemed to "pity" her barrenness by giving her children, when in fact they simply wanted to bring their children to a wealthy minder, to avoid expenses.

The importance of the social definition of the concept of "family size" is clear in this case: although this woman was biologically incapable of being a grandmother, she had more "granny children" to mind—including some who were not related to her—than most of her formerly fertile peers.

ADVANTAGES AND DISADVANTAGES TO CHILDREN IN BEING RAISED BY GRANNIES

The Mende have mixed feelings about sending their children to grannies. On the one hand, many people argue that grannies are the best caretakers for young children. Most grannies have had long experience in caring for their own children, and probably for others as well. Because of their age, they are said to have a wide knowledge of the foods considered proper for children of different ages and of herbal cures for childhood diseases. People also believe that grannies are more responsible than young women who have babies but· resent the time and energy necessary to care for them. Grannies are said to watch their small charges attentively and affectionately.

Grannies are also said to be aggressive food scroungers for the children they mind, even in times of hardship such as rainy season. Parents know that grannies beg food and money from other people, if they have to, including those they minded in the past, and use these resources to provide for their minded children. Hence, parents are eager to send their small children to grannies who have previously minded children. Moreover, despite a strong Mende ethic about sharing food, grannies are said to hide food for their grandchildren until everyone else leaves for the farm or other tasks, feed it to them quietly in the house, and remove traces of the meal by washing their hands and faces thoroughly before allowing them to go outside.

Even when their grandchildren eat from a large bowl with other children in the household of approximately the same age, as children usually do, grannies find ways to help the children they are minding. One young man related that he used to eat with three other boys his age in the household. One had a grandmother present as he did, but two had no relatives in the house. The two grandmothers took turns supervising the meals, ostensibly to ensure that each child got equal amounts of meat and sauce from the bowl they shared. But each, when it was her turn, made sure that the other three boys slowed down while she overlooked the rapid, greedy eating of her own grandchild. When the bowl was almost finished, she saved the rest and gave it secretly to her own grandson at night before bed, perhaps reserving a bit for his breakfast. No one did this for the two boys without grannies present.

Parents consider sending a child to its grandmother beneficial for ritual purposes as well. In every family, someone, usually an old woman, is in charge of the family guiding spirit, to which she makes sacrifices and in turn requests assistance for the family. If a child is staying with his granny, he is said to benefit immensely, because she will come to love him and will ask the spirit for special protection for him. In many ways, then, sending a young child to a granny is considered better than having the real mother raise it, despite the impoverished environments in which many grannies live.

The major problem, however, with allowing grannies to keep children, especially as the children get older, is that in the Mende view, grannies are notoriously lax with children. They are said to feed children upon demand and do not beat them or withhold meals from them for bad behavior or for failing to work or learn. Instead of demanding compliance, grannies are seen as using only rewards and no punishment—a socialization strategy that people believe can ultimately come to no good. Said one man about his 14-month-old son, whom his wife's stepmother had taken several months ago:

> I am not pleased, at times, with how they [the grandparents] treat him. They "pet" [spoil, pamper] him too much. Sometimes he will just remain in bed and they won't do anything with him. Most of these habits are very difficult to remove. She [the granny] doesn't punish him or anything! In fact, they [grannies] overfeed children! Even when I thought about my own experience [being raised by my granny] I didn't like the idea. My grandmother used to "pet" me. And I know very well that "petting" a child at that age [early school age] is not nice. I wouldn't want my own child to be raised in that way. Perhaps a bit of it is alright at an early age, but later on it is not good.

Children raised like this are said to grow up lazy and dishonest: since grannies try to lure them with rewards, they will take these luxuries for granted. They will also find that stealing desired things is easier than earning them. In the cultural view, moreover, children can even insult their grannies in play or in anger, as a child dare not do to his own parent or any other respected person. Such behavior, if retained in later life, renders a person vulnerable to devastating lawsuits.[4]

According to the Mende, children should experience hardship and discipline if they want to succeed in life, particularly in the modern world. In the Mende view, a child can attain competence in the setting in which he is born. But an older child who wants to advance beyond his family's current status in life, as its members urge him to do, must be prepared to undergo hardship and privation in the household of a prestigious patron who gives him an opportunity to go to a good school, but demands hard work and unquestioning obedience in return.[5]

Parents fear that a child raised to maturity by a granny will not be motivated to concentrate on his training and will grow up ignorant particularly of the modern world. He will be a lazy worker and disrespectful of authority figures—a tremendous liability within such a hierarchical patron-client system—whom he would rather insult than obey. Since he lacks discipline and respect for authority that are considered necessary to progress in life, he will inevitably lose his job, if indeed he gets one, and will not even be fit to work on the farm. One person explained:

> Parents will like to see the granny "pet" and joke with the grandchild, if it is underage. But if the child is bigger, like the ones who bring you water, the parents may get annoyed, and say the grandmother is trying to instill bad behaviors in the child. And if she is insulting the child and he is insulting her, they will say that when the child is grown up, he will insult outsiders like that also. So that will bring palaver [trouble, arguments] to the child.

Two Mende teachers amplified, arguing that children raised by grannies perform the most poorly in school. They attend only fitfully, because grannies are said to encourage them to stay home and avoid the rigors and discipline of the classroom. Later, if they have an opportunity to live with a guardian in a larger town to attend school after being raised by a granny, they have little self-discipline and lack any ability to endure hardship. They do not concentrate on the class work because they daydream about the food that is being prepared at their guardian's house. They are also said to be "ungrateful" to their guardian, complaining about hunger and overwork, thus angering him and making him send them back to the village, destroying their chances for success. Some concerned parents do not send children to grannies at all: not from fear of underfeeding (perhaps more the empirical reality) but of overfeeding and pampering.

Unless the granny is living in an area with a prestigious school that the child can attend, or is an important or educated woman herself who will train the child to be competent in this context, then being raised by a granny until maturity is a major embarrassment and hindrance, particularly for boys. It implies that a child has no educational or political potential worth developing. Or, if he is with an elderly woman from his mother's family, it suggests that his father suspects him to be the product of his mother's illegitimate love affair. To taunt a young adult by calling him a *mama-loi*, or "granny child," whether or not he actually was—is a serious insult and grounds for a lawsuit.

In the Mende cultural view, then, a child should be taken from a granny when he or she reaches the "age of sense," about 5 or 6, when the child is capable of performing small tasks or of learning in school or another endeavor.

Which Children are Sent to Grannies?

Cultural perceptions of grannies affect the kinds of children sent to grannies and when they are sent and withdrawn. Such differences entail issues of legitimacy, sibling order, sex, and age. First, people reported that children suspected by their mothers' husbands of being illegitimate are most likely to be sent to grannies (usually their mothers' mothers), although those considered legitimate are frequently sent as well. So are those whose parents are no longer married, either through divorce or death. Grannies are clearly preferred as child raisers to fathers' other wives.

Second are differences among which siblings are sent to grannies and how long they stay. In the past, people related, parents were pressured to send their first child to one or another granny, out of obligation to her for raising them. Nowadays, although a granny may still apply great pressure to take the first child, parents try to put her off, especially if it is a boy, because they want to educate him so he can help the rest of his siblings. However, this urgency declines with subsequent children and with girls. One father revealed that he had sent his first son and later his first daughter to his wife's mother when they were small, but had withdrawn them to enter school. Finally, he had sent his last child, a girl, to the granny to keep. He compared his feelings about sending the two girls:

> With the first daughter, I told the granny that when she was five I would go and collect her to attend school, and I did. But with the youngest daughter, I'm not bothered about her, although I visit them regularly. But I'm not bringing her (back) again. That's the granny's own child. [With] the first daughter, I said no. I said I would come and collect her at the age of five to come and attend school. But the last I said was the granny's own. Let her train her in the way she likes. But I have to train the first one in the way I like. So the first one was only with the granny for "caretaking." But with the second, [since she is there to stay] she can be trained for marketing [the granny's trade].

STRATEGIES OF CHILD-FOSTERAGE AMONG MENDE GRANNIES *457*

TABLE 10.2   Percent Distribution of In-Fosters' Ages, by Relationship
with Caretakers

Caretaker	Children's Ages					
	0–5		6+		Totals	
Granny	(11)	47.8	(19)	21.3	(30)	26.8
Other	(12)	52.2	(70)	78.7	(82)	73.2
Total	(23)	100.0	(89)	100.0	(112)	100.0

However, these worries made only small difference in which kinds of guardians boys had, compared to girls: seven (16 percent) of the forty-four fostered-in boys were with grannies, as were eight (22 percent) of the thirty-seven girls.

The most critical determinant appears to be age: it is most common to send children of weaning age to grannies. As we showed earlier, the Mende often send out very young children. Table 10.2 shows that compared to older children, a higher proportion of young ones go to "grannies." ("Grannies" are defined in these tables as women two generations removed from the children they are minding, and related to them through biological or marital ties. Most are actual mothers' mothers or fathers' mothers.)

The table shows that 27 percent of the in-fosters were with actual and classificatory grannies, while 73 percent are with "other" people such as relatives of the parents, older siblings, non-relatives, and so on. However, 48 percent of the young in-fosters were with grannies (mostly mothers' mothers), compared to 21 percent of the older children. (Analogously, about 38 percent of all out-fosters had been sent to grannies. But 44 percent of the young ones were with grannies, compared to 16 percent of the older ones.) As children get older, most of those remaining with grannies are those with parents not married to each other. In only two instances were any older children whose parents were still married—one boy and one girl—remaining with grannies. These children, however, were still relatively young (7 and 8, respectively), and both had come from small villages, the significance of which we discuss below. Moreover, even though the boy was with his grandmother, he was attending Arabic school in the bigger survey town and would later be taken for formal schooling. And the granny of the girl reported that the girl was to leave her soon to enter school.

Place of origin versus where the potential minder lives is also significant in decisions about sending children to grannies. Table 10.3 shows the sizes of settlements in-fosters are coming from and whether they now live with grannies or other minders. These are further broken down into the two age groups. (The categories of "rural," "semiurban," or "urban" origins were

TABLE 10.3   Percent Distribution of In-Fosters by Place of Mother's Residence and Child's Relationship with Caretaker

Current Caretaker		Mother's Residence							
		Rural (<2000)		Survey Town (4500)		Other Semiurb & Urban (>2000)		Total	
All Children									
Granny		(9)	30.0	(7)	23.3	(14)	46.7	(30)	100.0
Others		(50)	61.0	(10)	12.2	(22)	26.8	(82)	100.0
	Total	(60)	52.7	(17)	15.2	(36)	32.1	(112)	100.0
Children 0–5									
Granny		(0)	0.0	(5)	45.5	(6)	54.4	(11)	100.0
Others		(6)	50.0	(3)	25.0	(3)	25.0	(12)	100.0
	Total	(6)	34.8	(8)	34.8	(9)	39.1	(23)	100.0
Children 6+									
Granny		(9)	47.4	(2)	10.5	(8)	42.1	(19)	100.0
Others		(44)	62.9	(7)	10.0	(19)	27.1	(70)	100.0
	Total	(53)	59.6	(9)	10.0	(27)	30.3	(89)	100.0

constructed by matching towns from which in-fosters came with population figures from the 1975 census, as summarized by Thomas, 1983.)

As the table shows taking all in-fosters, 53 percent did come from rural areas (less than 2000). But these tended to be older ones (60 percent) rather than younger ones (26 percent) presumably because of the enhanced opportunities for advancement in a larger town.

When we look at the ages of children staying with grannies versus other minders, however, sharp regional differences appear. Although only 26 percent of the small children came from rural areas, none of those who were staying with grannies came from rural areas, compared to 47 percent of the older children, who had presumably come for training outside the home. Younger children came instead from semiurban to urban areas (54 percent) or from the survey town itself (46 percent). In all, 74 percent of the young children (35 percent + 39 percent) came from areas of 2000 or above (including the survey town), compared to only 40 percent of the older children (10 percent + 30 percent).

This means that childbearing women generally live in more urban areas and send a child back to granny or leave one behind before migrating. Alternatively, those women who do live in more rural areas send fewer small children to grannies living in more urban areas than older ones. Small chil-

TABLE 10.4   Percent Distribution of Out-Fosters by Destination and Caretakers

Current Caretaker		Destination							
		Rural (<2000)		Survey Town (4500)		Other Semiurb & Urban (>2000)		Total	
All Children									
Granny		(11)	47.8	(2)	8.7	(10)	43.5	(23)	100.0
Others		(19)	30.2	(4)	6.3	(40)	63.5	(63)	100.0
	Total	(30)	34.9	(6)	7.0	(50)	58.1	(86)	100.0
Children 0–5									
Granny		(7)	53.8	(1)	7.7	(5)	38.5	(13)	100.0
Others		(5)	41.7	(2)	16.6	(5)	41.7	(12)	100.0
	Total	(12)	48.0	(3)	12.0	(10)	40.0	(25)	100.0
Children 6+									
Granny		(4)	40.0	(1)	10.0	(5)	50.0	(10)	100.0
Others		(14)	27.5	(2)	3.0	(35)	68.7	(51)	100.0
	Total	(18)	29.5	(3)	4.9	(40)	65.6	(61)	100.0

dren staying with other people, on the other hand, are likely to come from more rural areas (50%), probably in preparation for school. Of course, those staying with grannies sometimes enroll in school, but children are rarely sent into more rural areas, particularly to grannies, for this purpose.

The data for out-fosters roughly parallel those for in-fosters.[6] Table 10.4 shows that most out-fosters go to semiurban or urban areas (58 percent), but older children comprise more of this number, proportionately (66 percent), than small children (40 percent). In contrast, 35 percent of out-fosters are living with people in rural areas (<2000), but these are mostly young children, proportionately (48 percent vs. 30 percent of older ones).

To summarize, the net migration of younger children is to more rural areas; that of older children is to more urban areas. This reveals potentially significant regional patterns of fosterage that go beyond usual interests in kinship correlates of fosterage. On the whole, children remain within rural areas or even move to areas more rural than those of their parents—where many grannies live—for the first few years of life. When they reach 6 or so, however, there is a reverse shift, as they come back to where their parents live, or even go on to more urban areas for training.

Because of the tendencies to move toward cities for better health, schooling, and employment possibilities, the fact that older children move toward more urban areas is not surprising. What is surprising is that any children would be sent to other places upcountry, or even to places more rural than their own home. Significantly, these are mostly younger children.

BENEFITS TO GRANNIES IN MINDING CHILDREN

The differences in characteristics of children in combination with regional patterns in their distribution point to some potentially important economic consequences for different kinds of children, such as illegitimate ones and those of divorced parents. However, since our present focus is caretakers, we restrict our discussion to them. We focus first on the advantages to grannies and then return to the implications of these regional patterns in terms of more macro-level patterns of distributing the costs and benefits of children.

Present Benefits to Grannies

When parents have little money or a young mother has no husband, a granny may reap little benefit from taking in children, at least in the short run. But in many cases, grannies benefit from minding children as soon as they get them. These benefits are diverse. Many grannies report emotional rewards. Commented one young man:

> Grandmothers love the grandchildren more than their children. Even with me, I love my grandmother! When I was coming on holidays from school, I would come and say, "Granny, I missed you!" When I would go, she would say, "Come, let me burp you. Come suck the breast." They will hold you, embrace you, put the breast [in your mouth]. [Grannies "burp" and "nurse" even adult grandchildren, in jest.]

Besides emotional rewards, grannies hope for economic ones. Among their immediate benefits is labor. Despite the view that grannies do not demand work of children, children as young as 4 or 5—particularly girls—are put to work for elderly women, bringing water, washing dishes, and running errands. Even grannies living with husbands or other kinsmen are anxious to mind small children for the labor they can derive. This means, however, that if parents take their child from a granny when it is ready for schooling, she loses the child's more productive labor years. One person explained:

> When the family comes to take the child away from the granny, she will get annoyed. She says the child is just getting old enough to run errands for her, fetch water and firewood, and so on, so she is being deprived of her young worker. However, the parents will talk to her nicely, perhaps giving her something nice like a new lappa cloth to carry a child, and give her a new child to raise until it too gets old enough to take away from her.

But the child's labor is only secondary to many grannies, compared to the support they hope to obtain from the children's parents, who might otherwise pay little attention to them. Parents know that one of the main reasons why grannies lobby for children is that they will soon begin asking the parents for food, clothes, and money which they would ordinarily have little leverage to demand. A man whose young child was with his wife's mother explained:

> In most cases, the demands are increased [when the granny has a grandchild]. Usually, when your child stays with them, you don't forget about them at all. You are always in close contact with them. Any time you go to them, you will tend to give them something. When you go, you buy a few provisions and present them. Sometimes, of course, the grandmother will remind you of your obligations. But if your child is not staying with them, you forget about them. So this is one reason why these old people try to get grandchildren to mind.

Another man explained that the elderly woman in whose house he was living (not his actual mother) was asking to take his two children when he went to college in Freetown. About his obligations to her, he said:

> When she takes all these children [his plus others], we just have to support the house, financially and otherwise. . . . When she takes all these children, in the future we have to take care of the house, because she will not go anywhere. She may only sit to take care of the children. We have to buy clothes, supply the house with food, and other things.

Most grannies are straightforward about their expectations. Said one old woman:

> Because of the good care and maintenance I take of the grandchildren, the children will visit me and send me things.

Elaborated another:

> If you are minding your child's own child, your child will love you too much [a lot] because of the children you are minding for her. Whatever the child gets, she will just take it to you in the name of the children you are minding. So whatever good or whatever progress or benefit you get from the child, it will be through the children you are minding. You will always be in the child's thoughts. Whenever he gets something, he will say, "OK, let me send this to Mother, who is minding my children." So when a granny has a child to mind, the connection between her and her child is much more smooth.

Minding a child also provides a granny with leverage to ask for money and supplies from other relatives of the child: not just the mother and father. One man reported that he regularly sent money to his mother, who was minding his sister's two sons, because his sister had little money.

Grannies, of course, appropriate many of the resources parents send on behalf of their children. One granny insisted that a young relative come to stay in her house with a new baby. From her vantage point, the granny could take possession of all the gifts of money and food that people gave on behalf of the new child. This included money from the young woman's husband. When the woman wanted to take the new baby to the clinic for a checkup, for example, the husband gave her enough money to cover the visit, but the granny took it, assuring him that her own herbal skills were sufficient to keep the newborn in good health.[7]

To insure that money and supplies keep coming, a granny usually couches her requests in terms of the child she is minding. According to one person, a granny will say:

> "We are hungry [his emphasis]. Why not send us a bag of rice?" Or, "We don't have kerosene tonight. We haven't had kerosene for weeks. The child will wake up at night and at times she will excrete in her clothes at night. She would like to go out at night to excrete while people are asleep, but it is dark." Similarly, "We need a new bucket so that I can bathe Boima [the minded child]." Or, "Boima needs a mosquito net. He gets bitten every night." [Note that minded grandchildren usually sleep with their grannies.]

Not surprisingly, parents frequently begin to feel that these demands are incessant and onerous. Grannies ask for as much as they think the parents will give, and step up their demands if the parents seem to comply with little protest. One man, a polygynist, was experiencing growing pressure from two grannies who were minding his children by different wives. Just as wives would get jealous if the husband gave one more money or a nicer lappa cloth than the others, the grannies also became jealous when each heard that the other got something from him that she did not. Consequently, their demands escalated rapidly.

All this suggests, contrary to a more standard kinship explanation—that grannies mind children because of their links to the children's parents—that the reverse is more accurate instead: grannies mind small children in order to strengthen their links to the parents of the grandchildren. One old woman even stated quite explicitly that minding small children, because of the resulting ties to the children's parents, was essential in order to subsist.

Of course, there is no guarantee that a granny will get whatever she asks from parents. In fact, parents can try to avoid economic demands imposed by grannies. If a man has a limited income or if he wants to use some of it for other purposes, he can construe his lack of support for the child as the granny's fault. One man confided:

> If I am not doing anything [economically] for the child [while it is with the granny], I will create a problem and put [blame] it on my wife. I will say it is because my wife has not been respectful, she has not been loyal to me [implying that she is promiscuous or insulting]. Because of the maltreatment she gave me, the problems at home, she is always bringing [court] cases. I settle cases, and by the time the month ends [and the paycheck comes], she comes with four or five cases which I settle. So I do not have extra to send for my child.

As this quote implies, the man indirectly put the blame on the granny herself, for not raising his wife to be better behaved. Hence, he claimed, the granny had no right to make these demands on him.

Since the possibility of support from children's fathers is critical, in grannies' assessments, this makes the issue of illegitimacy highly significant. In the Mende ideal a granny dearly loves her grandchild, even if he is the product of a love affair. The reality, however, is that many grannies discriminate against these children. Said one person:

> The mother's mother will have a biased mind toward the child, because there will be no responsible father to help with expenses while she is minding the child. Any support the child gets will be from the mother and not the father. So the granny will go out of her way less for the illegitimate child, provide fewer clothes, fewer books and other facilities for the child to go to school.

This occurs even when a man keeps his child from an illegitimate union, and the child's mother provides no support. Thus, despite the patrilineal ideology, which would assign children to the man's lineage, regardless of their maternal origin, one man related:

> I used to have another child in the house, by a girlfriend. My grandmother was very indifferent to this child. She used to give a bath to the others, but began to grumble and sometimes refused to give a bath to the other girl. Also with feeding: since my wife and I went to work every day, the granny was in charge of feeding. So the children of my wife got more food every day. And the other child's clothes were not washed or mended well. Even with munching [snacking], when my granny went to town and came back with things to eat between the meals, they were always given to the legitimate kids. When this other girl was here [until she was 7] she was also doing a lot of work around the house, sweeping, bringing water, etc. Of course, any child could do these things, but she was getting a lot of work piled on her. She probably did more, even, than the granny. [Despite this] the granny used to grumble that the child was in the house but not doing anything good [worthwhile], and it would have been better if the mother came and took her. The granny was also vexed because the mother was in [another city], working on her own, and not contributing toward the upkeep of the child, while we were struggling to keep her in the house. The granny [also] showed preference for my wife's children because my wife was working in the hospital and providing support for them. So she encouraged [nurtured, praised] this woman's children more than the one whose mother gave nothing to her.

Future Benefits for Grannies from the Children Themselves

A crucial reason that grannies want to mind children is to derive support from these children themselves in the future. The head of a mission hospital reported that when grannies bring in very sick children they are minding for treatment, they often say something like:

Try [hard] for me for this child. I have no other grandchild. It was given to me. This is the one that sleeps with me. This is the one that is going to take care of me when I am old.

Although it is easy to see why parents might worry about their future welfare in old age, it is more difficult at first to understand why people who are already old and presumably near death might have these worries. Hence, we usually look only at the transfer of wealth from an adult child to his or her own parent. However, many Mende grannies are only in middle age or even in early middle age. Having survived this long, grannies worry about who will take care of them when they are even older, "feeble old," as the Mende say, and can do little for themselves. In fact, grannies probably worry more about their futures than mothers, because in the event that they do survive, their incapacity is closer at hand. Minding a small child makes sense for a granny, because she may live until well into the child's adulthood, or even that of the next generation, and may derive benefits from these children when they mature.

Significantly, the term the Mende use for the granny caring for the grandchild, "minding," is also applied to the reverse situation: when the grandchild shall in turn take care of the granny in her "feeble old" age, perhaps even taking her with him to the city where he lives. As a young man explained:

The grandmother will bring [bath] water and warm it up for you, just for you to love her presently and in the future. Grandmothers want you to mind them or take care of them when they shall have grown too old. [Just as they took care of you], you will take care of them when they shall have grown too old. A *kpokui* is an old, old person who has gray hair, wrinkled body, can do nothing for themselves. Then you will take over. In fact, many grandchildren have their grandmothers with them, whether in [a nearby city] or wherever they might be.

A granny also may profit doubly from minding children. She may use the support she receives from former minded children to care for a child she is currently minding, in effect reinvesting these gifts in the present child, from whom she will in turn derive benefits.

It is important to stress that a granny need not have actually minded a child to feel justified in claiming rewards from him in the future. She can simply have fed him a meal or a tidbit when he was hungry. She need not have even done anything for him directly, but may claim to have performed services of dubious utility on his behalf. One young woman living in Freetown reported that every time she came back to her natal town, elderly female neighbors besieged her with requests for money, claiming, "We took care of your granny [her grandfather's wife, not her actual grandmother] in your absence."

MINDING CHILDREN IN ORDER TO ACQUIRE RESOURCES FROM THE MODERN WORLD

That grannies seek support for minding children, whether from the child's parents or the child himself after he grows up, points to some potentially important economic patterns, both in terms of individual benefits to grannies as well as in terms of broader economic patterns of distributing costs and benefits of children. This section will examine the local-level interests of grannies, and the next one will analyze the larger regional and economic implications of these patterns.

Grannies are always anxious for subsistence goods such as rice, particularly in the rainy season. But, as the previous section has suggested, they also value goods from the modern world that are hard to obtain: for example, cash, kerosene lamps, matches, soap, and cloth, and even commercially grown staples such as rice. One woman who was encountered in the local market reported that she was buying onions, bouillon cubes, palm oil, and commercially dried fish for her mother in a nearby rural village. She was on her way to visit her mother because she wanted to check on her 18-month-old son, who was with the granny. She pointed out that as expensive as these goods were for her, the granny would value them greatly because of their scarcity in the rural areas and because the granny herself had little cash.

Like other guardians, moreover, old women want patrons living in the modern world whom they can press for cash and other assistance. Besides food, money, and modern household amenities, a granny hopes for legal help to prevent financial and social ruin from lawsuits levied by rival neighbors. She also hopes for medical treatment and medicines from a doctor, a new house from a rich man, and so on. When asked what she wanted her children or grandchildren to become, one granny who spoke no English or Krio (the national lingua franca) and had never been to school said she preferred a lawyer, then a doctor, then a teacher, and so on.

As we noted in general for how grannies derive benefits from minding children, a granny seeks modern rewards first from the parents of the children she is minding and later from the children themselves.

Present Benefits

Minding a child is one of the most potent levers a granny can gain over the limited resources of a young cash earner, even if it is her own child. A granny with such a grandchild may come into town, saying she needs rice, kerosene, and money; and the parent of the child is likely to give her demands priority over those of other rural relatives and comply as best he can.

The extent to which a granny is able to attract these resources from her minded children's parents may invite the jealousy of her village neighbors, who may see her getting a sack of rice from the parents of the child she is minding. This can provoke bitter feelings, especially in the rainy season, if neighbors smell the granny's rice cooking in the lean-to kitchen behind the house.

Related jealousies can arise even between a child's mother and father, over whose relative gets their mutual child. Spouses realize that the granny who gets their child will have the best claims on whatever limited money and supplies the household can provide. Hence, the husband and wife frequently argue over to whose granny they are going to send the child.

Conflicts over whose granny will be supported through a minded child are paralleled by conflicts between cowives. Cowives argue among themselves about the fact that one's mother (or other relative) is getting support because of minding a child, while another's mother is receiving little support because she is not minding a child. This cowife conflict itself seems to lead to fosterage: a woman may give a child to her mother to even the score: the household's resources will go to her family as well as that of her rival cowife. Ultimately this may be to her own advantage: if she ever wants to divorce her husband, the money and goods her mother is able to build up through fostering her child will provide her some security.

So much do village people desire modern resources that those grannies who manage to acquire a child from parents living in urban areas are likely to encounter jealousy from their neighbors in the villages. This can turn into angry hostility, especially if benefits are not shared. People stated that small children from urban areas were often in grave danger of witchcraft because jealous neighbors of the granny would see these plump, well-dressed children and the rewards grannies were getting for minding them.

This has interesting implications for assumptions that individual parents are the only ones to consider in fertility decisions. Mende grannies levy great pressure even on young educated urban women to maintain high fertility rates and to begin bearing early. This pressure does not stem simply from a desire to increase the size of the kin group. Rather, it stems largely from grannies' desires for modern goods and services from parents of the children they mind. As one young woman complained:

> Whenever I come [to the rural area, from Freetown], they [my elderly kinswomen] keep talking about getting married and having kids. When I say I'm not interested in that now, they say, "Alright, just have the children and then send them to us to train." As long as you can send them support, they will be happy. Then you can have your child when you are ready.

Future Benefits

Besides seeking modern benefits from the parents of the children they are minding, grannies also seek modern benefits from the children themselves, when they grow up. One granny stated explicitly that when she minded a grandchild, she hoped for the future support from the modern world, when the child graduated and got a big job in an office. Although she herself had no children, she revealed that every Christmas vacation, she sees an influx of urban wage earners she had minded, some of them now quite prominent, who bring her things. To provide for herself during the hard weeks of one rainy season, however, she had a literate grandchild write a letter for her to one of the grandchildren she had minded who was now working in Freetown. She asked for a bag of rice and some money, and the man complied.

Given the particular regional patterns of dispersing children of different ages, then, grannies increasingly view fosterage as a way of acquiring benefits from the modern world. And since it is even more likely that these grandchildren, rather than their parents, will become educated or trained in occupational trades and will be more likely to live in areas where they have wage or trade jobs, it is not surprising that grannies devote much effort to obtaining benefits from the modern world from grandchildren, besides, or even instead of, children.

Of course, many obstacles can get in the way of future reciprocity from grandchildren to grannies, especially given that there are often great regional as well as cultural disparities between illiterate rural grannies and the educated civil servants they may have raised years ago. The actual value of what the granny gave a child under her care could soon be repaid, if the transaction were defined as an equal exchange. Moreover, wage earners frequently deny requests for assistance from rural kin and acquaintances, emphasizing that the costs of living in the city absorb what looks to villagers like exorbitant incomes. (However, rural people frequently complain that their young relatives and neighbors whom they claim to have raised and educated neglect them when they get jobs in the city.)

Finally, an adult's sense of obligation to a granny who raised him briefly in his childhood could dim over time. Such diminutions are reflected in Mende cultural beliefs that witches can damage relationships between people, including those between a child and his granny. Contemporary witches realize that one of the most devastating setbacks for a granny is to "convert the heart" of her grandchild to forget about her, keeping him from visiting her and bringing her things from the city. (Grannies sometimes employ countercharms themselves, to try to make grandchildren remember them.)

Many grannies, however, do surprisingly well in obtaining benefits from young urban relatives. One reason is that urban parents who work outside the home are particularly vulnerable if they have young children. Care of young children is an intensive endeavor, and one that the children themselves cannot yet mitigate by working in the household, hawking goods, and so on. Hence, grannies who take care of young children can argue that their child care efforts deserve bountiful rewards.

But grannies also seem to do well in obtaining benefits from children they minded long ago who now live in the city because of the apparently artless and altruistic ways in which they "pet" or pamper children that we noted earlier. Although "petting" undoubtedly stems from affection, it also stems from the prospect of future economic rewards. As one person explained, since most grannies have little to attract children in terms of advancement opportunities, they feel that "petting" is their best strategy. First, grannies apparently spoil children to lure them back to them—the grannies—in the future, rather than to their own parents, who would otherwise have first claims on their resources, but would probably demand work and obedience from the children during their stays.

Such patterns apply to children who are still going to school, as well as those who are employed. (To grannies, as to many rural people, anyone living in a big town must have cash. Therefore, even children attending school in big towns are asked for money.) Explained one young man, who found himself spending more time with his granny during the vacations than with his parents:

> On most of the holidays, the children go to the villages: to the grandmothers, not to the parents. They will leave the parents in Kenema or Bo [large regional cities]. They go [instead] to the villages. Because whenever they go, they get whatever they want. People in the villages know the school year. When school is coming to be closed, they will say, "*Oh, holidei wa*" ("the long vacation is coming"). So when the children come, the grandmother will be catering to them: rice flour, bananas, whatever food or thing she might get, to give it to the grandchild.

> With the parents [on the other hand], and here I am speaking from my own experience, you go to the parents to get school fees only! You have only a brief visit with them, because you don't expect them to give you pocket money, rice flour, and you won't get the desired treatment [pampering] from them. If you go to visit your parents, they will put you to work. But when you go to the grandparent, you will just be for yourself [free to do what you like].

More importantly, such visits lay the groundwork for future habits that grannies want to cultivate: when the adult children come back to visit from their jobs, their pockets will be laden with cash for the grannies who coddled them before, and will do the same for them now.

Second, spoiling places grandchildren under heavy moral obligations that demand gratitude and recompense. Some grannies construe their grandchildren as indebted because they insulted the grannies, even though in play, an act that normally provokes legal action. Grannies also remind the grandchildren about how they were "petted," and given abundant food, rest, and comfort. Grannies emphasize that their own wealth and comfort were sacrificed in the process. In fact, they construe their acts of sacrifice on behalf of the children as demanding *more* repayment, ultimately, than straightforward exchange transactions, because of the heavy moral debts that they claim are placed on grandchildren. Consequently, people who are accused of neglecting the grannies who helped raise them come under great pressure. These observations have further significance in terms of the mechanisms by which costs and rewards of children are assumed to be spread. Although social relationships such as "child" and "grandchild" are associated with particular kinds of behavior, such as providing support, they do not mechanically determine behavior. In the present case, grannies know that the formal expectations of assistance from grandchildren or their parents rarely produce the results of remittances and assistance that they desire, despite the culturally sanctioned norms. Hence, grannies seek to spoil grandchildren and later arouse feelings of obligation and guilt in order to evoke the desired responses.

THE SOCIAL AND REGIONAL SIGNIFICANCE OF GRANNIES FOSTERING YOUNG CHILDREN FOR SUPPORTING FERTILITY

The Mende fosterage material reveals that the costs and benefits of children are distributed on a scope much wider than theories of fertility usually encompass. First, they are adjustable postnatally, as people assess their current needs and problems. Second, these costs and benefits are spread among a wide range of people, not simply the reproductive couple. These costs and benefits are spread so widely, in fact, that some very important variations consist of economic and social relationships of a regional nature.

From young urban parents' perspectives, sending small children to rural grannies brings parents relief from many of the monetary and labor costs of high fertility[8] at times in their lives or family cycles when such costs are most burdensome. On the other hand, in the local view as well as in many academic descriptions, grannies are cast as archetypal preservers of tradition who are conservative and backward in their values, fear modern innovations, and find security in traditional beliefs and practices. Hence, it is no surprise that Mende grannies do in fact urge young people to have many children and to use most of their resources in support of the local villages where the grannies happen to live.

Yet, the grannies encountered during the study made it clear that they wanted the benefits of the modern world: cash, imported household and clothing items, access to modern legal help, and so on—benefits that are normally associated with reducing fertility in order to educate and otherwise enhance children's value.

Fosterage is a link that makes these goals consistent. Old women can attempt to gain economic and political benefits from the modern world from the parents of the children they mind, and, if they live long enough, from these children themselves. In fact, despite their illiteracy and inability to participate directly in the modern economy, rural grannies view fosterage as their most critical link to the benefits of modernization. As such, older women comprise one of the most incessant sources of pressure on young urban women to have children.

On a wider level, these local level strategies of parents and grannies create regional patterns in two types of flows: people and wealth. As we have shown, fosterage produces a flow of children generally toward areas more rural than those of their parents' homes for the first few years of life. When they reach 6 or so, there is a reverse shift as they come back to their parents' homes, or even go on to more urban areas for training.

There are also transfers of wealth from young parents to older grannies, a finding quite compatible with Caldwell's work. But whereas most analyses focus on relationships between the young and the old in single locations, the present study has focused on generational transfers of wealth that crosscut regional boundaries (see, however, Caldwell, 1980, as well as various discussions of labor migration remittances).

The data also reveal a complex picture of how wealth is transferred. Despite their illiteracy and lack of direct access to the wage economy, many rural grannies use fosterage to extract cash and other modern forms of wealth from the younger urban generation whose young children they mind. Ironically, one of the greatest modern innovations, by most accounts, has been the influx of modern medical facilities and programs aimed at children: maternal/child health programs, vaccination programs, and so on. However, from the point of view of older people in Sierra Leone, hardly any programs are aimed directly at geriatric problems. Because they feel excluded from privileged access to modern benefits, grannies must continue to rely on social institutions grounded firmly in indigenous family structures. Grannies correctly perceive that without institutions such as fosterage, they, and old rural people in general, would have much more tenuous links to the mobile, educated generation of wage earners and the benefits they can provide.

Nevertheless, we have identified substantial transfers of wealth—or, perhaps more accurately, support—from grannies to young parents and their children, which common assumptions about African family economics would not have predicted. It is clear that looking only at parent-child relationships cannot explain the complexities of how the costs of African children are absorbed. It is also clear that we must work harder to understand the subtleties of these exchanges, both between children and their sponsors, as well as among the sponsors themselves. The support that grannies, for example, provide for young children and, indirectly, their parents is comprised of rural labor and subsistence foods. Such support is easily overlooked in the analysis because of its non-cash nature. Nonetheless, it figures centrally in the relationship between the rural old and the urban young. This support may in turn affect fertility, since grannies provide it to reproductive people at times when it may most likely lessen their costs of fertility.

The regional consequence is that many of the costs of urban fertility are being absorbed by the rural subsistence sector,[9] as political economists might also argue. Thus, the labor and food which must be expended for the children of urban parents is relatively cheap in cash terms: a pattern similar to the colonial era in some African countries, in which authorities sought to restrict women and children to rural areas, while employing men in urban jobs. Only when children are older, usually, are they sent to more urban areas where educational and training facilities are better, but costs of rearing are more expensive. We suggest, therefore, that other regional strategies for spreading the costs and benefits of children besides fosterage merit closer attention: for example, when rural relatives send urban parents subsistence staples to substitute for expensive urban foods.

Finally, despite our emphasis on fosterage, the fact that so many young children are sent to rural grannies is an outcome of the basic economic fact to which we alluded earlier: that the urban sector remains dependent in fundamental ways on the rural sector. We described how rural family members are occasionally called upon to send farm-grown subsistence foods to hardpressed urbanites who may be unemployed or without paychecks for several months. Rural elders are also called upon to grant access to rural family lands, to which all family members should be entitled. If, however, rural family members believe that their younger urban members have not remitted enough benefits from the modern world back to them, they may deny them access to these lands or may assign land with little farming value. Sending a child to a granny is a key sign of good will: that the parent is willing to send back remittances to his rural elders, when he can. Refusing to send a child, on the other hand, implies that the urbanite considers himself independent enough to risk endangering these ties. Needless to say, this is seldom done.

The paradox, of course, is that if urbanization increases and the national economy continues to deteriorate, the institution of sending young children to rural grannies is likely to increase: not merely because it is an expeditious way of caring for young children, but because it is only one of several options for bolstering the security that rests or strong urban-rural ties.

ACKNOWLEDGMENTS

We are grateful to the residents of the town in Sierra Leone where the child fosterage study was conducted (which we have kept anonymous for reasons of informant protection), and to the research assistants who worked on the project. The Institute of African Studies at Fourah Bay College offered in-country sponsorship of the child-fosterage project, and Dr. C. M. Fyle provided prompt and courteous assistance during the research. The Ford and Rockefeller foundations, the National Science Foundation, and the Population Council have provided generous support for data gathering and analysis. Finally, members of the Population Studies Center at the University of

Pennsylvania have been extraordinarily generous in delegating time and resources to the analysis phase of the project. For this we thank particularly Sam Preston and Etienne van de Walle. For comments on the issues raised in the paper, we are grateful to Sandra Barnes, Pat Caldwell, Douglas Ewbank, Douglas Massey, Ann Miller, Phil Morgan, William Murphy, Sam Preston, and Etienne van de Walle.

NOTES

1. Adherents of the demand side argue that desires for children are a primary determinant of fertility/and that people will find ways to regulate their family sizes accordingly. In contrast, supply side adherents suggest that because the demand for children is infinite in many developing countries, differences in fertility rates are determined by factors affecting the supply of children such as the "proximate determinants" of fertility, child mortality, and so on. We acknowledge that, at least in Africa, there is generally infinite demand for children. However, we believe that institutions such as fosterage may provide important clues for the much larger issue of why the demand for children remains so high.

2. However, ethnographic observations and interviews suggest that in many cases, fertility is determined less by a mechanical biological sequence of events than by individuals' efforts to produce certain fertility outcomes by using biology as a tool. Hence, fosterage and high fertility may be associated less because fosterage automatically reduces the time before the next conception through the proximate determinants of fertility, than because the desire to have another child quickly induces women to send their young children away to resume sexual relations with men.

3. Since young children seem to be sent further upcountry to rural grannies, their health and nutritional conditions frequently suffer. Many grannies live in areas with untreated water supplies, diminishing supplies of animal protein and staple foods, and lack of access to clinics and immunization programs. Grannies may also breast-feed children (or claim to), or say they will feed the children tinned milk—the health consequences of which are sometimes questionable. (See Bledsoe et al., in press.)

4. The reality, of course, is often different, since many grannies do enforce tough discipline on children and do not tolerate insults. But the notion that grannies spoil children strongly affects people's decisions about when to withdraw children from grannies. In contrast, people do not worry about a grandfather spoiling a child. A grandfather is seen as a senior elder in the family with great status, and his relationship with his grandchildren is seen as warm but distant. One young man expressed this well:

> The grandfather will just treat you as your parents do. A grandfather doesn't really pet you. He will not cook for you to eat, he will not bring water for you. He will best you, but the grandmother won't, at all! So people have more love for their grandmothers.

5. Of course, parents are also likely to "pet" their own children. For this reason, people may advise them to send the children to other people who will enforce discipline on them, so they can be of future benefit to the family. People stress that a child

must get away from the warm nurturance—yet severe restriction—of his natal household if he is to "develop" and to benefit his family. These worries are compounded if a child is with his granny.

6. There were more older in-fosters, proportionally, than older out-fosters in the survey. This is because, apparently, the town surveyed has several schools that would attract older children. The town was also located near a sawmill and had thriving carpentry and masonry businesses, which took in apprentices.

7. As this suggests, children's health is sometimes endangered by grannies' usurpation of resources intended for their minded children. In another instance, a woman took her 18-month-old son to stay in a rural village with her mother while she took on a parttime job in the larger town. Receiving news that the boy had contracted malaria, diarrhea, and anemia, and was rapidly losing weight, the mother sent for him so she could bring him to the hospital clinic. When the messenger returned, however, he reported that the granny refused to bring the child. Knowing her mother's probable motive, the woman explained that the granny was afraid she would not bring the boy back. After two such attempts, the mother finally went for the boy herself and brought him to the clinic.

8. The costs of older children may be absorbed in different ways within the urban sector. But since many children are fostered, their costs are borne by nonnatal family members or friends who may be better able to accommodate them. They also may be borne by the children themselves, who work in their foster households, as well as by the society at large, since a great deal of what these children consume may be stolen in various ways (see Bledsoe, 1983).

9. Ann Miller (personal communication) describes analogous patterns in the United States, when young black adults left the south and migrated to the north to work. Although many were poorly educated and unskilled, the south basically bore the costs of producing this labor, from which the north benefited in revenues. Similarly, Phil Morgan (personal communication) reports complaints from southern counties that bore the burden of educating black children who stayed behind when their parents migrated north for work and paid no southern taxes that would have offset these costs.

BIBLIOGRAPHY

Bledsoe, C. 1983. Stealing food as a problem in demography and nutrition. Paper presented at the 1983 meeting of the American Anthropological Association, Washington, D. C.

———. (In press). The politics of polygyny in Mende education and child fosterage transactions. In *Gender hierarchies*, ed. Barbara D. Miller.

———. 1987. Tinned milk and child fosterage: side-stepping the post-partum sex taboo. Paper presented at the Rockefeller Foundation conference on Cultural Roots of African Fertility Regimes, University of Ife, Ife, Nigeria.

Bledsoe, C., D. C. Ewbank, and U. C. Isiugo-Abanihe. (In press). The effect of child fosterage on feeding practices and access to health services in rural Sierra Leone. *Social Science and Medicine.*

Cain, M. 1981. Risk and insurance: Perspectives on fertility and agrarian change in India and Bangladesh. *Population and Development Review* 7: 435–474.

Caldwell, 1977. The economic rationality of high fertility: An investigation illustrated with Nigerian survey data. *Population Studies* 31(1): 5–27.

———. 1978. A theory of fertility: From high plateau to destabilization. *Population and Development Review* 4(4): 553–557.

———. 1982. Fertility and the household economy in Nigeria. In: *Theory of Fertility Decline*. New York: Academic Press, 11–81.

———. 1980. The wealth flows theory of fertility decline. In *Determinants of fertility: Theories re-examined*, ed. C. Hohn and R. Mackensen. Liège: Ordina Editions, 171–188.

Davis, K. 1955. Institutional patterns favoring high fertility in underdeveloped areas. *Eugenics Quarterly* 2(1): 33–39.

Etienne, M. 1983. Gender relations and conjugality among the Baule. In *Female and Male in West Africa*, ed. C. Oppong. London: George Allen and Unwin, 303–319.

Fapohunda, E. 1978. Characteristics of women workers in Lagos. *Labour and Society* 3(2): 158–171.

Frank, O. 1984. Child-fostering in sub-Saharan Africa. Presentation for the Population Association of America, Minneapolis, Minn.

Goody, E. N. 1982. Parenthood and social reproduction: Fostering and occupational roles in West Africa. Cambridge: Cambridge University Press.

Goody, E. N., and C. M. Groothues. 1977. West Africans: The quest for education. In: *Between two cultures*, ed. J. L. Watson. Oxford: Basil Blackwell.

Isaac, B. R., & S. R. Conrad. 1982. Child fosterage among the Mende of Upper Bambara Chiefdom, Sierra Leone: rural-urban and occupational comparisons. *Ethnology* 21: 243–257.

Isiugo-Abanihe, U. C. 1983. Child Fosterage in West Africa. *Population and Development Review* 11(1): 53–73.

Oppong, C. 1973. *Growing up in Dagbon*. Tema: Ghana Publishing Corp.

Potash, B. 1986. *Widows in African societies: Choices and constraints*. Stanford: Stanford University Press.

Schildkrout, E. 1973. The fostering of children in urban Ghana: Problems of ethnographic analysis in a multi-cultural context. *Urban Anthropology* 2: 48–73.

Scrimshaw, S. 1978. Infant mortality and behavior in the regulation of family size. *Population and Development Review* 4(3): 388–403.

Thomas, A. C. 1983. The population of Sierra Leone: An analysis of population census data. Freetown, Sierra Leone: Demographic Research and Training Unit, Fourah Bay College.

CHAPTER ELEVEN

Social Organization, Economic Crises, and the Future of Fertility Control in Africa

Ron Lesthaeghe

INTRODUCTION

At the United Nations population conference of Bucharest in 1974, African governments were almost without exception highly critical toward family planning programs. They felt that deliberate fertility regulation was either against their interest or not a priority. Socioeconomic development would automatically take care of the population problem—if there was one—and family planning was essentially a Western invention that would be brought to Africa in the wake of neocolonial patronage.

Two major elements changed this attitude. First, it was realized that African societies have always had a marked pattern of child-spacing implemented through prolonged breastfeeding and postpartum abstinence, and that this long-standing tradition was being eroded rather than supported by increased education, rising income, and especially urbanization. Without a countervailing force capable of restoring the older patterns of child-spacing, it was feared that such a change could lead to a deterioration of maternal and child health, to a slowing down of the infant mortality decline, and possibly to a fertility bulge. It was clear, at least during an initial phase, that socioeconomic development was not automatically "the best contraceptive." From that point onward, forms of fertility regulation were much harder to categorize as Western inventions, and contraception achieved legitimation as a necessary corrective for the declining authentically African pattern of child-spacing.

The second series of events accounting for a changing policy climate has been the succession of ecological, agricultural, economic, and political crises. Obviously, the severity of these problems varies widely from region to region, but, during the second half of the 1970s and the 1980s, virtually all nations felt that they had had too great a share of them. Even countries with stable political regimes such as Senegal, the Ivory Coast, and Cameroon, or major oil-exporting countries such as Nigeria, faced declining commodity prices and dwindling oil revenues. As a consequence, crises were no longer viewed as being sporadic and isolated. Instead, they were a pan-African problem.

The second African population conference held in Arusha in 1984 and the resulting Kilimanjaro Program of Action constitute a major turning point with respect to African demographic policies (Karefa-Smart, 1986; Adepoju, 1986). Of the forty-four nations present, thirty expressed dissatisfaction with current rapid population growth and explicitly indicated a need for contraceptive information and dissemination.

The decisive change in policy climate during the decade between 1974 and 1984 is obviously a necessary condition, but by no means a sufficient one. What are the prospects for a real fertility transition in Africa and how can the use-effectiveness of contraception be enhanced? This brings us to two critical questions:

1. Is it conceivable that a genuine and sustained fertility decline can occur in a situation of relative deprivation and in response to economic hardship, that is, in contrast to the conventional wisdom of demographic transition theory which connects a fertility transition to increased prosperity and advancing structural transformation?
2. What are the best strategies for promoting family planning, considering that the patterns of African social organization are distinct from those found in other LDCs?

Any attempt to answer these questions contains of necessity a great deal of speculation. But the need for addressing them is inescapable.

THE CRISIS-LED TRANSITION

Economic and sociological theories of fertility transition deal with the calculus and strategies of individuals and groups directed at the improvement of the welfare of children, women, parents, and even grandparents in a variety of cultural and structural contexts. The interpretations of Dumont (1980), Sauvy (1960) and Ariès (1980), for instance, accentuate the preoccupation with the welfare of children: parents limit fertility in an altruistic attempt to raise "child quality." Several current American economic theories and sociological theories concentrating on gender stratification accentuate predominantly the welfare and aspiration of women against the backdrop of unfolding economic opportunities or constrained emancipation. Caldwell's theory (1976, 1978) concerns the welfare of the three generations at once and accentuates the structural shifts in their relative positions with respect to intergenerational patterns of exchange and support. Cain's explanation

(1984, 1985) concentrates on the parental preoccupation with old-age security in high-risk environments. But all these theories connect, each in its own
way, the onset of a fertility transition to elements of structural change, such
as rising standards of living permitting greater investment in "child quality"
rather than quantity, female schooling producing rising opportunity costs of
maternity, transformations of spousal and kinship relations, and the development of non-kinship-based systems of risk devolution.

Theoretically at least, the current economic situation in Africa is likely to
have serious adverse effects on schooling, opportunities, and standards of
living, which in their turn may result in a further postponement of the fertility transition. Admittedly, there exists an extensive historical record showing *temporary* declines in fertility in response to economic crises, but these are
clearly distinct from a *sustained* fertility transition. Hence, there are hardly
any examples of genuinely "crisis-led" transitions.

Despite this, there is speculation that Africa may constitute an exception.
We have already pointed out that the change in policy climate with respect to
fertility control is induced largely by crises and fear for the future. This parallels to some extent the current situation in Bangladesh or the Indian situation in the 1950s and 1960s, where the fear of continued economic problems
has been equally prominent in fostering support for fertility regulation. But
the arguments in favor of a crisis-led transition go well beyond those concerning national policy formulation. Boserup for instance argues that the African
crises are seriously shaking the postindependence aspirations and that growing economic constraints may have a considerable effect on the individual
calculus (1985, p. 391):

> The majority of Africans experienced little, if any, increase in income after
> independence. But most anticipated a brighter economic future and better con-
> ditions for rearing a large family. In subsequent years, however, both income
> and expectations changed for the worse. In most African countries, the opti-
> mism has been replaced by disappointment and pessimism over future pros-
> pects. It is feared that educated children may be unable to find jobs. With
> diminishing employment opportunities for educated children, salary differences
> by educational level are diminishing or likely to diminish in the future. . .
> These changes are likely to make more Africans, especially in urban areas,
> inclined to delay the next birth or to terminate child-bearing.

Further on, Boserup argues that the much higher contraceptive prevalence
rates in Ghana compared to those of Kenya, that is, comparing the two countries that have had a favorable policy environment the longest, are attributable to Ghana having been hit much earlier and much harder by economic
hardship.

The hypothesis of a crisis-led transition clearly relies on the argument of
frustrated aspirations brought by rising costs of childrearing, reduced
prospective utility of educated children, and declining opportunities for

adults in general. Locoh (1985) sees a similar evolution for southern Togo, an area which is economically in much better shape than neighboring Ghana or Benin. But, she makes the fertility-reducing effect of rising child expenditures contingent on the capacity of kinship networks to fulfill their traditional function of risk devolution. The same is argued by Frank (1985). Beyond this point, however, the arguments become speculative. Such networks are functionally diversified in urban and rural areas respectively (see Page's chapter on child circulation). The educational function of urban child-fosterage, for example, is likely to undergo the immediate effects of rising costs and diminishing prospective returns, since not only biological parents but the entire network is facing a reassessment of positions and strategies. At present, it is not at all clear whether the added strain leads to tighter solidarity and mutual sacrifice or to harder bargaining. Our guess would go in the direction of the latter as there are signs that child-fosterage is increasingly being monetarized, thereby replacing strictly particularistic transactions governed by allegiance to a lineage by more marketlike ones.

The ramifications of the economic crisis for the childrearing costs are manifold. Another significant element in the process is undoubtedly the trend toward greater dependency of children on female incomes. The evolution pictured by Graham and Timaeus for Lesotho and Botswana, although not generated by the recent economic recession, ranks among the most dramatic in this regard. But in many African countries, trends during the last two or three decades have followed a similar direction, often as a result of changing land-tenure systems, lagging female education, and various other disadvantages for women associated with both traditional and new forms of division of labor (Boserup, 1970; Safilios-Rothchild, 1985). Given reduced projected returns from child investments for mothers, the economic security function of children may now be outbalanced by the greater immediate demands of child-related costs on weakening female incomes, even in West African areas with long-standing traditions of female economic self-reliance. In such conditions, wives may resort to harder bargaining with husbands on the issue of more equitable sharing of child costs, but it is not at all evident that male positions are responsive.

A third feature directly associated with the economic recession is the reduced importance of the migration valve (Locoh, 1985; Ssennyonga, 1985). Most colonial regimes had strict policies on migration, which was planned according to specific agricultural and industrial needs and curtailed for the rest. Such restraints were lifted in the postcolonial era, resulting in large migration streams to areas that offered better opportunities. The possibilities associated with migration formed part and parcel of the postindependence "aspirations boom." Ssennyonga, for instance, argues that Kikuyu parents were, at least until recently, still expecting their sons to migrate to the former "White Highlands" in Kenya, although these niches were filled more than a decade ago. At present, however, the continent-wide economic recession is eliminating such expectations. Deportation of illegal aliens from Nigeria, for instance, came as a shattering blow to many residents of neighboring countries. The psychological impact of the closure of the migration valve is consequently another salient argument in favor of the hypothesis of a crisis-led transition.

There is, however, no shortage of counterarguments. First and foremost, the situation in many areas—often those affected by civil war or ecological disaster—seems so precarious that the old Malthusian "positive checks," that is, mortality and refugee migration, are taking the upper hand. In such situations with elementary nutritional and health conditions falling considerably short of minimum standards, there is no scope for modern fertility control. If anything, fertility in such areas falls as a result of spousal separation, increased widowhood, or outright famine-induced amenorrhea. As the total area affected by political instability and/or dwindling agricultural output seems to be growing (see southern Sudan, Mozambique), one can envisage a widening disparity between the prevailing demographic regimes of sub-Saharan regions.

The second major caveat with respect to the hypothesis of a crisis-led transition is that curtailment of aspirations may either produce a temporary fertility trough only or, at best, a partial fertility transition with fertility remaining well above replacement level. In the first instance parents would again resort to higher fertility as soon as opportunities stop shrinking or if they realize that the benefits of reduced fertility control are spread over too long a period and therefore hardly worthwhile. The second possibility is more likely to occur in the more developed parts of Africa and especially in urban areas. According to this scenario, a reduction in total fertility from six to eight children to four or five reflects a population's responsiveness to both higher child costs and the continued importance of the security function of children (see Cain, 1983; Bongaarts, 1986). This scenario would also be consistent with a contraceptive breakthrough, but one with an early leveling-off of contraceptive momentum. The value at which the rise in the effectiveness of contraceptive use would level off is not only a function of the utility of higher-parity children but also of family planning availability and accessibility of medical services. With a current per capita annual expenditure on health for the continent as a whole of less than U.S. $2, efficient hormonal contraception is still beyond the means of many. In addition, there is virtually no local pharmaceutical industry producing hormonal contraceptives or vaccines. In such conditions, declining foreign export earnings and inflation can result in exorbitant prices. If contraception joins the list of hard-to-get essentials such as fertilizers and mechanical equipment, then conditions are fulfilled to sustain high fertility, low agricultural output, deficient transportation, and poor health. The combination of these would undoubtedly act in favor of an even more rapid return of the old Malthusian checks.

Third, one should also be aware, as shown in several of the preceding chapters, that there is still substantial room for a rise in the level of natural fertility through further reductions in breastfeeding, postpartum abstinence, and infertility. The evolution of breastfeeding durations needs close attention, especially in the Islamized sahelian belt and the interlacustrine area (Kivu, Rwanda, Burundi), where lactational amenorrhea is at present the single most important fertility-reducing component. The change in postpartum abstinence is of particular importance for the other areas of West and Central Africa. In addition, it is not evident that the relatively slow nuptiality transition of the 1960s and 1970s will be sustained or accelerated, and one should be equally aware of the trend toward rising teenage fertility in areas where traditional social controls are weakest. Hence, rising contraceptive prevalence may not be directly and fully translated into a substantial fertility reduction, and any attempt to evaluate program performance must continue to take such counterbalancing features into account.

The fourth factor that may steer parts of Africa away from a classic fertility transition is the spread of AIDS. If the current WHO estimates are correct, 5 million persons in this region are carriers of the virus, which implies an expected death toll of 1.5 million for the next decade assuming that 30 percent of those exposed are expected to develop AIDS within this time period. The exposed population is rapidly expanding, and the percentage developing AIDS is likely to be in excess of 30 percent in the long term. If no adequate vaccine is developed, AIDS casualties are therefore likely to be well in excess of 1.5 million. There are at present only three major ways to limit the spread: generalized use of condoms, a drastic change in sexual mores, and a further curtailment of migration. As a consequence, the demand for condoms as a prophylactic may far outstrip the demand for any other type of contraception in these regions. In the process, AIDS would not only cause a rise in mortality and a drop in fertility associated with weakness among those displaying the symptoms, but also through greater use of condoms among the hitherto unaffected individuals and latent carriers. At this point, it is far too early to produce the demographic picture of AIDS-affected populations, but it is certain that a new, and far more dangerous, pathological regime is in the making than the one that was based on venereal diseases and which was responsible for the Central African infertility belt.

To sum up, the current economic, political, ecological, and health crises in Africa are likely to produce three dominant demographic regimes:

1. The recurrence of old Malthusian positive checks in areas of drought, and diminished agricultural output and military operations

2. A new AIDS-dominated regime with high mortality among both adults and infants, and presumably, also with lowered fertility

3. A partial fertility transition characterized by lowered desired family

size and increased contraception, but with ultimate fertility levels well above replacement level.

Combinations of regimes 1 and 2 or of 2 and 3 are obviously possible. In the first instance, growth rates are likely to fall as a result of increased mortality and pathologically reduced fertility, whereas in the second, fertility would drop but only partially in response to a pathological factor, the rest being the result of an incipient transition. If total fertility rates fall to approximately five children by the year 2000 and four children by 2010, the United Nations medium projections as assessed in 1984 would hold, but this could be just as much the result of pathological conditions (regimes 1 and 2) as of a partial, crises-led fertility transition in the more developed and the urban areas (regime 3). All three regimes responsible for a prospective slowing down of population growth are a far cry from the original optimistic assumption that the United Nations medium projection would be the outcome of general economic development and greater prosperity.

THE COMMUNITY PERSPECTIVE

Community participation theories of development basically have a populist concept at their core: the possibilities for development reside essentially in simple people and their collective traditions (Medley, 1986). As such, the key issues are the *mobilization* of indiviudals and groups for *self-help* and self-sufficiency through *participation* in decision making at the local level. On the one hand, the philosophy of grass-roots development has gained worldwide acclaim, not in the least because it draws support from sources as diverse as utopianism (e.g., Ghandi's legacy), missionary activities, Marxist doctrine concerning cooperatives, political mobilization in one-party systems, ideological and moral patronage in pluralist societies, United Nations and non-governmental organizations' basic needs programs, Western "postmaterialist" values, anthropological and general social science insights, and ecological concerns. On the other hand, the record of community participation contains numerous caveats: problems range from bureaucratic mismanagement, "muddling through," pseudo-participation (defined by Medley as the mere ratification of decisions taken by outside agencies), and political patronage and corruption, to community fragmentation by class, caste, ethnic, or religious interests, internal political strife, and conflicts of leadership. In short, external agencies have their own goals and hidden agenda, whereas the communities seldom display the ideal image of a fully integrated "organic entity." However, it would be grossly unfair to impute these drawbacks to community-based projects in general: the variation in performance is huge and the lessons learned from both successes and failures are invaluable.

It is not our aim to drum up a lengthy narrative on community-based projects and their performance history. Rather, we shall try to explore the a priori possibilities for sub-Saharan Africa with respect to family planning program organization. In doing so, we shall briefly review the interest of the demographic profession in community variables, draw on some Asian experience of community involvement in family planning, and on African experience with the closely related topic of maternal and child health. Finally, we shall discuss the functions of a variety of African associations since many of them have played historical roles in community development.

On the whole, the demographic profession has exhibited relatively little interest in variables concerning local aspects of social organization and their potential for action. The contrast with other "applied fields" like medicine or agriculture is often striking. In the 1960s, however, it seemed that the issue of family planning program diffusion was about to generate an active academic momentum for modeling diffusion and for studying network mechanisms and patterns of social integration (Retherford and Palmore, 1983). But such studies remained scarce and the field did not grow beyond a small set of sociometric studies, mostly conducted in Southeast Asia (e.g., Rogers, 1962, 1973; Rogers and Kincaid, 1981; Rogers et al., 1976; Palmore, 1968; Palmore et al., 1977; Kim and Palmore, 1978). Nevertheless, several of these studies highlighted the crucial role of the Korean mothers' clubs in the rapid spread of contraception in the rural parts of that country (see also Lee, 1977; Enea, 1985).

The directions indicated by these "network" studies were not followed. The background paper by Bulatao (1984) produced for the World Bank on policy levers, for instance, contains a framework that identifies two agents only: governments and individual households. There are no organizations or networks at the community level, there is no moral and social patronage, no leadership, not much of a diffusion process, in short, not much of a community. We suspect that part of a shift away from the analysis at the community level can be linked to the growing dominance of microeconomic theories of demographic behavior. Such models are primarily concerned with the calculus of *individuals* and assess utilities, disutilities, and strategies at this level only. There is often a total disregard for context and especially for patterns of social organization. In all fairness though, it should be mentioned that a more recent World Bank policy study, "Population Growth and Policies in Sub-Saharan Africa" (1986), redresses the balance and pays ample attention to the roles of churches and indigenous African organizations.

In the 1980s, another major think-tank was organized by the U.S. National Academy of Sciences, and a complete summary of research dealing with the determinants of fertility in LDCs was commissioned. The 840-page report (Bulatao and Lee, 1983) contains an analytic framework put together by six eminent specialists. This framework lists a set of "illustrative effects of major social institutions on fertility," but there is no mention of social organizational characteristics at the community level among them. Admittedly the initial framework is complemented by several chapters that could have treated the latter subject in greater detail, but only two of these chapters really discuss networks, local patterns of organization, and stratification variables as a central issue. None of the chapters discusses the issue of community organization in sub-Saharan Africa.

The third major demographic enterprise since 1975 is undoubtedly the World Fertility Survey. The WFS did construct a "community module" to serve along the individual-level data gathering, but the module's interest is almost exclusively directed at utilities and amenities such as piped water, electricity, sanitation, access to health facilities, schools, communication facilities, and roads. Nothing touches on the issues of local organization and their historical roots, or on older and contemporary functions of village organizations and urban neighborhood networks. Clearly, the information on utilities and amenities was gathered in the hope that such variables would provide convenient proxies for the degree of socioeconomic development or for the degree of integration into the wider economy and social life of the nation. But individual education does almost as well, if not better, in providing such a proxy. A subsequent seminar tried to put the findings into perspective, and Casterline (1985, p. 73) reports:

> Totalling up the statistically significant findings leaves one almost empty-handed. Measures of community development—agricultural modernization, non-agricultural economic activities, village modernization as measured by the presence of utilities and amenities—rarely show systematic relationships with fertility.

Casterline is careful enough to point out some exceptions, and so does Tsui in her review of sixteen earlier studies that included contextual variables; but Casterline reaffirms his pessimistic conclusion (1985, p. 73):

> Nevertheless, one cannot help but think that were community features—such as clinics, schools, availability of electricity and piped water or paved roads—influencing reproductive behaviour through some means, this fact would be more apparent in the results.

Somewhat akin to the WFS community-module approach are studies that pick specific "infrastructural" development projects (e.g., electrification, irrigation, and introduction of new plant varieties) and attempt to trace the ultimate effect on reproduction (e.g., Stoeckel and Jain, 1986, dealing with such projects in Asia). These attempts are more sophisticated in the sense that they offer a time perspective by sketching a historical chain of events and follow the "infrastructural" effect through intermediate variables such as schooling, health, female employment, or child labor. But several critical issues remain:

1. One can focus equally well on "infrastructural" projects that show either no effect or even a positive effect on fertility. Hence, a comparison of relative "failures" and "successes" seems necessary to throw light on crucial intervening variables, which are likely to be part of the social organizational environment.

2. Local groups are either interested in attracting, or alternatively, instrumental in rejecting development projects. The causality is now reversed: local patterns of social organization and village interest groups can also be considered as the initiating force rather than as mere mediating instruments.

Our survey of major recent conceptual frameworks (World Bank, U.S. National Academy of Sciences, WFS) that guided both research and policy formulation shows that the importance of local organizational parameters has been underdocumented and therefore undervalued. Such an underestimation, if continued, seems particularly lethal in the sub-Saharan context for reasons we shall now discuss.

IS THE ASIAN FAMILY PLANNING EXPERIENCE RELEVANT FOR SUB-SAHARAN AFRICA?

With the start of the fertility transition during the late 1970s in most non-Islamic Asian countries and in many Latin American ones, this question is obviously firmly on the agenda. Although most classic authors dealing with the conditions necessary for a demographic transition admit that there is no clearly delineated threshold in terms of levels of socioeconomic development beyond which a fertility decline starts, many still expect sub-Saharan Africa to go through its own fertility decline once improvements in child survival, school enrollment, urbanization, and income have been realized. The World Bank obviously leans towards this view (1986, pp. 12–13):

> The strength of traditional pronatalist attitudes in much of sub-Saharan Africa raises the question of whether they are unique to Africa or parts of Africa. The answer is, probably not. First, incomes are generally lower than in other countries, levels of education and health levels are poorer, and urbanization is less extensive; these factors help explain Africa's persistent high fertility. Secondly, much of the progress that has occurred in Africa—reduction in child mortality and improvements in life expectancy, increases in school enrollment and in urbanization, and improvements in status of women—is so recent that old attitudes have had little time to change. Parents may not fully recognize the improvements in health, for example, or they may not be convinced that they will last. Third, although traditional beliefs . . . reinforce pronatalist attitudes in much of Africa, such beliefs are not unique to Africa. Some religious leaders express reservations about family planning, but others, both inside and outside Africa, are supportive. The teachings of the Catholic Church on marriage and

sex have an influence in some African countries, but so do they elsewhere. It is likely that in Africa, as in other parts of the world, these views will change as development proceeds.

J. and P. Caldwell (1985) are considerably more cautious and consider the economic, political, and religious arguments in greater depth. Restricting the comparison to southern India and West Africa, the two areas they are most familiar with, they concentrate on important differences with respect to organizational context and policy levers. Among the contextual variables, attention is drawn to the almost diametrically opposed systems of traditional land tenure and social stratification, to the contrasts in family structure and intrafamilial decision processes, and finally to the different contents of religion. Among the policy variables, the difference in the role and especially the power of governments is stressed. In our opinion too, these are precisely the factors that are of greater importance than the classic structural indicators of development. Such organizational and political factors are responsible for the failure of any threshold hypothesis in accounting for the fertility transition. In addition, they are bound to shape the sub-Saharan family planning effort in a distinct way. The arguments advanced by the Caldwells require further elaboration.

1. The Caldwell analysis centers largely on the intrafamilial responsibilities and decision-making systems. These are indeed crucial for the adoption of family limitation and even for the specific contraceptive method-mix used. In the African context, husbands and wives, being members of different lineages and having numerous responsibilities to a variety of persons within their respective corporate kinship groups, are frequently in a bargaining position vis-à-vis each other. They often keep separate budgets and maintain a fairly large social distance. This system of diverging interests and loyalties contrasts with the much more unified and cohesive husband–wife dyad in Asian systems. In the latter, husbands are directly and fully responsible for their offspring on the basis of a pooled family budget stemming from relatively fixed familial land resources or from familial artisanal productivity. The family economy in Asia is consequently much more cohesively structured than the African one, where corporate allegiance and traditional corporate "ownership" of land resources with "fluid" individual usage have left a fundamental mark on the functioning of household and lineage economies. This structural difference between Asian and sub-Saharan families is used by the Caldwells in explaining the lack of interest in family limitation among African males as opposed to the much greater interest among Asian fathers, and for the African aversion toward male contraception as opposed to the central role played by vasectomies in India. The contrast outlined by the Caldwells may

be somewhat exaggerated. Their comparison involves predominantly examples from the Akan and Yoruba groups that are renowned for their typically Western African weak husband-wife dyad. Also, individual ownership of land has made serious inroads in Africa and this trend is the singularly most important factor that weakens lineage cohesion. Nevertheless, the presence of so many female-headed households, even in areas other than Southern Africa, and the gradual replacement of polygyny by "outside wives" in urban areas point in the direction of a continued weaker husband-wife dyad in Africa than in Asia. When the responsibilities of men toward their offspring is not enhanced, the myth of male virility, which existed everywhere, is also likely to have a longer life in Africa.

2. The Caldwells use the religious contrast and its social organizational basis in accounting for the Asian-African disparity with respect to the acceptability of abortion. As is well known, the Korean, Chinese, and Japanese fertility limitation programs at one point all relied on this method to a considerable extent. It is also well known that these populations resorted occasionally to infanticide of girls in the past. According to Arthur Wolf (1984), historical infanticide and female mutilations (e.g., bound feet) in the Far East are typical for societies where families tend to expand control over resources through the maximization of the number of sons. Families and households are essentially rivals, and daughters constitute merely a loss. Low female status, total female economic dependence, and customary female mutilation in the past have culturally facilitated recourse to abortion as a major family planning ingredient. The main obstacles to "programmatic" abortion in Asia have been Islam and Christianity (e.g., in the Philippines). The African religious system with its strong component of ancestral punishments is historically oriented toward protecting and expanding *corporate* lineage or tribal control over territories. The strategy does not oppose households but much larger entities. In this system both males and females are valuable and indispensable for the survival of the corporate group: males were protectors and potential conquerors of cattle and territory, females are procreators and agricultural producers. In other words, corporate groups are *collectively* preoccupied with demographic survival and fertility. Fertility impairments were always considered in Africa to be an ancestral curse, not only for the woman concerned but for her entire lineage. Polygyny and the occasional transfer of male sexual rights to someone other than the husband are typically African ways of coping with an infertility problem. In such a situation abortion and female sterilization are not likely to become major ingredients in any family planning program.

3. The third contrast stressed by the Caldwells pertains to the differences

in state formation, bureaucratic strength, and social stratification. These differences are not so much important for the contraceptive method-mix but for program implementation and design. Asian societies experienced state formation centuries before the colonial period and they have complex forms of class and caste stratification. Some of them developed large bureaucracies and intricate taxation systems. Furthermore, within the social stratification system there was often a group that specialized in theological and moral leadership (e.g., Hindu Brahmans, Buddhist monks, Confucian administrators), and this was combined with plain economic patronage over lower castes. Strong moral and administrative leverage was therefore already present well before family planning was an issue. Moreover, at a later stage, the family planning issue became a major element through which central governments strengthened their position and eliminated local oppositions. The Asian record in this respect is particularly striking: the family planning programs of India, Indonesia, Korea, Singapore, and above all of the People's Republic of China are the direct result of major governmental pressure and mass mobilization. Despite the fact that the opposition was sometimes strong (e.g., in India) and the stakes high, governments took family planning extremely seriously as their own authority had come to depend on it. The Indonesian case is rather illustrative of this (Warwick, 1986; van Norren, 1985). According to McNicoll and Singarimbun (1983), the 1965 coup led to a major strengthening of the central government and a weakening of the local traditionalist groups: "there was a sudden quieting, in fact virtual halting, of village politics" (p. 87), and "the depolitization of village life helped to ensure that there was no misapprehension about the government's programme goals in population, and that there were no attacks of any consequence on the programme on moral grounds (or on political grounds masquerading as moral)" (p. 87). The program in South Korea operated along more subtle lines, but the famous Korean mothers' clubs in the rural areas were essentially a government initiative and so are the obligatory periodic "neighborhood meetings" where individuals are supposed to discuss how government policies can be implemented locally. The other side of the coin is of course that oppositions also use the family planning issue and do not fail to point out its coercive aspects (see Warwick, 1986, on Indonesia). But the general lesson from the Asian family planning successes has been that they occurred when central governments were in a phase of strengthening their positions and were mastering greater control over virtually all matters of daily life. In short, family planning has been one of the vehicles of "nation building" as understood by central governments in Asia.

The African situation is at present far removed from these Far Eastern examples. Bureaucratic forms of control, even in the African examples of indigenous state formation, were never at par with the Indian, Indonesian, Chinese, Korean, or Japanese examples prior to the industrial revolution or the colonial period. Moreover, several African examples of early state-formation stem from Islamic conquests, and the rulers' legitimacy among the conquered was often tarnished by the practice of slavery. Colonial regimes were never experienced as legitimate. Postcolonial regimes, finally, are often besieged by rivalry between ethnic groups, and in some instances those who happen to be in command are viewed by others as intruders. Clearly, the nation-building record of African states is highly varied: the range spans cases of hitherto minimal ethnic tensions (e.g., the Ivory Coast), to cases of permanent experimentation (e.g., Nigeria), and ultimately to examples of outright failure (e.g., Uganda). Although state-sponsored family planning programs have been scarce in Africa, the few examples show the link with phases of nation building: the first family planning program on the continent, that is, Ghana's, lasted until the purges took place against the Akan elites that carried the country to independence, and the present, allegedly strong program performance in Zimbabwe is a part of the ZANU government extending and consolidating its control over the country. Hence, Caldwell's argument that the strength of a national government delineates a marked Asia-versus-Africa contrast in program performance seems highly valid. Hence, one can argue that the African national family planning efforts in the post-Arusha era are likely to be *intimately* linked with the further *political* developments of the nations that signed the Kilimanjaro declaration of 1984.

All of this constitutes a major departure from the too-facile extrapolations of the Asian experience to Africa performed on the basis of half a dozen international development indicators. Aside from the fact that the Asian contraceptive method-mix with its components of abortion and male and female sterilization cannot be grafted onto a sub-Saharan setting, the main difference seems to stem from the respective histories in state formation and from current levels of governmental leverage. With very few exceptions, African governments have neither the strength or audacity, nor the necessary means of totally committing themselves to a full-scale and nationwide family planning operation. African leaders may furthermore realize that family planning, if fostered too strongly and too fast, could be a rope they hang around their own neck. They will, as a consequence, have to follow a more subtle path, namely that of eliminating major obstacles and allowing more grassroot level organizations, whose legitimacy has been forged by virtue of a long-standing record of community service, to engage in the actual program implementation. This means encouragement and where possible also ad hoc subsidizing of women's associations, churches, and other NGOs involved in projects of maternal and child health, income generation, and family planning promotion.

THE GRASS-ROOTS: WHO ARE THEY?

As already mentioned, day-to-day activities and management with respect to social and economic aspects of development in sub-Saharan Africa are largely in the hands of numerous community networks. Several such networks existed in a traditional form before the colonial period, and they have gradually shifted their functions and orientations since then. Other organizations were brought in with the Islamic and colonial conquests, and the latest set is largely the product of the postcolonial era. Obviously, not all types of associations and networks reviewed here will be instrumental in family planning, and several may even vigorously oppose it. In fact, we know very little about membership, shifts in functions, and attitude toward fertility regulation. Large surveys of the WFS type would be ideally suited to collect membership data and to draft lists of local organizations with the aim of studying differential interest in and use of contraception in such networks. At present, however, such statistically representative data are extremely rare for all continents, not just for sub-Saharan Africa alone (for an exception see the study of mothers' clubs in Bangladesh by J. Akbar, 1985). Hence, not only is the field of inquiry wide open but, more importantly, we can at present offer only highly speculative comments drawing on a small set of examples, mainly described by anthropologists. We shall start with a discussion of the traditional organizations and proceed chronologically.

The first major set of traditional organizations belong, especially in West Africa, to what O'Barr (1984) calls the *dual sex system*. These organizations form an intricate cluster and are often to some degree a mirror image of male organizations at the various levels. The female branch of the dual system often starts with a female counterpart to a paramount chief or regional chief and descends to local female work parties. Typical examples of such an unfolding by sex from the top down are for instance found among the Bamileke of the Cameroon Highlands (see chap. 1), the Edo, Igbo, Yoruba and Nupe of Nigeria, the Akan groups in Ghana and the Ivory Coast, or the Mende of Sierra Leone. All these ethnic groups had a "queen," either at the summit of a cluster of clans or at the top of market women's associations (e.g., the Ashanti "Queen Mother," the Igbo Omu, the Nupe Sagi and Sonya, the Yoruba Iyalode, the Bamileke Mafo) (Awe, 1977; Okonjo, 1976; Wipper, 1984). Officers in these traditional organizations were often elected and decisions were frequently taken after consultation with the basis. Traditionally, such societies fulfilled four main functions: (1) they were legislative bodies, often with juridical power, (2) they organized community services and female work parties, (3) they had important ritual functions associated with initiation and burial, and (4) they protected women, either individually or as a group, against men, particularly when physical harm was inflicted or when political and economic interests of women were at stake. Protest actions could take the form of public manifestations, civic disobedience, or charivari (e.g., the "sitting on a man" practiced by Igbo women; see Van Allen, 1972; Okonjo, 1976).

In central, eastern, and southern Africa, both male and female branches of the "dual sex system" are much less developed. By contrast, the main traditional form of nonkinship solidarity among women in Eastern and Southern Africa is based simply on age grades and traditional work parties (which are not uncommonly structured by age grade). The relative importance of associations introduced during the colonial period has therefore been enhanced to a considerable extent. Networks associated with churches, both mainstream and syncretic, and associations sponsored by the governments of the postcolonial period have largely filled the original eastern and southern African vacuum.

The record and the potential of traditional, colonial, and postcolonial systems of mobilization will now be considered.

1. The most traditionalist of all original female associations are beyond doubt the *secret societies*. They are especially of importance in Guinea, Sierra Leone, Liberia, and the Southwest of the Ivory Coast. Female secret societies, commonly known in this region as the Sande or Bundu, have as main functions the education and initiation of girls (the "bush schools"), the creation of cohesion among women, and the strengthening of their own patterns of stratification (Wipper, 1984). These societies are commonly described as highly conservative forms of patronage of the poorer and younger women by the wealthy and older ones (Little, 1951, 1965; Hoffer, 1972; Bledsoe, 1980; Wipper, 1984). The ruling women of the Sande societies each have an area of special competence, and as such they control substantial segments of the educational system as an extension of their patronage over the former "bush schools." Traditional midwives, the Sowo, are also found at the top of the Sande hierarchy (McCormack, 1982; Wipper, 1984). Hence, such secret societies constitute powerful networks in matters concerning procreation, infant and maternal health, education, local politics, and ancestral religion. Despite their conservative image, Sande support has been obtained in health projects. Already in the 1940s the subsequent first prime minister of Sierra Leone, Dr. Milton Margai, managed to propagate modern methods of nursing and sanitation through the Sande bush schools (Kaplan, 1976). More recently, a regional Catholic hospital in Seratu (Southern Sierra Leone) used the Sande midwives and the male Poro secret societies, in a health project (Ross, 1979; Hardiman, 1986). The project goals were the reduction of the incidence of intestinal parasites, infant diarrhea, malnutrition, and tuberculosis through improvements in sanitation, hygiene, and immunization. The Seratu scheme operated through village health com-

mittees set up by the villagers themselves. As such the project came into direct contact with the Sande midwives and with the male Poro societies, whose traditional responsibilities include water supplies, rubbish removal, and defecation regulations. One of the results of the project is the virtual eradication of neonatal tetanus, which accounted previously for a quarter of all neonatal deaths, and widespread tuberculosis inoculation. The Seratu project illustrates how an existing and admittedly traditionalist network can be put to the advantage of a new idea, provided that support is mustered in the right way and at the right time. It is, furthermore, not difficult to imagine that any family planning effort in Liberia or Sierra Leone could run into serious trouble if its introduction were to ignore the Sande or to consider them a priori as a traditionalist counterforce.

2. As in the Asian setting, traditional birth attendants are also of major significance in Africa for all matters concerning procreation and infant health. The original link between their work and traditional religion has become weaker, and as a result traditional midwives are not always integrated into a larger female society. Nevertheless, they have remained persons with considerable authority within the villages or towns. Moreover, they form a very important profession numerically. The Danfa project in Ghana, for instance, enumerated 730 traditional midwives per 100,000 population against 9 medical doctors and 91 nurses. In the Machakos region east of Nairobi, there were 120 traditional birth attendants compared with 6 doctors and 77 nurses per 100,000 population (Family Health International, 1986). These figures are illustrative for much of Africa, and they clearly indicate that any maternal and child health or family planning project is unlikely to be met with success if this potential remains either unused or underutilized.

3. The second set of traditional networks is made up of *age grades* and local *work parties*. Age grades, or looser versions thereof, fulfilled essentially a socialization function. They can also continue to function as formal or informal adult groups or constitute the basis for other forms of organizations such as work parties or dance groups. In general, the functions of age grades have been considerably weakened by formal education and urbanization. The same also holds for traditional work parties as communities have become more heterogeneous ethnically and especially since land tenure has evolved toward private ownership. Nevertheless, the trust that members of such groups have in each other has facilitated the formation of *income-generating groups* and several of these are known to have developed into modern *producer cooperatives*. Another modern development grafted onto existing traditional work parties has been fostered by governments that have tried to set up and structure

new *self-help groups* (e.g., the Kenyan Harambee). Already in their traditional form, female work parties were confronted with the problem of child care, and more recent organizational forms stemming from them have often found better-structured solutions. Matters of child care and child health are hence very important issues in modern female income-generating groups. Benefits accruing to the group or cooperative rather than to the individual members are therefore commonly used to set up dispensaries or other communal health facilities.

4. The third type of traditional associations is *occupational*. By far the most important ones are the West African *market-women associations*. Over 80 percent of all petty and wholesale traders are women in southern Ghana and Southwest Nigeria; this figure is roughly 60 percent in the Dakar region and 50 percent in eastern Nigeria (Kaplan, 1971; Wipper, 1984). Their associations fulfill the following functions. First, they regulate prices and, on occasion, organize the black market (e.g., the Ghanaian "queen bees"). Second, they buy in bulk and make sure that a certain commodity is not traded by others, women or men. Third, they often have their mutual aid arrangements for important ceremonies, and last but not least, they often constitute the main form of female economic and political power. In East and Central Africa, on the other hand, trading is predominantly a male preoccupation and such powerful female occupational groups are lacking. Women's associations also exist in other occupations, but they never approach the West African market-women's associations in size and economic or political importance.

5. The fourth set of traditional associations is made up by *mutual aid societies* and *rotating credit networks*. Both initially provided group insurance against major expenditures such as those occasioned by marriages or burials. Group insurance is equally based on mutual trust and, as a result, such organizations can be grafted onto other sorts of networks based on neighborhood, occupation, ethnicity, or even entertainment clubs. The rotating credit system is found in virtually all regions of sub-Saharan Africa. Periodic contributions are made to a common fund and the individual members take turns in receiving the proceeds. A large advance can be given if a special need arises, for example, a burial or a substantial hospital bill. At present, however, rotating credit networks are often instrumental in financing hire-purchase. Mutual aid societies, *senso strictu*, do not necessarily involve rotating credit but merely spread the cost of a single event over all members. A typical example is the Swahili *lelemama* dance association along the Kenyan coast. The *lelemama* provide entertainment at weddings and at the same time organize mutual help for members by collecting money for funerals and festivities. The *lelemama*, however, did not develop any other

major economic or political functions, despite the fact that attempts were made to use them as a basis for more profound female solidarity (Strobel, 1974, 1976). In contrast to age grades, mutual aid societies and rotating credit networks seem to be flourishing in urban environments, not least because their fundraising system resembles that of a chain letter, which obviously thrives on the rapid growth of membership. Another reason for their popularity is that mutual aid societies based on ethnicity or region of origin provide means for migrant integration (Little, 1965, 1974; Kaplan, 1971; Nelson, 1974). *Urban migrant clubs* are also known to develop functions vis-à-vis the area of origin. The typical example of such a development is provided by the Igbo "Improvement Unions" (Nelson, 1972). These unions were predominantly made up of better-educated and wealthier migrants who not only sponsored infrastructural projects (schools, dispensaries) in the home town, but also provided fellowships and served as spokesmen for the "new ways." The typical term for this activity was to help one's community in "getting up." It is obvious that mutual aid societies and especially urban migrant clubs involved in similar activities for the benefit to communities of origin possess a considerable potential in legitimizing fertility control by discussing the issue and in spreading the acceptability to rural areas.

The colonial period is of course characterized by the addition of Western-style organizations often sponsored and run by Christian missions. Typical services concerned basic health and above all education. But, around these nuclei other organizations grew. They included youth organizations (such as Girl Guides and Boy Scouts, the YMCA, the YWCA, once Catholic youth clubs) and church women's groups (such as the Zimbabwean Mothers' Unions or Women's Fellowships [Muchena, 1982]). With the departure of Western missionaries, many of these organizations declined, but in Eastern and especially in Southern Africa, local black churches remained a vigorous source of political and social mobilization. Both local and mainstream Protestant churches are members of the World Council of Churches, and this organization has continued its sponsorship of development projects. Moreover, several Kenyan Protestant churches are at present directly involved in family planning. The Catholic church, by contrast, has been trailing behind with respect to the Africanization of its clergy (largely a consequence of imposed celibacy) and, of course, it still opposes any form of family planning through methods other than rhythm. Although local priests are often more tolerant than the church itself, Catholic networks are not likely to function openly as agents of family planning propagation. Moreover, the rhythm method is both unpopular and more often than not misunderstood. Finally, as the Vatican is unlikely to adapt its theological ruling whereas governments are currently reviewing and altering their policies, an important conflict between state and church is in the making (e.g., in Rwanda).

Other types of colonial initiative stemmed from white settlers and the colonial administration itself. Examples of such a development are the Kenyan *Maendeleo ya Wanawake* ("progress for women") and the Cameroon *corn mill societies*. The Maendeleo was organized initially by a small group of European women in the 1950s under the auspices of the colonial Department of Community Development and Rehabilitation. It was patterned after the Women's Institutes of rural Britain and its objectives were to improve African standards of living through instruction concerning farming methods, nutrition, hygiene, and handicrafts. This was done in combination with cultural and sports activities (Wipper, 1975, 1984). Shortly after independence, however, the Maendeleo went into decline as the movement's leadership was taken over by the new urban elite and as the rural members were alienated by unfulfilled promises, meagre financial support, and the lifestyles of their leaders (Wipper, 1975, 1984). More recently, however, there are signs that the Maendeleo is being reorganized and the promotion of family planning has been included among its goals. The Cameroon corn mill societies also stemmed from the ideals of the British Women's Institute in the 1950s (Wipper, 1984). The colonial Department of Education bought fifteen corn mills and made then available on loan to some 30 villages. These loans were paid off very quickly and more mills were purchased. The mill societies spread until they totaled 200 and other activities were added. First came classes in cooking, child care, hygiene, and nutrition. This was followed by agricultural improvements in cattle keeping, corn growing, and poultry farming. Finally village plots were reforested, water storage facilities were built, and cooperative stores were opened (Wipper, 1984).

As already indicated, traditional work parties have probably the greatest potential for developing into a broad network of self-help and cooperative associations, especially if such a movement is fostered by governments. Kenya's Harambee illustrates this grass-root effort. In the Kikuyu Central Province, and especially in the district of Murang'a, the initial mobilization took place through the *mabati*—work groups that were originally set up to provide corrugated iron roofing and were also involved in mutual assistance among women (Mønsted, 1978). In the Kamba area (Eastern Province), the roots were the *mwethya* groups that were involved in coffee plantation terracing since the 1950s (i.e., since the Swynnerton plan) and the clan-based *Mbai sya Eitu* ("girls' clans") which provided political support for local politicians in the 1961 election (Wipper, 1984). The Mbai sya Eitu furthermore raised a substantial amount of funding for self-help projects in the process. In 1976–1978 the Kenyan Women's Bureau, a governmental organization, carried out one of the very few surveys that provide statistics on the size and activi-

TABLE 11.1 Number of Women's Self-Help Groups and Membership, Kenya 1978

Province	Number of Groups	Average Membership	Total Membership	Total Membership Per 1000 Women 20+	District with Highest and Lowest Relative Membership
Central	2900	46	134 100	275	Muranga's (413), Nyeri (141)
Eastern	2840	30	105 200	191	Kitui (299), Isiolo (37)
Coast	330	55	18 150	64	Taita-Taveta (159), Mombasa (35)
Rift	855	35	29 900	58	West Pokot (130), Turkana (9)
Nyanza	770	30	24 600	37	Kisii (46), Kisumu (29)
Western	450	30	13 500	35	Busia (51), Kakamega (27)
Northeastern	30	30	900	14	Garissa (27), Mandera (6)
Kenya (excluding Nairobi)	8225	40	326 400	110	

SOURCE: M. Mønsted, 1978; Women's Bureau estimates based on 1976 survey.

ties of female income generation and self-help groups. The results, presented by province in table 11.1, indicate that the self-help groups could draw on the involvement of a quarter of all adult women in most of the districts inhabited by the Kikuyu, Kamba, and Meru-Embu, whereas the figures fall short of 5 percent in the other densely populated areas of Western and Nyanza provinces (Luhya, Luo, Kisii, and Kalenjin groups). Typical for the Rift Valley is also the greater support (10 to 15 percent) in districts with substantial Kikuyu settlements, that is, belonging to the former "White Highlands." Evidently, this regional pattern has been formed as a joint result of the prior existence of viable traditional work parties among agriculturalist populations and the presumably preferential channeling of funds to the ethnic groups that supported the government. Typical is also that pastoralists of the Rift Valley and Northern Kenya are hardly to be found in these statistics. Wipper (1984) considers this absence of viable modern self-help groups among pastoralists as a general feature and not as a specifically Kenyan pattern. Furthermore, she also indicates that the populations of the "labor reserve" areas in southern Africa exhibit such a contrast with the persistence of traditional forms of cooperative work in Kenya. This is obviouly related to the fact that agriculture is not thriving in the arid zones of Botswana, Lesotho, and the regions set aside as Bantu homelands in the RSA, to the strong dependence on male wages, and to the general breakdown of traditional structures caused by male and female labor mobility and resettlement.

The postcolonial era has been characterized by the formation of political organizations. A few have roots in the older forms and female networks (e.g., the Mbai sya Eitu among the Kamba), many grew during the struggle for independence, and almost all have become the instruments of the single-party system. As such, they have often regressed to public relations outfits for the production of folklore shows during diplomatic visits or they form the typical recruitment basis for the slots in international delegations. However, because of their closeness to the centers of power, leading political women have often been highly instrumental in altering the policy environment in favor of matters of direct importance to women. This includes the recent change in governmental policies with respect to family planning. But, the main problems arise when it comes to the relations with the population at large. The wide gap between elite urbanites and rural women is seldom bridged, as we have documented through Wipper's description of the Kenyan Maendeleo. The second example is provided by Swantz (1985) and Geiger (1982) for the Tanzanian Umoja wa Wanawake (UWT), organized in 1962. Its purpose was the provision of an umbrella for existing women's associations and the channeling of political support, readily given by women to the TANU party during the independence struggle, toward Ujamaa. But Swantz's account is so typical for female political organizations elsewhere that it is worth repeating once more (1985, p. 160):

It was overlooked at the time that women in villages and in the towns had their own forms of association not recorded anywhere, and that the services of the natural leaders of the social groups within the local structures were not asked for when the new structures were being created. . . . Thus, an opportunity to build on women's ways of linking up and acting together was missed. . . . When during our various studies ordinary women in villages and workplaces were questioned about the significance of UWT to them, their answers almost invariably had the tone: "We have not yet come so far."

But political control can be more deleterious than that if governments use their political organizations for squarely imposing centrally conceived plans, however well intentioned some of these may be. The *zemecha* policy of the revolutionary government of Ethiopia provides an illustration. The zemecha are a corps of 60,000 mostly urban-based students and officials who were deployed to take command over the 1974 agricultural reforms, which were indeed badly needed to replace the feudal system of the old regime. As such the zemecha were also put in charge of the new peasant associations (Abate and Teklu, 1982; Hall, 1986). In 4 years time 28,000 such associations were formed, officially covering 7.8 million households. But, as the zemecha remained in control and left very little initiative to the peasantry itself, absenteeism was rampant and the reformers often came to be viewed as intruders. The drama can be complete in settings of recurrent violence and political disintegration as for instance in Ghana, or even more so, in Uganda. Membership in a political association formed at the time of independence has put many persons in jeopardy when regimes were overthrown and ethnic rivalries turned into civil war. But also in settings of relative or apparent political stability, the possibilities of a violent coup and political reprisal are too important to ignore. Local associations have, therefore, not only an interest in coming to terms with current regimes (especially if some of their activities are sponsored by governments), but also an interest in never becoming too closely identified with the political powers of the moment. This obviously relates to our earlier opinion that the process of nation building is different in Africa than in Asia and that, as a result, the major role of African governments is to faciliate family planning or more general socio-economic development by providing a suitable climate and subsidies, but not to push it politically over the heads of local organizations. We fully realize that this constitutes the advocating of the slow approach in the face of an urgent problem but, in the current political context, any hurried approaches are likely to be inefficient as local resources would not be tapped adequately and, more dangerously, they are likely to backfire, which would put Africa even further behind schedule. The consensus-building approach with a major involvement of local networks is therefore an absolute priority, and whether one likes it or not, this is bound to involve a period of discussion and experimentation.

There is one final but important issue left for this discussion on the potential of grass-root associations with respect to family planning. Individual
involvement in development projects is of course positively rewarded by the
community. At present, the adoption of family planning is not: most acceptors hide their decisions, and knowledge of it by others is a cause of embarrassment. Kin and acquaintances offer their opinions very frankly and these
judgments matter tremendously. The report by Reyes and colleagues (1985)
on the community-based family planning and health projects in the areas in
and around Ibadan provides insights that are both typical and critical.
Adults are ashamed of buying condoms themselves for instance and perfer to
send children for them. Potential acceptors of other methods provided by the
family planning clinics frequently request, and obtain, that they be accompanied by their trusted local health worker on the journey to the delivery place.
Caldwell and Caldwell (1986) studied the community and kin opinions toward the small group that has attempted to limit family size in Ibadan, and
their compendium is a vivid illustration of the special importance of opinions
in African networks. This clearly indicates how deeply rooted threshold fears
are, even in an area of Nigeria, which, by most accounts, is easily among the
most developed of the country and of sub-Saharan Africa as a whole. It also
shows that the main function of grass-roots networks is to discuss the subject
and to legitimize contraception in the process, thereby eventually developing
their own referral system, more than in their direct financial sponsoring of
family planning clinics. Reliable services are of course needed, but *self-
confidence* among potential acceptors is of even greater importance at this
stage. The dynamics whereby acceptors can recruit others through such networks is a subject of study that is at the very least of an importance equal to
the organization of another round of fertility- or contraceptive-prevalence
surveys.

CONCLUSIONS

If we were to summarize the essence of what is presented in this volume, the
message would be that the reproductive regimes of sub-Saharan Africa are
still strongly attached to forms of social control prevailing in societies that
capitalize on corporate allegiance. The nonaccentuation of the husband-wife
dyad, the socialization of children by larger corporate units (e.g., in age
grades or through fosterage in lineages), the numerous kinship- and community-based networks, the stress on lineage membership, exogamy, circulation of wealth, corporate ownership of land, ancestral religion, and so forth,
are all ingredients of a particular form of social organization that sub-
Saharan Africa does not share with Asia or Latin America. Change has not
been lacking though. The privatization of land ownership, the growth of the
wage sector, urbanization or external cultural influences, all have altered the

landscape. But, even when it comes to the appropriation of a plot or to secur-
ing a job in the wage sector, the reliance on corporate kinship groups or other
particularistic networks reemerges with full force. Life is not easy, both in
urban and rural environments, and support from others is always wanted.
Also the imponderabilia of political life associated with the difficult process of
nation building and the extra stress produced by the current economic crisis
accentuate the importance of reliance upon and allegiance to trustworthy
solidarity networks. In short, survival strongly depends on what Ben Porath
(1980) calls "investment in identity." The complement of such an investment is of course the enhancement of moral patronage and social control
exerted by the protecting agencies. This provides the background against
which the stepwise format of the various changes in the reproductive regime
can be evaluated.

A remarkable feature in the pattern of adaptation of reproduction is
indeed its stepwise progression. The traditional pattern of child-spacing
through prolonged lactation and postpartum abstinence has eroded or is
currently eroding at a rather fast pace, thereby causing an initial fertility
increase. Changes in nuptiality or, more specifically, in age at first union
formation, proceed at a slower tempo. Parity-specific control is obviously
lagging. As several studies have shown, individuation with respect to curtailment of family size seems a particularly difficult process, even in urban areas.

The most logical explanation for this hitherto sequential progression of
reproductive adaptation is that the reduction in child-spacing has obviously
a fertility-increasing effect that is not likely to be met with hostility in strongly pronatalist societies for as long as infant survival is not endangered. And,
as the shortening of birth intervals has not generally been associated with an
increase in infant and child mortality as a result of other mortality-reducing
factors, the reduction in postpartum abstinence and greater reliance on
bottle-feeding are not considered to be immoral or dysfunctional. The weight
of traditional aspects of social organization on ages at first union formation is
firmer: polygyny in rural areas has not been reduced and female ages at first
marriage are only slowly increasing. Migration of men during the 1960s and
1970s and the current economic situation, however, have also served to keep
male ages at marriage high, so that the husband-wife age gap remains virtually intact in most of sub-Saharan Africa. Bridewealth is still commonly
exchanged, the sums involved are substantial, and the provision of bridewealth becomes more and more the exclusive responsibility of the individual
son (Isiugo-Abanihe, 1987). Parity-specific fertility limitation runs at present
directly counter to the cultural pattern. Pressure in favor of better spacing
and fertility control emerges, however, once individuals realize that there is
growing tension between a potential oversupply of children and aspirations
for "higher-quality" children. The hypothesis of a crisis-led transition argues
that this tension is now emerging more quickly and more sharply as a result

of frustrated aspirations and increased child costs, whereas the sequential transition theory is arguing the same point starting from the potential over-supply of surviving offspring. However, the utility of children, and especially their security function, is still likely to remain high for decades to come and, as a consequence, any future fertility decline is likely to lose momentum at average parities around four to five children. Much then depends on mortality levels in determining population growth rates. Finally, pathological demographic regimes are emerging in areas affected by AIDS, and if no vaccines are developed in the next decade, the spread of this threat can determine the future of many sub-Saharan regions in directions that were never envisaged.

The onset of the fertility transition will clearly be contingent on the format of family-planning implementation. As the process of nation building in Africa is strikingly different from that of the Asian countries that have provided the examples of rapid fertility declines and strong family planning programs, a different approach needs to be followed. National governments can certainly be instrumental in legitimizing and subsidizing the use of contraception, but little progress is to be expected if they act solely on their own. The moral attitudes and the shifts in functions of the numerous grass-roots networks have been considered in this chapter as equally crucial determinants. Particularly women's organizations and local Protestant church organizations can fulfill this catalytic role. Hence, the future map of the fertility transition in Africa is not only likely to follow the classic pattern with education, urbanization, size of wage sector, or evolution of income as major determinants, but equally likely to exhibit the impact of local social organizational features that either facilitate or hamper the legitimation of new forms of fertility control. Once again, leads and lags in the transition may prove to be as much a function of political and social organizational factors as of economic ones.

BIBLIOGRAPHY

Abate, A., and T. Teklu. 1982. Land reform and peasant associations in Ethiopia: A cast study of two widely differing regions. In: *Studies in rural participation*, ed. A. Bhaduri and M. Rahman. New Delhi: Oxford University Press, 58–59.
Adepoju, A. 1986. The population situation in Africa since Arusha. *Populi* 13(2): 31–35.
Akbar, J. 1985. Mothers' clubs of rural Bangladesh. Ann Arbor: Univeristy of Michigan, Department of Population Planning (mimeo).
Ariès, P. 1980. Two successive motivations for the declining birth rate in the West. *Population and Development Review* 6(4): 645–650.
Awe, B. 1977. The Iyalode in the traditional Yoruba political system. In: *Sexual stratification—A cross-cultural view*, ed. A. Schlegel. New York: Columbia Univeristy Press, 144–159.
Bascom, W. 1952. The Esusu—A credit institution of the Yoruba. *Journal of the Royal Anthropological Institute* 82(1): 63–69.

Ben Porath, Y. 1980. The F–connection: Families, friends and firms, and the organization of exchange. *Population and Development Review* 6(1): 1–30.

Bledsoe, C. 1980. *Women and marriage in Kpelle society.* Stanford: Stanford University Press.

Bongaarts, J. 1986. The transition in reproductive behavior in the third world. *Working Paper of the Center for Policy Studies*, no. 125. New York: The Population Council.

Boserup, E. 1970. *Women's role in economic development.* London: Allen and Unwin.

————. 1985. Economic and demographic interrelationships in sub-Saharan Africa. *Population and Development Review* 11(3): 383–398.

Bulatao, R., and R. D. Lee, eds. 1983. *Determinants of fertility in developing countries.* 2 vols. New York: Academic Press.

Bulatao, R. 1984. Reducing fertility in developing countries—A review of determinants and policy levers. *Working Paper of the World Bank Staff*, no. 680. Population and Development Series, no. 5. Washington, D.C.: The World Bank.

Cain, M. 1983. Fertility as an adjustment to risk. *Working Paper of the Center for Policy Studies*, no. 100. New York: The Population Council.

————. 1984. Women's status and fertility in developing countries: Son preference and economic security. *Working Paper of the Center for Policy Studies*, no. 110. New York: The Population Council.

————. 1985. The fate of the elderly in South Asia: Implications for fertility. *Working Paper of the Center for Policy Studies*, no. 116. New York: The Population Council.

Caldwell, J. C. 1976. Towards a restatement of demographic transition theory. *Population and Development Review* 2(3–4): 321–366.

————. 1978. A theory of fertility: From high plateau to destabilization. *Population and Development Review* 4(4): 553–557.

Caldwell, J. C., and P. Caldwell. 1985. ·Is the Asian family planning programme model suited to Africa? Paper presented at the IUSSP seminar on Societal Influence on Family Planning Programme Performance, National Family Planning Board of Jamaica, Ocho Rios, Jamaica.

————. 1986. The limitation of family size in Ibadan City, Nigeria—An explanation of its comparative rarity from in-depth interviews. Paper presented at the Conference on the True Determinants of Fertility in Africa, The Rockefeller Foundation and the University of Ife, Ife, Nigeria.

Casterline, J. 1985. Community effects on fertility. In *The collection and analysis of community data*, ed. J. Casterline. Voorburg, Netherlands: International Statistical Institute, 65–75.

Chioma-Steady, F. 1976. Protestant women's associations in Freetown, Sierra Leone. In: *Women in Africa—Studies in social and economic change*, ed. N. Hafkin and E. Bay. Stanford: Stanford University Press.

Cho, L. F., F. Arnold, and T. H. Kwon. 1982. *The determinants of fertility in the Republic of Korea.* Washington, D.C.: National Research Council, National Academy Press.

de Cour Grandmaison, C. 1972. *Femmes Dakaroises—Rôles traditionnels féminins.* Abidjan, Ivory Coast: Annales de l'Université d'Abidjan, série F, tôme 4.

Dumont, A. 1980. *Dépopulation et civilisation: Etude démographique.* Paris: Editions Lecrosnier et Babé.

Enea, S. 1985. Mothers' clubs and family planning: An international perspective. Washington, D.C.: International Statistical Programs Center, U.S. Bureau of the Census (mimeo).

Family Health International. 1986. *Network*. French ed., vol. 1. Research Triangle Park, N.C.: Family Health International, 12.

Fraenkel, M. 1964. *Tribe and class in Monrovia*. Oxford: Oxford University Press. (Esp. chap. 5: Churches and Societies)

Frank, O. 1985. The demand for fertility control in sub-Saharan Africa. *Working Paper of the Center of Policy Studies, no. 117*. New York: The Population Council.

Geiger, S. 1982. Umoja wa Wanawake wa Tanzania and the needs of the rural poor, *African Studies Review* 25(2–3): 45–69.

Hall, A. 1986. Community participation and rural development. In: *Community participation, social development and the state*, ed. J. Medley. New York: Methuen, 87–104.

Hardiman, M. 1986. People's involvement in health and medical care. In: *Community participation, social development and the state*, ed. J. Medley. New York: Methuen, 45–69.

Hecht, E. D. 1980. The voluntary associations and the social status of Harari women in Harar, eastern Ethiopia. Paper presented at the Sixth International Ethiopian Studies Conference, Tel Aviv. Nairobi: Institute of African Studies.

Hoffer, C. 1972. Mende and Sherbro women in high offices. *Canadian Journal of African Studies* 6(2): 151–164.

Isiugo-Abanihe, U. 1987. High bridewealth and age at marriage in Igboland. Paper presented at the Conference on the True Determinants of Fertility in Africa. The Rockefeller Foundation and the University of Ife, Ife, Nigeria.

Jeffreys, M. 1956. The Nyama society of the Ibibio women. *African Studies* 15(1): 15–28.

Jules-Rosette, B. 1981. Women in indigenous African cults and churches. In *The black women cross-culturally*, ed. F. Chioma-Steady. Cambridge, Mass.: Schenkman, 185–207.

Kaplan, I. ed. 1971. *Area handbook for Ghana*. Washington, D.C.: Government Printing Office.

Kaplan, I. ed. 1976. *Area handbook for Sierra Leone*. Washington, D.C.: Government Printing Office.

Karefa-Smart, J. 1986. Health and family planning in Africa. *Populi* 13(2): 20–29.

Kim, J. I., and J. Palmore. 1978. Personal networks and the adoption of family planning in rural Korea. Paper presented at the Fourth Annual Social Networks Colloquium, Honolulu, Hawaii.

Ladner, J. 1981. Tanzanian women and nation building. In *Black women cross-culturally*, ed. F. Chioma-Steady. Cambridge: Schenkman.

Lee, S. B. 1977. System effects on family planning innovativeness in Korean villages. Ph.D. dissertation. University of Michigan, Ann Arbor.

Leis, N. 1974. Women in groups: Ijaw women's associations. In *Women, culture and society*, ed. M. Zimbalist-Rosaldo and L. Lamphere. Stanford: Stanford University Press.

Lewis, B. 1976. The limitations of group action among entrepreneurs: The market women of Abidjan, Ivory Coast. In *Women in Africa—Studies in social and economic change*, ed. N. Hafkin and F. Bay. Stanford: Stanford University Press, 135–156.

———. 1982. Women in development planning: Advocacy, institutionalization and implementation. In: *Perspectives on power*, ed. J. O'Barr. Durham, N.C.: Duke University Press, 102–118.

Little, K. 1951. Cultural role of the Poro and other societies. In: *The Mende of Sierra Leone*, ed. K. Little. London: Routledge and Kegan Paul.

———. 1965. *West African urbanization—A study of voluntary associations in social change.* Cambridge: Cambridge University Press.

———. 1974. *Urbanization as a social process—An essay on movement and change in contemporary Africa.* London: Routledge and Kegan Paul.

Locoh, T. 1985. Les obstacles à l'acceptation de la planification familiale en Afrique de l'ouest. Paper presented at the IUSSP-seminar on Societal Influences on Family Planning Programme Performance, National Family Planning Board of Jamaica, Ocho Rios, Jamaica.

MacCormack, C. 1982. Health, fertility and birth in Moyamba District, Sierra Leone. In: *Ethnology of fertility and birth*, ed. C. MacCormack. London: Academic Press, 115–139.

McNicoll, G. 1983. Notes on the local context of demographic change. *Working Paper of the Center for Policy Studies*, no. 98. New York: The Population Council.

McNicoll, G., and M. Singarimbun. 1983. *Fertility decline in Indonesia—Analysis and interpretation.* Washington, D.C.: Committee on Population and Demography, National Research Council, National Academy Press.

Medley, J. 1986. *Community participation, social development and the state.* New York: Methuen, part 1, 13–44.

Mønsted, M. 1978. Women's groups in rural Kenya and their role in development. CDR-paper A78.2 (mimeo). Copenhagen, Denmark: Centre for Development Research.

Muchena, O. 1982. Women's organizations in Zimbabwe and assessment of their needs, achievements and potential. In *Women's programmes in Zimbabwe*, ed. K. Jorgersen. Copenhagen: Univeristy of Copenhagen Press, 31–71.

Nangawel, E., F. Shomet, E. Rowberg, T. McGinn, and W. van Wie. 1985. Community participation in health programs: Experiences from the Maasai health service project, Tanzania. *Working Paper of the Center for Population and Family Health*, no. 18. New York: Columbia University.

Nelson, H., ed. 1972. *Area handbook for Nigeria.* Washington, D.C.: Government Printing Office.

———. 1974. *Area handbook for the United Republic of Cameroon.* Washington, D.C.: Government Printing Office.

O'Barr, J. 1984. Women in politics and policy. In *African women south of the Sahara*, ed. M. Hay and S. Stichter. London: Longman, 140–155.

Okonjo, K. 1976. The dual-sex political system in operation: Igbo women and community politics in midwestern Nigeria. In *Women in Africa—Studies in social and economic change*, ed. N. Hafkin and E. Bay. Stanford: Stanford University Press.

———. 1981. Women's political participation in Nigeria. In *The black women cross-culturally*, ed. F. Chioma-Steady. Cambridge: Schenkman, 79–105.

Palmore, J. 1968. Awareness sources and stages in the adoption of specific contraceptive. *Demography* 5: 960–972.

Palmore, J., C. K. Cheong, K. C. Ahn, S. K. Park, and H. Y. Kwon. 1977. Interpersonal family planning communication in Korea, 1976: Opinion leadership, home visits by F. P. workers, and population problem groups. In: *Reducing problem groups in family planning IE & C program*, ed. D. W. Han, C. K. Cheong, and K. C. Ahn.

Seoul, Korea: Korean Institute for Family Planning, 79–105.

Parkin, D. J. 1966. Urban voluntary associations as institutions of adaptation. *Man* 1(1): 90–94.

Retherford, R., and J. Palmore. 1983. Diffusion processes affecting fertility regulation. In: *Determinants of fertility in developing countries*, ed. R. Bulatao and R. D. Lee. New York: Academic Press, vol. 2, 295–339.

Rogers, E. 1962. *Diffusion of innovations*. New York: The Free Press.

———. 1973. *Communication strategies for family planning*. New York: The Free Press.

Rogers, E., H. J. Park, K. K. Chung, S.-B. Lee, W. S. Puppa, and B. A. Doe. 1976. Network analysis of diffusion of family planning innovations over time in Korean villages: The role of mothers' clubs. In: *Communication for group transformation in development*, ed. G. C. Chu, S. A. Rahim, and D. Kincaid. Honolulu, Hawaii: East-West Communication Institute, 253–276.

Rogers, E., and D. Kincaid. 1981. *Communication networks: Toward a new paradigm for research*. New York: The Free Press.

Ross, D. 1979. The village health committee: A case-study of community participation in Sierra Leone. *Contact* 49: 1–9.

Safilios-Rothchild, C. 1985. Socioeconomic development and the status of women in the third world. *Working Paper of the Center of Policy Studies*, no. 112. New York: The Population Council.

Sauvy, A. Essai d'une vue d'ensemble. In *La prévention des naissances dans la famille: Ses origines dans les temps modernes*, ed. H. Bergues. Cahier de l'INED. Paris: Presses Universitaires de France, 375–391.

Ssennyonga, J. W. 1985. The human ecological context of family planning—The case of Kenya. Paper presented at the IUSSP seminar on Societal Influences on Family Planning Programme Performance, National Family Planning Board of Jamaica, Ocho Rios, Jamaica.

Standst, K. 1979. Women and participation in rural development—A framework for project design and policy oriented research. *Rural Development Committee, Occasional papers series*, no. 8. Ithaca: Cornell University.

Stoeckel, J., and A. Jain. 1986. *Fertility in Asia—Assessing the impact of development projects*. London: Frances Pinter Publishers.

Strobel, M. 1974. Sorority without solidarity. Paper presented at the UCLA colloquium on Women and Change in Africa, 1870–1970 (mimeo).

———. 1976. From Lelemama to lobbying: Women's associations in Mombasa, Kenya. In *Women in Africa—Studies in social and economic change*, ed. N. Hafkin and E. Bay. Stanford: Stanford University Press, 183–212.

Swantz, M.-L. 1977. Strain and strength among peasant women in Tanzania. *Research Paper of the Bureau of Resource Assessment and Land Use Planning*, no. 49. Dar Es Salaam, Tanzania: University of Dar Es Salaam.

———. 1985. *Women in development: A creative role denied? The case of Tanzania*. New York: St. Martin's Press.

Tsui, A. O. 1985. Community effects on contraceptive use. In: *The collection and analysis of community data*, ed. J. Casterline. Voorburg, Netherlands: International Statistical Institute, 76–99.

Van Allen, J. 1979. Sitting on a man—Colonialism and the lost political institutions of Igbo women. In: *Women in society*, ed. S. Tiffany. Montreal: Eden Press, 163–187.

van Norren, B. 1985. Socio-culturele structuur en innovatie: een structuurvergelijkend onderzoek naar adoptie van family planning in de periode 1969–73 door Sundanese echtparen in twee rurale gemeenschappen op West-Java. Ph. D. dissertation. Wageningen, Netherlands: Landbouwhogeschool.

Warwick, D. P. 1985. Culture and the management of family planning programs. Paper presented at the IUSSP seminar on Societal Influences on Family Planning Programme Performance, Family Planning Board of Jamaica, Ocho Rios, Jamaica.

————. 1986. The Indonesian family planning program: Government influence and client choice. *Population and Development Review* 12(3): 453–490.

Wipper, A. 1975. The Maendeleo ya Wanawake organization: The cooptation of leadership *African Studies Review* 18(3): 99–120.

————. 1984. Women's voluntary associations. In *African women south of the Sahara*, ed. J. Hay and S. Stichter. London: Longman, 69–86.

Wolf, A. 1984. Fertility in prerevolutionary China. *Population and Development Review* 10(3): 443–470.

World Bank. 1986. *Population growth and policies in sub-Saharan Africa*. Washington, D.C.: World Bank.

Appendixes

APPENDIX A Indicators of Social, Cultural, and Reproductive Regimes; 61 Ethnic Groups, WFS Surveys

	AGEMAR 25	SINGLE 15	MEDMAR	POLYG	PROWWID	PRODIV	REMAR	PIRBRFD	PIRAMEN	PIRABST	PIRNSP	PLETWOLF	PCON	CONPREV	KNOWIM	DESLT 6	XDESFAMS	ILLIT	XSCHOOL	XIAN	MUSLIM	TRADE	WEALTH	FEMROLE	TRADREL	NEGINT	CHILDN 9	STRATTOP	STRATSELF
SENEGAL*																													
Wolof, Lebu	16.3	48	16.4	55	8	19	88	20.1	13.6	2.3	14.0	12	1.9	1.7	26	18	7.5	84	1.0	0	100	8	4	0	0	4	4	13	68
Poular, Fula	15.2	29	15.4	42	11	21	92	20.3	13.7	5.2	14.2	17	3.3	3.1	16	18	7.6	89	.7	0	99	9	5	0	1	2	3	12	71
Manding	15.6	24	15.4	54	11	10	84	20.2	13.6	2.0	14.0	9	11.0	10.7	23	11	8.1	90	.6	0	98	3	3	0	2	4	11	18	72
Serer	16.6	45	16.8	43	7	23	92	21.5	14.8	2.3	15.1	10	1.1	1.0	21	9	8.0	89	.6	1	91	5	3	2	8	5	7	9	72
Diola, Balante	17.7	60	17.9	49	8	17	85	19.4	13.0	4.0	13.6	14	6.6	5.6	33	16	7.7	70	1.9	34	66	4	0	2	0	10	6	12	63
Other Mande	15.9	44	16.2	48	10	24	81	18.3	12.1	3.0	12.4	15	8.2	7.2	31	24	7.3	75	1.6	0	100	4	4	0	0	7	5	25	44
GHANA																													
Fante	18.9	68	18.7	29	5	35	75	15.8	11.9	8.8	13.1	12	9.7	8.9	79	45	5.7	54	4.0	84	7	36	2	3	9	7	12	24	41
Twi	18.0	75	18.3	28	3	27	67	18.6	14.3	9.0	15.1	10	11.1	10.2	72	45	5.8	36	5.5	85	3	24	2	3	12	8	14	31	41
Other Akan	17.8	55	17.5	38	5	41	68	18.5	14.1	9.2	15.3	11	5.3	4.9	80	38	5.8	69	2.6	77	3	24	2	3	20	14	16	17	56
Mole-Dagbani	17.2	43	17.4	49	3	9	85	27.9	19.2	24.4	26.1	13	2.0	1.8	30	14	7.4	88	1.0	13	31	32	1	3	56	8	9	6	72
Ewe	18.8	79	18.9	36	4	25	78	21.7	15.6	14.0	18.0	12	14.1	12.7	86	49	5.5	46	4.4	67	1	37	2	3	32	8	15	26	42
Ga-Adangbe	18.8	77	19.0	32	5	28	73	16.6	10.3	8.4	12.2	12	18.9	16.8	84	50	5.4	38	5.4	79	4	56	2	3	17	8	16	42	27
Guan	18.1	69	18.1	22	6	23	70	19.9	14.6	13.0	16.3	17	6.9	6.1	65	31	6.2	60	3.4	53	18	41	2	3	29	11	10	18	54
Other North	17.9	50	17.8	45	3	13	69	22.6	14.6	16.1	18.8	14	6.2	5.8	52	31	6.4	74	2.2	21	39	33	1	3	40	10	10	14	54
BENIN																													
Adja	17.7	49	18.0	42	7	9	96	24.2	15.5	15.3	19.0	5	1.6	11.8	66	9	8.0	96	.2	12	0	12	2	3	88	4	17	14	78
Fon	18.7	63	18.5	28	5	11	84	20.4	11.7	16.3	17.5	10	4.1	2.8	26	29	6.5	76	1.7	35	1	41	2	3	64	16	21	19	51
Yoruba	19.5	78	19.6	30	4	15	73	19.6	13.2	18.8	19.3	16	3.9	2.3	24	23	6.4	65	2.7	30	57	59	1	3	13	19	17	21	70
Goun	19.6	68	19.0	31	4	11	77	20.3	14.6	20.3	21.0	11	2.7	1.6	10	12	6.7	78	1.6	53	6	57	1	3	41	18	18	18	67
Nagot	19.7	68	19.3	32	2	9	80	21.7	15.2	19.9	20.1	26	1.7	1.2	19	10	7.2	88	.7	52	36	34	1	3	12	18	19	15	69
Other South & Central	18.9	46	18.6	30	3	12	88	19.7	12.1	14.6	16.6	9	8.6	5.3	30	15	7.4	88	.7	29	4	30	1	3	67	18	21	12	69
Dendi-Dittamari	16.9	32	17.3	46	10	18	83	21.7	13.4	20.8	21.3	10	4.5	2.9	69	15	7.7	87	.6	5	49	42	0	3	46	18	15	16	61
Bariba	17.1	30	17.1	43	7	27	89	24.3	16.7	23.5	23.7	14	1.3	.9	55	7	8.1	89	.5	4	34	74	0	3	62	20	23	17	72
Other North	17.6	36	17.7	41	9	17	88	22.5	16.1	22.5	23.2	25	2.0	1.2	52	11	8.0	94	.3	8	43	48	0	3	49	18	15	7	76

APPENDIX A continued

	AGEMAR 25	SINGLE 15	MEDMAR	POLYG	PROVWID	PROVDIV	REMAR	PIRBRED	PIRAMEN	PIRABST	PIRNSP	PLETWOLB	PCON	CONPREV	KNOWIM	DESLT 6	XDESFAMS	ILLIT	XSCHOOL	XIAN	MUSLIM	TRADE	WEALTH	FEMROLE	TRADRELI	NEGINT	CHILDIN 9	STRATTOP	STRATSELF
CAMEROON**																													
Bakosi, Bakundu	17.5	57	17.6	31	11	17	39	20.0	12.7	20.7	21.0	9	1.4	1.1	32	4	8.4	50	2.5	94	1	1	1	2	5	28	14	22	62
Ekoi, Mbembe	18.4	56	17.8	30	9	18	25	19.0	14.7	18.1	18.5	14	0.0	0.0	32	4	8.3	75	1.2	95	1	5	1	2	4	23	15	11	64
Duala	18.3	81	18.6	11	9	27	20	13.2	4.3	5.5	6.4	9	7.6	4.6	70	13	7.2	29	3.6	98		8	1	3	1	22	18	41	29
Bassa	18.5	70	18.8	24	12	21	40	13.5	9.2	9.2	12.3	25	2.9	1.9	59	15	7.2	41	3.0	98	0	6	1	2	2	26	16	26	27
Pangwe	18.9	74	18.6	37	10	24	80	17.3	12.6	16.0	16.9	39	5.3	3.6	83	20	6.7	37	3.2	98	1	1	0	2	1	44	7	19	61
Kaka	18.6	54	18.0	42	8	20	84	21.1	13.0	13.0	16.3	27	5.6	3.6	39	26	6.3	67	2.4	97	2	1	0	2	2	29	16	9	70
Maka	18.2	54	18.4	38	8	21	63	17.0	12.6	12.6	15.2	33	1.9	1.2	35	24	6.4	52	3.2	98	0	1	0	2	2	25	13	14	71
Yaounde	19.8	70	19.5	26	10	17	44	15.3	10.4	15.1	15.8	35	5.2	3.2	75	14	7.4	38	2.0	98	0	4	0	3	2	44	12	20	42
Other South	18.3	58	17.9	30	13	18	51	22.8	17.4	18.2	20.4	28	1.6	1.0	27	24	5.9	55	1.7	68	3	3	1	2	29	23	12	8	56
Bamenda	18.3	46	17.9	47	7	7	40	20.6	13.7	20.6	21.0	13	1.3	.9	46	4	8.4	66	2.7	91	3	3	1	1	6	22	21	17	62
Bamileke	18.0	62	18.1	48	7	7	39	20.9	14.1	19.5	20.4	11	1.9	1.3	34	5	8.3	47	1.7	87	3	7	1	3	12	11	16	18	50
Bamun	19.8	57	18.4	51	9	7	51	20.9	12.5	21.0	21.0	30	0.0	0.0	15	13	7.7	66	2.9	21	77	2	0	3	1	36	13	11	63
Bafia	18.2	67	18.6	32	10	10	44	18.0	12.6	15.8	17.0	14	1.9	1.3	54	11	7.5	41	1.6	97	2	4	0	2	1	23	14	20	54
Widekum	18.4	58	20.4	47	6	10	40	22.6	14.9	22.2	22.2	12	1.3	1.2	42	7	8.3	67		96	0	2	1	2	4	30	14	13	69
Tuburi, Gizega	15.3	19	15.5	43	4	18	97	22.1	15.9	14.2	18.0	26	0.0	0.0	10	18	7.0	90	.5	32	18	4	1	2	50	11	8	9	65
Chari-Logone	15.2	34	15.7	44	6	16	90	24.2	15.1	12.8	16.3	31	0.0	0.0	12	25	6.5	92	.4	39	34	6	0	2	27	18	6	5	64
Mandara, Wandala	15.9	18	15.4	45	3	16	83	20.8	15.8	15.0	17.4	33	.3	.2	7	17	7.2	96	.2	11	38	2	0	2	51	17	4	8	74
Peul	15.7	17	14.6	47	6	30	87	19.7	14.6	12.8	16.8	49	0.0	0.0	13	25	6.4	93	.3	2	98	7	5	2	0	13	6	20	63
Baya, Adamawa	17.5	24	15.7	43	8	19	83	20.0	11.8	12.1	15.0	47	3.9	2.3	36	25	6.3	78	.8	61	35	7	0	2	4	15	10	10	76
Choa Arabs Hausa	16.4	18	14.7	28	9	23	80	18.9	13.9	11.8	14.9	44	0.0	0.0	9	21	6.6	92	.4	6	94	5	5	1	0	13	2	10	80
LESOTHO																													
Sotho	18.4	69	18.2	8	8	7	19	21.8	11.4	18.0	19.3	20	5.2	4.1	65	47	5.8	8	5.0	82	0	4	2	1	18	5	8	3	3

APPENDIX A   *continued*

	AGEMAR 25	SINGLE 15	MEDMAR	POLYG	PROVWID	PROVDIV	REMAR	PIRBRFD	PIRAMEN	PIRABST	PIRNSP	PLETWOLB	PCON	CONPREV	KNOWIM	DESTL 6	XDESFAMS	ILLIT	XSCHOOL	XIAN	MUSLIM	TRADE	WEALTH	FEMROLE	TRADRELI	NEGINT	CHILDIN 9	STRATTOP	STRATSELF
KENYA																													
Kikuyu	18.4	85	19.4	12	5	10	23	15.1	10.8	3.6	11.5	7	12.1	11.0	92	27	6.9	32	4.3	96	1	1	0	1	3	28	25	22	32
Luo	16.5	58	17.0	43	5	7	64	18.1	11.5	3.2	12.2	12	5.6	5.0	89	32	6.6	45	3.4	98	1	1	1	1	1	14	18	23	28
Luhya	17.1	68	17.8	35	4	14	65	17.9	11.2	3.1	11.4	8	4.5	4.1	87	21	7.1	37	4.0	94	5	2	1	1	1	18	14	22	27
Kamba	18.2	84	19.4	27	6	20	53	19.6	11.9	3.7	12.5	8	8.0	7.1	89	21	7.1	41	3.6	94	1	2	0	2	5	26	20	21	25
Kissii	17.9	74	18.4	33	4	7	56	18.6	14.1	4.2	14.7	3	2.9	2.5	86	15	7.6	50	3.2	97	0	0	0	0	3	20	13	15	60
Meru, Embu	18.6	87	19.6	24	3	9	45	21.2	13.6	7.5	15.1	8	9.9	8.9	85	27	7.1	42	3.4	98	1	1	0	1	1	37	23	18	58
Mijikenda	16.1	43	16.5	41	6	20	76	23.1	15.5	3.7	15.8	20	2.1	2.1	81	16	7.7	82	1.1	19	47	1	0	0	34	18	13	12	46
Kalenjin	17.5	72	18.3	24	4	5	8	19.5	11.0	5.7	11.5	6	5.3	4.4	82	17	7.6	50	2.8	91	1	0	0	1	8	22	16	18	52
Other	16.8	58	17.4	37	3	14	53	18.3	11.4	7.8	13.4	14	6.0	5.5	87	21	7.3	55	3.0	66	17	0	0	1	17	17	17	21	37
IVORY COAST																													
Lagunaires	17.2	49	17.6	33	6	27	76	15.9	10.3	10.3	13.1	2	4.9	3.7	82	17	7.6	53	2.9	84	10	24	2	3	6	13	17	35	27
Agni	18.2	52	17.5	34	4	32	78	16.7	11.2	9.9	13.5	11	4.0	3.6	84	14	7.6	60	2.6	82	2	8	2	3	16	13	21	46	29
Baoule	19.7	63	18.9	38	6	32	80	17.4	12.5	14.7	16.8	16	2.1	1.8	86	14	7.8	80	1.3	26	3	13	1	3	71	13	14	28	38
Kru	16.9	53	17.0	40	4	32	84	16.9	12.1	16.6	17.6	13	7.3	6.7	89	16	7.7	55	2.8	68	1	13	0	3	31	13	16	33	31
Guéré	16.4	42	16.3	46	8	20	64	20.4	14.4	20.8	21.8	17	2.4	2.0	90	15	7.8	70	1.7	27	2	7	0	3	71	13	15	24	48
Malinke	17.0	41	17.0	54	9	10	81	21.9	14.4	19.5	20.7	12	1.2	1.0	87	12	8.0	91	.6	0	98	37	3	2	2	7	15	14	64
Kulango & Senufo	17.4	47	17.5	47	8	14	85	23.1	14.7	19.1	20.3	12	1.7	1.5	67	15	7.8	92	.5	15	38	18	1	2	47	9	14	17	60
Guro, Yacuba	16.9	40	16.5	44	9	22	83	21.4	14.7	19.9	20.4	13	4.7	4.4	89	18	7.7	82	1.0	10	9	13	0	3	81	11	13	21	57

*PIRABST for Senegalese populations are from B. Ferry. The senegalese surveys, in *Child-spacing in tropical Africa: traditions and change*, ed. H.J. Page and R. Lesthaeghe (1981), table 3, p. 269, and pertain to the period 1963–1968. PIRAMEN values are calculated on the basis of PIRBRFD and the Bongaarts relationship between the mean duration of lactational amenorrhea (Ā) and the mean length of breastfeeding (B̄): $\bar{A} = 1.753 \exp(0.1396\bar{B} - 0.001872\bar{B}^2)$.

**REMAR values for five small Cameroon ethnic groups (Other South, Bamun, Widekum, Chari-Logone, Duala) are estimates obtained through the relationship with POLYG and comparison with culturally related neighboring groups; see text. SINGLE 15: the value for Ekoi, Mbembe is estimated from the regression with MEDMAR. These estimates are considered better than the default option for missing values, which is the insertion of the overall sample mean for the sixty-one ethnic groups.

APPENDIX B Socioeconomic Development Scores (Factor I of Table 2.9) for 61 Ethnic Groups; (WFS Data)

1. *Senegal*			5. *Cameroon*	
Wolof, Lebu	−.61		Bakosi, Bakundu	.17
Poular, Fula	−.68		Ekoi, Mbembe	−.77
Manding	−.76		Duala	1.96
Serer	−1.05		Bassa	1.64
Diola	−.76		Pangwe	.20
Mande groups	.48		Kaka	−.96
			Maka	−.48
2. *Ghana*			Yaunde	.61
Fante	.86		Other South & Central	−.38
Twi	1.46		Bamenda	−.33
Other Akan	−.01		Bamileke	.36
Mole-Dagbani	−1.09		Bamun	−.57
Ewe	1.16		Bafia	.31
Ga-Adangbe	2.24		Widekum	−.65
Guan	.34		Tuburi, Gizega	−1.01
Other North	−.21		Chari-Logone	−1.38
			Mandara, Wandala	−1.47
3. *Benin*			Peul	−.32
Adja	−.91		Baya, Adamawa, Benue	−1.23
Fon	.23		Choa Arabs, Hausa	−1.02
Yoruba	−.08			
Goun	−.30		6. *Kenya*	
Nagot	−.85		Kikuyu	1.07
Other South & Central	−.78		Luo	.97
Dendi, Dittamari	−.61		Luhya	1.12
Bariba	−.66		Kamba	.93
Other North	−1.35		Kissii	−.17

4. *Ivory Coast*	
Lagunaires	1.50
Agni	1.71
Baoule	.55
Kru	1.11
Guere	.26
Malinke	−.65
Kulango, Senufo	−.61
Guro, Yacuba	−.21

Meru-Embu	.13
Mijikenda	−.55
Kalenjin	.11
Other Kenya	.45
7. *Lesotho*	
Sotho	1.64

NOTE: The signs have been reversed to obtain a scale running from low development to high (Factor I in table 2.9 goes the other way around).

APPENDIX C Contextual Background Variables for 33 WFS Regions

REGION	% Women Muslim	% Women Christian	% Women Traditional Religion	% Women in Trade	% Women Illiterate	Average Female Schooling	% Husbands Professional, Clerical, Employers of Wage Labor	% Husbands Self-Employed without Wage Labor	% Husbands Wage Earners Other Sectors	Development Score
1 Nairobi (Kenya)	1	96	3	4	20	6.2	49	7	44	2.30
2 Central & Eastern	0	96	4	1	37	3.7	20	41	39	0.60
3 Rift Valley	1	90	9	1	44	3.3	19	37	44	0.47
4 Coast	37	40	23	2	69	2.2	20	40	40	−0.06
5 Nyanza & Western	3	96	1	1	46	3.2	19	40	41	0.39
6 West & Central (Ghana)	9	78	13	34	60	3.2	17	46	37	0.09
7 Greater Accra & East	7	75	18	41	37	5.6	34	29	37	1.38
8 Volta	9	67	24	31	46	4.5	23	50	27	0.57
9 Ashanti & Brong-Ahafo	11	75	14	26	43	4.8	30	44	26	0.88
10 North & Upper	19	11	70	27	93	.6	6	68	26	−1.32
11 Lowlands (Lesotho)	0	86	14	4	4	5.6	4	3	93	1.57
12 Rest, Lesotho	0	78	22	4	11	4.6	3	4	93	1.27
13 Central–South & East (Cameroon)	4	94	2	2	53	2.2	12	63	25	−0.34
14 Littoral & Southwest	1	96	3	5	53	2.3	16	54	30	−0.12
15 West & Northwest	14	73	13	2	69	1.5	13	72	15	−0.77
16 Yaounde & Douala	4	93	3	12	29	3.8	33	18	49	1.28
17 North	54	19	27	5	91	.4	13	71	16	−1.23
18 Atacora & Borgou (Benin)	41	8	51	56	89	.6	14	70	16	−1.14

19	Central & South	7	28	65	33	88	.7	12	70	18	−1.15
20	Cotonou	8	67	25	53	43	4.2	46	21	23	1.39
21	Cap Vert, Thiès (Senegal)	93	7	0	9	71	2.0	18	48	34	−0.28
22	Central	98	1	1	4	93	.4	8	80	12	−1.48
23	Casamance	87	13	0	3	89	.6	11	78	11	−1.31
24	Fleuve & Senegal Oriental	99	1	0	10	91	.5	17	64	19	−1.04
25	Abidjan (Ivory Coast)	38	40	22	31	65	2.5	25	17	58	0.45
26	Forest Urban	45	36	19	40	68	2.2	28	32	40	0.21
27	Savannah Urban	49	25	26	43	76	1.6	24	33	43	−0.09
28	Forest Rural	23	37	40	10	82	.9	28	49	23	−0.44
29	Savannah Rural	44	6	50	10	95	.3	12	76	12	−1.39
30	Khartoum (Sudan)	96	4	0	0	57	2.7	31	25	44	0.60
31	North & East	99	1	0	1	79	1.0	23	28	49	−0.19
32	Central	99	1	0	1	79	.9	26	33	41	−0.22
33	Kordofan & Darfur	98	0	2	0	89	.6	15	56	29	−0.93

NOTE: No missing values.

APPENDIX C *continued*   Contraceptive Use-Effectiveness and Mean Duration of Breastfeeding (AFT Estimates) by Age and Schooling Level, WFS regions

	Contraceptive Use-Effectiveness								X̄ Duration of Breastfeeding in Months							
	illit 15–24	illit 25–34	illit 35–49	1–4 15–24	1–4 25–34	5+ 15–24	5+ 25–34	All currently Married Women	illit 15–24	illit 25–34	illit 35–49	1–4 15–24	1–4 25–34	5+ 15–24	5+ 25–34	All Ever-Married Women
REGION																
Nairobi (Kenya)	3	6	6	7	15	10	29	15	14	15	19	13	15	13	14	14
Central & East	3	4	4	1	9	8	12	7	18	18	20	17	17	15	15	17
Rift Valley	1	3	4	5	6	3	10	5	18	19	19	15	19	15	16	17
Coast	1	3	2	0	0	8	15	4	24	21	26	22	21	15	13	20
Nyanza & Western	1	1	3	0	3	5	7	3	19	20	22	17	18	16	17	19
Western & Central (Ghana)	0	3	1	0	15	4	15	4	17	18	15	16	16	14	13	15
Greater Accra & East	2	5	5	3	9	10	17	9	19	18	19	19	18	17	16	17
Volta	0	3	3	0	19	5	14	6	23	21	26	99	99	20	18	22
Ashanti & Brong-Ahafo	0	2	4	3	6	8	16	6	20	20	22	21	20	18	17	19
North & Upper	0	1	0	0	0	99	99	1	36	32	34	99	99	99	99	33
Lowlands (Lesotho)	0	0	9	1	5	3	10	6	99	99	99	23	99	21	21	22
Rest, Lesotho	2	0	1	4	2	1	4	3	23	23	21	22	24	21	21	22
Central–South & East (Cameroon)	4	4	2	4	1	3	6	3	21	20	20	19	18	17	16	18
Littoral & Southwest	0	0	0	2	3	3	5	1	22	21	21	20	21	16	15	19
West & Northwest	0	0	0	0	0	2	1	1	24	23	24	23	21	20	19	22
Yaounde & Douala	0	1	1	5	3	5	10	6	21	18	17	20	18	16	14	16
North	0	0	0	0	0	2	8	0	22	20	21	20	18	17	15	20
Atacora & Borgou (Benin)	1	2	1	0	5	99	99	2	25	24	24	21	20	99	99	24
Central & South	3	5	4	9	5	99	99	4	21	21	23	20	19	99	99	21

Cotonou	3	5	6	10	13	99	99	8	17	17	18	16	17	99	99	17
Cap Vert & Thiès (Senegal)	0	0	0	0	6	7	16	2	20	19	20	17	16	99	99	19
Central	0	0	0	0	0	0	21	0	22	20	23	18	16	99	99	21
Casamance	0	0	0	0	0	4	12	0	23	23	27	19	20	99	99	23
Fleuve & Senegal Orient.	0	1	0	0	0	1	0	0	19	21	21	99	99	99	99	19
Abidjan (Ivory Coast)	1	2	0	0	3	6	10	2	19	19	21	15	14	14	14	18
Forest Urban	0	1	0	5	0	5	9	2	19	19	20	99	99	14	14	18
Savannah Urban	0	0	0	0	0	2	99	1	16	21	21	99	99	13	17	18
Forest Rural	0	0	0	0	3	1	0	0	23	23	23	19	18	18	18	22
Savannah Rural	0	0	0	0	0	0	99	0	24	24	28	99	99	99	99	25
Khartoum (Sudan)	5	4	6	8	33	99	99	13	19	16	20	20	16	14	12	17
North & East	0	3	0	5	7	99	99	3	17	17	19	16	15	15	15	17
Central	0	4	4	14	28	99	99	7	18	20	18	16	18	99	99	18
Kordofan & Darfur	0	1	0	9	14	99	99	2	17	18	18	17	18	15	16	18

NOTE: 99 = missing value; illit = 0 yrs of schooling or Koranic only.

APPENDIX C continued   Mean Durations of Postpartum Amenorrhea and Postpartum Abstinence by Age and Schooling Level, WFS Regions (AFT Estimates)

REGION	X̄ Duration Postpartum Amenorrhea in Months								X̄ Duration Postpartum Abstinence in Months							
	illit 15-24	illit 25-34	illit 35-49	1-4 15-24	1-4 25-34	5+ 15-24	5+ 25-34	All Ever-Married Women	illit 15-24	illit 25-34	illit 35-49	1-4 15-24	1-4 25-34	5+ 15-24	5+ 25-34	All Ever-Married Women
Nairobi (Kenya)	8	10	10	9	11	7	8	8	4	4	3	4	4	3	3	3
Central & Eastern	11	12	15	10	11	9	10	12	3	4	6	3	4	2	3	4
Rift Valley	11	14	13	10	12	8	10	11	6	6	9	4	5	4	4	6
Coast	14	15	25	11	12	9	10	15	2	4	6	2	3	3	4	4
Nyanza & Western	12	14	13	12	14	9	10	12	3	4	4	3	3	3	3	3
West & Center (Ghana)	12	13	12	12	13	10	11	12	7	7	8	8	8	8	7	7
Greater Accra & East	11	12	14	12	13	10	11	12	10	9	9	9	9	8	8	9
Volta	17	14	19	99	99	15	13	15	19	17	19	99	99	15	13	17
Ashanti & Brong-Ahafo	14	14	15	15	15	13	13	14	10	8	9	9	6	8	6	8
North & Upper	19	18	21	99	99	99	99	19	27	29	34	99	99	99	99	29
Lowlands (Lesotho)	99	99	99	9	13	8	11	11	99	99	99	18	17	17	16	17
Rest, Lesotho	9	11	15	9	11	10	11	11	19	19	22	19	18	18	18	19
Central–South & East (Cameroon)	12	15	15	11	13	11	13	13	13	14	18	13	14	13	14	15
Littoral & Southwest	14	13	14	13	13	10	9	13	19	19	23	18	18	14	14	18
West & Northwest	16	16	18	14	14	12	12	12	24	23	24	21	21	20	19	22
Yaounde & Douala	9	11	9	9	11	8	9	15	17	16	17	17	14	12	10	12
North	14	14	15	10	10	9	9	14	16	12	16	16	14	12	11	14

Region																
Atacora & Borgou (Benin)	16	17	18	12	13	99	99	16	24	23	23	23	22	99	99	23
Central & South	12	14	15	8	10	99	99	13	16	16	20	17	17	99	99	17
Cotonou	8	8	15	7	8	99	99	9	11	12	14	10	10	99	99	11
Cap Vert & Thiès (Senegal)	14	13	14	11	10	99	99	13	99	99	99	99	99	99	99	99
Central	15	14	16	12	10	99	99	14	99	99	99	99	99	99	99	99
Casamance	16	16	19	13	14	99	99	16	99	99	99	99	99	99	99	99
Fleuve & Senegal Orient.	13	14	14	99	99	99	99	13	99	99	99	99	99	99	99	99
Abidjan (Ivory Coast)	12	12	11	11	11	9	9	11	15	14	17	16	14	11	10	14
Forest Urban	10	11	11	99	99	8	8	10	16	15	22	99	99	8	7	14
Savannah Urban	9	13	12	99	99	7	10	11	13	18	15	99	99	11	16	15
Forest Rural	12	15	14	11	14	10	13	13	16	17	18	15	16	13	14	16
Savannah Rural	13	15	19	99	99	13	99	15	19	19	24	99	99	99	99	20
Khartoum (Sudan)	11	11	8	11	10	7	6	9	5	3	6	3	2	2	1	3
North & East	11	13	12	8	10	4	5	11	5	5	5	2	3	2	2	4
Central	13	15	12	9	10	99	99	12	2	4	4	2	3	99	99	3
Kordofan & Darfur	13	15	13	10	12	8	9	13	3	2	2	3	2	1	1	3

NOTE: 99 = missing value; illit = 0 yrs of schooling or Koranic only.

APPENDIX c *continued*   Mean Durations of Postpartum Nonsusceptible
Period by Age and Schooling Level, WFS Regions (AFT Estimates)

$\bar{X}$ *Duration Postpartum Nonsusceptible Period in Months*

REGION	15–24 illit	25–34 illit	35–49 illit	15–24 1–4	25–34 1–4	15–24 5+	25–24 5+	All Ever-Married Women
Nairobi (Kenya)	9	10	11	9	11	7	9	9
Central & Eastern	12	13	16	10	12	9	11	13
Rift Valley	12	14	15	11	14	9	11	12
Coast	14	15	25	11	12	10	11	15
Nyanza & Western	12	14	14	13	14	10	11	13
West & Central (Ghana)	12	13	14	13	15	11	12	13
Greater Accra & East	13	14	14	12	13	12	12	13
Volta	24	19	24	99	99	19	15	20
Ashanti & Brong-Ahafo	16	15	16	17	16	14	13	15
North & Upper	29	30	35	99	99	99	99	30
Lowlands (Lesotho)	99	99	99	19	19	18	17	19
Rest, Lesotho	20	20	24	19	19	18	19	20
Central–South & East (Cameroon)	16	17	20	16	17	15	16	17
Littoral & Southwest	19	20	23	19	19	15	15	19
West & Northwest	24	23	25	21	21	20	20	23
Yaounde & Douala	19	17	17	18	16	13	12	14
North	18	16	18	17	16	13	12	17
Atacora & Borgou (Benin)	24	23	24	22	22	99	99	23
Central & South	18	18	21	17	18	99	99	18
Cotonou	12	12	19	12	12	99	99	13
Cap Vert & Thiès (Senegal)	15	14	15	12	11	99	99	14
Central	16	15	17	13	11	99	99	15
Casamance	17	17	20	14	15	99	99	17
Fleuve & Senegal Orient.	14	15	15	99	99	99	99	14
Abidjan (Ivory Coast)	18	16	18	18	17	13	12	16
Forest Urban	17	16	21	99	99	11	10	16
Savannah Urban	14	19	19	99	99	12	17	17
Forest Rural	18	19	20	16	18	15	16	18
Savannah Rural	19	21	25	99	99	99	99	22
Khartoum (Sudan)	12	11	9	12	11	7	7	10
North & East	11	14	13	9	11	5	7	12
Central	13	16	13	9	11	99	99	13
Kordofan & Darfur	13	15	13	10	12	8	9	14

NOTE: 99 = missing value, illit = 0 yrs of schooling or Koranic only.

APPENDIX D Comparison of Regional Estimates of Spacing Variables Obtained through Accelerated Failure Time Models (AFT) and Prevalence-Incidence Ratios (P/I) from 8 WFS surveys

Country & Region	Breastfeeding			Abstinence			Amenorrhea			Nonsusceptible Period		
	AFT (a)	P/I (b)	(a) – (b)	AFT (a)	P/I (b)	(a) – (b)	AFT (a)	P/I (b)	(a) – (b)	AFT (a)	P/I (b)	(a) – (b)
KENYA												
Whole Country	17.7	17.8	–.1	4.0	4.1	–.1	11.6	11.7	–.1	12.3	12.4	–.1
Nairobi	13.9	14.4	–.5	3.4	4.1	–.7	8.1	8.8	–.7	8.6	9.3	–.7
Central, Eastern	17.3	17.5	–.2	4.1	3.9	.2	11.7	11.7	0.0	12.5	12.4	.1
Rift	17.2	17.3	–.1	5.5	5.8	–.3	11.4	11.8	–.3	12.2	12.6	–.4
Coast	20.2	20.3	–.1	3.5	3.7	–.2	14.7	13.4	1.4	14.9	14.3	.6
Nyanza, Western	18.8	18.7	.1	3.2	3.2	0.0	12.0	12.1	–.1	12.5	12.6	–.1
GHANA												
Whole country	19.8	20.2	–.4	12.1	12.4	–.3	13.8	14.6	–.8	16.5	16.8	–.3
Western, Central	15.2	15.7	–.5	7.4	8.3	–.9	11.6	12.3	–.7	12.8	13.6	–.8
Accra, Eastern	17.2	18.2	–1.0	8.7	9.7	–1.0	11.8	12.8	–1.0	12.9	13.9	–1.0
Volta	22.0	22.9	–.9	16.5	17.2	–.7	15.4	16.9	–1.5	19.7	20.3	–.6
Ashanti, Brong-Ahafo	19.2	19.6	–.4	8.1	8.9	–.8	13.8	14.6	–.8	14.9	15.6	–.7
Northern, Upper	32.5	28.3	4.2	28.8	25.6	3.2	18.7	18.8	–.1	30.0	26.1	–3.9
LESOTHO												
Whole country	21.7	21.8	–.1	18.0	18.0	0.0	11.0	11.4	–.4	19.3	19.3	0.0
Lowlands	21.7	21.7	0.0	17.3	17.2	.1	10.6	10.9	–.3	18.7	18.7	0.0
Foothills, Orange River Valley, Mountains	21.7	22.3	–.6	18.5	18.3	.2	11.3	11.4	–.1	19.7	19.5	.2

CAMEROON												
Whole Country	19.1	19.5	–.4	16.0	16.2	–.2	12.8	13.3	–.5	17.7	17.9	–.2
Center South, East	18.2	17.5	.7	14.5	15.5	–1.0	12.9	12.6	.3	16.8	17.0	–.2
Coast, Southwest	18.9	18.8	.1	17.8	17.9	–.1	12.2	12.5	–.3	18.6	18.7	–.1
West, Northwest	22.4	22.0	.4	22.2	21.4	.8	15.1	15.1	0.0	22.6	21.9	.7
Yaounde, Duala	15.5	14.8	.7	12.3	11.8	.5	8.9	8.1	.8	13.8	12.9	.9
North	20.3	20.4	–.1	13.5	12.9	.6	13.9	14.2	–.3	16.7	16.2	.5
BENIN												
Whole Country	21.3	21.4	–.1	18.3	18.2	.1	13.5	13.7	–.2	19.4	19.4	0.0
Atacora, Borgou	23.5	22.9	.4	23.0	22.3	.7	16.3	15.9	.4	23.3	22.8	.5
Atlantic, Mono, Oueme, Zou	21.2	21.3	–.1	17.0	17.1	–.1	13.1	13.4	–.3	18.4	18.5	–.1
Cotonou	17.1	17.3	–.2	11.4	12.3	–.9	8.8	9.6	–.8	13.2	14.1	–.9
IVORY COAST												
Whole Country	21.0	19.7	1.3	16.3	16.5	–.2	12.7	13.0	–.3	18.1	18.1	0.0
Abidjan	17.6	17.3	.3	13.9	14.2	–.3	10.8	10.9	–.1	16.1	16.2	–.1
Urban Forest	18.3	17.8	.5	14.2	14.6	–.4	10.2	10.9	–.7	15.8	16.2	–.4
Urban Savannah	18.3	16.8	1.5	15.2	14.8	.4	10.6	10.2	.4	16.5	16.1	.4
Rural Forest	21.9	20.4	1.5	16.4	16.5	–.1	13.3	13.7	–.4	18.2	18.3	–.1
Rural Savannah	24.9	22.6	2.3	20.2	20.2	0.0	15.3	15.9	–.6	21.6	21.3	.3

SENEGAL												
Whole Country	20.4	20.5	-.1	—	—	—	—	—	—	—	—	—
Cap Vert, Thiès	18.7	19.1	-.4	—	—	—	—	—	—	—	—	—
Diourbel, Sine												
Saloum, Louga	21.2	21.0	.2	—	—	—	—	—	—	—	—	—
Casamance	23.1	22.9	.2	—	—	—	—	—	—	—	—	—
Oriental, Fleuve	19.4	19.9	-.5	—	—	—	—	—	—	—	—	—
SUDAN												
Whole Country	17.6	17.3	.3	2.9	3.2	-.3	11.8	12.1	-.3	12.3	12.6	-.3
Khartoum	16.8	17.1	-.3	3.0	3.3	-.3	9.4	9.7	-.3	10.0	10.3	-.3
Northern, Eastern	17.3	17.1	.2	4.2	3.6	.6	10.7	10.1	.6	11.9	11.2	.7
Central	18.4	19.1	-.7	3.2	3.3	-.1	12.4	13.0	-.6	12.8	13.4	-.6
Kordofan, Darfur	17.6	18.5	-.9	2.5	3.0	-.5	13.4	14.2	-.8	13.5	14.4	-.9

SOURCE: Eelens and Donné, 1985, p. 101.

Region	Percent Illiterate	Average Schooling Duration	Percent Husbands as:		Socioeconomic Development Score
			Clerical, Professional, Employer of Wage-Earning Employees	Self-Employed Farmer, Artisan, Trader without Wage-Earning Employees	
KENYA					
Nairobi	20%	6.2 yrs	49%	7%	2.30
Central, Eastern	37	3.7	20	41	0.60
Rift Valley	44	3.3	19	37	0.47
Coast	69	2.2	20	40	−0.06
Western, Nyanza	46	3.2	19	40	0.39
GHANA					
West, Central	60	3.2	17	46	0.09
Accra, Eastern	37	5.6	34	29	1.38
Volta	46	4.5	23	50	0.57
Ashanti, Brong-Ahafo	43	4.8	30	44	0.88
Northern, Upper	93	0.6	6	68	−1.32
LESOTHO					
Lowlands	04	5.6	4	3	1.57
Foothills, Orange River Valley Mountains	11	4.6	3	4	1.27
CAMEROON					
Central-South, East	53	2.2	12	63	−0.34
Littoral, Southwest	53	2.3	16	54	−0.12

West, Northwest	69	1.5	13	72	-0.77
Yaounde, Douala	29	3.8	33	18	1.28
North	91	0.4	13	71	-1.23
BENIN					
Atacora, Borgou	89	0.6	14	70	-1.14
Atlantic, Mono, Oueme, Zou	88	0.7	12	70	-1.15
Cotonou	43	4.2	46	21	1.39
SENEGAL					
Cap Vert, Thiès	71	2.0	18	48	-0.28
Central	93	0.4	8	80	-1.48
Casamance	89	0.6	11	78	-1.31
Fleuve, Oriental	91	0.5	17	64	-1.04
IVORY COAST					
Abidjan	65	2.5	25	17	0.45
Forest Urban	68	2.2	28	32	0.21
Savannah Urban	76	1.6	24	33	-0.09
Forest Rural	82	0.9	28	49	-0.44
Savannah Rural	95	0.3	12	76	-1.39
SUDAN					
Khartoum	57	2.7	31	25	0.60
North, East	79	1.0	23	28	-0.19
Central	79	0.9	26	33	-0.22
Kordofan, Darfur	89	0.6	15	56	-0.93

APPENDIX F   Age and Education contrast with Respect to Spacing Variables and Distribution Characteristics for Regions in WFS Countries

Contrasts	Breastfeeding	Postpartum Abstinence	Postpartum Nonsusceptible	Current Use Contraception
Value Illiterate Women minus Value Women 1–4 yrs of Schooling				
Age group 15–24	$\bar{X}$ = 1.7 mos.	0.6 mos.	1.3 mos.	−2.0%
	σ = 1.5	1.3	1.5	3.4
	N = 26	23	26	33
Age group 25–34	$\bar{X}$ = 1.3	0.7	1.0	−4.5
	σ = 1.5	1.1	1.7	7.1
	N = 26	23	26	33
Value Illiterate Women minus Value Women 5+ yrs of Schooling				
Age group 15–24	$\bar{X}$ = 3.7	2.5	3.5	−3.5
	σ = 1.8	2.3	1.7	2.7
	N = 22	22	22	25
Age group 25–34	$\bar{X}$ = 3.7	2.4	3.3	−9.0
	σ = 1.6	2.1	1.8	6.1
	N = 22	22	22	23
Value Illiterate Women 35–49 minus Value Illiterate Women 15–24	$\bar{X}$ = 0.9	1.9	2.3	+1.1
	σ = 2.1	2.4	2.8	2.1
	N = 32	28	32	33

	$\bar{X} = 4.6$	4.0	5.6	−2.4
Value Illiterate Women 35–49 minus	$\sigma = 2.5$	3.1	2.9	2.7
Value Women 15–24 with 5+ yrs of Schooling	$N = 22$	22	22	25

NOTE: —No data on postpartum abstinence durations in Senegalese regions.
—N = number of regions.

APPENDIX G Education-Related Differences in Child-Spacing; Measurement of Combined Effect of Postpartum Nonsusceptibility and Contraceptive Use-Effectiveness through Bongaarts Indices; Results for Women Aged 15–24

	Illiterate			1–4 Yrs Schooling			5+ Yrs Schooling			$\Delta(0,5+)$	$\Delta(0,1-4)$	$\Delta(1-4,5+)$
	C_c	C_i	$C_c \cdot C_i$	C_c	C_i	$C_c \cdot C_i$	C_c	C_i	$C_c \cdot C_i$			
KENYA												
Nairobi	.968	.739	.715	.924	.739	.683	.892	.795	.709	.006	.032	−.026
Central, East	.968	.669	.648	.989	.714	.706	.914	.739	.675	−.027	−.058	.031
Rift	.989	.669	.662	.946	.691	.654	.968	.739	.715	−.053	.008	−.061
Coast	.989	.629	.622	1.000	.691	.691	.914	.714	.653	−.031	−.069	.038
Nyanza, West	.989	.669	.662	1.000	.648	.648	.946	.714	.675	−.013	−.026	−.027
GHANA												
West, Central	1.000	.669	.669	1.000	.648	.648	.957	.691	.661	.008	.021	−.013
Greater Accra, East	.978	.648	.634	.968	.669	.648	.892	.669	.597	.037	−.014	.051
Volta	1.000	.484	.484	1.000	—	—	.946	.547	.517	−.033	—	—
Ashanti; Brong Ahafo	1.000	.593	.593	.968	.577	.559	.914	.629	.575	.018	.034	−.016
North, Upper	1.000	.434	.434	1.000	—	—	—	—	—	—	—	—
LESOTHO												
Lowlands	1.000	—	—	.989	.547	.541	.968	.562	.544	—	—	−.003
Other	.978	.533	.521	.957	.547	.523	.989	.562	.556	−.035	−.002	−.033
CAMEROON												
Central-South, East	.957	.593	.568	.957	.593	.568	.968	.611	.591	−.023	.000	−.023
Littoral Southwest	1.000	.547	.547	.978	.547	.535	.968	.611	.591	−.044	.012	−.056
West, Northwest	1.000	.484	.484	1.000	.520	.520	.978	.533	.521	−.037	−.036	−.001
Yaounde, Douala	1.000	.547	.547	.946	.562	.532	.946	.648	.613	−.066	.015	−.081
North	1.000	.562	.562	1.000	.577	.577	.978	.648	.634	−.072	−.015	−.057

BENIN												
Atacora, Borgou	.989	.484	.479	1.000	.508	.508	—	—	—	—	-.029	—
Central, South	.968	.562	.544	.903	.577	.521	—	—	—	—	.023	—
Cotonou	.968	.669	.648	.892	.669	.597	—	—	—	—	.051	—
SENEGAL												
Cap Vert, Thiès	1.000	.611	.611	1.000	.669	.669	—	—	—	—	-.058	—
Center	1.000	.593	.593	1.000	.648	.648	—	—	—	—	-.055	—
Casamance	1.000	.577	.577	1.000	.629	.629	—	—	—	—	-.052	—
Fleuve, Oriental	1.000	.629	.629	1.000	—	—	—	—	—	—	—	—
IVORY COAST												
Abidjan	.989	.562	.556	1.000	.562	.562	.935	.648	.606	-.050	-.006	-.044
Urban Forest	1.000	.577	.577	.946	—	—	.946	.691	.654	-.077	—	—
Urban Savannah	1.000	.629	.629	1.000	—	—	.978	.669	.654	-.025	—	—
Rural Forest	1.000	.562	.562	1.000	.593	.593	.989	.611	.605	-.043	-.031	-.012
Rural Savannah	1.000	.547	.547	1.000	—	—	—	—	—	—	—	—
NORTHERN SUDAN												
Khartoum	.946	.669	.633	.914	.669	.611	—	.795	—	—	.022	—
North, East	1.000	.691	.691	.946	.739	.699	—	.860	—	—	-.008	—
Central	1.000	.648	.648	.849	.739	.627	—	—	—	—	.021	—
Kordofan, Darfur	1.000	.648	.648	.903	.714	.645	—	.766	—	—	.003	—

NOTES: Δ(illit., lit.) = C_cC_i (illiterate) − C_cC_i (literate); positive values of Δ imply that an overall increase in child-spacing is associated with a rise in female education.

APPENDIX H Education-Related Differences in Child-Spacing: Measurement of Combined Effect of Postpartum Nonsusceptibility and Contraceptive Use-Effectiveness through Bongaarts Indices; Results for Women Aged 25–34

	Illiterate			1–4 yrs of Schooling			5+ yrs of Schooling					
	C_c	C_i	$C_c \cdot C_i$	C_c	C_i	$C_c \cdot C_i$	C_c	C_i	$C_c \cdot C_i$	$\Delta(0,5+)$	$\Delta(0,1-4)$	$\Delta(1-4,5+)$
KENYA												
Nairobi	.935	.714	.668	.838	.691	.579	.687	.739	.508	.160	.089	.071
Central, East	.957	.648	.620	.903	.669	.604	.870	.691	.601	.019	.016	.003
Rift	.968	.629	.609	.935	.629	.588	.892	.691	.616	−.007	.021	−.028
Coast	.968	.611	.591	1.000	.669	.669	.838	.691	.579	.012	−.078	.090
Nyanza, West	.989	.629	.662	.968	.629	.609	.924	.691	.638	−.016	.013	−.029
GHANA												
West, Central	.968	.648	.627	.838	.611	.512	.838	.669	.561	.066	.115	−.049
Greater Accra, East	.946	.629	.595	.903	.648	.585	.816	.669	.546	.049	.010	.039
Volta	.968	.547	.529	.795	—	—	.849	.611	.519	.010	—	—
Ashanti, Brong-Ahafo	.978	.611	.598	.935	.593	.554	.827	.648	.536	.062	.044	.018
North, Upper	.989	.429	.424	1.000	—	—	—	—	—	—	—	—
LESOTHO												
Lowlands	1.000	—	—	.946	.547	.517	.892	.577	.515	—	—	.002
Other	1.000	.533	.533	.978	.547	.535	.957	.547	.535	.010	−.002	.012
CAMEROON												
Central-South, East	.957	.577	.552	.989	.577	.571	.935	.593	.554	−.002	−.019	.017
Littoral, Southwest	1.000	.533	.533	.968	.547	.529	.946	.611	.578	−.045	.004	−.049
West, Northwest	1.000	.496	.496	1.000	.520	.520	.989	.533	.527	−.031	−.024	−.007
Yaounde, Douala	.989	.577	.571	.968	.593	.574	.892	.669	.597	−.026	−.003	−.023
North	1.000	.593	.593	1.000	.593	.593	.913	.669	.611	−.018	.000	−.018

BENIN

Atacora, Borgou	.978	.496	.485	.946	.508	.481	—	—	—	—	.004	—
Central, South	.946	.562	.532	.946	.562	.532	—	—	—	—	.000	—
Cotonou	.946	.669	.633	.860	.669	.575	—	—	—	—	.058	—

SENEGAL

Cap Vert, Thiès	1.000	.629	.629	.935	.691	.646	—	—	—	—	-.017	—
Center	1.000	.611	.611	1.000	.691	.691	—	—	—	—	-.080	—
Casamance	1.000	.577	.577	1.000	.611	.611	—	—	—	—	-.034	—
Fleuve, Oriental	.989	.611	.604	1.000	—	—	—	—	—	—	—	—

IVORY COAST

Abidjan	.978	.593	.580	1.000	.577	.577	.892	.669	.597	-.017	.003	-.020
Urban Forest	.989	.593	.586	.968	—	—	.903	.714	.645	-.059	—	—
Urban Savannah	1.000	.547	.547	1.000	—	—	—	.577	—	—	—	—
Rural Forest	1.000	.547	.547	.968	.562	.544	1.000	.593	.593	-.046	.003	-.049
Rural Savannah	1.000	.520	.520	1.000	—	—	—	—	—	—	—	—

NORTHERN SUDAN

Khartoum	.957	.691	.661	.644	.691	.445	—	.795	—	—	.216	—
North, East	.968	.629	.609	.924	.691	.638	—	.795	—	—	-.030	—
Central	.957	.593	.568	.719	.691	.497	—	—	—	—	.071	—
Kordofan, Darfur	.989	.611	.604	.849	.669	.568	—	.739	—	—	.036	—

NOTE: Δ(illiterate, literate) = C_cC_i (illiterate) − C_cC_i (literate).

APPENDIX I   Variations of Ratio of Ever-Married Women to Ever-Married
Men in Response to Change in Rate of Increase

The following derivation demonstrates how the ratio of the number of ever-married women to the number of ever-married men (Z) varies in response to changes in the rate of increase which result from changes in the underlying fertility schedule. Consider female and male stable age distributions (of the form $Be^{-rx}l_x$) with a rate of increase (r), a sex ratio at birth (males per female) of S, and respective life tables l_x^f and l_x^m. Under the assumption of fixed ages at marriage of women and men of a_f and a_m respectively,

$$Z = \frac{\# \text{ ever-married women}}{\# \text{ ever-married men}} = \frac{\int_{a_f}^{\omega} e^{-rx}\, l_x^f\, dx}{S \int_{a_m}^{\omega} e^{-rx}\, l_x^m dx} \qquad \text{Eq. A1}$$

Note that we can ignore the number of female births B, since it acts as a multiplier for both numerator and denominator. The effect of a change in r (due to a change in fertility) on the ratio Z can be determined by evaluating the derivative of the logarithm of Z with respect to r:

$$\frac{d\,ln\,Z}{dr} = \frac{\dfrac{d[\int_{a_f}^{\omega} e^{-rx}\, l_x^f\, dx]}{dr}}{\int_{a_f}^{\omega} e^{-rx}\, l_x^f\, dx} - \frac{\dfrac{d[\int_{a_m}^{\omega} e^{-rx}\, l_x^m\, dx]}{dr}}{\int_{a_m}^{\omega} e^{-rx}\, l_x^m\, dx} \qquad \text{Eq. A2}$$

[Note that S disappears from the above equation since $d[ln\,S]/dr$ equals zero.]

If we let μ_f and μ_m denote the mean ages of ever-married women and ever-married men respectively,

$$\mu_f = \frac{\int_{a_f}^{\omega} xe^{-rx}\, l_x^f dx}{\int_{a_f}^{\omega} e^{-rx}\, l_x^f\, dx} \quad \text{and } \mu_m = \frac{\int_{a_m}^{\omega} xe^{-rx}\, l_x^m dx}{\int_{a_m}^{\omega} e^{-rx}\, l_x^m\, dx}$$

then equation A2 can be rewritten as

$$\frac{d\,ln\,Z}{dr} = -\mu_f + \mu_m = \mu_m - \mu_f.$$

or $\qquad \dfrac{\dfrac{dZ}{dr}}{Z} = \mu_m - \mu_f.$ Eq. A3

Expressing the derivatives in terms of small differences Δr and ΔZ, we have

$$\frac{\Delta Z}{Z} \approx \Delta r (\mu_m - \mu_f).$$ Eq. A4

In words, equation A4 indicates that the percentage change in the ratio Z as a result of a small change in r is directly proportional to the difference in the mean ages of ever-married men and of ever-married women in the population. We can view this comparison of ratios either as one between two stable populations, one with a slightly higher rate of growth than the other, or as one between an original stable population and an eventual new one which results from a small change in r.

Since the above equations incorporate the mean ages of ever-married persons, μ_f and μ_m, rather than the ages at marriage, a_f and a_m, the effects of changes in the age difference at marriage on Z and on dZ/dr are not obvious. Because male mortality rates at the older ages generally exceed female rates at the older ages by a considerable amount, overall male age distributions tend to be younger than those of females. This need not be true, however, of the age distributions of ever-married persons because of sex differences in age at marriage. If males marry at considerably older ages than females, μ_m will exceed μ_f; a further increase in the age difference (with males marrying at older ages) will increase the value of $(\mu_m - \mu_f)$. However, for very small age differences—such as men marrying at an age one or two years older than women—the difference $(\mu_m - \mu_f)$ will be very small or even negative. For the range of mortality being considered in this paper (a life expectancy of approximately 50 years), about a two year age difference in marriage produces equal values of μ_f and μ_m. For example, in the stationary population described by the Coale and Demeny West life table 13 (life expectancy for women and men of 50 and 47.1 years respectively), the mean ages of *all* females and males equal 33.9 and 32.6 respectively—i.e., men are younger by slightly over a year, on average. An age difference at marriage of two years equalizes the average ages of ever-married women and men: the mean age of women over 20 in this stationary population is 45.6, a value just equal to the mean age of men over 22.

Figure 5.1 demonstrates how the sign and magnitude of dZ/dr vary according to the age difference at marriage. For age differences above two or three years (positive values of $\mu_m - \mu_f$) increases in r result in increases in Z. The larger the age difference (with men marrying at ages 5, 10, and 15 years older than women), the greater the impact of a given absolute change in r on Z. For an age difference of about two years $(\mu_m \approx \mu_f)$, a change in r

has almost no effect on Z; with a zero age difference (for which $(\mu_m - \mu_f)$ is negative), an increase in r results in a *decrease* in the ratio Z. Not shown in the figure is the result of men marrying at successively younger ages than women—for example, values of $(a_m - a_f)$ of -2, -5 and -10 years. The result would be a mirror image of the top part of the figure: a given absolute change in r would result in successively larger changes in Z but in a negative direction—increases in r would decrease the ratio Z.

APPENDIX J Percentage of Currently Married Women *Not* Reporting Their Husband's Age by Type of Marriage

	Monogamous	Polygynous	
		First Wife	Junior Wife
Cameroon	49.9	65.4	63.7
Ghana	0.1	0.1	
Ivory Coast	64.2	68.7	73.8
Kenya	.6	0.4	0.7
Lesotho	1.4	3.9	2.9
Senegal*	56.1	36.9	44.1

*A question on husband's age was *not* included in the Senegal individual questionnaire. Instead, we used household interview records to match currently married women with their husbands, in an attempt to determine husband's current age. The percentages for Senegal in this table represent the proportion of women who were successfully matched with a husband whose age was reported on the household schedule. The total percent successfully matched for each marriage type was 47 percent monogamous, 67 percent polygynous first wives, and 61 percent second and higher order wives.

APPENDIX K   Association between Marriage Type or Other Characteristics
and the Probability of Conception, Hazard Model Coefficients and
t-statistics, Kenya WFS Data*

	Model			
Polygynous senior wife	−.190	−.188	−.182	−.178
	(2.54)	(2.51)	(2.43)	(2.38)
Polygynous junior wife	−.146	−.142	−.055	−.059
	(2.90)	(2.83)	(1.00)	(1.07)
Wife's age 35+	−.366	−.353	−.284	−.297
	(4.90)	(4.69)	(3.62)	(3.69)
Marriage duration	−.032	0.45	−.024	.037
less than 5 years	(.30)	(.39)	(.23)	(.34)
5–15 years	−.222	−.130	−.191	−.142
	(2.11)	(1.23)	(1.82)	(1.27)
15+ years	−.612	−.529	−.539	−.528
	(5.13)	(4.42)	(4.44)	(3.85)
Still breastfeeding at:				
0 months**		−1.00		−.995
		(1.70)		(1.69)
3 months		−1.381		−1.382
		(5.31)		(5.31)
6 months		−1.552		−1.555
		(8.73)		(8.72)
9 months		−1.149		−1.144
		(8.32)		(8.29)
12 months		−.453		−.446
		(5.67)		(5.58)
18 months		−.568		−.558
		(5.54)		(5.79)
24 months		−.258		−.241
		(2.47)		(2.31)
36 months		−1.195		−1.168
		(2.64)		(2.58)
48 months		−.857		−.857
		(.85)		(.85)
Husband age				
40–54			−.145	−.138
			(2.65)	(2.49)
55+			−.341	−.322
			(3.65)	(3.41)
Coresides with husband				.042
				(.87)
Children ever born at				.011
start of observation				(.96)

APPENDIX K   *Continued*

	Model			
Duration Constants:				
0–2 months	−4.554	−3.659	−4.559	−3.719
	(30.48)	(6.24)	(30.50)	(6.32)
3–5 months	−4.072	−2.877	−4.077	−2.928
	(30.28)	(10.96)	(30.29)	(11.01)
6–8 months	−3.733	−2.481	−3.737	−2.532
	(29.30)	(13.46)	(29.31)	(13.36)
9–11 months	−3.311	−2.506	−3.314	−2.560
	(27.51)	(16.75)	(27.51)	(16.46)
12–17 months	−2.564	−2.305	−2.566	−2.359
	(23.98)	(19.35)	(23.97)	(18.67)
18–23 months	−2.486	−2.368	−2.484	−2.418
	(22.84)	(21.27)	(22.81)	(20.40)
24–35 months	−2.612	−2.628	−2.605	−2.673
	(24.06)	(23.70)	(23.98)	(22.65)
36–47 months	−3.024	−3.047	−3.015	−3.089
	(24.52)	(24.57)	(24.43)	(23.63)
48–59 months	−3.372	−3.438	−3.367	−3.481
	(23.05)	(23.38)	(23.01)	(22.80)
Log-likelihood	−11295.6	−11184.5	−11287.5	−11177.3

*Sample size is 5648 open and last closed birth intervals. 617 intervals in which contraception was used are excluded.

**This variable indicates whether a woman ever breastfed in this interval.

APPENDIX L   Association between Marriage Type or Other Characteristics
and the Probability of Conception: Hazard-Model Coefficients and
t-statistics, Ivory Coast WFS Data*

	Model				
Polygynous senior wife	−.101	−.092	−.095	−.094	−.085
	(1.63)	(1.48)	(1.53)	(1.52)	(1.37)
Polygynous junior wife	−.196	−.186	−.176	−.178	−.166
	(3.51)	(3.33)	(3.09)	(3.19)	(2.90)
Wife's age 35+	−.583	−.571	−.570	−.565	−.552
	(7.07)	(6.91)	(6.89)	(6.83)	(6.14)
Marriage duration	.038	−.045	.040	.029	.038
less than 5 years	(.40)	(.48)	(.42)	(.31)	(.40)
5–15 years	−.050	−.002	−.043	−.029	.010
	(.53)	(.03)	(.45)	(.30)	(.10)
15+ years	−.291	−.024	−2.76	−.262	−.218
	(.255)	(2.06)	(2.38)	(2.29)	(1.73)
Still breastfeeding at:					
0 months**		−3.061			4.064
		(.45)			(.36)
3 months		−1.873			−1.780
		(5.19)			(4.66)
6 months		−1.694			−1.395
		(6.44)			(4.70)
9 months		−1.187			−.807
		(5.84)			(3.76)
12 months		−.776			−4.88
		(6.66)			(3.90)
18 months		−.826			−7.19
		(8.50)			(6.95)
24 months		−.424			−.423
		(5.14)			(4.82)
36 months		−.408			−.413
		(1.13)			(1.14)
48 months		−.374			.345
		(.37)			(.34)
Still abstaining at:					
3 months				−.895	−.404
				(2.03)	(.87)
6 months				−1.017	−.597
				(4.25)	(2.22)
9 months				−1.129	−.943
				(6.12)	(4.84)
12 months				−.781	−.642
				(7.50)	(5.74)

APPENDIX L *Continued*

	Model				
18 months				−.631	−.337
				(5.29)	(2.66)
Husband's age					
40–54				−.073	−.004
				(.75)	(.04)
55+				−.300	−.243
				(1.10)	(.89)
Age unknown				−.118	−.059
				(2.19)	(1.09)
Coresides with husband					−.020
					(.024)
Children ever born at start of observation					−.001
					(.04)
Duration Constants:					
0–2 months	−5.304	−8.386	−5.231	−5.318	−9.338
	(27.31)	(1.23)	(26.55)	(27.39)	(.83)
3–5 months	−5.037	−3.417	−4.963	−4.243	−3.081
	(28.40)	(10.39)	(27.50)	(10.15)	(6.74)
6–8 months	−4.482	−3.079	−4.408	−3.789	−2.863
	(30.23)	(12.77)	(28.99)	(18.64)	(10.96)
9–11 months	−3.862	−2.913	−3.788	−3.283	−2.680
	(30.46)	(14.93)	(28.86)	(22.62)	(12.66)
12–17 months	−3.278	−2.688	−3.202	−2.900	−2.544
	(32.06)	(20.18)	(29.67)	(26.22)	(16.16)
18–23 months	−2.803	−2.453	−2.726	−2.664	−2.368
	(28.48)	(23.57)	(26.11)	(26.51)	(17.75)
24–35 months	−2.580	−2.463	−2.502	−2.597	−2.412
	(27.70)	(25.61)	(25.11)	(27.86)	(18.93)
36–47 months	−2.956	−2.971	−2.880	−2.975	−2.923
	(27.56)	(27.49)	(25.53)	(27.72)	(21.35)
48–59 months	−3.486	−3.526	−3.409	−3.505	−3.479
	(24.01)	(24.13)	(22.85)	(24.12)	(20.64)
Log-likelihood	−8460.1	−8531.1	−8457.3	−8386.3	−8315.0

*Sample size is 4412 open and last closed birth intervals.
**This variable indicates whether a woman ever breastfed in this interval.

Subject Index

Author Index

Ethnic Group Index

Geographical Index

Designer: U.C. Press Staff
Compositor: ASCO Trade Typesetting Ltd.
Text: 10/12 Baskerville
Display: Baskerville
Printer: Edwards Bros., Inc.
Binder: Edwards Bros., Inc.